HANDBOOK OF

Primary Care Medicine

Second Edition

HANDBOOK OF

Primary Care Medicine

Second Edition

Editor
Dale D. Berg, M.D.
Teaching Attending, Framingham Union Hospital
Boston, Massachusetts

Contributing Editors
Katherine Worzala, M.D.
Fellow, General Internal Medicine
Boston University Medical School
Boston, Massachusetts

Robert W. Pachner, M.D.
Assistant Professor
Department of Family Medicine
University of Wisconsin
Assistant Director, Residency Program
Milwaukee, Wisconsin

James L. Sebastian, M.D.
Associate Professor of Medicine
Medical College of Wisconsin
Milwaukee, Wisconsin

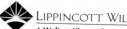 LIPPINCOTT WILLIAMS & WILKINS
A **Wolters Kluwer** Company

Philadelphia · Baltimore · New York · London
Buenos Aires · Hong Kong · Sydney · Tokyo

Acquisitions Editor: Richard Winters
Developmental Editor: Erin O'Connor
Manufacturing Manager: Dennis Teston
Production Manager: Robert Pancotti
Production Editor: Jonathan Geffner
Cover Designer: Karen Quigley
Indexer: Nancy Newman
Compositor: PRD Group, Inc.
Printer: R. R. Donnelley, Crawfordsville

Printed in the United States of America

9 8 7 6 5 4 3 2

Library of Congress Cataloging-in-Publication Data

Handbook of primary care medicine / editor, Dale D. Berg; contributing editors, Katherine Worzala, Robert W. Pachner, James L. Sebastian. — 2nd ed.
    p. cm.
    Includes bibliographical references and index.
    ISBN 0-7817-1431-1
    1. Primary care (Medicine)—Handbooks, manuals, etc. I. Berg, Dale.
    [DNLM: 1. Family Practice handbooks. 2. Primary Health Care handbooks. WB 39 A23656 1998]
    RC55.H28 1998
    616—dc21
    DNLM/DLC
for Library of Congress   97-48991
                                              CIP

Contents

C H A P T E R 4

Pulmonary Diseases   196

C H A P T E R 5

Hematology/Oncology   253

C H A P T E R 6

Infectious Diseases   312

C H A P T E R 7

Musculoskeletal Disorders   358

CHAPTER 8

Dermatology   413

CHAPTER 9

Endocrine Disorders   464

CHAPTER 10

Male Genitourinary Tract   516

C H A P T E R 15

Psychiatry 679

C H A P T E R 16

Prevention 703

Subject Index 713

Preface

Primary care medicine is perhaps the quintessential discipline of medicine. The prototypic general practice physician was the turn-of-the-century country doctor who had an unflappable personality, enormous quantities of empathy, a great deal of common sense both in medicine and in life, and the zeal and overriding concern for and of his or her patients. Although a powerful force for good, the general practice physician was able to intervene only minimally against many of the common disease entities of that time.

As medicine has evolved scientifically, new treatment modalities have been developed, many of which have prolonged the length and improved the quality of life. These modalities, including coronary angioplasty and bypass grafting, organ transplantation, and antineoplastic chemotherapy, have impacted significantly on health care. This component in medical evolution and development, however, involved a subspecialization in medicine in which physicians became experts in one endeavor or specific field of medicine, but potentially allowed other medical skills to atrophy.

Although this subspecialization has been positive for health care overall, it has come at some expense. These potential expenses include, but are not limited to, a loss of the art of medicine, a decrease in the empathetic nature of the physician, a fragmentation of care with a built-in inefficiency both in time and financially, a decrease in emphasis on prevention, and, finally, some would submit, a loss of the common sense inherent to being a physician and not a technician. Medicine, however, has continued to evolve in such a way that therapeutic advances can now be administered by nonspecialists, i.e., primary care providers. The role of a primary care physician will continue to evolve but will clearly continue to be the central component in health care delivery in this and the next millennium.

Based on the above discussion, primary care physicians must have a model to approach a diverse set of medical problems; know how to recognize, evaluate, and manage common problems; have a sense of when to consult other physicians and whom to consult; recognize when patients should be admitted to an inpatient service; and have references in the literature to support these models.

This book is designed with the following features to assist in easy utility:

1. The format is reproducible from section to section.
2. Boxes outlining the overall approach to common problems appear in each section. These boxes are designed to provide a readily accessible source of focused, on-your-feet type of information. They are meant to complement, not supplant, the text and discussion.
3. Bibliographies on each major topic are provided at the end of each chapter.
4. Each section ends with an outline of when and with whom to consult. In this section "elective" means as necessary, "required" means within the next month, "urgent" means within the next 24 hours, and "emergent" means within the next hour.
5. At the end of each section is an outline of indications for admission to an inpatient setting.

Chapter 1

Cardiology

Atherosclerotic Heart Disease: Risk Factor Modification

I. Risk factors

The **risk factors** for the development of atherosclerotic disease, especially coronary arterial atherosclerotic disease, include the following:

A. Cigarette smoking

B. Hypertension, if uncontrolled

C. Diabetes mellitus, both insulin-resistant and insulin-dependent

D. Obesity (exacerbates other risk factors)

E. Family history of premature atherosclerotic disease in a first-degree relative

F. Hyperlipidemia (Box 1-1)

G. Microalbuminuria of >40 mg/24 hr: This is a risk factor for accelerated atherosclerotic heart disease (ASHD) independent of non–insulin-dependent diabetes mellitus (NIDDM)

H. Vitamin B_{12} deficiency with resultant homocystinemia

I. Low levels of aerobic exercise

Of these risk factors, the only one that cannot be modified is a family history of premature heart disease. All of the other factors can and should be modified. Modification of risk factors slows the development and progression of atherosclerotic disease.

Strategies for modifying several of these risk factors are discussed in other chapters (cigarette-smoking cessation, Chapter 16; hypertension, Chapter 3; diabetes mellitus, Chapter 9).

II. Consultation

Problem	Service	Time
Severe diabetes mellitus	Endocrinology	Elective
Refractory hyperlipidemia	Endocrinology	Required

III. Indications for admission: None

B O X   1-1

Overall Evaluation and Management of the Hyperlipidemias

1. Assess the **risk-factor** profile of the patient for accelerated ASHD.
2. Hyperlipidemia is often **asymptomatic,** for accelerated ASHD and its detection requires screening.
   a. National Institutes of Health (NIH) recommendations for screening for hyperlipidemia: In every individual older than 20 years, a random, nonfasting total cholesterol level should be determined every 5 years.
      i. If the value is >240 mg/dL, a full cholesterol evaluation is warranted (see the following).
      ii. If the value is 200–239 mg/dL and two or more risk factors are present, a full cholesterol evaluation is warranted.
      iii. If the value is <199 mg/dL, the test is repeated in 5 years.
   b. The full cholesterol evaluation includes:
      i. Looking for secondary causes of hyperlipidemias
         (a) Diabetes mellitus (fasting blood glucose)
         (b) Nephrotic syndrome (urinalysis to check for proteinuria)
         (c) Hypothyroidism (thyroid-stimulating hormone [TSH])
         (d) Cholestatic jaundice (total bilirubin, alkaline phosphatase)
      ii. Measuring fasting plasma triglyceride (TG), high-density lipoprotein (HDL), and total cholesterol (TC) levels to calculate the low-density lipoprotein (LDL). The equation used to calculate this value is:

      $$LDL = TC - (HDL + TG/5).$$

      iii. A **physical examination** to look for goiter, peripheral signs of hypothyroidism, xanthomas (nodules in the skin), or xanthelasma (yellow streaking in the infraorbital skin). Xanthomas or xanthelasma may be indicative of cholesterol deposition.
   c. The goals of the full cholesterol evaluation include looking for any secondary causes, assessing

   (continued)

B O X 1-1 *(continued)*

the degree of lipid elevation, and categorizing the type of hyperlipidemia (see Table 1-1).
3. Therapeutic intervention: Goals
   a. If hyperlipidemia is the only cardiac risk factor, keep LDL <160 mg/dL.
   b. If hyperlipidemia is one of many cardiac risk factors, keep LDL <130 mg/dL.
   c. If documented coronary artery disease (CAD), keep the LDL to <100 mg/dL.
   d. Decrease levels of TC, TG, and LDL overall.
   e. Increase levels of HDL overall.
4. Therapeutic intervention: Methods
   a. Dietary changes (see Table 1-2)
   b. Exercise: Increase aerobic exercise, especially walking, swimming, or jogging.
   c. Drug therapy (see Table 1-3)

Chest Pain

Chest pain is a common problem with many possible causes. Assessment and diagnosis can be difficult. Because several of the underlying causes are disorders that can result in imminent death, any individual with chest pain requires an intensive evaluation to determine its cause. Diagnosis begins with deciding whether the chest pain is of cardiac or noncardiac origin.

I. **Types of chest pain by origin**
   A. **Cardiac origin**
      Chest pain of cardiac origin is clinically assessed to be the result of cardiac ischemia. This type of chest pain is also referred to as angina pectoris (see Box 1-2).
      1. **Typical or true angina pectoris** is characterized by a squeezing sensation that is retrosternal, is reproducibly precipitated or exacerbated by exercise, and is relieved with rest or sublingual nitroglycerin. Typical angina pectoris is easily diagnosed from a thorough history and is virtually diagnostic of atherosclerotic heart disease (i.e., Heberden's angina pectoris).
      2. **Atypical chest pain** has some features of angina but other features that are quite different from the classic description. In patients with atypical cardiac chest pain, no other noncardiac cause of the pain can be demonstrated, although one might exist. Atypical cardiac chest pain may result from coronary arterial spasm (Prinzmetal's angina), from a diabetic neuropathy,

T A B L E 1-1
Classification of Hyperlipidemia

Type	Lipoprotein	Elevated Lipid	Incidence (%)	Manifestations	Secondary Causes
I	Chylomicrons	TG	<1	Pancreatitis Eruptive xanthomas Lipemia retinalis	Diabetes mellitus
IIa	LDL	Chol.	10	Premature ASHD Tendinous Xan- thoma Xanthelasma	Hypothyroidism Nephrotic syndrome Biliary obstruction
IIb	LDL + VLDL	TG + chol.	40	Premature ASHD	Same as for IIa
III	IDL	TG + chol.	<1	Premature ASHD Tuberous Xanthomas	Hypothyroidism Ethanolism Diabetes mellitus
IV	VLDL	TG + chol.	45	Premature ASHD	Diabetes mellitus Ethanolism Estrogens/steroids
V	VLDL + chylomicrons	TG + chol.	5	Pancreatitis Eruptive xanthomas Lipemia retinalis	Diabetes mellitus Ethanol

T A B L E 1-2
American Heart Association's Dietary Therapy for Hyperlipidemia

Dietary Component	AHA Step 1 Diet	AHA Step 2 Diet
Total fat	<30% of total calories	Same
Saturated fatty acids	<10% of total calories	<7% of total calories
Polyunsaturated fatty acids	≤10% of total calories	Same
Mono-unsaturated fatty acids	10%–15% of total calories	Same
Carbohydrates	50%–60% of total calories	Same
Protein	10%–20% of total calories	Same
Cholesterol	<300 mg/day	<200 mg/day
Total calories	To achieve and maintain a desirable weight	Same
Ethanol	Maximum 1–2 beverages/day	Same

which may mask the symptoms of cardiac chest pain, or from nonischemic cardiac causes (e.g., pericarditis).

3. **Atypical chest pain in women** deserves special discussion. Several recent studies demonstrated that in the evaluation of atypical chest pain in women, the presence of multiple risk factors for the development of ASHD is far more powerful in predicting the presence of significant CAD than it is in men. This is particularly true in young women. Caveats to chest pain specific to women include:

   a. A decrease in HDL is more important as a risk factor than is an increase in LDL.

   b. Hypertension in a premenopausal woman increases her risk 10-fold relative to sex- and age-matched normotensive individuals.

   c. The presence of uncontrolled diabetes mellitus is a more powerful risk factor than it is in men.

   d. In postmenopausal women, no hormone replacement markedly increases the risk.

B. **Noncardiac-origin chest pain** is assessed to be from a discrete noncardiac source. Some of the more common causes of noncardiac chest pain are listed in Table 1-4.

T A B L E 1-3
Drug Therapy for Hyperlipidemias

Bile Acid–Binding Agents (Cholestyramine, Colestipol)

Effect: Reduces LDL levels
Dose: Cholestyramine 4 g b.i.d., increasing to 4 g q.i.d., and q HS (max: 20 g/day)
Side effects: Constipation, bloating, excess flatulence. May interfere with absorption of other drugs. Can cause hypertriglyceridemia

Gemfibrizol

Effect: Reduces serum triglycerides (also tends to reduce LDL cholesterol and increase HDL)
Dose: 600 mg p.o. b.i.d.
Side effects: Transient increase in transaminase levels. Less frequent side effects include nausea, diarrhea, gallstones, alopecia, and muscle weakness with an elevated CPK
Note: Use with caution when combined with HMG CoA reductase inhibitors (see below) because of reports of an increased incidence of myositis

HMG CoA Reductase Inhibitors (Lovastatin)

Effect: Reduces LDL cholesterol and plasma triglycerides, midly elevates HDL
Dose: 20–40 mg p.o. once or twice daily
Side effects: Transaminase elevations and increased CPK levels in a few patients

Nicotinic Acid

Effect: Reduces cholesterol and triglyceride levels, increases HDL cholesterol levels
Dose: 500–1,500 mg t.i.d.
Side effects: Flushing, which can be minimized by pretreatment with aspirin. Can also increase uric acid levels, cause mild hepatitis, and increase plasma glucose levels in diabetic patients. Rarely may produce a dermatologic manifestation, acanthosis nigricans

---

II. **Diagnosis**

Typical and atypical cardiac chest pain are clinical diagnoses (see Box 1-2, page 7). Once the chest pain has been categorized (see I, above), further evaluation and management are necessary.

The **specific evaluation and management** of angina pectoris include determining if the angina is stable or unstable or if it is the manifestation of an acute MI.

B O X 1-2

Overall Evaluation and Management of Chest Pain

Evaluation

1. Take a thorough history to document the nature of the chest pain. Typical ischemic chest pain has an onset with exertion, is relieved with rest, is squeezing and oppressive in nature, is substernal in location, often radiates to the left chest, jaw, and/or upper extremity, and often is accompanied by dyspnea, diaphoresis, and lightheadedness. Further historic data include the patient's profile of risk factors for the development of ASHD. Recall that angina pectoris in women is often atypical and that the clinician must rely more on risk factors in women than on the characteristics of the chest pain. See text for specifics.
2. Perform a physical examination with emphasis on vital signs. An S_4 gallop can be indicative of cardiac ischemia.
3. Obtain a 12-lead electrocardiogram (ECG), looking for any ischemic changes (e.g., flipped T waves) or evidence of acute injury (i.e., localized ST-segment elevation) or of old myocardial infarction (MI; i.e., Q waves).
4. Determine electrolytes, blood urea nitrogen (BUN), creatinine, glucose, and CBC for baseline purposes.
5. Monitor O_2 saturation. If <90%, obtain arterial blood gas values and give patient oxygen, 2 L/min, delivered by nasal cannula.
6. Obtain chest radiographs, posteroanterior (PA) and lateral, to look for any cardiomegaly, any pulmonary vascular redistribution, or any potential noncardiac causes of the chest pain (e.g., an infiltrate indicative of pneumonitis).
7. Obtain enzymes: lactate dehydrogenase (LDH) and CPK levels. If the LDH is increased, the LDH_1/LDH_2 is flipped, and the CK is increased with an increase in the CK-MB fraction, there is convincing evidence that myocardial necrosis has occurred. (DIAGNOSIS)
8. CK-MB subforms in the first 6 hours after the onset of chest pain. If the $CK\text{-}MB_2$ is >1.0 U/L and if the $CK\text{-}MB_2/CK\text{-}MB_1$ is >1.5, this is highly sensitive and specific for myocardial necrosis. If the values are <1.0 and 1.5 they are normal (i.e., no myocardial necrosis). (DIAGNOSIS)

(continued)

B O X   1-2 *(continued)*

9. Troponin-T is a marker for prognosis after an MI. The troponin-T is a tropomyosin-binding protein in myocytes that is spilled out after the death of cells; if troponin-T is elevated, the prognosis is poorer. There is a direct correlation between level of troponin-T elevation and the risk of death. (PROGNOSIS)

Management

1. Based on results of the evaluation, categorize the chest pain as being cardiac, atypical, or noncardiac in origin.
   a. If cardiac in origin, intervention with aspirin, antianginal agents (see Table 1-7, page 13), and cardiac catheterization is indicated. If there is any evidence that the chest pain is unstable or potentially an MI, admission for aggressive intervention is mandatory. See text and Table 1-8 (page 14) for details.
   b. If atypical in nature, give the patient aspirin, 325 mg p.o. q.d., and nitroglycerin, 1/150 gr sl prn and perform a noninvasive test for cardiac ischemia (i.e., a symptom-limited stress test, sestamibi stress test, or persantine sestamibi stress test). Refer to Table 1-5 (page 10) for specific test characteristics. If one of these noninvasive tests is positive for coronary arterial disease, referral to a cardiologist for cardiac angiography is indicated.
   c. If noncardiac in nature, treat the underlying cause. Musculoskeletal chest pain responds well to a nonsteroidal antiinflammatory agent (e.g., ibuprofen, 400–600 mg p.o., t.i.d.).
2. Assess the functional capacity of the patient. One method is to use the Canadian Cardiovascular Grading System (Table 1-6) (page 12). This provides a powerful baseline for future reference and assessment of therapy.
3. Long-term therapy for stable angina is discussed in the text (see III. Management, page 6).
4. The short-term management of unstable angina and other acute coronary syndromes is described in the text (see III. Management, page 6).

Referral

Referral to a cardiologist is indicated for all patients with cardiac-origin or atypical chest pain.

T A B L E 1-4
Some Causes of Noncardiac Chest Pain

Skin lesions
  Trauma to the skin
  Herpes zoster
Chest-wall trauma
Pulmonary embolism/infarction
Pneumothorax
Pneumonitis
Dissecting thoracic aortic aneurysm
Peptic ulcer disease
Costochondritis (Tietze's syndrome)

III. Management

A. Stable angina pectoris

Stable angina pectoris is present in a patient who has a history of ASHD and chest pain that is not increasing in frequency, duration, or intensity. The **specific management** includes the initiation of aspirin, 325 mg p.o., every morning, and antianginal agents from one or more of the following categories: nitrates, β-blockers, and/or calcium channel blockers (see Table 1-7).

Coronary angiography is indicated if the coronary anatomy is not known. Surgical intervention with bypass grafts is indicated in patients with stable angina who have left main coronary arterial disease or three-vessel ASHD, especially if there is evidence of ventricular dysfunction, as evidenced by a decreased ejection fraction. The **goals** of treatment are to minimize the episodes of angina and to prolong life; the combination of medical and surgical interventions will help achieve those goals. Recent studies have demonstrated that percutaneous transluminal coronary angiography (PTCA) and coronary artery bypass graft (CABG) are effectively equivalent therapies save for two caveats: (a) the patient may need a CABG in the future, and (b) in patients with diabetes mellitus, CABG is clearly superior.

B. Unstable angina pectoris

If the angina is of new onset (i.e., began within 6 weeks of presentation) or has been increasing in frequency, duration, or intensity, it is, by definition, unstable angina pectoris. Unstable angina requires therapy with antiplatelet agents (i.e., aspirin, 325 mg p.o., q.d.) and nitrates (e.g., 1 inch of nitroglycerin ointment q.6hr). Other modalities include β-blockers, calcium channel blockers (see Table 1-7), and oxygen.

Admission to a cardiology service is indicated.

If the patient has severe angina that is refractory to first-line therapy, the initiation of intravenous nitroglycerin

T A B L E 1-5
Noninvasive Tests for Atherosclerotic Heart Disease

Reference standard is coronary angiography.
Significant disease is defined as a >50% defect in the lumen of a coronary artery.
Sensitivity/specificity: determined when a heart rate >85% of the target heart rate is reached.

Test	Description and Procedure	Indications	Results/Sensitivity/Specificity
Symptom-limited stress test (SLST)	The patient is placed on a treadmill or bicycle to exercise. Parameters monitored include rhythm, ECG, blood pressure, and development of symptoms attributable to coronary arterial disease (i.e., angina pectoris). The exercise is conducted by using a standardized protocol, the most commonly used protocol being that described by Bruce. These protocols allow reproducible tests and the measurement of aerobic respiration (O_2 consumption) in units of METs (metabolic equivalents). One MET = 3.5 mL O_2 consumed/kg/min.	Diagnosis of atypical chest pain Diagnosis of Q-wave MI 6 wk after episode. Cannot be performed if any of the following contraindications exist: Aortic stenosis Asymmetric septal hypertrophy MI in past 6 wk Unstable angina pectoris Decompensated CHF	Diagnosis of ASHD >2 mm ST-segment depression: Sensitivity: 95% Specificity: 95% 1–2 mm ST-segment depression: Sensitivity: 25%–40% Specificity: 85% Indications to stop SLST Hypotension ST-segment depression Severe dysrhythmias Angina pectoris

Stress thallium or sestamibi test	Same as the SLST, plus the administration of a radioisotope, either thallium or Tc-sestamibi, in a fixed dose at the peak of exercise. Normally perfused and functioning cardiac myocytes take up the radioisotope; however, nonviable or underperfused areas will not take up the radioisotope. Scintigraphy is performed at the time of initial administration and 3 hr later.	Same as for SLST except that the patient has an abnormal resting ECG; women <45 years even with a normal resting ECG.	A *fixed defect*—i.e., one that remains constant at rest—is consistent with nonviable myocardium. A *reversible defect*—i.e., one that resolves at rest—is consistent with hypoperfusion (i.e., ASHD) in the vessel supplying that area. Sensitivity: 84% Specificity: 87% Fixed and reversible defects are as defined above. Sensitivity: 85% Specificity: 82%
Dipyridamole thallium or sestamibi stress trest	Instead of exercise, the agent dipyridamole is used. This agent causes coronary vasodilation and when used with the radioisotope thallium or Tc-sestamibi can scintigraphically assess for uptake. A scintigraphic picture is taken at the time of administration of the radioisotope and 3 hr later.	Same as for SLST except that the patient cannot exercise.	

T A B L E   1-6
**Canadian Cardiovascular Society Grading Scale for
Angina Pectoris**

Class I	Ordinary physical activity does not cause angina: no angina occurs when walking or climbing stairs; angina does occur with strenuous or rapid or prolonged exertion at work or recreation
Class II	Slight limitation of ordinary activity: angina occurs when walking or climbing stairs rapidly, walking uphill, walking or stair climbing after meals, in the cold, in the wind, under emotional stress, or only during the first few hours after awakening; walking more than two blocks on the level and climbing more than one flight of ordinary stairs at a normal pace and in normal conditions
Class III	Marked limitation of ordinary physical activity: angina occurs when walking one or two blocks on the level and climbing one flight of stairs in normal conditions and at a normal pace
Class IV	Inability to carry on any physical activity without discomfort. Anginal symptoms may be present at rest

and/or anticoagulation with heparin (see Table 1-8) is indicated.

In all cases of unstable angina, coronary angiography is indicated and will provide a basis for a decision on intervention with angioplasty or surgery.

C. **Myocardial infarction**
   Angina that is not relieved with nitroglycerin, is present for >15 minutes, and is accompanied by ST-segment elevation is an MI. If there is no contraindication, emergency thrombolysis with streptokinase or tissue plasminogen activator (tPA) and admission to an intensive care unit (ICU) is indicated (see Table 1-8). Primary angioplasty in myocardial infarction (PAMI) has demonstrated that there is a better outcome (decreased mortality, increased left ventricular function, and decreased reinfarction rate) in patients who receive emergency PTCA compared with acute emergency thrombolysis, especially in acute anterior wall MI. The concurrent administration of vitamin E (α-tocopherol), 400–800 IU q day p.o., decreases nonfatal MIs in patients with significant ASHD. Further acute management schemas are beyond the scope of this text.

T A B L E 1-7
Antianginal Agents

Class	Agent/Dose	Mechanism of Action	Side Effects
Antiplatelet	Aspirin, 325 mg p.o. q. A.M. *or*	Inhibits platelet aggregation	Gastric erosions
	Ticlopidine, 250 mg p.o. b.i.d.	Inhibits platelet aggregation (ADP-related)	Neutropenia, must check CBC q 2 wk for the first 2 mo of therapy
Nitrates	Isordil, 10 mg p.o. t.i.d. to 40 mg p.o. q.i.d. *or*	Decreases preload, dilates capacitance vessels	Hypotension, headaches
	Nitropaste, 1–2 inches q.6hr		
β-Blockers	Atenolol (Tenormin), 25–100 mg p.o. q.d. *or*	Decreases heart rate and contractility, therefore decreasing myocardial oxygen demand	AV nodal block, exacerbation of bronchospasm, hypotension, exacerbation of heart failure
	Metoprolol (Lopressor), 50–150 mg p.o. b.i.d. *or*		
	Propranolol (Inderal), 10–40 mg p.o. t.i.d. to q.i.d.		
Calcium channel blockers	Diltiazem (Cardiazem), 30–120 mg p.o. q.i.d.	Decreases preload, mildly decreases heart rate, moderate vasodilator	Hypotension; diltiazem can exacerbate AV nodal blocks and heart failure
		Decreases preload, moderate vasodilator	

TABLE 1-8
Thrombolytic and Adjunctive Drug Therapy for Acute Myocardial Infarction

Agent	Contraindications	Initial Dose	Maintenance Dose	Study
Streptokinase	Active bleeding Hypersensitivity Major surgery in previous 6 wk Cerebrovascular accident in previous 6 wk Use within previous 6 mo	1.5 million units i.v. bolus over 60 min	Concurrent use of heparin, dose below Concurrent use of ASA 325 mg q.d.	
Tissue plasminogen activator	Active bleeding Major surgery in previous 6 wk Cerebrovascular accident in previous 6 wk	6 mg bolus i.v., then 54 mg i.v. over 1 hr 20 mg i.v. over 2nd hr; 20 mg i.v. over 3rd hr	Concurrent use of heparin in dose below Concurrent use of ASA 325 mg p.o. q.d.	GUSTO
Heparin	Active bleeding History of heparin related thrombocytopenia Major surgery in previous 6 wk Cerebrovascular accident in previous 6 wk	5,000–10,000 units i.v. bolus	1,000 units i.v./hr Target a PTT: 45–60 sec	

β blockers: atenolol, metoprolol	Asthma, reversible airway disease High degree AV block, without pacemaker Severe systolic heart failure	Atenolol 5 mg i.v. q.5 min × 2 doses then 50 mg p.o. Metoprolol 5 mg i.v. q.5 min × 3 doses then 50 mg p.o. q.6hr × 4	Atenolol 100 mg p.o. q.d. Metoprolol 100 mg p.o. b.i.d.	ISIS-4 TIMI-IIB MIAMi
Ace inhibitors in myocardial infarction	Captopril-cough Angioedema	Captopril 6.25 mg p.o., then 12.5 mg p.o. at 2 hr, then 25 mg p.o. at 12 hr, then 50 mg p.o. b.i.d. *or* Lisinopril 5 mg p.o. q.d.	Captopril 50 mg p.o. b.i.d. *or* Lisinopril 10 mg p.o. q.d.	ISIS-4 GISSI-3
ACE inhibitors in left ventricular failure	Captopril-cough Angioedema	Captopril 6.25 mg p.o., then 12.5 mg p.o. at 2 hr, then 25 mg p.o. at 12 hr, then 50 mg p.o. b.i.d.	Captopril 50 mg p.o. b.i.d.	ISIS-4 GISSI-3

ISIS, International Study of Infarct Survival; MIAMI, Metoprolol in Acute Myocardial Infarction; TIMI, Thrombolysis in Myocardial Infarction; GISSI, Gruppo Italiano perlo Studio della Sopravzenzanell' Infarcto Miocardio; SAVE, Survival and Ventricular Enlargement; and GUSTO, Global Utilization of Streptokinase versus TPA for Occluded Coronary Arteries.

IV. Consultation

Problem	Service	Time
Stable angina	Cardiology	Required
Unstable angina	Cardiology	Urgent/Emergent
Myocardial infarction	Cardiology	Emergent

V. **Indications for admission:** Any degree of instability or any evidence of MI. The patient is admitted to the ICU.

Heart Failure

The heart is a pump that provides the flow of blood and therefore oxygen and nutrients to the vital tissues and organs of the body. If the heart fails in its mission, the flow of blood, nutrients, and oxygen to the tissues is markedly decreased. Therefore, failure of the heart will result in failure, to various degrees, of all of the organs, including the brain.

The **overall manifestations** of heart failure are quite diverse and are best categorized by grouping them into those that are the result of **backward failure** (i.e., pulmonary congestion) versus those that are the result of **forward failure** (i.e., low output). Heart failure of any cause can have any of these manifestations, but quite often the manifestations of backward or forward failure will predominate. The overall manifestations are given in Table 1-9.

   I. Categorization of congestive heart failure (CHF) by **overall manifestations**
      A. **Backward failure**
         The manifestations of backward failure (i.e., resulting from pulmonary congestion) include dyspnea, tachypnea, orthopnea, paroxysmal nocturnal dyspnea, an S_3 gallop, bilateral crackles, and right-sided failure findings: ascites, bipedal pitting edema, and distended neck veins.
      B. **Forward failure**
         The manifestations of forward failure (i.e., resulting from pump failure) include hypotension, confusion, lethargy,

T A B L E 1-9
Overall Manifestations of Congestive Heart Failure

Paroxysmal nocturnal dyspnea or orthopnea
Rales/crackle
Laterally displaced PMI
S_3 gallop
Jugular venous distention
Hepatojugular reflux
Dependent edema (ankle most common)
Nocturnal cough
Dyspnea on exertion
Hepatomegaly
Tachycardia, rate >120 beats/min

renal dysfunction, tachycardia, and cool, clammy skin and extremities.

Another method of categorizing heart failure that is central to the pathophysiology and management of this syndrome is by **systolic versus diastolic dysfunction.** Distinguishing systolic from diastolic dysfunction is difficult when only clinical methods such as the history, physical examination, electrocardiography, and chest radiograph are used.

II. Categorization of CHF by pathophysiology

A. Systolic dysfunction

Systolic dysfunction is characterized by reduced contractility, a decreased ejection fraction, and left ventricular dilation. It is the most common pathogenesis of heart failure. The most common causes of systolic heart failure include cardiomyopathy and ischemic heart disease. Cardiomyopathy results in a global defect; ischemia usually results in a local defect.

B. Diastolic dysfunction

Diastolic dysfunction is a common clinical problem, occurring in 30%–40% of patients referred for evaluation for CHF. The **underlying pathogenesis** of primary diastolic dysfunction is usually associated with left ventricular hypertrophy (LVH) normal or supernormal, contractility, and normal to increased ejection fraction. There is an increased end-diastolic pressure in a patient with normal ventricular-chamber size. There is increased resistance to diastolic filling resulting from increased left ventricular wall thickness and/or subendocardial ischemia, which is often present in patients with LVH. The increased resistance to filling results in an elevated end-diastolic (filling) pressure, which is transmitted to the pulmonary capillaries and causes pulmonary congestive manifestations.

One of the most common causes of diastolic heart failure is a hypertrophied left ventricle, usually as the result of long-standing, severe hypertension.

C. Mixed systolic/diastolic dysfunction

There is overlap between the two categories. Most patients have components of both; the clinician must determine which is predominate.

III. Management of heart failure by clinical category

The various clinical categories of CHF are referenced to the site of the predominant pathology: the endocardium, the pericardium, and the myocardium. Myocardial causes are subgrouped into systolic versus diastolic dysfunction.

A. Endocardial (valvular) failure

Evaluation of the endocardium is quite useful in documenting the significance of a murmur appreciated clinically. Manifestations are specific to the valve involved.

1. **Aortic stenosis**
   a. **Manifestations**

   Aortic stenosis manifests with a systolic murmur at the base with radiation into the carotids, a decrease in the pulse pressure, and a carotid pulsation that is slow and low (pulsus parvus et tardus). Secondary manifestations include LVH, an S_4 gallop, and syncope.

   b. **Evaluation and management**

   The **specific evaluation and management** of aortic stenosis include the steps described in Box 1-3. Echocardiography should be performed with Doppler studies. The normal valve size is >2.0 cm^2. A valve <2.0 cm^2 is considered stenotic, a valve <1.0 cm^2 is severely stenotic, and a valve <0.5 cm^2 is critically stenotic. **Referral** to a cardiologist for cardiac angiography and ventriculography should be performed in preparation for aortic-valve replacement. Antibiotic prophylaxis is required for any procedure (see Table 6-4, page 342).

2. **Aortic insufficiency**
   a. **Manifestations**

   Aortic insufficiency manifests with a diastolic murmur at the base with an increase in pulse pressure and the development of bounding "Corrigan's" or "water hammer" pulses. Secondary manifestations include LVH, an S_4 gallop, and syncope.

   b. **Evaluation and management**

   The specific evaluation and management of aortic insufficiency include the steps listed in Box 1-3. Echocardiography should be performed with Doppler studies. The echocardiogram will confirm the insufficiency. The use of nifedipine, 20 mg p.o., b.i.d., appears to delay the need for aortic-valve replacement in patients with moderate to mild aortic insufficiency. **Referral** to a cardiologist for cardiac angiography and ventriculography should be performed in preparation for potential aortic-valve replacement. Antibiotic prophylaxis is required for any procedure (see Table 6-4, page 342).

3. **Mitral regurgitation**
   a. **Manifestations**

   Mitral regurgitation (MR) manifests with a systolic murmur at the apex. Although many patients have benign mitral insufficiency, acute mitral insufficiency that has been acquired from an MI as the result of dysfunction or rupture of the papillary muscles may manifest with pulmonary edema, hypotension, and a loud murmur (i.e., one with an associated palpable thrill).

BOX 1-3

Overall Evaluation and Management of Congestive Heart Failure

Evaluation

Two questions are integral to the approach, evaluation, and management of heart failure: Why is the patient in heart failure (i.e., what is the etiology)? Why is the patient worse now? The evaluation is designed to answer these questions.

1. History, including onset of symptoms and the presence of backward or forward manifestations of failure (see text).
2. Physical examination for vital signs, crackles, the presence of an S_3 gallop, and to assess the severity of the failure.
3. A 12-lead ECG to look for any acute changes consistent with acute ischemia: any Q waves, indicative of old infarctions and therefore more systolic dysfunction or LVH, consistent with diastolic dysfunction.
4. Chest radiography (Fig. 1-1), PA and lateral, to look for an enlarged heart. A ratio of heart size to chest size >0.5 is a marker of cardiomegaly. In addition, there is often pulmonary vascular redistribution and a right pleural effusion.
5. Attempt to categorize the heart failure as being predominantly backward or forward, systolic versus diastolic in nature, and whether the site of failure is endocardial, pericardial, or myocardial. The most powerful tools to assist in such a grouping are the physical examination and echocardiography.

Management

1. Acute intervention in a patient with florid pulmonary edema includes administration of the following agents:
   a. Oxygen, to keep $P_{a_{O_2}} >60$ mm Hg.
   b. Morphine sulfate, 2 mg i.v., to decrease preload, to decrease any chest pain, and to decrease anxiety. This agent is underused in the acute management of heart failure.

(continued)

B O X   1-3 *(continued)*

   c. If no pericardial process is suspected and if the systolic blood pressure is >100 mm Hg, the clinician can administer nitroglycerin paste, 1 inch, to decrease preload, and a loop diuretic (e.g., furosemide [Lasix], 20 mg i.v.).

2. Admit patient to inpatient service.
3. See page 17 (III. Management of CHF by clinical category) for long-term management schemas.

  b. **Evaluation and management**

    The **specific evaluation** and management of mitral regurgitation include the steps listed in Box 1-3. Echocardiography should be performed with Doppler studies. Of note is that significant MR will result in a falsely elevated ejection fraction on multiple-gated acquisition (MUGA) or echocardiogram. The echocardiogram will reveal the mitral insufficiency and, quite often, an area of inferior wall hypokinesis.

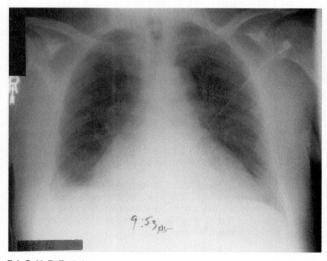

F I G U R E   1-1
AP chest: Cardiomegaly and pulmonary vascular congestion of pulmonary edema.

Referral to a cardiologist for cardiac angiography and ventriculography should be performed in preparation for potential mitral-valve replacement. Antibiotic prophylaxis is required for any procedure (see Table 6-4, page 342).

    4. **Failure of replacement valve**
        a. **Manifestations**
            The **specific manifestations** include the insidious onset of pulmonary edema with a slow increase in the intensity of regurgitant murmurs: aortic regurgitation (diastolic) in a failing aortic-valve replacement, or mitral insufficiency (systolic) in a failing mitral-valve replacement. This occurs in xenografts (e.g., the Hancock or Carpentier modified porcine valves) an average of 8–12 years after replacement.
        b. **Evaluation and management**
            The **overall evaluation and management** include making the clinical diagnosis by routine scheduled physical examination and echocardiography. The auscultation is for any regurgitant murmurs, and the echocardiogram, to confirm the diagnosis of any regurgitation. If there is any significant evidence of valve failure, **referral to** a cardiologist for cardiac catheterization and potential valve replacement is indicated.

B. Pericardial dysfunction
    1. **Manifestations**
        The **specific manifestations** of a pericardial effusion include those of low-output failure: hypotension, an elevated jugular venous pressure, and peripheral edema. The heart tones are usually quite distant, and on the ECG, there often is the unique phenomenon of electrical alternans (i.e., there is a 2- to 3-mA difference in the amplitude of QRS complexes). Chest radiography will show a large cardiac shadow.
    2. **Evaluation and management**
        The **specific evaluation and management of** pericardial disease include the steps listed in Box 1-3 and admission to an ICU if the patient is unstable. The echocardiogram will reveal a large pericardial effusion with end-diastolic collapse of the right ventricle. Therapy includes draining the pericardium and determining the underlying cause. Referral to a cardiologist for pericardiocentesis is indicated on an emergency basis.

C. Myocardial dysfunction
    1. **Manifestations**
        The **specific manifestations** and pathogenesis are those described in Box 1-3 and the preceding discussion. The history, physical examination, and echocardiogram will assist in categorizing the failure into predomi-

nantly systolic versus predominantly diastolic. The echocardiogram is pivotal in this differentiation. Although the measurement of ejection fraction is less accurate and precise with echocardiography than with nuclear cardiography (MUGA), echocardiography provides an excellent opportunity to visualize the myocardium in action. One can easily differentiate a predominantly systolic (low-contractility) process from a predominantly diastolic (poor filling, good-to-excellent contractility) process.

2. **Evaluation and management**

   The **specific evaluation and management** of myocardial etiologies of heart failure include the steps described in Box 1-3 and admission to the inpatient service if the failure is of new onset, is worsening, or is associated with any dysrhythmias, chest pain, syncope, or ECG changes.

3. **Management**

   a. **Systolic dysfunction:** Objectives in management and specifics in methods to achieve those objectives

      i. **Decrease pulmonary edema by** decreasing preload and improving oxygenation
         - Diuretics, especially loop diuretics [e.g., furosemide (Lasix), 20 mg, i.v.)
         - Nitrates (e.g., isosorbide dihydrate (Isordil), 10 mg p.o., q.i.d., or nitropaste
         - Oxygen supplementation

      ii. **Increase myocardial contractility** to increase cardiac output
         - Digoxin, 0.125–0.250 mg, p.o. q day;
         - If severe and end stage, i.v. dobutamine may be of benefit

      iii. **Decrease afterload** (i.e., systemic resistance) to assist the ventricle in pumping effectiveness and to prolong life
         - Angiotensin-converting enzyme (ACE) inhibition
            - Captopril (range, 6.25–150 mg) p.o. t.i.d.; titrate to blood pressure and to a dose of $\geq$50 mg, p.o. t.i.d., the target dose for survival benefit
            - Lisinopril (range, 2.5–40 mg) dosed q day
            - Quinipril (range, 5–20 mg) dosed b.i.d.
         - Angiotensinogen II receptor blocker
            - Valsartan, 80 mg p.o. q day (maximum, 160 mg, p.o. q day)
         - Carvedilol (novel agent: β-blocker, α_1-blocker, antioxidant) decreases mortality and sudden cardiac death
            - Carvedilol, 25–50 mg, p.o. b.i.d.

iv. **Determine the underlying origin**
Referral to a cardiologist for assessment of the underlying cause of the systolic failure, usually by coronary angiography, is indicated.

b. **Diastolic dysfunction**
The **management objectives** for diastolic dysfunction are similar to those for systolic dysfunction, with the following caveats:

i. Diuretics and nitrates should be used judiciously. Overuse may exacerbate this type of failure by decreasing preload and embarrassing the filling of the ventricles.

ii. Digoxin and other inotropic agents are relatively contraindicated.

iii. Optimal control of hypertension is necessary. The best agents to use are β-blockers or ACE inhibitors in the doses and goals listed previously. β-Blockers control hypertension and decrease the heart rate, affording an increase in ventricular filling. This is particularly true if the patient has concurrent ischemic heart disease. Calcium channel blockers, in addition to the effects described for β-blockers, may assist in ventricular relaxation. Refer to Table 3-3 (page 152) for dosing details.

iv. As with systolic dysfunction, referral to a cardiologist for assessment of the underlying cause, usually with coronary angiography, is indicated.

IV. **Consultation**

Problem	Service	Time
Any new heart failure	Cardiology	Required
Valvular disease	Cardiology and cardiovascular surgery	Required
Pericardial effusion	Cardiology	Emergent

V. **Indications for admission:** Any new-onset heart failure, any acute decompensation of chronic heart failure, any concurrent unstable angina pectoris, or any syncope or hemodynamically unstable tachydysrhythmias or bradydysrhythmias.

Syncope

Syncope is defined as transient, sudden loss of consciousness that resolves spontaneously. Because there are many potential causes for syncope in adults, it is important to approach this problem systematically with an appreciation for the various pathophysiologic mechanisms that might be involved in producing an individual patient's manifestations.

The critical question to address in patients with syncope is whether or not the syncope appears to be associated with a cardiac cause. Such patients tend to have a worse prognosis than patients with syncope not associated with cardiac causes or those with syncope of undetermined origin. The latter group may compose ≤50% of all patients with syncope evaluated in some large series.

I. **Differential diagnosis** (Table 1-10)

The most common causes of syncope, although multiple and varied, can be categorized into vasovagal causes, cardiac causes, orthostatic hypotension, neurologic causes, and electrolyte disturbances.

A. **Vasovagal causes**

Vasovagal reactions, also known as a simple faint, are a specific, quite common cause of syncope. The underlying pathogenesis of this entity is a massive surge in the parasympathetic system, resulting in transient hypotension and syncope. Carotid sinus hypersensitivity (CSH) may also result in syncope.

Specific manifestations include a preceding emotionally traumatic event with the patient spontaneously and very transiently having a complete loss of consciousness. There are no associated symptoms or any signs on physical examination.

B. **Cardiac causes**

The cardiac causes of syncope are quite diverse. The underlying **pathogenesis** is a decrease in the ability of the heart to perfuse the brain, resulting in syncope. Categories of etiologies include those associated with rhythm disturbances and those associated with structural cardiac abnormalities. The rhythm disturbances include bradycardias (e.g., third-degree AV nodal block) and tachycardias (e.g., atrial fibrillation or ventricular tachycardia). The structural abnormalities include aortic stenosis, asymmetric septae hypertrophy (ASH), and ventricular dysfunction as a result of ischemic heart disease.

C. **Orthostatic hypotension**

Orthostatic hypotension is one of the most common causes of syncope. The underlying **pathogenesis** is either a marked decrease in the intravascular volume or loss of the sympathetic tone necessary to maintain the actions of the vascular system. The most common causes of volume loss include gastrointestinal losses from vomiting or diarrhea, gastrointestinal bleeding, and excessive urinary losses, usually as the result of iatrogenic overzealous diuresis. The most common causes of sympathetic dysfunction include neuropathies due to diabetes and the use of β-blockers.

Specific manifestations include, for volume depletion, a source of the volume loss and an appropriate increase in heart rate when determining orthostatic parameters, and for autonomic dysfunction, an inappropriate lack of increase in heart rate.

T A B L E 1-10
Differential Diagnosis of Syncope

Vasovagal/Carotid Sinus Hypersensitivity

A. Faint, emotion or pain-related
B. Vasodepressor type CSH
   Nonbradycardic hypotension
C. Cardioinhibitory type CSH
   Bradycardic hypotension

Cardiac Causes

A. *Structural pathology*
   Inflow-track pathology
      Atrial myxoma
      Mitral stenosis
   Outflow-track obstruction
      Aortic stenosis
      Asymmetric septal hypertrophy
B. *Dysrhythmia*
   Tachydysrhythmia
      Ventricular tachycardia
      Atrial flutter/fibrillation
   Bradydysrhythmia
      Third-degree heart block
C. *Ischemic heart disease*
   Anginal equivalent
   Myocardial infarction

Orthostatic Hypotension

A. Intravascular volume depletion
B. Autonomic dysfunction

Situational Syncope*

A. Posttussive
B. Postmicturation
C. Postdefecation

Neurologic Causes*

A. Vertebrobasilar insufficiency
B. Subclavian steal syndrome

Metabolic Causes*

A. Hypoglycemia

_____

* Not discussed in text.

II. **Specific evaluation and management** of syncope, by cause
    A. **Vasovagal causes**
       Make the clinical diagnosis and reassure the patient. The
       natural history of the disorder is uniformly benign. If ca-

TABLE 1-11
Bradycardias

Type	ECG Findings	Manifestations/Etiologies	Treatment (see Table 1-15)
First-degree AV block	PR interval >0.20 sec No dropped QRS Intermittent bradycardia	Minimal, few/ Normal variant Medication related: a) Digoxin b) β-blockers c) Calcium channel blockers	Observe and modify medication:
Mobitz I Second-degree AV block (Wenckebach)	PR interval >0.20 sec Dropped QRS with grouped beating a) In each group: (QRS = P − 1) b) The PR interval increases with each beat until QRS is dropped Narrow QRS (0.08–0.10 sec)	Few/ Inferior wall ischemia Digoxin toxicity	Observation Modify medications Temporary VVI pacemaker, if hypotensive

Mobitz II Second-degree AV block	PR interval >0.20 sec Dropped QRS without grouped beating Widened QRS	Hypotension/ Senile atrophy of the conduction system (e.g., Lev's and Lenegre's) Anterior wall or inferior wall myocardial infarction	Temporary VVI pacemaker Permanent pacemaker
Third-degree AV block	AV dissociation Wide QRS, usually ventricular escape rhythm	Syncope (Stokes/Adams/Morgagni) Hypotension Senile atrophy of the conduction system (e.g., Lev's and Lenegre's) Anterior wall or inferior wall myocardial infarction	Permanent pacemaker
Cardioinhibitory bradycardic syncope	Intermittent first-degree, second-degree, or even third-degree AVB	Intermittent syncope	Permanent pacemaker

rotid sinus hypersensitivity (CSH) is suspected, a tilt-table examination may be indicated. If the syncope is severe and disabling, cardiac pacing may be of benefit; in addition, a trial of β-blockers may reverse the syncope, especially in vasodepressor CSH.

B. Cardiac causes (see also Table 1-12, pacemakers/brady-cardias)

The **specific evaluation and management** of cardiac syncope include that described in Box 1-4 and referral to a cardiologist. If the underlying cause is bradycardia (Table 1-11), either cardiac or bradycardia due to carotid sinus hypersensitivity (Table 1-12) is usually required. If the underlying cause is supraventricular tachycardia, treatment with an antidysrhythmic agent is indicated; if the underlying cause is ventricular tachycardia, electrophysiologic studies and potentially an automatic implantable cardiac defibrillator are indicated (Tables 1-13 and 1-14). Any ischemic coronary arterial disease will require cardiac angiography and intervention.

The **natural history** of cardiac syncope shows a poor prognosis; therefore, evaluation and intervention must be inpatient and aggressive (Box 1-4).

C. **Orthostatic hypotension**

The **specific evaluation and management** of orthostatic syncope includes the steps listed in Box 1-4 and defining whether the patient is volume depleted or has autonomic dysfunction. If the patient is **volume depleted,** replete the fluids. If i.v. repletion is necessary, normal saline is the fluid of choice. Furthermore, the underlying origin of the

---

B O X   1-4

Overall Evaluation and Management of Syncope

Evaluation

1. ABCs as outlined by basic and advanced life support.
2. Perform a thorough history, looking for information on the activity or situation antecedent to the event. Further data include the use of any mood-altering agents, including ethanol; the use of medicinal agents; and any history of cardiac or seizure activity. Witnesses to the event may provide powerful historic data, including observation of any convulsive activity consistent with a seizure and the duration of the episode.

(continued)

B O X 1-4 *(continued)*

3. The physical examination includes looking for any signs of trauma resulting from the syncopal episode, and:
   a. Vital signs, including orthostatic blood pressure and pulse, looking for any evidence of intravascular volume depletion or any hemodynamically compromising tachydysrhythmia or bradydysrhythmia.
   b. Cardiac examination, looking for any significant murmurs and/or gallops. A systolic murmur at the base with decreased carotid pulsations is consistent with aortic stenosis or asymmetric septal hypertrophy (ASH). A diastolic murmur at the apex is consistent with mitral stenosis or an atrial myxoma. An S_3 gallop is consistent with left ventricular heart failure.
   c. Neurologic examination, looking for any new focal motor or sensory deficits that might be consistent with a cerebrovascular accident or, in the postictal state, a Todd's paralysis. Focal deficits bespeak an focal intracranial origin.
4. 12-lead ECG with rhythm strip, looking for ischemic cardiac changes and/or atrioventricular (AV) nodal block.
5. Telemetry and/or Holter monitoring. These tests are used to monitor the patient's rhythm over a finite period. Telemetry entails monitoring while the patient is in the hospital. A Holter recording is a 24- or 48-hour recording of the patient's rhythm. To increase the specificity of this test, instruct the patient to record any symptoms and then correlate the symptoms with any rhythm disturbances.
6. Laboratory examinations
   a. Serum glucose (hypoglycemia).
   b. Serum electrolytes (baseline purposes).
   c. Serum BUN and creatinine. If both are elevated, with BUN greater than creatinine, the clinical picture is consistent with dehydration.
   d. Plasma levels of any antiseizure medication levels, if indicated.
   e. Hematocrit.
7. If there is any murmur or any evidence of heart failure, echocardiography should be performed to look at the valves and myocardial wall.

(continued)

B O X 1-4 *(continued)*

8. If the patient has no carotid bruits and there is no other cause noted, one can perform carotid sinus massage, which entails gentle massage of one of the carotid arteries and concurrent monitoring the blood pressure and rhythm strip. An abnormal response is hypotension, which may be due to or independent of a bradycardia.

9. If no cause is determined and there are no contraindications (e.g., aortic stenosis), a symptom-limited stress test looking for ischemia is indicated.

10. If there is any evidence that the patient has ventricular tachycardia (e.g., nonsustained ventricular tachycardia on Holter monitoring), signal-averaged ECG can be performed to look at the terminal aspect of the QRS complex. A normal test decreases the risk of sustained ventricular tachycardia; an abnormal test puts the patient at higher risk, and therefore further evaluation with electrophysiologic studies is indicated.

11. If no diagnosis has been made for the syncope by using these modalities, an upright tilt-table test is indicated. This test is used to detect any autonomic dysfunction that might cause syncope. Further details of this test are beyond the scope of this text.

12. No routine computed tomography (CT) scans of the head or electroencephalograms are indicated unless there is evidence from the history or physical examination of a seizure disorder or intracranial event.

Management

1. If the patient has depleted intravascular volume, replete fluids either enterally or parenterally.

2. The specific management depends on the underlying cause (see text and references for specifics).

Referral

1. If a cardiac cause is suspected, referral to a cardiologist is indicated.

2. If a neurologic cause (e.g., seizure disorder) is suspected, referral to a neurologist is indicated.

volume loss should be defined and treated. Any diuretic therapy should be temporarily discontinued.

Autonomic dysfunction is more difficult to treat and includes the following simple measures:

T A B L E 1-12
Indications for Pacemakers

1. Cardioinhibitory vasovagal
2. Third-degree AV block
3. High-grade second-degree AV block
4. Recurrent torsades de pointes (prolonged QTc)

    1. Arising slowly or with assistance from a supine position.
    2. Use of above-knee support stockings.
    3. Use of a nonsteroidal antiinflammatory agent, as these agents will cause volume retention and alleviate orthostatic hypotension.

III. **Consultation**

Problem	Service	Time
Any cardiac etiology	Cardiology	Required
Seizure disorder	Neurology	Urgent

IV. **Indications for admission:** Virtually all patients with syncope should be admitted. Exceptions are those who have had a vasovagal episode (fainting) or who have evidence of intravascular volume depletion that has resolved with fluid repletion.

Peripheral Vascular Disease of the Lower Extremities

The anatomy of the peripheral vasculature to the lower extremities is quite simple. The **arterial system** is a high-pressure system that supplies oxygen- and nutrient-rich blood to the lower extremities. The femoral artery enters the thigh immediately deep to the inguinal ligament and gives off several perforating branches into the thigh, including the profunda (deep) femoris artery. The femoral artery becomes the popliteal artery in the popliteal fossa. The popliteal artery then divides into the anterior and posterior tibial arteries and the anterior and posterior peroneal arteries. The anterior tibial artery gives off the dorsalis pedis artery. The clinically palpable arteries include:

1. The femoral artery: Palpable and auscultable at the level of the inguinal ligament.
2. The popliteal artery: Palpable and auscultable in the popliteal fossa.
3. The dorsalis pedis artery: Palpable on the proximal medial dorsal aspect of the foot.
4. The posterior tibialis artery: Palpable on the posterior aspect of the medial malleolus.

T A B L E 1-13
Cardiac Dysrhythmias

Rhythm	ECG Manifestations	Physical Manifestations	Causes	Therapy and Further Evaluation
Atrial fibrillation	No discrete P-waves Narrow-complex QRS Narrow-complex QRS	Irregularly irregular rhythm Ventricular response is usually fast Hypotension Heart Failure Unstable angina pectoris Any gallop ausculted must be an S_3; atrial fibrillation precludes the development of an S_4 gallop	Hyperthyroidism Valvular disease a) aortic b) mitral Hypertension with secondary cardiac damage Ischemia	Slow the rate with: a) Digoxin, 0.25 mg i.v. (see Table 1–14) b) Verapamil, 5 mg i.v. (see Table 1–14) If unstable, electrically cardiovert emergently, perform ACLS protocol (see Table 1–15) Once rate is controlled (i.e., <90 beats/min at rest): a) Determine the underlying etiology b) Continue digoxin 0.125–0.250 mg p.o./day c) Consider anticoagulation; warfarin should be initiated to obtain an INR of 2.0–3.0 in any patient who is at risk for emboli (i.e., with poor

left ventricular function, mitral stenosis, paroxysmal atrial fibrillation, or desire to cardiovert the patient)

d) All other patients should receive aspirin, 325 mg p.o. q.d., or ticlopidine 250 mg p.o. b.i.d.

e) Concurrent use of a β-blocker or calcium channel blocker will further control the rate (see Table 1-14)

f) Amiodarone or sotalol are excellent for long term control of rate and maintenance of sinus rhythm

(continued)

33

Rhythm	ECG Manifestations	Physical Manifestations	Causes	Therapy and Further Evaluation
Atrial flutter	P waves are large, best seen in lead II, and have a rate of 280–300 beats/min Narrow-complex QRS at a rate of 150 beats/min (2:1 conduction), 100 beats/min (3:1)	Regular rhythm Palpitations Heart failure Unstable angina pectoris Syncope Invariably there is a structural heart defect, present usually ASHD Other factors, those which precipitate atrial fibrillation exacerbate atrial flutter	Invariably there is a structural heart defect present, usually ASHD Other factors, those which precipitate atrial fibrillation exacerbate atrial flutter	Same as for atrial fibrillation, except: a) Always requires echocardiography and evaluation, after control of ventricular rate, for ASHD (e.g., a stress test) b) Anticoagulation is not necessary
Paroxysmal supraventricular tachycardia	Hypotension Discrete P-waves Narrow-complex QRS complexes	Palpitations Hypotension Chest pain	Ethanol Caffeine Ischemic heart disease (ASHD)	a) Minimize ethanol and caffeine ingestion b) Same as for atrial fibrillation c) Anticoagulation not necessary

Ventricular tachycardia	AV dissociation Wide QRS tachycardia Left axis deviation	Hypotension Sudden cardiac death Chest pain	ASHD, ischemia Hypokalemia Hypomagnesemia Hypoxemia Prolonged QTc syndromes as a result of medications (phenothiazines, tricyclic antidepressants), which predisposes patient to torsades du pointes	a) ACLS protocol with emphasis on electrical cardioversion if the patient is unstable b) Lidocaine, 75 mg i.v. bolus and a 2 mg/min i.v. drip c) Correct any hypokalemia and/or hypomagnesemia d) Determine the underlying cause and attempt to reverse e) Admit and refer to a cardiologist for SA ECG and/or electrophysiologic study; excellent negative predictive value; poor positive predictive value f) A further discussion of chronic antiventricular tachycardia agents is beyond the scope of the text, but includes AICD, amiodarone, or sotalol g) If torsades du pointes, overdrive pacemaker

T A B L E 1-14
Medications for Tachydysrhythmias

Agent	Atrial Fibrillation	Atrial Flutter	Paroxysmal Supraventricular Tachycardia	Ventricular Tachycardia
Propranolol	Acute: 0.5–2.0 mg i.v. bolus, rate of bolus infusion not to exceed 1 mg/min Chronic: 10 mg p.o. q.i.d. to 40 mg p.o. q.i.d.	Acute: same as for atrial fibrillation Chronic: same	Acute: same as for atrial fibrillation Chronic: same	No indication
Esmolol	Acute: 500 μg/kg over 1 min i.v., then 50–200 μg/kg/min IV drip Chronic: no indication	Acute: same as for atrial fibrillation Chronic: no indication	Acute: same as for atrial fibrillation Chronic: no indication	No indication Chronic: no indication
Verapamil	Acute: 0.075–0.15 mg/kg over 2 min IV; can repeat q. 15 min × 2 Chronic: 80 mg p.o. t.i.d. to 120 mg p.o. t.i.d.	Acute: same as for atrial fibrillation Chronic: same	Acute: same as for atrial fibrillation Chronic: same	No indication

Diltiazem	Acute: 0.25–0.35 mg/kg over 2 min i.v. Chronic: 30 mg p.o. q.i.d. to 120 mg p.o. q.i.d.	Acute: same as for atrial fibrillation Chronic: same	Acute: same as for atrial fibrillation Chronic: same
Digoxin	Acute: 0.25 mg i.v. now, repeat in 30 min × 1, then repeat q,6h. × 2 Chronic: 0.25–0.375 mg p.o. q. A.M.	Acute: same Chronic: same	Acute: same Chronic: same
Adenosine	Acute: 6.0 mg i.v., can repeat in 15 min × 1	Acute: same	Acute: same
Lidocaine	No indication	No indication	No indication
Sotalol	40 mg p.o. b.i.d., increase slowly to 80 mg p.o. b.i.d.	Same	Same
Amiodarone	Loading: 800 mg q.d. p.o. for 2 weeks then 400–600 mg q.d. p.o.	Same	No indication

(Lidocaine: No indication — Acute: 75 mg i.v. bolus with a concurrent 2 mg/min i.v. drip)

T A B L E 1-15
Cardioversion: Indications and Contraindications

Indications

Atrial fibrillation/flutter of recent onset (i.e., <3 days) with or
without anticoagulation
Atrial fibrillation/flutter of any duration if adequately anticoag-
ulated with warfarin for >3 wk
No contraindications
Emergently if the patient is unstable

Contraindications to Elective Cardioversion

Any known or suspected intracardiac thrombus
TIA, recent CVA, or cerebrovascular disease
Recent MI (relative contraindication)
Uncertain duration of adequate anticogulation (i.e., >3 wk of
warfarin with an INR of 2.0–3.0)
CHF (relative contraindication)
Electrolyte imbalance, especially hypokalemia
Digitalis toxicity

The **venous system** parallels the arterial system, but with more
individual variation. The venous system is a low-pressure system
that returns oxygen-poor and waste-containing blood to the inferior vena cava. A major contribution to venous return is provided
by extrinsic compression by the lower-extremity musculature.

The venous system can be divided into the **deep** and **superficial
venous systems.** The deep venous system accounts for >90% of
the venous drainage. The deep system includes the anterior and
posterior peroneal veins and the anterior and posterior tibialis
veins of the calf, all of which drain into the popliteal vein. The
popliteal vein then drains into the superficial femoral vein, which
then drains into the inferior vena cava. The profunda (deep) femoral vein drains the thigh into the femoral vein.

The **superficial venous system** drains <10% of the blood from
the lower extremities. The system consists of the greater (medial)
and lesser (lateral) saphenous veins.

I. **Manifestations of lower extremity vascular disease**
   A. **Arterial disease**
      The **specific manifestations** of arterial vascular disorders
      in the lower extremities are all attributable to ischemia in
      the affected lower extremity. These include claudication,
      that is, the development of pain, often crampy in nature,
      on exercise of the lower extremity (e.g., while walking).
      There can be, and often are, bruits over the femoral artery;
      decreased pulses in the popliteal, dorsal pedis, and poste-
      rior tibialis arteries in the affected lower extremity; and
      a cool extremity with an increased capillary-refill time.

Capillary refill is measured by palpating over the distal toe, blanching the skin, and observing the amount of time for it to return to its baseline pink color.

Risk factors for the development of lower extremity arterial disease include hypertension, diabetes mellitus, smoking, hyperlipidemia, and obesity.

The **natural history** is one of progression to symptomatic claudication, a manifestation that can severely limit the patient's activities; ulcers in the skin; cellulitis; and gangrene.

B. Venous disease

Many problems can develop in the low-pressure venous system. The vast majority of these problems are benign and cosmetic; however, some entities, if untreated, are potentially mortal.

1. **Varicosities.** The **specific manifestations** of varicose veins include the presence of tortuous, dilated, enlarged, nontender veins within the skin of the lower extremities. Usually the process affects both lower extremities. The lesions are usually asymptomatic.

   Risk factors for the development of varicosities include obesity, inactivity, wearing tight clothes about the waist/abdomen, and wearing girdles.

   The **natural history** is benign, with occasionally an episode of superficial thrombophlebitis.

2. **Venous stasis.** The **specific manifestations** of venous stasis include bilateral lower extremity edema that may be worse in the evenings and resolves overnight when the patient sleeps in a recumbent position. There often are concurrent lower extremity varicosities.

   The **risk factors** are quite similar to those described in the development of varicose veins. However, one additional risk factor plays a role in development: damage to the venous valves, most commonly as the result of a past episode of DVT (the postphlebitic syndrome).

   The **natural history** is usually benign, but complications can develop. These complications include changes in the overlying skin, such as increased pigment and skin breakdown, and therefore an increased risk of cellulitis. The risk of cellulitis is particularly high in patients who have a concurrent risk factor (i.e., neuropathy resulting from diabetes mellitus, or arterial insufficiency).

3. **Superficial thrombophlebitis.** The **specific manifestations** include an acute onset of pain, swelling, erythema, and warmth in one of the lower extremities. The patient often has a palpable cord, which represents the thrombosed vein itself. These manifestations are quite similar to those of DVT.

   Risk factors for the development of superficial thrombophlebitis include varicosities, trauma to the area, the placement of i.v. catheters, and, as with deep venous thrombophlebitis, immobilization and hypercoagulable states.

The **natural history** of this entity is quite benign, with no risk of systemic embolization.

4. **Deep venous thrombophlebitis.** The **specific manifestations** include an acute onset of pain, swelling, erythema, and warmth in one of the lower extremities. There can be various degrees of warmth, redness, tenderness, and swelling in the affected lower extremity. Risk factors for the development of DVT include hypercoagulable states, inflammation, and immobilization.

The **natural history** of DVT depends on the location of the thrombosis, either distal (inferior to the popliteal space) or proximal (in and superior to the popliteal space). Distal thrombus rarely embolizes to the pulmonary bed, whereas proximal thrombus is at high risk for embolizing to the pulmonary bed with resultant morbidity and mortality. Because distal thrombus can, over time, propagate proximally, repeated imaging is necessary to follow the thrombus.

II. **Specific evaluation and management**

A. **Arterial disease**

The **specific evaluation and management** include that described in Box 1-5, and if the distal pulses are nonpalpable, determining the ABI to assess the degree of obstruction to arterial flow. If the patient has a history of arterial thrombosis at other sites (i.e., cerebrovascular accident, upper extremity ischemia) or is in the rhythm of atrial fibrillation, perform echocardiography to look for intracardiac thrombus.

The **specific management** depends on the underlying pathogenesis.

1. If the underlying pathogenesis is **atherosclerotic disease,** the **risk factors** for the development of atherosclerotic disease must be modified, aspirin, 325 mg/day, p.o., should be initiated, and a referral to a vascular surgeon for arterial bypass surgery should be made.

2. If the patient has any evidence that the underlying pathogenesis is one of **arterial thrombotic events** (i.e., the patient is in atrial fibrillation, or has a dilated cardiomyopathy, or has thrombus in the ventricle demonstrated with echocardiography), admit the patient and provide anticoagulation on a long-term basis with warfarin (Table 1-17). The target international normalized ratio (INR) is 2.0–3.0, except in patients with a prosthetic heart valve, in whom the target INR is 3.0–4.2. Referral to vascular surgery is also indicated in the acute setting, as surgical removal of the thrombus may be of acute benefit.

B O X 1-5

***Overall Evaluation and Management of Lower
Extremity Vascular Disease***

Evaluation

1. Take a history, focusing on:
   a. Claudication (i.e., the development of pain in one
      or both lower extremities on exercise, indicative
      of decreased arterial flow.
   b. Risk factors for the development of atheroscle-
      rotic disease, which are the same as those de-
      scribed on page 1, this chapter.
   c. Any history of arterial or venous thrombotic
      events.
   d. The time of onset of lower extremity swelling and
      whether it is unilateral or bilateral.
   e. Concurrent symptoms, including pain in the af-
      fected lower extremity.
   f. Risk factors for the development of venous throm-
      botic disease:
      i. Recent immobilization
      ii. Any inflammation in one or both lower extrem-
          ity(ies), including any infectious process
      iii. Hypercoagulable states, as manifested by a
           history of deep venous thrombosis (DVT); this
           might indicate a deficiency in one of the nor-
           mally present proteins of anticoagulation (e.g.,
           protein C, protein S, antithrombin III), homo-
           cystinemia, and factor V Leiden or the revers-
           ible hypercoagulable state of pregnancy
2. Perform a physical examination, including:
   a. Auscultating for bruits over the femoral artery.
   b. Palpating for pulses over the popliteal artery, dor-
      salis pedis artery, and posterior tibialis artery.
      If the pulses are nonpalpable, perform a Dopp-
      ler-flow study of the lower extremity arteries. This
      examination determines the ratio of flow in the
      lower extremity arteries relative to flow in the ar-
      teries of the upper extremity (arterial blood ratio,
      ABI). The ratio is normally 1; any ratio <0.5 is in-
      dicative of significant obstructive lower extremity
      arterial disease.
      If there is any evidence of swelling or edema in
      the lower extremities, determine whether there is

(continued)

BOX 1-5 (continued)

>   any asymmetry by measuring calf and thigh circumferences.
>   c. Looking for concurrent signs of inflammation [i.e., redness (rubor), tenderness, warmth (calor), and any areas of skin breakdown].
>
> *Management*
>
> Based on the history and physical examination results, determine whether the process is predominantly arterial or venous.
>
> 1. If the process is arterial, check for and modify any risk factors in the development of atherosclerotic disease; initiate aspirin, 325 mg p.o./day (unless contraindicated*); and refer the patient to vascular surgery (see text).
> 2. If the process is venous and asymmetric, rule out DVT by imaging techniques (see text and Table 1-16). If DVT in the proximal venous system is diagnosed, admission and the initiation of heparin are mandated (see Chapter 4, page 227).
>
> *Referral*
>
> Referral to a vascular surgeon is necessary for any patient with lower extremity arterial disease.
>   The overall manifestations of and approaches to lower extremity vascular problems are quite diverse and are best categorized by the underlying pathogenesis (i.e., according to whether the arterial or venous system is predominantly affected).
>   *If contraindicated: Ticlopidine, 250 mg, p.o. b.i.d.

  B. **Venous disease**
    1. **Varicosities.** The specific evaluation and management include making the clinical diagnosis by performing a thorough history and physical examination (see Box 1-5) and preventing further progression of the process. The patient should be instructed to lose weight, wear loose-fitting clothes, not to cross the legs, to increase exercise, and not to wear girdles. The use of above-knee elastic hose is of benefit in prevention. If the varicosities are of significant concern to the patient, referral to a vascular or general surgeon for sclerotherapy is indicated.

2. **Venous stasis.** The specific evaluation and management of venous stasis include making the clinical diagnosis by performing a thorough history and physical examination, as described in Box 1-5, and preventing further progression of the disease. The patient should be instructed to lose weight, wear loose-fitting clothes, not to cross the legs, to increase exercise, and not to wear girdles. The use of above-knee elastic hose and elevating the lower extremities when sitting are also of benefit in prevention. There is no indication for diuretic therapy in a patient with edema due to venous stasis. Any cellulitis should be aggressively treated (see section on Bacterial Skin Disease, Chapter 6, page 312).

3. **Superficial thrombophlebitis.** The specific evaluation and management of superficial thrombophlebitis include that described in Box 1-5 and ruling out any concurrent DVT by the imaging techniques described in Table 1-16. Specific management includes rest, lower extremity elevation, initiation of a nonsteroidal antiinflammatory agent (see Table 7-8, Musculoskeletal Disorders, page 393), and the application of local heat.

4. Deep venous thrombosis. The specific evaluation and management of DVT include making the diagnosis and defining the thrombus as being distal or proximal, by using the information detailed in Box 1-5 and Table 1-16. The specifics in management include:

   a. **Superficial thrombophlebitis**
      Evaluation and management are described in preceding paragraph 3.

   b. **Conclusively distal DVT**
      Manage the patient conservatively with leg elevation and initiation of a nonsteroidal antiinflammatory agent. A noninvasive imaging study (see Table 1-16) should be repeated in 3–5 days. If there is any propagation of the thrombus proximally, it must be treated as a proximal DVT.

   c. **Proximal DVT**
      The thrombus is at high risk for embolizing. For all intents and purposes, thrombosis in the deep venous system is the same disease process as pulmonary thromboembolic disease.

      (See pulmonary chapter, pleuritic chest pain; pulmonary thromboembolic disease; page 224)

III. Consultation

Problem	Service	Time
Recurrent venous disease	Hematology	Elective
Arterial thrombotic disease	Hematology	Required
Arterial thrombotic disease	Vascular surgery	Urgent
Intermittent claudication	Vascular surgery	Required
Varicosities	Vascular surgery	Elective

TABLE 1-16
Imaging Techniques for the Lower Extremity Venous System

Test	Procedure Description	Results/Sensitivity/Specificity
Compression ultrasound	Segments of the proximal deep venous system are imaged on ultrasound; direct pressure is applied to the veins by the examiner: If compressible, indicative of no luminal defects; therefore, no thrombus If not compressible, consistent with thrombus	Proximal: Sensitivity: 89% Specificity: 97%
Doppler ultrasound	The Doppler probe measures flow within the vessel itself. Spontaneous flow and augmented (i.e., by compressing the vessels distal to the proble level) flow are measured. If flow in the vessel is not compromised and if there is an increase in flow on augmentation, no thrombus is present. A decrease in flow and a decrease in augmented flow are consistent with thrombus	Proximal: Sensitivity: 84% Specificity: 87%

| Impedance plethysmography (IPG) | This procedure is based on the facts that proximal thrombus will decrease the flow of blood from the distal bed and that the blood flow can be measured by measuring the impedance to the flow of AC current through an extremity. The procedure is performed by placing a blood pressure cuff around the proximal thigh and applying 50 mm Hg pressure. The flow will slowly decrease, as measured by the impedance. When a plateau is reached, the cuff is deflated with, in the normal setting, a rapid flow from the distal to proximal systems, as reflected by a marked and rapid decrease in impedance. If proximal thrombus is present, there is minimal flow into the proximal system and therefore a blunting of the normal rapid change in impedance | Proximal: Sensitivity: 96%–100% Specificity: 94% |
| Contrast venography | Intravenous contrast dye is injected into the venous system of the lower extremity via a foot vein. This invasive procedure remains the reference standard with which all other procedures are compared. It can result in phlebitis and even anaphylaxis and is no longer the first-line procedure; essentially it is used for those cases in which DVT is suspected even with a negative noninvasive imaging study | Proximal: Sensitivity: 95% Specificity: 95% |

T A B L E 1-17
Indications for Oral Anticoagulation (Warfarin)

Indications	Target INR	Duration of Anticoagulation
Atrial fibrillation, especially if Left ventricular failure Embolic CVA Rheumatic fever Mitral stenosis Left atrial dilation	2.0–3.0	Long term
Cardioversion of atrial fibrillation Chemical Electrical	2.0–3.0	3 wk before and after the cardio-version
Mechanical/prosthetic valves St. Jude's Björk–Shiley Starr–Edwards	3.0–4.2	Lifelong
First deep venous thrombosis/pulmonary thromboembolic disease	2.0–3.0	3–6 mo
Recurrent deep venous thrombosis/pulmonary thromboembolic disease or a hypercoagula-ble state, or both	2.0–3.0	Lifelong *or* Duration of the hypercoagulable state
Large myocardial infarction, especially if ante-rior wall with thrombous formation	2.0–3.0	6 mo

Problem	Risks/Tests for Risk Stratification	Prophylaxis	Diagnosis, If Prophylaxis Failed

Deep venous thrombosis	Factors associated with an *increased* risk
	a) Any procedure that results in >24 hr of immobilization, e.g.,
	  Pelvic surgery
	  Gynecologic
	  Prostate
	  Hip replacement
	  Knee replacement
	b) Concurrent malignant neoplasm
	c) History of DVT/PTE
		a) Early ambulation, if possible *and*
		b) Intermittent compression devices; N.B. difficult to use in fractures
		  or
		c) Enoxaparin 30 mg s.c. q12 (commence 12 hr before surgery);
		  or
		d) Low-molecular-weight heparin, 75 IU/kg s.c. q12 (commence 12 hr before surgery);
		  or
		e) Heparin, 5,000 units s.c. q12 (commence 12 hr before surgery);
		  or
		f) Adjusted-dose heparin, 3,500–5,000 units s.c. q8 hr, goal aPTT is 31–36 sec.
		  or
		g) If high risk: Warfarin, 5 mg PO q HS to achieve a goal INR of 2.0–3.0. (refer to Table 1-17)
			1. Clinical suspicion
			2. Duplex (ultrasound and Doppler)
			Sensitivity is only fair in this setting as acute thrombus here is nonocclusive, thereby decreasing the detection rate of the test [i.e., 65%-70% as opposed to the high (95%) sensitivity] of the study in outpatients

(continued)

47

T A B L E 1-18 *(continued)*

Problem	Risks/Tests for Risk Stratification	Prophylaxis	Diagnosis, If Prophylaxis Failed

Perioperative myocardial infarction	Clinically assess the risk to the patient; one method is the Goldman criteria (see Table 1-19) and stratify the patient to one of four risk factor categories (I, II, III, IV)
	
	a. If *no ischemic heart disease* known and patient has a good exercise tolerance (Category I):
	  1. ECG, 12-lead
	  2. Chest radiograph PA and lat
	
	b. If *ischemic heart disease* is known and patient is at *low risk* (i.e., a category I or II)
	  1. ECG, 12-lead
	  2. Chest radiography, PA and lat
		Control glucoses in patient with diabetes mellitus
		Maintain an adequate P_aO_2 (>70 mm Hg) and hematocrit ($>30\%$)
		If ECG changes, evaluate as for category III, IV below
			As for routine diagnosis of myocardial infarction
			Troponin-T-1 is highly specific for cardiac muscle (especially because CK and MB are elevated after trauma and surgery, leading to false positives)

c. If *ischemic heart disease known and patient is at high risk*, (i.e., category III or IV or has a poor functional status)
   1. ECG, 12-lead, and
   2. Chest radiograph

      and

   3. SLST

      or

   4. Persantine ST

      or

   5. Dobutamine echocardiograph

   Routine, as above, and
   If SLST or PST or dobutamine echocardiogram indicate ischemia, postpone surgery, and perform cardiac angiogram
   Control any heart failure
   Arterial-line monitoring
   Swan–Ganz monitoring

d. If *unstable angina*:

   a) Smoking history
   b) Arterial blood gas on room air
      P_aO_2 <60 mm Hg
      O_2 sat <90%

   Cancel surgery
   Treat as described in Chapter 1, page 9
   Cardiac angiogram
   a) Discontinue smoking
   b) Incentive spirometry
   c) Optimize β agonism (Albuterol MDI) and topical ipratropium (Atrovent MDI)

COPD

(continued)

Problem	Risks/Tests for Risk Stratification	Prophylaxis	Diagnosis, If Prophylaxis Failed
	c) Pulmonary-function tests FEV1 <1.5 L indicates significant embarrassment FVC: If low, demonstrates restrictive disease d) Chest radiograph and physical examination		
Blood loss	a) Trauma b) Hip replacement c) Prostate surgery d) Coronary bypass grafting	a) Cell saver in the surgical suite b) Autologous transfusion (may donate <2 units if an elective procedure) c) $FeSO_4$ after the procedure	a) Monitor hematocrits
Hypothyroidism	a) Poor compliance with medications b) Hypothyroidism	a) Diagnose hypothyroidism clinically and confirm with an elevated TSH (see chapter 9, page 507) b) May hold levothyroxine 7 days without replacement c) If needs to be held 7 days, replace at 1/2 dose intravenously	a) Clinical b) Elevated TSH

Primary adrenal insufficiency	a) Adrenal insufficiency b) Poor response to an ACTH cosyntropin (Cortrosyn) stimulation test (page 496)	a) Stress doses of steroids in the IV route (i.e., 50–100 mg IV hydrocortisone q6 hr)	a) Clinical, including perioperative hypotension b) Hyperkalemia
Chronic glucocorticoids	a) Long-term use of glucocorticoids b) Poor response to metyrapone stimulation test	a) Stress doses of steroids in the IV route (i.e., 50–100 mg IV hydrocortisone q6 hr)	a) Clinical, including perioperative hypotension b) Hypoglycemia
Medications	a) Use of aspirin b) Antihypertensives	a) Hold dose for 7 days before the scheduled surgery a) Change from oral route to Nitropaste IV labetalol see Table 3-3, page 152	a) Increased bleeding time a) Hypotension b) Hypertension
Hemophilia: see section on excessive bleeding, chapter 5, page 268			

T A B L E   1-19
Goldman Criteria for Preoperative Cardiac Assessment

Finding	Points
S₃ gallop or increased JVP on examination	11
Q wave or non–Q-wave myocardial infarction in the past	10
More than 5 PVC/min	7
Rhythm other than sinus or PACs	7
Age older than 70 years	5
Emergency procedure	4
Surgery of aorta/intrathoracic/intraperitoneal site	3
Aortic stenosis	3
Poor general medical condition	3

Class I, 0–5 points; class II, 6–12 points; class III, 13–25 points; and, class IV, >26 points.

IV. Indications for admission: Development of a significant cellulitis, gangrene, acute arterial thrombosis, and all cases of proximal DVT.

Preoperative Assessment

The primary care physician may be called on to render opinions on perioperative management of individual patients. The majority of such issues are cardiovascular, so it is included in this chapter (see Tables 1-18 and 1-19)..

Bibliography

Hyperlipidemia
Alpert JS, et al: Update in cardiology. Ann Intern Med 1996;125:40–46.
Gotto AM, ed: Dyslipoproteinemia education program: clinician's manual. London: Science Press Limited, 1991.
Grundy SM, Denke MA: Dietary influences on serum lipids and lipoproteins. J Lipid Res 1990;31:1149–1172.
Grundy SM, et al: The place of HDL in cholesterol management. Arch Intern Med 1989;149:505–510.
Hunninghake DB, et al: The efficacy of intensive dietary therapy alone or with lovastatin in outpatients with hypercholesterolemia. N Engl J Med 1993;328:1213–1219.
Manson M, et al: The primary prevention of myocardial infarction. N Engl J Med 1992;326:1406–1416.
Report of the national educational program expert panel on detection, evaluation, and treatment of high blood cholesterol in adults. Arch Intern Med 1988;148:36–71.

Chest Pain

Abrams J: A reappraisal of nitrate therapy. JAMA 1988;259:396–401.

Alpert JS, et al: Update in cardiology. Ann Intern Med 1996;125:40–46.

Bingle JF, Mayhew HE: Outpatient management of coronary artery disease. Am Fam Physician 1987;36:191–200.

Bypass Angioplasty Revascularization Investigation (BARI) investigators: Comparison of coronary bypass surgery with angioplasty in patients with multivessel disease. N Engl J Med 1996;335:217–225.

Campeau L: Grading of angina pectoris [Letter]. Circulation 1976;54:522–523.

Diamond GA, Forrester JS: Analysis of probability as an aid in the clinical diagnosis of coronary artery disease. N Engl J Med 1979;300:1350–1358.

Douglas PS, et al: The evaluation of chest pain in women. N Engl J Med 1996;334:1311–1315.

Epstein S, ed: Highlights of the 66th Scientific Sessions of the American Heart Association. J Myocard Ischem 1994;6:9–32.

Evans CH, Karunaratne HB: Exercise stress testing for the family physician: part I. Performing the test. Am Fam Physician 1992;45:121–132.

Goldman L, Lee TH: Noninvasive tests for diagnosing the presence and extent of coronary artery disease. J Gen Intern Med 1986;1:258–264.

Hennekens CH, et al: Adjunctive drug therapy of acute myocardial infarction: evidence for clinical trials. N Engl J Med 1996;335:1658–1667.

Kotler TS, Diamond GA: Exercise thallium-201 scintigraphy in the diagnosis and prognosis of coronary artery disease. Ann Intern Med 1990;113:684–702.

Lewis HD, et al: Protective effects of aspirin against acute myocardial infarction and death in men with unstable angina pectoris. N Engl J Med 1983;309:396–403.

Ohman EM, et al: Cardiac troponin T levels for risk stratification in the acute myocardial ischemia. N Engl J Med 1996;335:1333–1342.

Packer M, et al: The effect of carvedilol on morbidity and mortality in patients with chronic heart failure. N Engl J Med 1996;334:1349–1355.

Physicians' Health Study Research Group: Final report on the aspirin component of the ongoing Physicians' Health Study. N Engl J Med 1989;321:129–135.

Pryor DB, et al: Estimating the likelihood of significant coronary artery disease. Am J Med 1983;75:771–780.

Stephens NG, et al: Randomized controlled trial of vitamin E in patients with coronary artery disease: Cambridge Heart Antioxidant Study (CHAOS). Lancet 1996;347:781–786.

Veterans Administration Cooperative Group: Comparison of medical and surgical treatment for unstable angina pectoris. N Engl J Med 1987;316:977–984.

Heart Failure

Alpert JS, et al: Update in cardiology. Ann Intern Med 1996;125:40–46.

The Captopril–Digoxin Multicenter Research Group: Comparative effects of therapy with captopril and digoxin in patients with mild and moderate heart failure. JAMA 1988;259:539–544.

Chia-Sen Lee D, et al: Heart failure in outpatients. N Engl J Med 1982;306:699–705.

Cohn J: The management of chronic heart failure. N Engl J Med 1996;335:490–498.

The Criteria Committee of the New York Heart Association: Nomenclature and criteria for diagnosis of diseases of the heart and great vessels, 8th ed. New York: New York Heart Association/Little, Brown, 1979.

Deedwania PC: Angiotensin-converting enzyme inhibitors in congestive heart failure. Arch Intern Med 1990;150:1798–1804.

Harizi RC, et al: Diastolic function of the heart in clinical cardiology. Arch Intern Med 1988;148:99–108.

Packer M: Comparison of captopril and enalapril in patients with severe chronic heart failure. N Engl J Med 1986;315:847–853.

Packer M, et al: Influence of renal function on the hemodynamic and clinical responses to long-term captopril therapy in severe chronic heart failure. Ann Intern Med 1986;104:147–154.

Pfeffer MA, et al: Effect of captopril on mortality and morbidity in patients with ventricular dysfunction after myocardial infarction. N Engl J Med 1992;327:669–677.

SOLVD Investigators: Effect of enalapril on mortality and development of heart failure in asymptomatic patients with reduced left ventricular ejection fractions. N Engl J Med 1992;327:685–691.

Syncope/Cardiac Dysrhythmias

Alpert JS, et al: Update in cardiology. Ann Intern Med 1996;125:40–46.

Benditt DG, et al: Cardiac pacing for prevention of recurrent vasovagal syncope. Ann Intern Med 1995;122:204–209.

Brugada P, et al: A new approach to the differential diagnosis of a regular tachycardia with a wide QRS complex. Circulation 1991;83:1649–1659.

DiMarco JP, et al: Adenosine for paroxysmal supraventricular tachycardia: dose ranging and comparison with verapamil. Ann Intern Med 1990;113:104–110.

Ganz LI, et al: Supraventicular tachycardia. N Engl J Med 1995;332:162–173.

Hohnloser SH, et al: Sotalol. N Engl J Med 1994;331:31–38.

Jalal S, et al: Role of electrophysiologic testing after MI. J Myocard Ischem 1994;6:30–40.

Kapoor WN: Diagnostic evaluation of syncope. Am J Med 1991;90:91–106.

Kutalek SP, McCormick DJ: Classification of antiarrhythmic drugs. Am Fam Physician 1988;38:261–266.

Mason JW: Amiodarone. N Engl J Med 1987;316:455–465.

The Stroke Prevention in Atrial Fibrillation investigators: Predictors of thromboembolism in atrial fibrillation. Ann Intern Med 1992;116:1–5.

Tonnessen GE, et al: The value of tilt table testing with isoproterenol in determining therapy in adults with syncope and presyncope of unexplained origin. Arch Intern Med 1994;154:1613–1617.

Wellens HJ, et al: The value of the electrocardiogram in the differential diagnosis of a tachycardia with a widened QRS complex. Am J Med 1978;64:27–33.

Peripheral Vascular Disease

Becker DM: Venous thromboembolism. J Gen Intern Med 1986;1:402–411.

Doyle DJ, et al: Adjusted subcutaneous heparin or continuous intravenous heparin in patients with acute deep vein thrombosis. Ann Intern Med 1987;107:441–445.

Huisman MV, et al: Management of clinically suspected acute venous thrombosis in outpatients with serial impedance plethysmography in a community hospital setting. Arch Intern Med 1989;149:511–513.

Pedersen OM, et al: Compression ultrasonography in hospitalized patients with suspected deep venous thrombosis. Arch Intern Med 1991;151:2217–2220.

PIOPED Investigators: Value of the ventilation/perfusion scan in acute pulmonary embolism. JAMA 1990;263:2753–2759.

Wheeler HB: Diagnosis of deep vein thrombosis: Review of clinical evaluation and inpedence plethysmography. Am J Surg 1985;150:7–13.

Wheeler HB, Anderson FA: Diagnostic approaches for deep vein thrombosis. Chest 1986;89:407S–412S.

Preoperative

Adams JE, et al: Diagnosis of perioperative MI with measurement of cardiac tropinin I. N Engl J Med 1994;330:670–674.

Cygan R, et al: Stopping and restarting medications in the perioperative period. J Gen Intern Med 1987;2:270–282.

Goldman L: Cardiac risks and complications of noncardiac surgery. Ann Intern Med 1983;98:504–513.

Hull RD, et al: Prophylaxis of venous thromboembolism: an overview. Chest 1986;89:374s–383s.

Kearon C, Hirsch J: Starting prophylaxis for venous thromboembolism post-operatively. Arch Intern Med 1995;155:366–371.

Levine MN, et al: Prevention of deep vein thrombosis after elective hip surgery. Ann Intern Med 1991;114:545–551.

Manago DT, Goldman L: Preoperative assessment of patients with known or suspected coronary disease. N Engl J Med 1995;333:1750–1756.

Mangano DT, et al: Effect of atenolol on mortality and cardiovascular morbidity after noncardiac surgery. N Engl J Med 1996;335:1713–1720.

NIH Consensus Conference: Prevention of venous thrombosis and pulmonary embolism. JAMA 1986;256:744–749.

—D.D.B.

Gastrointestinal Medicine

Abdominal Pain: Overall Approach

The abdomen is a large anatomic region that contains many diverse structures, including those of the urinary system, the gastrointestinal system, and the reproductive system. Any dysfunction, trauma, or inflammation of any of these specific structures can and will manifest with abdominal pain. In addition to intraabdominal structures, any structure adjacent to the abdomen may result in referred abdominal pain.

Although most abdominal pain syndromes are self-limited and benign, in certain cases, abdominal pain can be a manifestation of a severe, even life-threatening process. Therefore the approach to the evaluation and management of abdominal pain must be thorough and reproducible (Box 2-1).

This section provides an overview of definitions, the differential diagnosis, evaluation, and management of abdominal pain, followed by a quadrant approach to abdominal pain. Specific common syndromes are discussed in subsequent sections.

I. **Definitions**

Definitions that are reproducible and workable are extremely important in the assessment of abdominal pain. Some of the most salient definitions include those listed subsequently.

A. **Pain versus tenderness**

Pain is a subjective manifestation, whereas tenderness is an objective finding that the examiner elicits. Tenderness is the reproduction of the pain symptoms in the course of performing an activity—usually palpation or pressing on the symptomatic area.

B. **Direct versus rebound tenderness**

Direct tenderness is pain elicited by palpating over an area; rebound tenderness is pain elicited on rapid release of the palpation and is indicative of peritoneal irritation and/or inflammation.

B O X 2-1

Overall Evaluation and Management of Abdominal Pain

Evaluation

1. Obtain a thorough history of the pain.
   a. Determine when the pain started, its location, its intensity, what makes it worse (exacerbating factors), what makes it better (alleviating factors), and for how long it has been present (duration).
   b. Obtain a history of any process that can produce pain. These processes include diverticulosis, urinary tract infections, cholelithiasis, choledocholithiasis, and nephrolithiasis.
   c. Additional historic data of importance include the menstrual history in women, the sexual history, the use/abuse of medications, the use of ethanol, recent or distant history of trauma to the abdomen, and recent or distant history of abdominal surgery.
   d. Document the presence or absence of associated features such as nausea, dysuria, pyuria, vomiting, diarrhea, constipation, fevers, loss of or decrease in flatus, hematemesis, or melena.
2. Perform a thorough physical examination to define any areas of tenderness and any associated, objective findings.
   a. Determine the presence and location of direct tenderness, the presence and location of rebound tenderness, and whether guarding is present.
   b. Determine vital signs, including orthostatic parameters. This information is important in determining volume status and whether fever is present.
   c. Assess bowel-sound activity and quality. If bowel sounds are hypoactive, the picture is usually consistent with ileus (the temporary loss of bowel activity). If bowel sounds are hyperactive, it can be the result of a partial or complete small- or large-bowel obstruction.
   d. Perform a pelvic examination in all women and a scrotal and penile examination in all men, looking for any discharge, tenderness, or masses.

(continued)

B O X 2-1 *(continued)*

    e. Perform a rectal examination. Note the color and guaiac response of the stool specimen. Melena (black, tarry stools) and hematochezia (red stools) are associated with GI bleeding, whereas a light, clay-colored stool is often associated with hepatic dysfunction and/or hepatic biliary obstruction.

    f. If possible, perform deep palpation of the abdomen to determine the presence and quality of masses (i.e., whether they are pulsatile, tender, or contiguous with normal structures).

    g. Determine the size of the liver by the scratch test, percussion, and palpation. If the liver is enlarged, note the presence or absence of tenderness.

    h. Perform percussion over the costovertebral angles. Tenderness elicited by light percussion or palpation over the costovertebral angle is consistent with pyelonephritis or nephrolithiasis.

    i. Determine the presence of abdominal distention by observation and palpation of the abdomen. A distended abdomen without shifting dullness but with tympany to percussion is consistent with increased gas in the bowel and therefore with obstruction. A distended abdomen with shifting dullness and a hyporesonant (i.e., dull) percussion note is consistent with ascites.

    j. The clinician must perform serial examinations, as results will change as the underlying process evolves or resolves.

3. Rule out pregnancy with a urine pregnancy test in all women of childbearing age with an intact uterus.

4. Test the guaiac response of stool to evaluate for occult GI bleeding.

5. Obtain an abdominal radiograph series (rule out pregnancy before performing this study in women). The series consists of four views of the abdomen, including a cross-table lateral view. Particular attention should be focused on the following:

    a. The presence of free air (i.e., air outside the bowel itself), which is indicative of perforation (Fig. 2-1).

    b. Any areas of distended bowel, small or large. A distended bowel is consistent with obstruction or

(continued)

B O X 2-1 *(continued)*

ileus. The small bowel can be differentiated from the large bowel in that the radiographic markings in the small bowel appear to extend across the width of the lumen (plicae semicircularis), whereas the radiographic markings in the large bowel appear not to extend across the entire lumen (haustra) (Fig. 2-2).
  c. The presence of air–fluid levels in the small bowel, which would be indicative of obstruction.
  d. The presence of calcified areas within the gallbladder, indicative of cholelithiasis. However, fewer than 15% of stones in the gallbladder are calcified.
  e. The presence of calcified areas within the renal pelvis, indicative of nephrolithiasis. More than 90% of urinary tract stones are calcified.
  f. The presence of calcifications in the area of the pancreas, indicative of chronic pancreatitis.
  g. The presence of large amounts of stool in the large bowel.
  h. The size of the large bowel if the abdomen is distended. Specifically, if the cecum is >13 cm in diameter, there is an increased risk of perforation.
     Caveat: The KUB (abdominal flat plate) study, although more convenient to obtain, is inferior to the abdominal series in demonstrating potential pathologic conditions.
 6. Obtain an ultrasound (US) examination of the kidneys, pancreas, gallbladder, and liver. Note the size of aorta, if it is >3.0 cm above the bifurcation, aneurysmal; if it is >5.0 cm, resection is indicated; if 4–5 cm, watchful waiting, i.e., repeat ultrasound in 3 months, is indicated.
 7. Withhold oral intake (NPO), at least initially.
 8. Provide fluid repletion and then maintenance. Normal saline (0.9) is usually the most appropriate fluid, especially if vomiting is present.
 9. Perform urinalysis with microscopic examination to reveal any hematuria, crystals (see Fig. 3-1, page 163), or pyuria (see Fig. 3-2, page 174).
10. Contrast studies, such as an air-contrast barium enema examination or an upper GI series with barium, should be reserved for the patient who is stable, is experiencing subacute or chronic pain, and in whom there is little risk of perforation.

(continued)

B O X   2-1 *(continued)*

11. If there is evidence of GI blood loss (i.e., anemia, iron deficiency, hematemesis, melena, hemato-chezia), refer to Box 2-9 and Table 2-13.
12. Based on these studies, formulate a clinical diag-nosis (Table 2-1) as to the location, by quadrant, and the severity of the pain. Further evaluation and management will be based on these two clinical assessments.
13. If the cause of the pain is still undetermined after these examinations, surgical referral and a potential for exploration with a laparoscope may be indicated. This is often superior to an explor-atory laparotomy.

Management

Specific management of abdominal pain-producing syn-dromes is given in subsequent sections of this chapter. **Emergent surgical consultation** is mandated for an acute abdomen, small-bowel obstruction, or bowel per-foration.

    C. **Guarding**

       Guarding is the voluntary or involuntary contraction of all or portions of the abdominal wall. Whereas voluntary guarding can be a nonspecific manifestation, involuntary guarding is quite often associated with peritoneal irrita-tion and therefore is more indicative of a pathologic process.

    D. **Acute abdomen**

       An acute abdomen, also known as a "surgical abdomen," denotes abdominal pain and associated peritoneal signs that required emergency surgical intervention. Examples include appendicitis, bowel obstruction, and perforation of the gastrointestinal (GI) tract.

  II. **Abdominal pain syndromes, by quadrant**

      Common abdominal pain syndromes and their characteristic features are described in Table 2-1. A reproducible categoriza-tion is to stratify abdominal pain syndromes into four groups based on location by abdominal quadrant. The **differential diagnosis** of pain in each quadrant is distinct (Table 2-2), and thus allows the clinician to focus the evaluation and management on the more likely causes of pain at a given lo-cation.

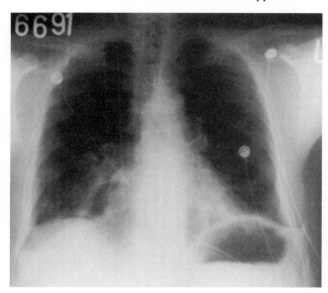

F I G U R E   2-1
AP chest radiograph showing free air under the right hemidiaphragm in a patient with a perforated duodenal ulcer.

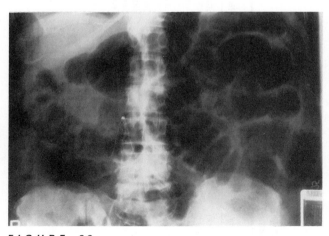

F I G U R E   2-2
Distal large bowel obstruction. Note loops of distended small and large bowel. Incidental finding of a Greenfield filter in IVC.

T A B L E 2-1
Characteristics of Abdominal Pain Syndromes

Syndrome	Location	Exacerbating Factors/ Alleviating Factors	Risk Factors	Associated Features
Peptic ulcer disease	Left upper quadrant; epigastric	Exacerbating: fasting, ethanol Alleviating: food, antacids	Ethanol NSAID's Past history of PUD	Afebrile No leukocytosis UGI bleeding Perforation of ulcer
Pancreatitis	Left upper quadrant	Exacerbating: ethanol Alleviating: fasting	Ethanol Cholelithiasis Choledocholithiasis High triglyceride	Low-grade fever Leukocytosis without left shift hypoxemia Elevated amylase and lipase
Cholecystitis	Right upper quadrant	Exacerbating: fatty meals Alleviating: fasting	Obesity Female sex Use of oral contraceptives	Low grade to spiking fever Mild leukocytosis Murphy's sign present Elevated alkaline phosphatase and total bilirubin levels Icterus Bilirubinuria
Appendicitis	Right lower quadrant	Exacerbating: none Alleviating: extension of the thigh with flexion of the knee	None	Low-grade to spiking fever Leukocytosis with left shift Peritoneal signs present Rovsing's sign

	Location of pain	Exacerbating/Alleviating	History/Risk factors	Clinical findings
Diverticulitis	Right lower quadrant	Exacerbating: none Alleviating: none	Low-fiber diets Constipation Irritable bowel Straining upon bowel movements	Low-grade fever Mild leukocytosis May have hematochezia if diverticulitis is present If complications, i.e. perforation of the diverticulum, obstruction of the large bowel or abscess formation, occur: can have leukocytosis, peritoneal signs, and/or fevers
Pelvic inflammatory disease	Right or left lower quadrant pain	Exacerbating: none Alleviating: none	Past history of STD Multiple sexual partners	Low-grade to spiking fever Leukocytosis with left shift Purulent discharge from cervix and vagina Tender adnexal mass
Ruptured ectopic pregnancy	Right or left lower quadrant pain	Exacerbating: none Alleviating: none	Past history of PID Tubal ligation	Low-grade fever Leukocytosis with left shift Adnexal mass Orthostasis Positive pregnancy test No intrauterine products of conception visualized with pelvic ultrasound
Nephrolithiasis	Right or left upper quadrant pain	Exacerbating: none Alleviating: none	UTI with *Proteus* Hypercalcuria Use of high dose vitamins C or D	Low-grade fever Leukocytosis, no left shift Hematuria
Abdominal aortic aneurysm (AAA)	Midabdomen with low back pain	Exacerbating: none Alleviating: none	Risk factors for atherosclerotic disease: Hypertension Diabetes mellitus Obesity Hyperlipidemia	Flank pain, may be severe Aneurysmal if at or above bifurcation >3 cm If size is 4–5 cm in diameter: consider surgical repair If size if >5 cm in diameter, surgical repair is indicated

T A B L E 2-2
Differential Diagnosis of Abdominal Pain

Right Upper Quadrant
Cholecystitis
Cholelithiasis
Hepatitis
Peptic ulcer disease
Pancreatitis
Pyelonephritis
Appendicitis (especially in pregnancy)
Fitz–Hugh–Curtis syndrome
Left Upper Quadrant
Peptic ulcer disease
Pancreatitis
Pyelonephritis
Splenic trauma/rupture
Pneumonitis
Angina pectoris
Pericarditis
Right and/or Left Lower Quadrant
Appendicitis
Diverticulitis
Nephrolithiasis
Pyelonephritis
Inflammatory bowel disease
Gastroenteritis
Ruptured ectopic pregnancy
Pelvic inflammatory disease
Ovarian cyst, especially if ruptured
Mittelschmerz (pain on day 14 of menstrual cycle, indicative
    of a normal ovulation)
AAA

III. Consultation

Problem	Service	Time
Any acute abdomen	General surgery	Emergent
Adnexal mass, nontender, negative pregnancy test	Obstetrics/Gynecology	Urgent
Adnexal mass, tender, or positive pregnancy test	Obstetrics/Gynecology	Urgent
Bowel obstruction	General surgery	Emergent

IV. **Indications for admission:** Any evidence of an acute abdomen, any GI bleeding, any signs of infection or impending sepsis, any significant intravascular volume depletion, fever, bowel obstruction, biliary tree obstruction, worsening of pain or tenderness during serial examinations, or the presence of an adnexal mass.

Cholelithiasis and Choledocholithiasis

(see Box 2-2)

The **anatomy** of the biliary tree is quite simple: it is a duct system that drains bile and secretions from the liver into the small intestine. The system has a reservoir, the gallbladder, attached to it by the relatively narrow-caliber cystic duct.

Biliary stones can be defined by their location within the biliary tree. In cholelithiasis, stones are located within the gallbladder itself. In choledocholithiasis, stones may be located anywhere within the biliary tree, from the intrahepatic ducts to the cystic duct to the common hepatic duct to the ampulla of Vater.

I. Pathogenesis

The **underlying pathogenesis** of stone formation, irrespective of location, is based on the fact that there are two different stone types, cholesterol stones and bilirubin stones.

A. Cholesterol stones

Cholesterol stones are by far the more common form of biliary tract stones. These stones result from supersaturation of cholesterol in the biliary contents; the cholesterol can precipitate with calcium and oxalate ions to form stones. Thus the chemical composition of cholesterol stones includes a complex mixture of cholesterol and cholesterol salts.

Specific **risk factors** for the development of these stones include the following:

1. Use of oral contraceptives
2. Moderate to morbid obesity
3. Female sex
4. History of multiple pregnancies
5. Older than 40 years
6. Native American ancestry

B. Bilirubin stones

Bilirubin stones are relatively uncommon. They result from excess amounts of conjugated bilirubin within the biliary tree due to the catabolism of hemoglobin derivatives in the liver. As with cholesterol biliary stones, there are specific **risk factors** for their development. The most common risk factor is an antecedent, concurrent, or chronic extravascular hemolytic process. These stones are not uncommon in patients with hereditary spherocytosis, SC hemoglobinopathy, or SS hemoglobinopathy.

II. Natural history

The **natural history** of cholelithiasis can be clinically divided into three distinct subsets.

A. Asymptomatic biliary stone disease

The natural history of asymptomatic cholelithiasis discovered surreptitiously is quite benign. This conclusion is based on a retrospective autopsy study by Wenckert et

B O X 2-2

Overall Evaluation and Management of Suspected Symptomatic Gallstone Disease

Evaluation

1. Take the history and perform a physical examination as described in Box 2-1 and in preceding sections.
2. Obtain the complete blood cell count to look for any leukocytosis.
3. Perform liver-function tests (LFTs) to determine the total bilirubin, direct bilirubin, alkaline phosphatase, γ-glutamyl transferase (GGT), aspartate aminotransferase (SGOT), and alanine aminotransferase (SGPT) levels. These determinations are made to look for extrahepatic dysfunction or obstruction. In extrahepatic processes, alkaline phosphatase, GTT, and total bilirubin levels will be elevated to a greater degree than transaminase levels. Also an amylase should be obtained, as a common bile duct stone may result in an elevated amylase level.
4. Obtain an abdominal radiograph series looking specifically for any radiopaque stones within the gallbladder or any concurrent manifestations (ileus, small-bowel obstruction, perforation). Only bilirubin stones and calcified cholesterol stones are radiopaque.
5. Perform US of the biliary tree. The US can detect stones >1–2 mm, will demonstrate the diameter of the common bile duct, and will demonstrate any thickening of the gallbladder wall. Biliary tree US is pivotal: it defines the anatomy of the biliary tree, demonstrates any extrahepatic biliary duct dilation, and shows the location of stones in cholelithiasis/choledocholithiasis. The common bile duct diameter is normally 5 mm.
6. Other imaging techniques may be of value in certain patients and in defined settings.
   a. Radionuclide imaging. The PIPIDA scan entails injection of a radiolabeled derivative of a molecule that is normally excreted through the biliary tree. The rate of excretion of the molecule from the liver into the small intestine is measured. A delay in the excretion time of this molecule is consistent with an obstructive process. If the liver is se-

(continued)

B O X 2-2 (continued)

verely damaged or if the obstruction is nearly complete, both as manifested by a significant increase in total bilirubin, the test will be essentially useless. Thus this specific evaluation tool is useful in diagnosing biliary obstruction if the total bilirubin is <10.0 mg/dL. This examination has a 95% sensitivity for acute cholecystitis.

Management

See text (IV. Specific management).

---

al. in which the records of all patients with cholelithiasis found at autopsy were retrospectively reviewed for any evidence of symptoms attributable to gallstone disease. Very few (18%) had pain in life suggestive of biliary dysfunction.

B. **One episode of pain**

Symptomatic gallstone disease. Up to 50% of patients will have recurrence of pain or will develop complications of cholelithiasis. The complications include ascending cholangitis, sepsis, pancreatitis, biliary obstruction, and death.

C. **Recurrent episodes of pain**

Recurrently symptomatic gallstone disease. The vast majority of patients will develop significant, potentially life-threatening complications in the near future.

III. **Manifestations**

The **specific manifestations** of biliary stone disease depend more on the location of the stone than on the chemical composition of the stone. Although the vast majority of patients are asymptomatic, biliary stones can and do produce symptoms, especially when they develop or as they pass from the gallbladder through the biliary tree itself. If they are within the biliary tree, they cause manifestations of biliary obstruction (see Box 2-2, page 66).

A. **Acute manifestations**

Acute manifestations include the acute onset of right upper quadrant pain. The pain is usually sharp, exacerbated by the ingestion of fatty foods, and relieved when the patient is fasting. Pyrosis may be present, as may intermittent nausea and vomiting. The patient may report a yellow discoloration to the eyes and clay-colored stools, all results of obstruction to bile flow.

B. Examination findings

On examination, the patient may be febrile, icteric, tender to deep palpation over the right upper quadrant, have Murphy's sign (i.e., pain in the right upper quadrant when attempting to inspire while the examiner palpates over the right upper quadrant), a normal liver span, and a hypopigmented, guaiac-negative stool in the rectal vault.

IV. Specific management

The **specific management** schemas for gallstone disease are based on the natural history and are different for each subset.

A. Asymptomatic cholelithiasis

Because asymptomatic gallstones that are discovered incidentally on another evaluative test have a benign natural history, intervention and therapy entail observation.

1. The risk of elective surgery (cholecystectomy) outweighs the risk of the asymptomatic cholelithiasis; therefore, conservative expectant therapy is indicated.

2. Watch the patient closely for the development of symptoms referable to biliary obstruction.

3. Risk-factor modification includes losing weight and discontinuing oral contraceptives.

B. Symptomatic cholelithiasis/choledocholithiasis

Therapeutic intervention is based on the natural history of the disease.

1. **Risk-factor modification** is necessary and includes weight loss and discontinuation of oral contraceptives.

2. Because of the natural history of the disease, the risks of recurrent symptoms and even complications are quite significant and outweigh the risk of surgery. In these cases, surgical intervention with cholecystectomy and biliary tree exploration, on an urgent or even emergency basis, is indicated.

3. **Laparoscopic cholecystectomy.** This novel surgical approach may be effective in high-risk patients with either cholesterol or bilirubin stones. The operation entails laparoscopically directed exploration of the gallbladder and biliary tree, removal of the gallbladder through the scope, and placement of a drainage tube (T-tube) from the biliary tree to the skin. This procedure has the advantage of limiting the incision size and therefore decreases the risk of traditional surgery.

4. If the stone is in the common bile duct, endoscopic retrograde choleangiopancreatography (ERCP), is indicated for papillomatomy and basket stone removal.

V. Complications of symptomatic cholecystitis

A. Pancreatitis

Biliary stone disease is one of the most common causes of pancreatitis worldwide. This form of pancreatitis is reversed when the underlying cholelithiasis is treated with ERCP or by surgical intervention.

B. **Ascending cholangitis**

Ascending cholangitis is one of the most severe complications of cholelithiasis. The **underlying pathogenesis** includes the obstruction and pooling of biliary secretions within the biliary tract. Obstruction is a prerequisite for the development of an infection in the biliary tree. The infection begins distally and ascends the biliary tree, with resultant hepatic abscess formation and severe hepatic infection. The **most common pathogens** in ascending cholangitis include group D streptococci (i.e., the enterococci), the Enterobacteriaceae (e.g., *Escherichi coli* and *Klebsiella* spp.), and the anaerobes (e.g., *Bacteroides* spp.).

The **specific management** of this life-threatening sequela of gallstone disease includes i.v. fluids, consultation with GI and surgery, and parenteral antibiotic administration to cover these pathogens.

C. **Sepsis**

Sepsis is of special concern in patients with ascending cholangitis or a gangrenous gallbladder. Pathogens and management are the same as those described for ascending cholangitis (see the preceding).

VI. **Consultation**

Problem	Service	Time
Symptomatic cholelithiasis	Surgery	Urgent
Complicated cholelithiasis	Surgery	Emergent
Gallstone pancreatitis	GI/ERCP	Urgent

VII. **Indications for admission:** Intravascular volume depletion, fever, intractable vomiting, any evidence of biliary obstruction, the development of acute pancreatitis, or suspicion of ascending cholangitis.

Acute and Chronic Pancreatitis

The pancreas is located immediately posterior and inferior to the duodenum and therefore is mainly in the epigastric and left upper quadrant of the abdomen. The pancreas has both exocrine and endocrine functions. The exocrine portion of the gland produces potent proteolytic enzymes, including trypsin and chymotrypsin, that are secreted into the intestine via the ducts of Santorini and Wirsung into the ampulla of Vater. In the normal setting, these proteolytic enzymes from the exocrine pancreas digest the ingested proteins. The endocrine portion of the gland consists of islets of cells within the gland. The alpha islet cells produce glucagon, whereas the beta cells produce insulin. Both glucagon and insulin have profound effects on glucose utilization and, therefore, on cellular function.

I. **Pathogenesis of pancreatitis**

The **underlying pathogenesis** is autodigestion of the gland itself by the abnormal release of the intrinsic proteolytic enzymes. If the pancreas is damaged, it releases and activates these enzymes within the gland itself, with resultant pancreatic damage, damage to the adjacent tissues, and eventually, both exocrine and endocrine pancreatic insufficiency.

II. Precipitants

Precipitating agents in the **pathogenesis** of pancreatitis include significant ethanol ingestion, the most common cause in the United States; choledocholithiasis (stones in the biliary tree), the most common cause worldwide; a duodenal ulcer that penetrates through the posterior wall of the duodenum; type I hyperlipidemia, which is associated with recurrent pancreatitis; medication-related [e.g., the use of didanosine (ddI) or azathioprine]; chronic hypercalcemia of any cause; congenital (i.e., anatomic) dysfunction of the duct system; and idiopathic causes, which must be a diagnosis of exclusion, as the vast majority of cases of pancreatitis do have a discernible cause.

III. Natural history

Recurrent attacks of acute pancreatitis, with resultant partial destruction of the gland each time, eventually lead to insufficiency of the exocrine and endocrine functions of the gland. Reflecting this natural history, the following discussion is divided into acute pancreatitis and the chronic pancreatic insufficiency state.

IV. Acute pancreatitis

A. Manifestations

The **specific manifestations** of acute pancreatitis include the acute onset of epigastric and left upper quadrant pain that is usually greater after oral intake and is associated with nausea, vomiting, and orthostatic dizziness. Often the precipitant can be easily determined from the history (e.g., a recent binge with ethanol). Examination usually discloses intravascular volume depletion, diffusely hypoactive bowel sounds, deep and rebound tenderness in the epigastrium and left upper quadrant, and guaiac-negative stool in the rectal vault. Fever is not uncommon.

B. Evaluation

The **specific evaluation** of acute pancreatitis includes making the clinical diagnosis with the evaluation steps described in Box 2-3. Further specific evaluative tests include the following:

1. **Serum amylase determination.** The enzyme amylase, which is normally produced in the exocrine pancreas, is abnormally elevated in acute pancreatitis. The sensitivity of this test is limited by the fact that in patients who have already had significant pancreatic destruction, amylase levels may not be elevated. The specificity is limited by the fact that dysfunction or diseases of other organs can cause amylase elevations, including renal insufficiency, diabetic ketoacidosis, inflamma-

B O X 2-3

Overall Evaluation and Management of Suspected Pancreatitis

1. Take the history and physical examination as described in Box 2-1, Abdominal Pain section, and in text.
2. Perform levels of serum LFTs (total bilirubin, direct bilirubin, alkaline phosphatase, GGT, SCOT, and SGPT) and levels of serum pancreatic enzymes (amylase and lipase). The transaminases will be elevated if there is concurrent ethanol-related hepatitis, whereas the alkaline phosphatase and bilirubin will be elevated if the pancreatitis is the result of choledocholithiasis. The amylase and lipase are consistent with acute pancreatitis.
3. A baseline ethanol level is of use if there is any suspicion of ethanol use/abuse.
4. Plasma lipid panel is of interest, as profound hyperlipidemia may be the cause of pancreatitis.
5. Obtain radiographs; if calcifications are found in pancreas, it is consistent with chronic pancreatitis.
6. US of the abdomen to image the pancreas and look for stones, pseudocyst, ascites, and concurrent hepatic or gallbladder findings.
7. If ethanol-related, treat the ethanol and ethanol-withdrawal manifestations as necessary (see Table 15-4).
8. Obtain a baseline set of Ranson's criteria (i.e., for prognostic significance):
   - Serum calcium: Assess for hypocalcemia
   - Hematocrit: Assess for profound anemia
   - O_2 saturation: Assess for hypoxia
   - Volume status: Assess for volume depletion
   - White blood count: Assess for leukocytosis
9. Repleted any volume deficit with D_5W 0.9 NS; Maintenance fluids of D_5W 0.45 NS
10. Pain relief, meperidine (Demerol), 25–50 mg i.m., i.v., may be of benefit.
11. Admit to inpatient service.
12. If no cause demonstrated or if there are stones in the ducts, GI consult for ERCP.

T A B L E 2-3
Chronic Pancreatitis: Constellation of Manifestations

Category	Pathogenesis	Manifestations	Evaluation and Management
Exocrine insufficiency	Destruction and loss of the exocrine gland (i.e., the acini producing lipase, amylase, trypsin, chymotrypsin), thereby decreasing digestion with resultant malabsorption	Steatorrhea Malabsorption of vitamins A, D, and K Decreased albumin Increased bleeding trauma Decreased weight Edema, including anasarca	Increased PT Decrease in albumin Replace the vitamin K with 10 mg p.o. q.d. Replace vitamins A and D Pancrelipase (pancreatic trypsin, lipase, amylase) 1–3 capsules 1 hr before meals
Endocrine insufficiency	Destruction of alpha (glucagon) and beta (insulin) cells from the islets of the pancreas	Insulin-dependent diabetes mellitus Very labile glycemic control as the result of a loss of glucagon concurrently	Fasting blood sugar Management of diabetes mellitus (see Chapter 9, page 464)
Pain syndrome	Idiopathic	Chronic, intractable abdominal pain	Analgesia, may even need morphine sulfate Celiac plexus block may be necessary

tion or destruction of the salivary glands, or ischemia of the gut itself.

2. **Serum lipase determination.** The enzyme lipase, which is normally produced in the exocrine pancreas, is abnormally elevated in acute pancreatitis. This test has a higher specificity than serum amylase determination because lipase is produced almost exclusively within the pancreas. This test can confirm the diagnosis when clinical suspicion is present and the serum amylase test is equivocal.

3. **Abdominal US.** This imaging technique of the gallbladder, biliary tree, liver, and pancreas is a simple and reasonable, cost-effective modality to visualize the structures and rule out any biliary obstruction and choledocholithiasis. If any abnormalities are demonstrated, computed tomography (CT) of the area is indicated.

4. **Abdominal CT.** Abdominal CT is not routinely indicated in all cases. It is indicated when no cause can be discerned after a thorough evaluation, when any complication is suspected, or if any abnormality is demonstrated on US.

C. **Management** (see Box 2-3)

V. Chronic pancreatitis: See Table 2-3

VI. Consultation

Problem	*Service*	*Time*
Any complications	GI	Required
	Surgery	Elective
Choledocholithiasis	GI	Urgent
	Surgery	Urgent
Idiopathic	GI	Required

VII. Indications for admission: Intravascular volume depletion, acute pancreatitis, any evidence of a complication to the pancreatitis.

Peptic Ulcer Disease, Duodenal or Gastric

The anatomy of the upper stomach and duodenum is pivotal to an understanding of peptic ulcer disease (PUD). The stomach is immediately inferior to and connected with the esophagus. It consists of three anatomic portions: the cardia, which is superior, the body, which is the largest portion of the stomach, and the pylorus, the narrowing of the stomach as it becomes contiguous with the duodenum. The transition between the body and the pylorus is called the antrum. The pylorus empties into the relatively narrow C-shaped first portion of the small intestine, the duodenum. All of these structures are lined with mucosa consisting of simple columnar epithelium.

I. **Pathophysiology**
   There are three major pathophysiologic mechanisms in the development of PUD. There are the use of nonsteroidal antiinflammatory drugs (NSAIDs), the hypersecretion of acid in the gastrinoma syndrome, and infection of the mucosa with the bacterium, *Helicobacter pylori.*

   A. **NSAID-related gastropathy** is the result of the overall decrease in the effectiveness of the mucosal barrier of mucus and bicarbonate. Acid secretion is usually low to normal and thus is not a major factor here. The NSAIDs, by virtue of their systemic inhibition of prostaglandin production, especially in the prostaglandin E (PGE) group, are effective antiinflammatory agents; however, this decreases the PG at the level of the gastric mucosa and may result in:
      1. A decreased secretion of HCO_3
      2. A decreased production of mucus, and
      3. A decreased mucosal blood flow,
         all resulting in a particularly fertile environment for erosion and ulcer formation.

   B. *Helicobacter pylori:* This is an etiologic agent in the vast majority of peptic ulcers in general and duodenal ulcers in particular. There is an increased risk of non-Hodgkin's lymphoma of the GI tract in these patients. There is compelling evidence to support this, including the fact that the vast majority of patients with PUD are infected with *H. pylori* and that patients treated to eradicate the *H. pylori* with antibiotics have a markedly decreased rate of recurrence relative to those treated with standard, traditional means (i.e., solely with antisecretory agents).

   C. **Other factors include:**
      1. **Ethanol** and nicotin. Both act via mechanisms analogous to NSAID-related disease.
      2. **Hypersecretion of acid.** This is the result of rare tumors of the pancreas, which result in stimulation of the parietal cells to release increased quantities of acid, thereby insulting the integrity of the mucosa. Diffuse uclers occur.

II. **Manifestations**
   The **specific manifestations** of PUD are quite similar, regardless of the underlying pathophysiology. Symptoms usually include an acute onset of epigastric pain that is exacerbated by fasting and relieved by food or antacid ingestion. Other historic features include a history of PUD or similar manifestations in the past that spontaneously resolved.

   Nausea and vomiting are not uncommon. The specific manifestation of postprandial vomiting usually is a result of ulcer-induced swelling and obstruction, especially when the ulcer is in the pylorus. The patient can have hematemesis ("coffee-ground" emesis) or melena (black tarry stools), both indicative of significant bleeding. Risk factors for the development of PUD are often present.

   On examination, there often is tenderness to deep palpation in the epigastrium, usually without rebound; a guaiac-positive stool in the rectal vault; and, at times, signs and symptoms of intravascular volume depletion.

III. **Specific evaluation and management** include that described in Box 2-4 and the following specific to the presumed underlying pathogenetic etiology:

   A. **NSAID-related disease:** Discontine all NSAIDs, nicotine, and ethanol. If the patient is bleeding or is unstable, admit; if the patient is stable, perform an upper GI radiographic study or an EGD. If the upper GI reveals a gastric ulcer, an EGD must be performed for biopsies; therefore, in most cases, EGD is the best first test. **Specific management** items include the use of antisecretory agents (e.g., the H_2 antagonist ranitidine, 150 mg p.o., b.i.d. or the proton-pump inhibitor, omeprazole, 20 mg p.o. q day for 8–10 weeks. Antacids (e.g., Maalox or Mylanta) may provide palliation but have no impact on the natural history. Prevention is by those methods described in Table 2-4.

   B. **Helicobacter pylori–related ulcers:** Discontinue all NSAIDs, nicotine, and ethanol. If the patient is bleeding or is unstable, admit; if the patient is stable, perform an upper GI radiographic study or an EGD. In most cases, EGD is the best first test, as the diagnoses of *H. pylori* may require invasive testing. Those tests that provide a diagnosis of *H. pylori* include:

      1. EGD with biopsy of the ulcer looking for the bacterium.
      2. Culture of the biopsy site/tissue.
      3. CLO test on the tissue specimen. This is the application of a dye to detect urea in the tissue specimen. The

T A B L E 2-4
Prevention of NSAID-Induced Gastropathy

---

1. Use other therapeutic modilities if possible, including
   Physical therapy
   Intraarticular steroids
   Nonacetylated salicylates (e.g., Disalcid)
   Acetaminophen
2. Limit NSAID therapy if possible
3. Take the NSAIDs on a full stomach
4. Discontinue cigarette smoking
5. Limit ethanol ingestion
6. For prevention, sucralfate possibly is the optimal pharmacologic agent because of its efficacy and minimal side effects
7. If the disease occurs treat as described in Box 2-4 and the text, page 76

B O X   2-4

***Overall Evaluation and Management of
Peptic Ulcer Disease***

Evaluation

1. Take a thorough history and perform a physical examination (see Abdominal Pain: Overall Approach, and as described previously).
2. Determine orthostatic vital-sign parameters.
3. Determine a baseline complete blood cell count to look for anemia.
4. Determine the platelet count and coagulation parameters [activated partial thromboplastin time (aPTT), prothrombin time (PT)] if there is any evidence of a coagulopathy.

Management

1. Instruct the patient to discontinue all NSAIDs and to discontinue ethanol and cigarette smoking.
2. If the patient is severely symptomatic or if there is evidence of bleeding, the clinician must:
   a. Admit the patient, preferrably to an intensive care unit (ICU)
   b. Place two large-bore (18- or 16-gauge) i.v. catheters, each with 0.9 NS
   c. Type and cross-match for packed RBCs
   d. Emergently consult GI service directly to image the area with a esophagogastroduodenoscopy (EGD)
   e. See section on gastrointestinal bleeding, page 110 for further details.
3. If the patient is stable, mildly symptomatic, not acutely bleeding, and not anemic, image the area radiographically with an upper GI series or consult a gastroenterologist for an EGD. If an upper GI series is performed and a gastric ulcer is demonstrated, EGD with biopsies of the ulcer crater is indicated to rule out a malignant gastric ulcer. If a duodenal ulcer is demonstrated, EGD with biopsies or a urea breath test (see text) are indicated.
4. Treat for *H. pylori* with antibiotics [e.g., amoxicillin/ metronidazole for 14 days and omeprazole (Prilosec) for 6 weeks. See text.]

presence of urea in tissue bespeaks the presence of a bacterium with urease activity (i.e., *H. pylori*).

Two noninvasive tests are the breath test and serology assessment, which may decrease the need for invasive procedures. The *H. pylori* serology is excellent before any treatment is initiated; it is a simple immunoassay with senstivity and specificity of >90%. The Breath Urea Test involves the oral administration of ^{14}C-radiolabeled urea. If *H. pylori* is present, it breaks down the urea by its urease activity, which results in the production of radiolabeled CO_2, which is exhaled and measured in the breath.

The **specific management** includes treating the ***H. pylori*** infection with antibiotics and antisecretory agents. Appropriate effective regimens include (both with an eradication rate >90%):

1. Amoxicillin, 1,000 mg p.o., b.i.d., for 14 days
   -and-
   clarithromycin, 500 mg p.o., b.i.d., for 14 days
   -and-
   omeprazole, 20 mg p.o., b.i.d., for 8 weeks
   -or-
2. Clarithromycin, 500 mg p.o., b.i.d., for 14 days
   -and-
   metronidazole, 500 mg p.o., b.i.d., for 14 days
   -and-
   omeprazole, 20 mg p.o., b.i.d, for 8 weeks.

If there is recurrent disease, performance of another EGD and treatment with an alternate regimen are indicated. Furthermore, long-term treatment with an antisecretory agent (e.g., ranitidine, 150 mg p.o. q HS) may be of benefit.

C. If **hypergastrinemia** is suspected, discontinue all NSAIDs, nicotine, and ethanol. If the patient is bleeding or is unstable, admit; if the patient is stable, perform an upper GI radiographic study or an EGD. In most cases, EGD is the best first test and will reveal multiple ulcers and erosions. The serum gastrin level will be markedly elevated. Long-term high-dose antisecretory therapy is indicated (e.g., omeprazole, 20 mg p.o., b.i.d., or ranitidine, 150 mg p.o., b.i.d.). If the gastrinoma is a definable tumor demonstrated in the pancreas, referral to a surgeon with expertise in endocrine tumors is indicated.

IV. **Complications**

The complications of PUD can include the following, all of which require admission and surgical intervention:

A. **Upper GI bleeding**

The bleeding can be mild to exsanguinating and usually is a function of the depth and location of the ulcer crater. Specifically, a duodenal ulcer can erode anteriorly into the anterior gastroduodenal artery and cause massive, even exsanguinating hematemesis (see section on Gastrointestinal Bleeding, page 110).

B. Perforation of the gastric or duodenal wall

Any ulcer can extend through the entire wall and result in perforation. Perforation invariably has the associated comorbidities of peritonitis, acute abdomen, and even death (see section on Abdominal Pain: Overall Approach, page 56).

C. Pancreatitis

This complication occurs when a posterior duodenal ulcer erodes through the wall and into the head of the pancreas. It is usually associated with severe pain and signs of an acute abdomen (see section on Abdominal Pain: Overall Approach, page 56).

D. Obstruction

This complication is associated with recurrent PUD with inflammation and fibrotic changes. It is most commonly associated with distal gastric (i.e., antral) ulcer disease with resultant symptomatic pyloric narrowing.

V. Consultation

Problem	Service	Time
Any complications	General surgery	Urgent/emergent
Any complications	GI	Urgent/emergent
Elevated gastrin level	Endocrinology	Elective

VI. Indications for admission: Development of any of the complications of PUD (i.e., obstruction, upper GI bleeding, perforation, intractable pain, or severe nausea and vomiting requiring parenteral fluid repletion) or acute pancreatitis.

Anorectal Dysfunction

Although many patients are embarrassed by pain or problems in the anal area and thus attempt to self-treat or to minimize the problem, anorectal problems can cause significant discomfort, anxiety, and even morbidity. As several infections may result in anorectal dysfunction, including anal warts and other sexually transmitted diseases (STDs), please refer to Chapter 8 for specifics.

I. Specific anorectal pathologic entities (see Box 2-5)

A. Hemorrhoids

Hemorrhoids are abnormally dilated veins within the venous network of the anus. These lesions can be minimally symptomatic or can, on a recurrent basis, cause severe pain and bleeding.

Hemorrhoids are classified by severity and location. The classification by severity is:

First degree, slight bleeding;

Second degree, prolapsed but easily reducible; and

Third degree, prolapsed, nonreducible, usually recurrent.

B O X 2-5

*Overall Evaluation and Management
of Anorectal Disorders*

Evaluation

1. Perform a digital rectal examination.
2. Visualize the area internally with an anoscope.

Management

Management is described under specific entities in the text.

The classification by location—either external or internal—is relative to the dentate line. The following discussion is organized according to this classification.

1. **External hemorrhoids**
   a. An external hemorrhoid is any hemorrhoid distal to the dentate line. The **specific manifestations** in the chronic setting include purple-colored skin tags in the anal area that are nontender and nonbleeding but can result in mild soiling of underpants and intermittent mild anal pruritus. These are old external hemorrhoids that have scarred and are now fibrosed asymptomatic lesions. In an acute exacerbation or acute development of external hemorrhoids, there is usually an acute onset of anal pruritus, which can be quite severe. Furthermore, there often is the presence of a prolapsed mildly tender mass. Finally, underwear may be soiled by stool.
   b. The two **acute complications** of external hemorrhoids are thrombosis and rupture.
      i. Thrombosed hemorrhoids are exquisitely painful and tender, with concurrent bluish swelling of the hemorrhoid. Pain and induration develop acutely.
      ii. Rupture of an external hemorrhoid occurs concurrent or concomitant with the development of thrombosis. When rupture occurs, a significant amount of bright red blood can be passed rectally; pain may also be relieved.
   c. **Risk factors** for the development or recurrence of external hemorrhoids include pregnancy, parturition, a history of straining during defecation, and occupations requiring sitting for prolonged periods.

    d. The **evaluation and management** of this entity include making the clinical diagnosis and performing anoscopy. Acute management entails application of a cold pack to the site for first hour, and then warm sitz baths 2–3 times a day for 3–5 days. In addition, topical steroids (e.g., Anusol HC cream b.i.d. or Proctofoam b.i.d. to t.i.d.) are of benefit. A thrombosed hemorrhoid is easily excised by direct incision and drainage.

        Chronic management and prophylaxis include the use of stool softeners or increased dietary fiber, exercise, and, if the condition is recurrent, possibly surgical removal or removal via infrared coagulation or laser therapy. Referral to gastroenterology in these cases is indicated on an elective basis.

2. Internal hemorrhoids

    a. Internal hemorrhoids are hemorrhoids that are proximal to the dentate line. The **specific manifestations** in the acute or chronic setting include bright red blood passed rectally, prolapse of a nontender mass through the anus, and virtually no pain or tenderness. The bleeding, which is intermittent, can be quite significant.

    b. The major **risk factor** for the development of internal hemorrhoids is hepatic portal venous hypertension. These lesions can be concurrent with external hemorrhoids.

    c. The **evaluation and management** include making the clinical diagnosis, performing anoscopy, and looking for other manifestations of portal venous hypertension (see section on End-Stage Hepatic Dysfunction). The specific management includes the local control of any bleeding, usually by applying direct pressure, and outpatient referral to gastroenterology.

B. Fissure-in-ano

Fissure-in-ano is the development of a superficial longitudinal laceration of the distal anus, usually as a result of trauma, usually while straining.

    1. Specific manifestations include an acute onset of severe pain in the anal area. The patient usually relates that the pain was precipitated by straining during a bowel movement and was exacerbated by each subsequent bowel movement. A small amount of bright red blood may be passed rectally.

    2. Risk factors for the development of fissure-in-ano include straining during bowel movements, constipation, and anal intercourse.

    3. The **evaluation and management** of this entity include making the clinical diagnosis and performing anoscopy. Acute management entails application of a cold pack to the site for first hour, and then warm sitz baths two to three times a day for 3–5 days. Chronic management includes the use of stool softeners and increased dietary fiber, exercise, and abstinence from receptive anal intercourse. Referral to gastroenterology in recurrent cases is indicated on an elective basis.

C. Fistula-in-ano

A fistula-in-ano develops between the anal lumen at the base of a crypt of Morgagni (i.e., the papilla of Morgagni) and the perianal skin.

1. **Specific manifestations** include the acute onset of pain in the anal or perineal area and a mass in the perineal area deep to the skin with associated discharge of liquid, at times purulent, material from an area immediately adjacent to the anus. This entity can develop into a perirectal abscess.

2. **Risk factors** for the development of fistula-in-ano and the differential diagnosis of entities associated with this entity include Crohn's disease, carcinoma, lymphogranuloma venereum (LGV), past rectal irradiation, and immunocompromise. Fistula-in-ano or a perirectal abscess must always be considered in an immunocompromised patient with rectal or anal pain.

3. The **evaluation and management** of this entity include making the clinical diagnosis and performing anoscopy. The perirectal tissues are examined for any tender masses, which may be perirectal abscesses. The fistula is examined from the internal side to the skin side. Usually the fistula must be surgically closed. If an abscess is found in the adjacent tissues, it must be incised and drained, with the concurrent initiation of antibiotics to cover anaerobic and gram-negative bacillary bacteria. Referral to surgery is indicated.

D. Pinworm

Pinworm is a common helmintic parasite ("worm") that is noninvasive and benign, but quite contagious.

1. **Specific manifestations** include the onset of severe anal pruritus that is especially severe at night. Usually pinworm occurs in children, but adults can contract the infection from children.

2. **Risk factors** for the development of pinworm include having children in the family and poor hand-washing practices by family members.

3. The **evaluation and management** include making a clinical diagnosis from a thorough history and physical examination. As part of the examination, a length of Scotch tape is placed on the perianal skin, then re-

moved, and helminths are sought in the residue on the tape. **Management** includes treating the patient and entire family with pyrantel pamoate (Antiminth), 11 mg/kg p.o. of body weight. Before treatment, one must document a negative pregnancy test on all fertile family members, as this agent is a teratogen.

II. **Consultation**

Problem	Service	Time
Hemorrhoids	GI (IRC/laser)	Elective
Fistula-in-ano	Surgery	Required
Perirectal abscess	Surgery	Urgent

III. **Indications for admission:** Bleeding internal hemorrhoids in a patient with coagulopathy, or a perirectal abscess.

Dysphagia and Odynophagia

The esophagus is a tubelike structure that connects the posterior oral cavity (i.e., the oropharynx) with the stomach. It is ~25 cm long and is lined by stratified squamous epithelium.

I. **Overall manifestations**

Dysphagia is defined specifically as difficulty is swallowing. The patient usually reports that the bolus of food or liquid "gets caught" or sticks while swallowing. Odynophagia is defined specifically as pain on swallowing. Pyrosis, i.e., heartburn, especially when the origin is gastroesophageal reflux disease (GERD), is common. In addition, postprandial vomiting, halitosis, and a recent cerebrovascular accident may be associated or concurrent processes. A final feature is one of weight loss. If the process is so significant as to result in unintentional weight loss, it indicates a more malignant process (see Box 2-6).

II. **Differential diagnosis** (See Table 2-5)

III. **Consultation**

Problem	Service	Time
Any esophageal motor disorder	GI (manometry)	Required
Any mechanical disorder	GI (EGD)	Urgent
Any esophagitis	GI (EGD)	Urgent
	ID	Required
Malignant stricture	Surgery	Urgent

IV. **Indications for admission:** Any evidence of aspiration pneumonia, of esophageal rupture, upper GI bleeding, intractable vomiting, or any evidence of malnutrition due to dysphagia or herpes simplex virus (HSV) esophagitis.

B O X 2-6

Overall Evaluation and Management of Dysphagia and Odynophagia

Evaluation

1. Take a thorough history and perform a physical examination, specifically querying the patient regarding the items listed under Overall Manifestations. In addition, ascertain whether the patient has any of the following:
   a. History of chronic smoking or ethanol abuse.
   b. History of immunocompromise [acquired immunodeficiency syndrome (AIDS), chemotherapy].
   c. Any evidence of vesicular lesions in the oropharynx, common with herpes simplex, or thrush in the oropharynx, consistent with candidal infection.
   d. Examination of cranial nerves IX and X, testing the gag reflex and swallowing mechanism.
2. Image the oropharynx and esophagus.
   a. If there is evidence of a recent cerebrovascular accident or of swallowing weakness, perform a "swallow study." This test, which uses either barium or Gastrografin as the contrast agent, is performed under fluoroscopy to demonstrate the swallowing mechanism itself.
   b. If there is no evidence of vesicular lesions or of a poor gag reflex, the clinician may perform an upper GI radiographic study by using barium or Gastrografin as the contrast agent to look for any functional or anatomic lesion in the esophagus.
   c. If there is evidence of vesicular lesions or any anatomic lesion, perform EGD for direct imaging and biopsy.

Management

The specific management of entities producing dysphagia or odynophagia is given in the text and Table 2-5.

T A B L E 2-5
Dysphagia and Odynophagia Syndromes

Diagnosis	Manifestations	Pathogenesis	Evaluation	Management
Diffuse esophageal spasm	Odynophagia and dysphagia to liquids and solids Symptoms worsen over time	Primary motor disturbance of the entire esophagus	*Upper GI barium study:* Increase in diffuse peristaltic activity throughout the esophagus *Manometry:* Diffuse increase in the amplitude and duration of peristaltic contractions in esophagus	Calcium channel blocker (e.g., Nifedipine, 60 mg XL q.d.
Achalasia	Odynophagia and dysphagia to liquids and solids Symptoms worsen over time	Primary neuron defect with localized loss of myenteric neurons in distal esophagus Chagas disease	*Upper GI barium study:* dilated esophagus with a narrowed distal esophagus; barium is retained in the esophagus for long periods *Manometry:* High-amplitude, repetitive tertiary contractions in the proximal esophagus. Base-line pressures are very high	Calcium channel blocker (e.g., Nifedipine 60 mg XL q.d.) or Intrasphincteric botulinum toxin
Oropharyngeal dysfunction	Mild to moderate dysphagia to liquids and solids No odynophagia	Brainstem infarction; damage to brainstem nuclei involved in mastication and deglutination	*Upper GI barium study:* defect in swallowing in real time is demonstrated EGD, manometry, and upper GI series are unnecessary	Refer to speech therapy Modify diet or place G-tube to prevent aspiration pneumonitis

	Clinical features	Etiology / anatomic findings	Diagnostic evaluation	Treatment
Bulbar: LMN Pseudobulbar: UMN	Associate features a) Dysarthria b) Dysphonia c) Passage of oral contents into the nose and nasopharynx on swallowing		*CT of head* and neurologic examination to look for CVA or bulbar palsy are necessary	Monitor for aspiration pneumonitis
Anatomic disorders	Slow, progressive worsening of dysphagia solids then liquids Patient often vomits 5–10 min after swallowing food Rare odynophagia	Ususally the distal aspect of the esophagus is involved a) Peptic stricture, secondary to GERD b) Squamous cell carcinoma, associated with smoking/ethanol c) Adenocarcinoma, associated with Barrett's esophagitis d) *Schatzi's ring*: A submucosal ring of tissue in mid/distal esophagus	*Upper GI barium study*: demonstrates the lesion, high sensitivity, low specificity Esophagogastroduodenoscopy (EGD) is the most important study in evaluation Biopsy of any suggestive lesion(s) is mandatory	Referral to GI for EGD for biopsy If *benign structure*, direct dilation and treat GERD, see page 125 Omeprazole, 20 mg p.o. q.d. If *malignant stricture*, resection or dilation If *Schatzi's ring*, direct dilation
Esophagitis	Subacute/acute onset of symptoms Significant odynophagia and mild dysphagia	Increased in immunocompromised patients: CMV Herpes simplex Candida Other etiologies include GERD Medications (e.g., tetracycline)	HIV serology *Upper barium study*: little assistance in diagnosis EGD is best, biopsy any lesion suggestive Examine mouth for yeast/candida	If *candida*, Fluconazole, 200 mg, q.A.M. *and* Clotrimazole (Mycelex) troches 5 times per day p.o. If *HSV*: Acyclovir, p.o./i.v. (see Table 6-6, page 332) If *CMV*: DHPG (ganciclovir) i.v. (see Table 6-6, page 332)

Diarrheal States: Acute, Recurrent, or Chronic

Diarrhea is a common problem worldwide. The approach to diarrhea entails making several basic distinctions, listed below.

1. **Quantity of stool.** Stool volume is one of the most important features in describing and defining diarrheal states. Therefore it is of utmost importance to set specific objective criteria, of which volume is the most reproducible and valuable. The number of stools and the qualitative consistency of the stool are of limited importance and are inferior to the volume of stool in terms of defining diarrhea. Diarrhea is defined as a stool weight >200 g/24 hr on a low-fiber diet.
2. **Bloody versus nonbloody diarrhea.** Bloody diarrhea bespeaks an origin of infection of inflammation.
3. **Acute versus chronic condition.** By convention, any diarrhea ≤2 weeks in duration is acute, whereas any diarrheal state of >2 weeks' duration is chronic.
4. **Extraintestinal manifestations.** These manifestations are important in determining the underlying cause of the diarrhea; especially if the diarrhea is chronic. These manifestations can be a direct result of the diarrhea or its pathogenesis. Examples include intravascular volume depletion from water loss, macrocytic anemia from malabsorption of folate and/or vitamin B_{12}, and the extraintestinal manifestations of inflammatory bowel disease (uveitis, ankylosing spondylitis, sclerosing cholangitis).
5. **Immunocompromised versus immunocompetent host.** The approach to immunosuppressed patients, including those undergoing chemotherapy, those with AIDS, and those with other immunocompromised states, differs significantly from the approach to immunocompetent patients. The underlying causes, evaluative procedures, and management are different for the two populations.
6. **Locally acquired versus traveler's diarrhea.** Diarrhea that began while the patient was in the local environment (at home) or during a trip to another location, either in the United States or elsewhere in the world.

I. **Diagnosis**

The **differential diagnosis** of diarrhea includes a number of extremely diverse entities. A general scheme for grouping the diarrheal syndromes is given subsequently; this scheme follows the qualifying features described in the general discussion of diarrhea. Acute diarrhea is discussed in Tables 2-6 through 2-9, and chronic diarrheal states are summarized in Table 2-10.

A. Acute, domestic (i.e., endemic to the United States) diarrhea; patient is immunocompetent (see Table 2-6).

B. Acute, nondomestic (i.e., not endemic to the United

States) **diarrhea;** patient is immunocompetent (see Table 2-7).

This form of diarrhea is often referred to colloquially as "traveler's diarrhea," "Montezuma's revenge," or "Turista." It is a common problem in persons traveling outside of the United States and Canada, and it is best treated with prevention. Effective methods of prevention include drinking only bottled water or water that has been boiled at a temperature >200°F for >10 minutes, and ingesting only completely cooked foods. This includes completely cooking any and all fresh vegetables. If fresh vegetables are used, they must be peeled before eating them. They must not be washed in water unless the water has first been boiled. The most common organisms that cause traveler's diarrhea include *Escherichia coli*, *Shigella*, *C. jejuni*, *Salmonella*, and *Giardia*. The most useful regimen for treatment is ciprofloxacin, 500 mg p.o., b.i.d.; start at outset of nausea and cramping symptoms. If greasy stools and no response to ciprofloxacin, consider it *Giardia lamblia* and treat as such. Refer to Tables 2-7 and 2-8 for the diagnosis and treatment of traveler's diarrhea.

C. **Immunocompromised patient, acute or chronic diarrhea.** The differential diagnosis includes, in addition to any and all of the causes listed earlier, those described in Table 2-9.

D. **Drug-induced diarrhea**
   1. **Antibiotic-associated diarrhea**
      a. The **specific manifestations** of this form of diarrhea include an onset of symptoms 2–10 days after initiation of antibiotics. The diarrhea can begin after completion of a course of antibiotics. Symptoms include a moderate amount of watery, nonbloody diarrhea with nausea, vomiting, and abdominal cramping, which may lead to modest intravascular volume depletion. The duration of symptoms and signs is variable but can extend until treatment is started.
      b. The **underlying pathogenesis** is a change in the normal colonic flora or the inappropriate growth of *Clostridium difficile* as a side effect of a systemic antibiotic. *C. difficile* is a gram-positive bacillus that can be present in small amounts in the normal colonic flora. Its growth is suppressed and held in check by the rest of the normal colonic bacterial flora. When this balance is disturbed, as when some of the other bacterial flora are suppressed by systemic antibiotics, *C. difficile* or other organisms can inappropriately dominate.
         i. *C. difficile* is enterotoxic to the GI mucosal cells, with resultant mucosal dysfunction.

T A B L E 2-6
Acute Domestic Diarrhea Syndromes

Organism	Manifestations/Mode of Transmission	Toxic Mechanism	Treatment
Viral agents (Norwalk agent, etc.)	Begins 6–12 hr after exposure Duration: 24–96 hr Nonbloody, watery diarrhea, usually with minimal concurrent vomiting except in children Transmitted by fecal–oral route	Enterotoxic to mucosal cells	Supportive (see Box 2-7)
Staphylococcus aureus food poisoning	Begins 2–6 hr after ingestion of food Duration: 18–24 hr Acute onset of large amounts of watery, non-bloody diarrhea; concurrent abdominal cramping and vomiting are common Acquired by ingestion of improperly stored pre-pared meats or custard-filled pastries	Enterotoxic to mucosal cells; gram-positive cocci	Supportive (see Box 2-7)
Clostridium perfringens food poisoning	Begins 8–20 hr after ingestion of food Duration: 12–24 hr Acute onset of large amounts of watery, non-bloody diarrhea; concurrent abdominal cramping and vomiting are common Acquired by ingestion of contaminated food from a buffet or smorgasboard, often food that has been steamed	Enterotoxic to mucosal cells; gram-positive rods	Supportive (see Box 2-7)

Salmonella spp. food poisoning	Begins 12–24 hr after ingestion of food Duration: 12–24 hr Acute onset of moderate to large amounts of non-bloody diarrhea; can progress to bloody diarrhea in a minority of cases; concurrent abdominal cramping and vomiting are common Acquired by ingestion of contaminated food, poorly cooked poultry or eggs, or foods washed in water contaminated with this organism	Enterotoxic to mucosal cells; gram-negative rods	Supportive (see Box 2-7)
Shigella spp.	Begins 12–30 hr after exposure Duration: 3–7 days Acute onset of moderate to large amounts of bloody diarrhea; concurrent abdominal cramping and vomiting are very common Transmitted by fecal–oral route; endemic in areas of poor sanitation	Enteroinvasive to the mucosa; gram-negative rods	See Box 2-7 and initiate antibiotics (Table 2-8)
Campylobacter jejuni	Begins 3–5 days after exposure Duration: 3–7 days Acute onset of moderate amounts of bloody diarrhea Transmitted by fecal–oral route; can be spread from a household pet, which can act as a reservoir for infection Highest incidence occurs in summer and early fall	Enteroinvasive to the mucosa; gram-negative rods, "seagull-wing" shaped	See Box 2-7 and initiate antibiotics (Table 2-8)

T A B L E 2-7
Acute, Nondomestic Diarrhea

Organism	Manifestations/Mode of Transmission	Toxic Mechanism	Treatment
E. coli	Begins 8–18 hr after ingestion of contaminated food or water Duration: 24–48 hr Acute onset of moderate to large amounts of nonbloody diarrhea; concurrent abdominal cramping and vomiting are common Transmitted by fecal-oral route; spread by contaminated water or incompletely cooked food that was cleaned in contaminated water	Enterotoxic to the mucosa; gram-negative rods	See Box 2-7 and text
Shigella spp. Salmonella spp.	See text and Table 2-6 See text and Table 2-6		
Entamoeba histolytica	Begins 12–24 hr after ingestion of contaminated food or water Duration: 3–7 days Acute onset of large amounts of bloody diarrhea; concurrent abdominal cramping and vomiting are common Indirect hemagglutinin assay (IHA) on the patient's serum will reveal antibodies against E. histolytica. A titer >1:128 is positive	Enteroinvasive to the mucosa; parasitic infection	See Box 2-7 and initiate antibiotics (Table 2-8)

Organism	Clinical Features	Pathophysiology	Treatment
Giardia lamblia	Begins 24–72 hr after ingestion of contaminated food or water Duration: 3–7 days Subacute onset of mildly blood, greasy/"frothy," and mucus-containing diarrhea Concurrent mild nausea and abdominal cramping are common Transmitted by fecal–oral route and by ingestion of contaminated ground water. Outbreaks have been described in St. Petersburg, Russia, and the Rocky Mountain states of North America Patients at highest risk are those with an IgA deficiency Highest incidence occurs in summer and early fall	Unknown; highest concentration in the distal duodenum and proximal jejunum	See Box 2-7 and initiate antibiotics (Table 2-8)
Vibrio cholerae	Begins 8–24 hr after ingestion of contaminated food or water Duration: 3–5 days Acute onset of large amounts of nonbloody diarrhea; concurrent abdominal cramping and vomiting are very common Transmitted by fecal–oral route, via ingestion of contaminated water, improperly cooked foods washed with contaminated water, or contaminated seafood (e.g., sushi, salmon, oysters)	Enterotoxic to the mucosa; gram-negative rods	See Box 2-7 and initiate antibiotics (Table 2-8)

T A B L E 2-8
Antibiotic Treatment of Specific Infectious Diarrheal States

Organism	Antibiotic
Campylobacter jejuni	Erythromycin, 500 mg p.o. q.i.d. for 7–10 days
Clostridium difficile	*Metronidazole, 500 mg p.o. q.i.d. for 7 days
	Vancomycin, 125 mg p.o. q.i.d. for 7–10 days
	Adjunctive therapy:
	Cholestyramine, one packet (4 grams) p.o. q.i.d. for 5–7 days
Cryptosporidium spp.	*Paromomycin 500 mg p.o. q.i.d. for 14 days
	and
	Infectious Diseases consult
Isospora belli	TMP–sulfa (Bactrim DS), one tablet p.o. q.i.d. for 10 days, then one tablet p.o. b.i.d. for 21 days
	and
	Infectious Diseases consult
Traveler's diarrhea	Pepto-Bismol, 60 mL p.o. q.i.d.
	and/or
	Ciprofloxacin 500 mg p.o. b.i.d., start at first sign of symptoms for 5–7 days
Shigella spp.	Ampicillin, 500 mg p.o. q.i.d. for 7–10 days
	or
	TMP-sulfa (Bactrim DS) one tablet p.o. b.i.d. for 7–10 days
Entamoeba histo-lytica	*Metronidazole, 750 mg p.o. q.d. for 7 days
	and
	*Diiodohydroxyquin, 650 mg p.o. t.i.d. for 21 days
Giardia lamblia	*Quinacrine, 100 mg p.o. t.i.d. for 5–7 days
	or
	*Metronidazole, 250 mg p.o. t.i.d. for 5–7 days
	or
	Furazolidone 100 mg p.o. q.i.d. for 7–10 days

* Contraindicated in pregnancy.

TABLE 2-9
Immunocompromised Patient, Chronic Diarrheal Etiologies

Organism	Manifestations/Mode of Transmission	Toxic Mechanism/Organism	Treatment
HIV-related enteropathy	Insidious onset, recurrent Large amounts of watery, nonbloody diarrhea; mild to moderate concurrent nausea and vomiting Transmission is discussed in Chapter 6	Direct infection of mucosal cells and neuronal cells in GI system; enterotoxic	Supportive (see Box 2-7)
Cryptosporidium spp.	Recurrent episodes Variable amounts of watery, nonbloody diarrhea; the quantity can be massive—8 L/day Transmitted by fecal–oral route in immunocompromised patients, either by ingestion of contaminated water or by direct oral–anal contact	Enterotoxic to mucosal cells; protozoan parasite	Supportive (see Box 2-7) and initiate antibiotics (Table 2-8)
Isospora belli	Recurrent episodes Variable amounts of watery, nonbloody diarrhea; the quantity can be massive—≤8 L/day Transmitted by fecal–oral route in immunocompromised patients, either by ingestion of contaminated water or by direct oral–anal contact	Enterotoxic to mucosal cells; protozoan parasite	Supportive (see Box 2-7) and initiate antibiotics (Table 2-8)
Mycobacterium avium-intracellulare	Recurrent episodes Variable amounts of watery, nonbloody diarrhea; the quantity can be massive—≤8 L/day Transmitted by fecal–oral route in immunocompromised patients, either by ingestion of contaminated water or by direct oral–anal contact	Enterotoxic to mucosal cells; protozoan parasite	Supportive (see Box 2-7) and initiate antibiotics (Table 2-8)

      ii. Any and all systemic antibiotics can cause antibiotic-related diarrhea in general, and *C. difficile* colitis, in specific.

      iii. A significant complication of this entity is the development of the ulcerative inflammatory colonic process, pseudomembranous colitis.

    c. **Evaluation** includes making the clinical diagnosis and performing the overall evaluation and management, as described in Box 2-7. A stool culture that yields *C. difficile* and toxin clinches the diagnosis.

    d. The **specific management** includes supportive therapy and, if possible, limiting the duration of systemic antibiotics (usually not possible). The clinician must concurrently initiate and administer antibiotics by mouth. Two antibiotics effective in the treatment of antibiotic-related diarrhea are vancomycin, 125 mg p.o., q.i.d., for 7–10 days, or metronidazole, 250–500 mg p.o., q.i.d., for 7–10 days (metronidazole is contraindicated in pregnancy). A further modality is to administer cholestyramine, two packets t.i.d. orally, for a duration of 3–5 days. This agent decreases the diarrhea by decreasing the quantity of toxin in the lumen of the colon.

2. **Diarrhea due to other agents**

    a. The **specific manifestations** of this type of diarrhea include the onset of watery diarrhea while the patient is taking a specific agent. Many forms of diarrhea, both acute and chronic, can result from or be exacerbated by medications the patient is taking, either prescribed or over the counter (OTC). Therefore, in all cases of significant diarrhea, the history of medication use—prescribed, illicit, or OTC—must be obtained. The duration is usually quite dependent on the duration of use of the agent.

    b. The **underlying pathogenesis** is usually either an osmotic-type diarrhea or one resulting from intestinal hypermobility. Osmotic diarrheal entities result from an abnormal increase in the water content of the stool. This can be due to many different, quite diverse agents, from the overuse of dietary fiber products, from lactulose, and from the use of magnesium-containing antacids. Hypermobility diarrhea is a result of increased peristalsis and therefore decreased transit time of the stool in the colon. The faster the transit time, the less water is absorbed from the stool, and therefore the more fluid is the stool. Hypermobility diarrhea can be caused by overindulgence in caffeinated beverages, excessive ethanol use, and the use of phenolphthalein or other laxatives, cathartics, or stool softeners. There is a

B O X   2-7

Overall Evaluation and Management of Diarrhea

Evaluation

1. Take a thorough history, with specific note of the qualifying features listed in the text in the introductory discussion of diarrhea.
2. Perform a physical examination, looking specifically for orthostatic changes, fever, and any abdominal findings, all of which portend a more acute and potentially malignant course necessitating a more aggressive evaluation. The physical examination includes a rectal examination directly to visualize the stool, to guaiac test the stool for occult blood, and to palpate the rectal mucosa for lesions.
3. If an infectious cause of the diarrhea is suspected (e.g., after antibiotic use, the patient is febrile, the diarrhea is bloody), place the patient on enteric precautions.
4. Perform stool studies on a freshly collected sample as soon as possible. These studies include:
   a. Gram stain, looking for white blood cells and bacteria, which are normally not present in the stool, or
   b. Leukocyte stain (Loeffler's methylene blue stain) looking for white blood cells, which are normally not present in the stool.
   c. Microscopic examination of fresh stool for ova and parasites. The clinician must inform the laboratory if any unique protozoa are suspected.
   d. Bacterial cultures for enteric pathogens (i.e., *Salmonella, Shigella,* and *Campylobacter*). Cultures are mandatory if there is any evidence of concurrent leukocytes or blood in the stool, or if the patient is febrile.
5. Obtain blood cultures if the patient is febrile. Any of the enteric pathogens can invade the bowel, and therefore bacteremia is potentially a sequela.
6. Determine serum electrolyte, blood urea nitrogen (BUN), and creatinine levels as part of the baseline evaluation.
7. Assay for *Clostridium difficile* toxin, and culture the stool. *C. difficile* is a gram-positive anaerobic rod; toxin B is the one measured by the assay. This is mandatory if the patient is taking or has recently completed a course of antibiotics.

(continued)

B O X   2-7 (continued)

8. Determine the complete blood cell count with differential, for baseline purposes and to document any leukocytosis.
9. If there is evidence of intravascular volume depletion, rehydrate the patient either intravenously or orally.
   a. Intravenous rehydration: dextrose 5% in 0.9 normal saline is the fluid of choice and can easily be given in the outpatient setting.
   b. Oral rehydration: if indicated or attempted, use solutions containing glucose, sodium chloride, citrate, and potassium, such as Pedialyte or water with the WHO oral rehydration packet or Gatorade.
10. Alkalinize a sample of the stool with NaOH. If the stool turns pink, it is indicative of phenolphthalein use or abuse. Phenolphthalein is a commonly used over-the-counter (OTC) laxative and cathartic agent; it is the active ingredient in Ex-Lax.
11. Perform a Sudan stain for fat in the stool. This is a good screening test for steatorrhea (i.e., fat malabsorption).
12. Consider colonoscopy or flexible proctosigmoidoscopy with biopsies of the mucosa if the stool is bloody, the patient is febrile, the diarrhea is severe, the diarrhea represents an acute exacerbation of a chronic diarrheal state, or the patient is immunocompromised.
13. Initiate antidiarrheal agents on the following schedule:
   a. Kaopectate, 15–30 mL p.o., q4–6h prn, or
   b. Pepto-Bismol (bismuth subsalicylate), 15–30 mL p.o., q4–6h prn, and/or
   c. Lomotil (diphenoxylate plus atropine), 2.5 mg p.o., q6h prn.
      NOTE: Use extreme caution when using narcotic-type antidiarrheal agents in infectious or inflammatory bowel diarrhea.
14. Use antibiotics cautiously. In general, there are very few indications for antibiotics, even in infectious diarrhea. See Table 2-8.

significant amount of overlap between these two mechanisms.

    c. The **specific evaluation and management** include making the clinical diagnosis and performing the overall evaluation and management, as described in Box 2-7. Invariably, withdrawing the agent and/or modifying the habits of the patient will result in resolution of the diarrhea in 1–3 days. If there is no resolution, other causes must be explored.

  II. Chronic diarrheal states
    Refer to Table 2-10.

  III. Consultation

Problem	Service	Time
Immunocompromised patient with diarrhea	Infectious diseases	Urgent
Chronic diarrhea	Gastroenterology	Required
Acute, bloody diarrhea	Gastroenterology	Urgent

  IV. Indications for admission: Severe intravascular volume depletion, any evidence or suspicion of an acute abdomen, any fevers or manifestations of septicemia, or any lower GI bleeding with a decrease in the hematocrit.

End-Stage Hepatic Dysfunction

End-stage hepatic dysfunction is a syndrome that results from the permanent loss of liver tissue and therefore of liver function. The manifestations and prognosis are virtually the same, irrespective of the underlying cause, and therefore this diagnosis supplants those previous diagnoses. The classic, virtually synonymous term is cirrhosis.

The **physiologic functions** of the liver include but are not limited to the following:

1. **Protein anabolism.** The liver produces proteins, including many of the coagulation factors (i.e., factors II, V, VII, IX, and X). The liver also produces albumin, a major determinant in the maintenance of intravascular colloid oncotic pressure and thus of keeping fluids within the intravascular system.
2. **Draining of venous blood from the GI tract.** Venous blood is drained from the GI tract via the hepatic portal system. Blood rich with nutrients is absorbed in the small intestine and delivered to the liver, where the nutrients are processed into usable substrates for energy and anabolism.
3. **Detoxification.** The liver helps maintain the physiologic milieu by detoxifying the body fluids of toxic substances.

TABLE 2-10
Features of Chronic Diarrheal Syndromes

Syndrome	Mechanism	Clinical Features	Diagnostic Tests/Treatment
Irritable bowel syndrome	Undefined motility disorder of the GI tract	Afebrile Mucous diarrhea alternating with periods of constipation No weight loss	Diagnosis of exclusion Treatment: a) Predominant manifestation is constipation, fiber (Metamucil) b) Predominant manifestation is diarrhea, Loperamide c) Predominant manifestation is pain, spastic, especially if post-prandial pain, Dicylomide, 10–20 mg p.o. t.i.d.
Diabetic enteropathy	Autonomic neuron dysfunction/destruction with an overall decrease in motility and, potentially, bacterial overgrowth	Nocturnal diarrhea Postprandial vomiting Malabsorption, especially of fats No improvement with fasting Concurrent other autonomic dysfunction	Diagnosis of exclusion in a diabetic patient Treatment: a) Prevention b) Diphenyoxylate and atropine (Lomotil) q.6hr p.o. PRN

Carbohydrate malabsorption	Either as a result of a decrease in the absorptive brush border, and/or as a relative or absolute deficiency in disaccharidases (most commonly lactase)	Bloating Increased flatus Diarrhea Improves with fasting Exacerbated by ingestion of specific disaccharide (e.g., lactose)	Resolution of symptoms on a diet low in the offending sugar (e.g., a no-dairy-product diet: decrease lactose); this is both diagnostic and therapeutic H_2 breath test: Excessive H_2 production by bacteria in the colon if undigested disaccharide (lactose, etc.) is present; hydrogen is measured in air exhaled by the patient Treatment: Modify diet to exclude offending sugar
Fat malabsorption	A decrease in bile salts, pancreatic enzymes, and/or ileal surface area DDX: a) small-bowel disorder or b) pancreatic insufficiency	Steatorrhea Malodorous stools Improves with fasting Greasy stools Vitamin K deficiency Vitamin A and D deficiencies	72-hr collection of stool for fecal fat on a 100-g fat diet KUB: to look for pancreatic calcifications, indicative of chronic pancreatitis Treatment: a) If small bowel, find and treat the underlying cause b) If pancreatic insufficiency, pancreatic enzyme replacement (e.g., Pancrease, 2 packets before meals)
Zollinger–Ellison syndrome	Hypersecretion of gastrin due to a gastrinoma, resulting in hypersecretion of acid and GI hypermotility	Watery diarrhea No improvement with fasting Recurrent gastric or duodenal ulcers or both	Gastric acid measurements Serum gastrin levels (off of H_2 blockers) Treatment: a) H_2-receptor blockers (e.g., ranitidine, 150 mg p.o. b.i.d.)

(continued)

Syndrome	Mechanism	Clinical Features	Diagnostic Tests/Treatment
			or
			b) H-K ATPase inhibitors (omeprazole, 40 mg p.o. q.d.)
			c) Surgical resection
			d) Somatostatin
Carcinoid	An intestinal or extraintestinal tumor producing bradykinins, prostaglandins, and/or serotonin	Watery diarrhea If a primary bronchial carcinoid and/or if hepatic metastases are present, a syndrome occurs of: Pulmonic valve stenosis Flushing of skin Watery diarrhea Bronchospasm	24-hr urine collection for 5-HIAA (catabolite of serotonin) Chest radiography CT scan of liver Treatment (beyond scope of text): Somatostatin Treat tumor
Crohn's disease	Unknown	Fevers Bloody diarrhea No improvement with fasting Transmural lesions Involvement throughout GI tract	Colonoscopy with biopsies UGI with small bowel follow-through Treatment: a) Sulfasalazine, 500–1000 mg p.o. q.i.d. b) Acute flares: steroids (e.g., methylprednisolone, 80 mg i.v. q 8 hr)

Disease	Etiology	Clinical features	Diagnosis/Treatment
		Malabsorption Sacroiliitis Uveitis Pyoderma gangrenosum Erythema nodosum Fistulas/strictures	c) Limit surgical procedures d) No clear efficacy of metronidazole
Ulcerative colitis	Unknown	Fevers Bloody diarrhea No improvement with fasting Mucosal lesions Proctitis/colitis Weight loss Increased risk of colon carcinoma	Colonoscopy with biopsy Treatment: a) Sulfasalazine, 500–1000 mg p.o. q.i.d. b) For acute flares and/or severe disease: steroids (prednisone, 60 mg p.o. q.d., or methylprednisolone, 80 mg i.v. q.8h.) c) Hydrocortisone enema, 50–100 mg retention enema q.h.s., especially effective in the treatment of proctitis d) Opiate agents can be used with caution in patients with chronic findings (Lomotil), one tablet p.o. q.6–8h., or loperamide (Imodium), 2–4 mg p.o. q.6–8h. e) Surgical intervention f) Mesalamine (Asocal) 800 mg t.i.d. p.o. for 6 wk also is effective g) 6-mercaptopurine (6-MP) 50 mg/day p.o. is also good in refractory ulcerative colitis

I. Manifestations of hepatic insufficiency (see Box 2-8)
The overall manifestations of hepatic insufficiency are directly related to a want of the normal physiologic functions performed exclusively by the liver. Problems that can and will develop include coagulopathy, ascites, edema, portal hypertension with potential for bleeding, and mental-status changes [i.e., encephalopathy as a result of toxin accumulation in the blood and central nervous system (CNS)]. The manifestations, pathogenesis, evaluation, and management of each of these problems are discussed subsequently.

B O X 2-8

Overall Evaluation and Management of Hepatic Insufficiency

Evaluation

1. Follow up on a regular basis, such as every 3–6 months, the following parameters:
   a. AST and total bilirubin.
   b. Prothrombin time (PT) and albumin, to monitor the synthetic function of the liver.
   c. CBC count, to monitor for anemia and thrombocytopenia.
   d. Electrolytes, BUN, creatinine, and glucose.
2. Determine the Child–Turcotte class of the patient (see Table 2-11).

Management

1. Instruct the patient to discontinue all ethanol use.
2. Administer the Pneumovax polyvalent vaccine at the time of presentation.
3. All hepatotoxic agents are contraindicated (e.g., ethanol, acetaminophen).
4. Instruct the patient to avoid the use of agents catabolized in the liver, such as benzodiazepines and acetaminophen. If use is necessary, the agents should be used with great caution and, if possible, close monitoring of plasma levels.
5. The patient should take a multivitamin pill orally once daily.
6. Administer an influenza vaccine every fall.
7. Salicylates are contraindicated, especially if there is any evidence of a coagulopathy.
8. The only curative modality for end-stage liver disease in liver transplantation.

T A B L E 2-11
Child–Turcotte Classification

Parameter	Class		
	A	B	C
Serum bilirubin (mg/dL)	<2.0	2.0–3.0	>3.0
Serum albumin (g/dL)	>3.5	3.0–3.5	<3.0
Ascites	None	Easily managed	Refractory
Encephalopathy	Absent	Mild	Severe
Nutritional status	Good	Fair	Poor

Other examination findings include icterus, both scleral and skin; a small liver [i.e., a span of <6 cm; palmar erythema (i.e., a diffuse redness of the palms and soles); and spider angiomas (i.e., red spiderlike lesions on the skin of the upper trunk and arms, which are thought to be a result of excess estrogens)]. Of interest, these lesions occur only in the distribution of the superior vena cava. Finally, male subjects may exhibit decreased testicular volume and impotence, along with bilateral gynecomastia, all as a result of excess estrogens (Fig. 2-3).

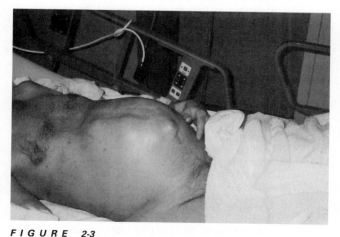

F I G U R E 2-3
End-stage liver disease. Note the ascites, umbilical hernia, and edema on this patient with liver disease as the result of ethanol-related cirrhosis.

II. **Complications of hepatic insufficiency**
Specific complications include the following:
  A. **Coagulopathy**
    1. The **specific manifestations** of coagulopathy include a subacute onset of easy bruisability, purpura, recurrent ecchymoses, epistaxis, and gingival bleeding. The patient may report uncontrolled bleeding after minor trauma.
    2. The **underlying pathogenesis** involves a deficiency in the coagulation factors produced by the liver. These coagulation factors include II, V, VII, IX, and X (i.e., those of the extrinsic coagulation cascade). This arm of the coagulation cascade is measured by using the PT. These factors, with the exception of factor V, are also vitamin K dependent, and therefore vitamin K deficiency can manifest with similar findings. Vitamin K deficiency is often present concurrent with the liver disease and thus must be ruled out in the evaluation.
    3. **Evaluation** entails determining PT, aPTT, platelet count, and ruling out any concurrent process that may exacerbate the bleeding disorder. Examples of reversible exacerbating factors include the use of salicylates, a deficiency in vitamin K, and a consumptive coagulopathy [disseminated intravascular coagulopathy (DIC)]. For example, an isolated elevation of PT can reflect either vitamin deficiency or liver disease.
    4. The **specific management** includes proscribing the use of aspirin and attempting to correct the elevated PT with vitamin K. The dose of vitamin K is 10 mg subcutaneously, once daily for 3 days, and then orally, or 10 mg p.o., once daily from the outset. If a surgical procedure is planned, fresh frozen plasma (FFP) should be administered before the procedure to attempt to normalize the elevated PT, or, at minimum, to decrease it to <15 seconds during the procedure.
  B. **Variceal bleeding** (refer to GI bleeding section).
    1. The **specific manifestations,** in addition to those accompanying any other upper GI bleeding (see section on Gastrointestinal Bleeding, page 110), include other findings of portal hypertension, among them distended superficial abdominal veins, including the specific sign of caput medusae (i.e., distended cutaneous veins radiating from the umbilicus); internal hemorrhoids; guaiac-positive stools; hematemesis; melena; and hematochezia. The patient may be intravascularly volume depleted and hemodynamically unstable at the time of presentation. Variceal bleeding must always be considered in the differential diagnosis of GI bleeding in any patient with hepatic dysfunction.

2. The **underlying pathogenesis** involves hypertension in the portal venous system, which results in significant congestion and dilation of the veins in the portal system—the veins of the GI tract. The dilated portal veins usually form in the distal esophagus but can form anywhere in the GI tract. They are easily traumatized and therefore bleed, with resultant massive GI hemorrhages.

3. **Evaluation** entails making the clinical diagnosis and emergency management of active bleeding.

4. **Management**
   Emergency consultation with gastroenterology for emergency EGD is indicated for potential sclerotherapy of the varices. Further treatment is beyond the scope of this text.

5. **Long-term therapy and prophylaxis**
   The long-term therapy and prophylaxis of variceal bleeding, especially esophageal variceal bleeding, includes the following:

   a. Checking the hematocrit frequently (i.e., q 1–2 months).

   b. Instructing the patient to watch for the development of melena.

   c. **Sclerotherapy** as a prophylactic modality by the gastroenterology service is probably effective in decreasing the number of upper GI bleeding episodes but has not been demonstrated to prolong life. In fact, one recent study demonstrated an increased mortality in the group receiving prophylactic variceal sclerotherapy. Therefore, it is not at present a recommended procedure for prophylaxis.

   d. Some recent studies demonstrated a positive effect of **β-blockers** (e.g., propranolol, 10–20 mg p.o., t.i.d.) in decreasing the magnitude of portal hypertension, thus potentially decreasing the risk of variceal development and bleeding. β-Blockers can be used only in patients without contraindications to them, and frequent follow-up is necessary to monitor blood pressure and vital signs. In addition, nitrates (e.g., isordil, 10 mg p.o., t.i.d.) may be of benefit to decrease the portal pressures and may be used in the stead of β-blockers in those patients who have contraindications to β-blockers or as adjunctive therapy in addition to β-blockers.

   e. Placement of a **portosystemic shunt** (e.g., a TIPS (transjugular portosystemic shunt) should be considered, especially in young patients of Child–Turcotte class A or B (see Table 2-11). This procedure shunts blood from the portal to the systemic venous circulation, thus bypassing the liver and decreasing portal hypertension. Shunt placement decreases the risk of recurrence of upper GI hemorrhage due to varices but has not increased the life expectancy of patients. This is also an invasive procedure with inherent morbidity, an increased incidence of encephalopathy, an increased risk of infection, and even mortality.

C. **Encephalopathy**

1. The **specific manifestations** of this not uncommon sequela of hepatic insufficiency include asterixis (i.e., bilateral involuntary flapping of the hands at the wrist when the patient is instructed actively to extend the hands); confusion (delirium); and lethargy.

2. The **underlying pathogenesis** is an increase in the level of nitrogenous wastes in the bloodstream, which in turn results in deterioration of brain function. A marker for this process is the serum ammonia level, which is elevated in encephalopathy but is not directly correlated with the degree of encephalopathy. Usually the encephalopathy is exacerbated by ingestion of proteinaceous foodstuffs, constipation, GI bleeding, intravascular volume depletion, and sepsis.

3. **Evaluation** entails making the clinical diagnosis and, at the outset, determining the serum NH_4 level. In addition, any concurrent process that might cause mental-status changes must be ruled out, and underlying, precipitating, or exacerbating factors must be sought and treated.

4. The **specific management** in the acute setting includes the initiation of lactulose and/or neomycin. Lactulose is a complex carbohydrate that increases colonic motility and results in diarrhea. The dose for lactulose is 15–30 mL p.o., q4–12hr. Neomycin is a nonabsorbable antibiotic that works well in the acute setting, especially when used with lactulose. This antibiotic is thought to be bactericidal for many of the bacterial flora that produce diarrhea and also decrease nitrogenous waste production by the bacteria in the distal small bowel and colon. The dose for neomycin is 500–1,000 mg p.o., b.i.d. The dose is titrated to symptoms and the number of bowel movements per day. The optimal number of bowel movements is two or three per day. Finally, central to management is limiting protein consumption to 40 g/day. To meet this goal, a dietary consultation is highly recommended.

D. **Ascites**

1. The **specific manifestations** of this quite common sequela of hepatic insufficiency reflect excess fluid within the peritoneal cavity. The patient will relate

that the pants feel tight or that the waist size of clothing has been increased to accommodate the increased abdominal girth. There is often concurrent edema in dependent areas (feet if ambulatory, back if bedridden) of the body. Examination often discloses abdominal distention, a shifting dullness in the distended abdomen, and a fluid wave. Unless infection exists concurrently, there usually is no tenderness to deep or rebound palpation. Ascites can spontaneously become infected, usually with bacteria that are normally present in the GI tract; thus, one must always be concerned that this has occurred when a patient has concurrent pain or tenderness or an increase in the quantity of peritoneal fluid.

2. The **underlying pathogenesis** of ascites is multifactorial but includes underlying portal hypertension with congestion of fluids in the portal system and concurrent moderate to profound hypoalbuminemia, all of which result in edema and leakage of fluids into the peritoneal cavity. In addition to these mechanisms, a secondary hyperaldosteronism develops, resulting in further sodium and water retention.

3. **Evaluation** entails making the clinical diagnosis. If there is any question as to its presence, abdominal US will clearly demonstrate it. Because ascites can become infected and result in potentially mortal infections and because other conditions can exacerbate ascites, all new cases of ascites and all patients with an increase in ascites or any abdominal tenderness to palpation mandate paracentesis. The evaluative studies that should be performed on the ascitic fluid are listed in Table 2-12.

4. **Management**
   The **specific management** of ascites is divided into short- and long-term management.
   a. Short-term management is necessary if the ascites is infected or is causing distress for the patient, especially if it is causing respiratory compromise.
      i. If there is any evidence of peritonitis, acute administration of antibiotics is mandatory. Regimens to cover the most common organismal causes (i.e., the gram-negative bacilli, anaerobes, and group D streptococci) include:
      Ampicillin, 2 g q.4–6hr i.v.
      -and-
      Clindamycin, 900 mg i.v., q.8hr
      -and-
      Aminoglycoside, i.v.
      -or-
      Unasyn, 3.0 g i.v., q.6hr

T A B L E   2-12
Diagnostic Examination of Ascites

1. **Albumin gradient:** Calculate gradient via serum albumin–ascitis-fluid albumin
   If the gradient is >1.1 g/dL, consistent with portal hypertension
   If the gradient is <1.1 g/dL, consistent with an underlying pathogenesis not related to portal hypertension
2. **Cell count in the ascitic fluid:** If the total WBC count is >500/mm^3 or the total polymorphonuclear cell counts is >250/mm^3, the result should be interpreted as and must be treated as bacterial peritonitis
   If the pretest probability for peritonitis is high (i.e., the presence of peritoneal signs), any PMNs in the fluid result in a positive test. Thus the threshold for positive changes based on the pretest probability
3. Amylase: If increased rule out pancreatic pseudocyst and pancreatic ascites
4. Gram stain
5. AFB smear.
6. Cultures of the ascitic fluid
7. Triglycerides, especially if the fluid appears milklike, to evaluate for chylous ascites
8. Cytologic examination if neoplastic process is suspected

---

  ii. If there is a large quantity of ascites resulting in respiratory compromise, one can remove the fluid. The traditional modalities of fluid restriction and bedrest are of minimal efficacy. A highly effective modality is to perform high-volume paracentesis (HVP). This is accomplished by removing 3–4 L of fluid in the standard manner. Concurrent with any HVP therapy, the initiation of diuretics for long-term therapy is indicated. Two different diuretics can be of clinical use.

  (a) Potassium-sparing diuretics are very effective in that they decrease aldosterone levels and thereby reverse secondary hyperaldosteronism, one of the basic pathophysiologic mechanisms leading to ascites. The initial dose is spironolactone, 25 mg p.o., t.i.d., which can be slowly increased to a maximum of 300 mg p.o. in a 24-hour period.

(b) Loop diuretics (e.g., furosemide, 20 mg p.o., q.d.) are excellent as adjunctive therapy to the potassium-sparing diuretics and may, especially if given early in the course of therapy, effect a more productive diuresis.

b. **Long-term therapy** is for patients who have already received acute intervention or who have an asymptomatic transudative fluid. The **specific management** includes monitoring for the development of subacute bacterial peritonitis, effectively treating the underlying condition if possible, and titrating diuretics (potassium-sparing or loop diuretics) to minimize the ascites without causing hyperkalemia or intravascular volume depletion. Instruct the patient to modify the diet to limit salt intake. It is essential to attempt to restrict the patient to a diet containing <2 g of sodium per day. The dietary service should be consulted to aid in this instruction.

   i. Parameters that must be followed include weight, creatinine, orthostatic measurements, and urine sodium. If the urine sodium is <10 and/or if there is evidence of volume contraction, may need to decrease the diuretic therapy.

E. **Hepatorenal syndrome**

Hepatorenal syndrome is the development of renal failure as a result of or concurrent with severe hepatic dysfunction. The process is usually precipitated by intravascular volume depletion, as a result either of upper GI hemorrhage or of overzealous diuresis. The renal failure is irreversible, and once present, this syndrome has a grave prognosis. The best method of treatment is prevention. Renal consultation should be obtained.

III. **Prognosis**

The overall prognosis for patients with end-stage liver disease is quite bleak. Even with abstinence from ethanol and other hepatotoxic agents and with supportive care, the 2-year survival rate is <50%. Some hope in the treatment of this disorder has arisen from transplants, but this modality, at least in its present form and for the immediate future, will be of benefit for only a small minority of patients. The potential for transplantation should be explored in all patients, and referral to gastroenterology for this purpose should be performed.

The **Child–Turcotte classification** scheme for hepatic dysfunction is given in Table 2-11. A study by Christensen et al. demonstrated a correlation with overall prognosis: as the class goes from A to B to C, the life expectancy dramatically decreases from years to months.

IV. **Consultation**

Problem	Service	Time
Variceal bleeding	GI	Urgent/emergent
Variceal bleeding	Surgery	Urgent/emergent
TIPS	Radiology	Elective
For low-salt diet and low-protein diet	Dietary	Elective

V. **Indications for admission:** Fever, upper GI bleeding, new or exacerbation of encephalopathy, intravascular volume depletion, presence or clinical suspicion of spontaneous bacterial peritonitis, or massive ascites that restricts respiratory function.

Gastrointestinal Bleeding

The **overall manifestations** of GI bleeding are quite variable and are related to the site, duration, acuity, and intensity of the bleeding. They include hematemesis (coffee-ground–type emesis, if the site is in the upper GI area) and melena (black, tarry stools) as a result of blood passing through the GI tract and into the stool. Black stools may result from upper GI bleeding, lower GI bleeding (i.e., from the colon, especially if the transit time across the colon is long), the use of $FeSO_4$, or the use of bismuth subsalicylate (Pepto-Bismol). A further manifestation is hematochezia—bright red blood passed rectally—which may be indicative of a lower GI source or of a massive upper GI hemorrhage.

Other manifestations may include intravascular volume depletion with accompanying symptoms and signs, a pale skin and conjunctivae, guaiac-positive stool (the guaiac test is negative in black stool caused by $FeSO_4$ or bismuth), and epigastric pain or tenderness. The patient may have a history of PUD, of hepatic disease with or without varices, of recent ethanol use, or of recent NSAID use.

Other, nongastrointestinal sites of bleeding can occasionally manifest with melena or what is presumed to be hematemesis. The most common of these conditions are epistaxis and hemoptysis. At the outset, the clinician must attempt to differentiate these causes from the history and physical examination findings (Box 2-9; Table 2-13).

II. **Consultation**

Problem	Service	Time
Any GI bleed requiring admission	Surgery GI	Urgent Emergent
Acute abdomen	Surgery	Emergent
Adenocarcinoma in stomach/colon	Surgery	Urgent

B O X 2-9

*Overall Evaluation and Management
of Gastrointestinal Bleeding*

Evaluation

1. Evaluate ABCs and perform ACLS protocol as necessary.
2. Take the history and perform a physical examination, looking for the features described in the introductory section.
3. Determine the complete blood cell count with differential to determine the degree of anemia present at the time of presentation.
4. Type and cross-match blood for 4 units of packed red blood cells so that the blood is ready when needed for transfusion.
5. Determine the platelet count and coagulation parameters, including PT and aPTT, at baseline to rule out any exacerbating or concurrent coagulopathy.
6. Determine electrolytes, BUN, creatinine, and glucose levels as part of the baseline evaluation.
7. Obtain a 12-lead ECG as part of the baseline evaluation.
8. LFTs, including albumin, are important, for if there is any evidence of hepatic dysfunction, one must include variceal bleeding in the differential diagnosis.

Management

1. Place the patient on NPO orders at the outset in all cases.
2. Discontinue all NSAIDs for the short and intermediate term, as these agents can be the underlying cause of the bleeding.
3. Establish i.v. access with two large-bore i.v.s (≥18-gauge) or a central venous catheter so that large volumes of blood or fluids can be easily administered.
4. Initiate i.v. fluids (normal saline or dextrose 5% in 0.9 normal saline) at 250–300 mL/hr, or faster if clinically indicated.
5. Correct any coagulopathies with platelet and FFP infusions to keep the platelet count >50,000 and the PT <15 seconds.

(continued)

B O X   2-9 *(continued)*

> 6. Transfuse packed RBCs to keep the hematocrit >30%.
> 7. Administer H_2-receptor blockers (e.g., cimetidine, 300 mg i.v., q.6hr, or ranitidine, 50 mg i.v., q.8hr).
> 8. Consultation with gastroenterology and surgery is mandatory.
> 9. Admission to an ICU usually indicated.
> 10. After initial stabilization, direct invasive imaging by EGD, if an upper GI source is suspected, or by colonoscopy, if a lower GI source is suspected, is indicated.
> 11. See each diagnosis (Table 2-13) for specific considerations and/or management schemae.

Problem	Service	Time
Any evidence of ruptured viscus	Surgery	Emergent
Bloody diarrhea	GI	Urgent/emergent
Epigastric pain with normal Hct/guaiac-positive stools	GI	Required

III. **Indications for admission:** Intravascular volume depletion, melena, significant hematochezia, hypotension, any evidence of peritoneal signs or the clinical suspicion of an acute abdomen, any anemia requiring transfusion, or the development or exacerbation of angina pectoris.

Hepatitis

Hepatitis is nonspecific inflammation of the liver. The inflammation can lead to various acute and chronic manifestations and sequelae, which may be potentially life-threatening of themselves.

I. **Pathogenesis**

The liver detoxifies internally produced, biological (usually catabolic) agents and ingested agents, either biochemical, chemical, or biological, that are toxic to human cells. In the process of detoxification, the liver itself can be damaged. Damage occurs as a result of a direct effect of the toxin on the hepatocytes or as a result of the inflammatory infiltrate that usually develops concurrent with the toxin-related insult. These two mechanisms produce hepatocyte dysfunction and even acute hepatocyte necrosis.

T A B L E 2-13
Causes of Gastrointestinal Bleeding

Etiology	Pathogenesis	Specific Manifestations	Specific Evaluation and Management
Peptic ulcer disease	NSAID-related *Helicobacter pylori* Hyperacidemia/gastrinoma	Epigastric pain, decreased after food ingestion; increased with fasting Melena	See PUD, page 73 and Boxes 2-4 and 2-9

Hemorrhagic gastritis	The diffuse, often marked, superficial breakdown of the gastric mucosa with erosions
	May increase risk of ulcer development
	Risks
	  Ethanol
	  NSAID-gastropathy
		Use of NSAIDs
		GI bleeding
		Epigastric pain with fasting
		Use/abuse of NSAIDs
		Use/abuse of ethanol
		Melena
			Box 2-9
			and
			Initiation of antisecretory agents (e.g., H₂ antagonists)
			or
			Omeprazole 20 mg p.o. q.d.
			Discontinue aspirin and NSAIDs
			Refer to GI
			If the patient needs an NSAID
			  a) Restart NSAID in 4–6 wk
			  b) Concurrent sucralfate may be of benefit
			If patient needs an antiplatelet agent
			  a) Change to ticlopidine, 250 mg p.o. b.i.d.

(continued)

Etiology	Pathogenesis	Specific Manifestations	Specific Evaluation and Management
Gastric malignancy	Lymphoma, especially non-Hodgkin's may be associated with *Helicobacter pylori* infection Adenocarcinoma, risks include, ? nitrite in the diet	Upper GI bleed is a late manifestation Weight loss Early satiety "B" symptoms Fever Decreased weight Night sweats	Box 2-9 -*and*- Referral to surgery and oncology
Mallory–Weiss tear	Longitudinal tear in the mucosa of the distal esophagus and proximal gastric cardia. Majority of tear is on the gastric side Precipitated by severe retching and vomiting Bulimia is a risk factor, binge vomiting, & retching Normal mucosa	Hematemesis Initial emesis of food and food stuff, then coffee grounds/bright red blood in the emesis	Box 2-9 *and* EGD Antisecretory agents
Esophageal varices	Portal hypertension with resultant increase in veins in the distal esophagus Bleeding from the enlarged, plump, thin-walled veins	Hematemesis Ascites Increased veins on abdominal wall Other manifestations of end-stage hepatic disease	Box 2-9 *and* Treatment of underlying cause (see text) Correct any coagulopathy No aspirin

Diverticular disease	Small, acquired herniation of the colonic mucosa through the wall of the colon. May occur any place in the large intestine, but usually in the sigmoid colon. Risks include increasing age and straining Types: a) *Diverticulitis:* The tics are inflammed b) *Diverticulosis:* The tics erode into the adjacent vessels and bleed; little inflammation	Hematochezia, especially with diverticulosis Tenderness, pain, nausea in lower quadrants, especially with diverticulitis	Box 2-9 *and* Colonoscopy No known benefit of a proscription of berries, nuts, popcorn; therefore, unnecessary Increase fiber in diet If severe and recurrent, refer to surgery
Angiodysplasia	Arteriovenous malformation, multiple and increasing with age; may be associated with Osler–Weber–Rendu	Hematochezia Multiple angiomas in the nasal and oral mucosa	Colonoscopy Direct cautery of AVMs and angiomata
Colon polyps/adenocarcinoma	Villous or adenomatous polyps (i.e., premalignant) *or* Hyperplastic polyps *or* Polyposis syndromes (Table 5-5)	Intermittent hematochezia Intermittent melena Paucity of manifestations Increasing constipation and fatiguability Iron-deficiency anemia See colon carcinoma section	Box 2-9 *and* Colonoscopy Referral to surgery See colon carcinoma See Screening
Ischemic bowel	Acute hypoperfusion of the bowel, either as the result of atherosclerotic disease of the bowel arteries with profound hypotension *or* Thromboembolic disease	Diffuse bloody diarrhea Significant abdominal pain out of proportion to objective findings Mortal sequelae and outcome	Box 2-9 *and* Free air in the wall of GI tract (pneumatosis cystoides intestinalis) Colonoscopy: friable mucosa Admit, surgical consult
Hemorrhoids	See section, page 78		
Bloody diarrhea	See section, page 86		

II. Acute manifestations

The overall **acute manifestations** of hepatitis, irrespective of cause, include an acute to subacute onset of mild to moderate nausea, vomiting, and malaise. The patient often describes clay-colored stools; the light or clay color occurs as a result of an abnormally decreased secretion of bile into the GI tract with a resultant decrease in pigment in the stool itself. Patients often relate a sensation of abdominal fullness, especially in the right upper quadrant, as a result of hepatomegaly. The patient may also have severe pruritus as a result of the elevated bilirubin level. Pruritus can be so severe as to be the presenting complaint of the patient. Finally, the patient may relate a history, in the recent or distant past, of transfusions of blood or blood products, the ingestion of toxic agents (e.g., ethanol or acetaminophen), or the use of intravenous drugs.

Examination invariably discloses icterus that is especially prominent in the sclerae, mucous membranes, and skin. The icterus occurs as a result of an increase in bilirubin within the body due to a decrease in normal secretion or excretion from the liver. Icterus is usually correlated with a serum bilirubin level >3.0 mg/dL. Right upper quadrant tenderness with hepatomegaly is often present. The normal liver span is 6–12 cm in width and has a smooth, nontender edge on palpation; in acute hepatitis, the liver is enlarged and tender. A **further manifestation** is darkened urine as a result of excretion of urobilinogen and bilirubin in the urine instead of in the biliary tree or GI tract. The increased urobilinogen is associated with an increase in plasma conjugated bilirubin, whereas the increased bilirubin in the urine is associated with an increase in the unconjugated bilirubin in the plasma.

III. Hepatitis entities

A. Ethanol-related hepatitis

1. The **specific manifestations** of ethanol abuse, a common cause of acute hepatitis in the United States, include those described in the overall preceding discussion. Associated manifestations include gynecomastia, palmar erythema, spider angiomas, testicular atrophy, and Dupuytren's contracture of the digits. Dupuytren's contractures are bilateral acquired flexion contractures of the digits as the result of idiopathic fibrosis of the palmar fascia.

2. The **underlying pathogenesis** entails direct hepatocyte damage by ethanol, which results in fatty changes in the liver itself. The inflammatory response is modest and thus plays a negligible role in the overall pathogenesis.

3. **Evaluation** entails making the clinical diagnosis according to the steps listed in Box 2-10. Whereas all of the transaminase enzymes can be and often are ele-

B O X 2-10

*Overall Evaluation and Management
of Suspected Hepatitis*

Evaluation

1. Take a thorough history and perform a physical examination based on the previous discussion and that described under Abdominal Pain: Overall Approach.
2. Determine liver-function parameters, including AST, ALT, LDH, GGT, alkaline phosphatase, total bilirubin, and direct bilirubin. In acute hepatitis, all of these parameters may be elevated, but the transaminase levels (i.e., AST, ALT, and GGT) are all elevated to a greater degree than the alkaline phosphatase and total and direct bilirubin levels.
3. Determine serum albumin level and prothrombin time. Although they are normal in most cases of acute hepatitis, a decreased albumin level or an increased PT can occur as a result of superimposed chronic hepatic dysfunction and may portend a more malignant course.
4. Further tests to aid in evaluating the underlying cause include determining ethanol and acetaminophen levels and a hepatitis A and B panel. Further tests may include hepatitis C, ASMA (anti–smooth muscle antibody) and ANA for autoimmune hepatitis; serum Fe, transferrin saturation for hemochromatosis; antimitochondrial antibody for primary biliary cirrhosis; ceruloplasmin for Wilson's disease; and α_1-antitrypsin for α_1-antitrypsin deficiency. See Table 2-14 for serologic tests of viral hepatitis.
5. Perform urinalysis to test for the presence of bilirubin or urobilinogen in the urine.
6. Consider imaging studies. US of the liver and biliary tree demonstrates liver size and any concurrent obstructive findings.
7. If there is any evidence of ethanol abuse, administer 100 mg of thiamine p.o. or i.m. to prevent the development of Wernicke's encephalopathy.
8. Screen for hemochromatosis: Transferrin saturation of >60% in male and >50% in female patients, consistent with hemochromatosis; if increased, check the ferritin; if the ferritin is increased, consider liver biopsy.

(continued)

B O X 2-10 *(continued)*

Acute Management

1. Instruct the patient on safe sexual practices (use of condoms, abstinence, etc.).
2. Encourage good nutrition: Encourage intake of fluids p.o. or, if the patient is intravascularly depleted and vomiting, parenterally.
3. Instruct the patient to discontinue any agents that may exacerbate the hepatitis or the hepatic dysfunction (i.e., ethanol, oral contraceptives, acetaminophen) and, if possible, other agents that are potentially hepatotoxic, such as the phenothiazines.
4. If the pruritus is severe, initiate cholestyramine, two packets p.o., q.12hr prn for itching.
5. If a viral cause is suspected or documented, notify the Public Health Service.
6. If the patient is cytomegalovirus (CMV) negative and if transfusions of blood or blood products are necessary, the transfused substances should, if possible, be CMV negative.
7. Monitor LFT results, glucose, and PT closely longitudinally, as any decrease in glucose or increase in PT is a harbinger of a fulminant, quite malignant clinical course.
8. If acetaminophen, administer *N*-acetylcysteine loading dose of 140 mg/kg p.o. or per NG. See text for specifics.

---

vated in ethanol-related hepatitis, the classic pattern is GGT ≫ AST (SGOT) > ALT (SGPT). If the acute hepatitis is severe, there can be a concurrent significant increase in the bilirubin with resultant icterus.

4. The **specific management** of ethanol-induced hepatitis includes the steps listed in Box 2-10 and monitoring the patient for the development of withdrawal from ethanol—delirium tremens. Furthermore, it is of paramount importance to monitor the patient's nutritional status closely, as many of these patients are malnourished and can develop symptomatic refeeding hypophosphatemia. An additional note is the potential initiation of therapeutic steroids with severe acute ethanol-related hepatitis. A recent study demonstrated an overall better outcome in patients with severe ethanol-induced hepatitis who received steroids, relative to the

T A B L E 2-14
Serologic Tests for Viral Hepatitis

Acute Hepatitis
A: IgM anti-HA
   IgM antibody against hepatitis A:
     Acute hepatitis A infection
B: IgM anti-HB c:
   IgM antibody against the core antigen of Hepatitis B:
     Acute hepatitis B infection
C: None for hepatitis C
Chronic Hepatitis
A: None necessary
B: HBs Ag: Hepatitis B surface antigen in the patient
   HBe Ag: Indicative of patient's being highly infectious
   Anti-HBe IgG: Recovery, no chronic disease
   Anti-HBs IgG: Recovery, no chronic disease
C: Anti-HCV IgG: After exposure and probable infection of patient with Hep C, patient probably is infectious
Postvaccine vs. Infection for B
Postvaccine
   Anti-HBs IgG: Present
   Anti-HBc IgG: Absent
Infection
   Anti-HBs IgG: Present
   Anti-HBc IgG: Present

control group. Severe was defined as an increased PT, increased bilirubin, severe transaminase elevations, and encephalopathy. The dose of steroids is either prednisone, 40–60 mg p.o., once daily, for 3–7 days, or methylprednisone, 40 mg i.v., q.8hr, for 4–7 days. Finally, consultation with an addiction specialist should be made in an expedient fashion. Refer to the section on Substance Abuse Syndromes in Chapter 15 (page 689).
  B. **Acetaminophen-related hepatitis**
    1. The **specific manifestations of** this entity, which is a not uncommon cause and/or exacerbating factor of acute hepatitis in the United States, include those described in the preceding overall discussion. Acetaminophen can cause significant and severe hepatitis after ingestion of large quantities, either accidentally or in a suicide attempt. The specific manifestations of hepatic damage usually occur 36–48 hours after the ingestion.
    2. The **underlying pathogenesis** involves the production of toxic catabolites. In therapeutic doses and in the normal state, acetaminophen is catabolized by the liver

into several inactive components that are excreted into the biliary system. The usual pathway produces a catabolite that is conjugated with sulfate or glucuronide and is uniformly nontoxic. However, when a large amount of acetaminophen is ingested and in need of excretion, an alternative pathway must be used. This alternative pathway involves the cytochrome P-450 (2E1) system and produces a catabolite that is a highly toxic oxidizing agent and damages the hepatocytes.

In normal hepatocytes, there is a concurrent safety mechanism to inactivate any oxidizing agents. This agent is the reducing agent glutathione, which will inactivate any oxidizing agent in general and the toxic catabolite of acetaminophen specifically. Glutathione occurs in limited quantity within the hepatocyte, and in large acetaminophen ingestions, the supply is exhausted.

Risk factors for acetaminophen hepatotoxicity include:

a. Anything that activates the P-450 (2E1) system (e.g., ethanol, barbiturates), thereby increasing the production of the toxic catabolite.

b. Chronic ethanol ingestion, which decreases the stores of the reducing agent glutathione.

c. Large doses of acetaminophen taken over a short period.

As with ethanol, the effect is direct hepatotoxicity. The inflammatory response is modest.

3. **Evaluation** entails making the clinical diagnosis according to the steps described in Box 2-10. It is of tremendous importance to ascertain the quantity of acetaminophen taken, the specific time it was taken, and the acetaminophen level at the present time. By knowing the two parameters, acetaminophen level and time since ingestion, one can determine the risk for acute hepatotoxicity. Plasma acetaminophen levels of >200 μg/mL at 4 hours, 100 μg/mL at 8 hours, or 50 μg/mL at 12 hours are highly correlated with hepatotoxicity.

4. The **specific management** includes, in addition to that described in Box 2-10, management for any ingestion includes the administration of charcoal, 50 g given enterally (p.o. or NG), to decrease absorption. If the level of acetaminophen is in the toxic range or unknown, the immediate initiation of *N*-acetylcysteine (Mucomyst) enterally is mandated. A loading dose of 140 mg/kg p.o. or per nasogastric tube is followed by a maintenance dose of 70 mg/kg q.4hr p.o. or by nasogastric tube for 17 doses over 3 days (72 hours). This

agent decreases toxicity by acting as a reducing agent for the toxic catabolites of acetaminophen. A further therapeutic intervention is the initiation of H_2-receptor antagonists. These agents decrease the activity of the cytochrome P-450 (2E1) system and thus decrease the production of the toxic catabolite. In all cases, admission and referral to gastroenterology and to psychiatry are indicated.

C. **Viral hepatitis A**
 1. The **specific manifestations** of this type of hepatitis, in addition to those described in the section on Acute Manifestations, are based on the biology, pathogenesis, and natural history of the virus itself.

   The **organism** that causes this quite common form of hepatitis is an RNA virus that is transmitted by the fecal–oral route. Epidemics can occur in areas of poor sanitation or by infected patients intimately interacting with others.

   The **natural history** includes an incubation period (duration of time from exposure to onset of manifestations) of 2–6 weeks. The patient usually has a 1- to 2-week prodrome of nausea and vomiting, followed by several weeks of mild right upper quadrant pain and mild jaundice. There is usually a fever, but no lymphadenopathy. The disease is virtually always self-limited and thus without major acute or long-term complications. It may be asymptomatic.

 2. **Evaluation** includes making the clinical diagnosis and performing the tests listed in Box 2-10. The hepatitis A immunoglobulin M (IgM) serology will be positive (Table 2-14).

 3. The **management** of this self-limiting disorder is as listed in Box 2-10 and consists mainly of support and reporting the case to the Public Health Service. The patient should not be allowed to work in any occupation involving contact with foodstuffs until the hepatitis has resolved.

 4. **Prevention:** Before exposure, hepatitis A vaccine i.m. >2 weeks before travel to an area where disease is endemic; after exposure: 0.02 mL/kg of immunoglobulin i.m. once.

D. **Viral hepatitis B**
 1. The **specific manifestations** of viral hepatitis B, in addition to those described in the section on Acute Manifestations are based on the biology, pathogenesis, and natural history of the virus itself.

   The **organism** that causes this quite common form of hepatitis is a DNA virus that is transmitted in blood and body fluids. Specific risk factors include i.v. drug abuse, blood transfusions with contaminated blood, and promiscuous sexual habits, but never through insect bites or fecal–oral routes.

The **natural history** of this entity include an incubation period that is quite long and variable, lasting 6–20 weeks after exposure to the agent. The patient usually has a prodrome of nausea, vomiting, urticaria, and arthralgias that can last for 2–3 weeks, followed by significant icterus. The icterus can be quite severe and associated with pruritus and tender hepatomegaly. There is a 1%–2% acute mortality for this infection. This form of viral hepatitis, unlike hepatitis A, can have several severe and potentially mortal complications (see 4. Potential sequelae).

2. **Evaluation** includes making the clinical diagnosis as described in Box 2-10. The hepatitis B surface antigen serology assay will be positive (Table 2-14).

3. The **management** of this self-limited disorder is as listed in Box 2-9 and consists of supportive care, watching for any sequelae, and prophylaxis of contacts.

4. **Potential sequelae of viral hepatitis B and C**
   a. **Fulminant hepatitis.** This severe and usually fatal sequela can occur during the acute infection or as a "flare" in patients with chronic active hepatitis B infection. This complication occurs in <5% of cases but is quite dramatic when it does occur. The patient usually has tremendous increases in transaminases, encephalopathy, coagulopathy, and, most ominously, hypoglycemia. Mortality can be as high as 80%. The underlying pathogenesis of this massive necrosis of the liver is thought to be concurrent infection with hepatitis D (formerly known as the delta agent), an RNA virus that parasitizes the DNA hepatitis B virus (HBV). Whereas hepatitis B is the highest risk of developing fulminant hepatitis, any type can have a fulminant course.
   b. **Chronic active hepatitis.** This development occurs in 2% of all cases of hepatitis B. It can also occur in hepatitis C and other non-A, non-B hepatitides. The patient remains HBsAg-positive for an extended, indefinite period and has chronic significant elevations of the hepatic transaminases. A liver biopsy is required for definitive diagnosis and completely to differentiate this condition from chronic persistent hepatitis. The biopsy will demonstrate a diffuse mononuclear infiltrate that extends from the entire lobule and has associated bridging across the entire lobule and concurrent "piecemeal" necrosis of the hepatic tissue.

c. **Chronic persistent hepatitis.** This condition occurs in 5%−10% of all cases of hepatitis B. The patient remains HBsAg-positive for an extended, indefinite period but has no resultant elevations of transaminases. This condition has a better prognosis than chronic active hepatitis and should be differentiated from it. Because there is a significant amount of clinical overlap between these two sequelae, liver biopsy is indicated. Biopsy demonstrates a mononuclear infiltrate in the periportal area but not extending across the entire lobule, and virtually never with any necrosis. There is a long-term HbsAg and HbeAg positivity.

d. **Cirrhosis.** This is the result of any chronic, severe insult to the liver, irrespective of the cause. Although this diagnosis can usually be made clinically (see section on End-Stage Hepatic Dysfunction, page 97), it truly can be diagnosed only from liver biopsy results. In patients with chronic active hepatitis, the incidence of cirrhosis is 40%, whereas in chronic persistent hepatitis, it is much lower, ~5%−10%.

e. **Primary hepatocellular carcinoma.** This sequela may occur in association with any chronic or recurrent hepatic insult, but it most commonly occurs as a result of chronic infections with HBV.

f. **Immune-mediated processes,** including cryoglobulinemia and polyarteritis nodosum, are not uncommon.

g. **In hepatitis C, B-cell lymphoma.**

   The evaluation and management of these complications usually requires consultation with gastroenterology, preferably with a hepatologist. Often a liver biopsy is indicated, and empiric initiation of α-interferon can be considered (see section on End-Stage Hepatic Dysfunction, page 97, for a discussion of cirrhosis).

5. **Prevention**

   a. Infants and children <11 years, HbsAg-negative mother: 2.5 μg of recombivax HB i.m. or 10 μg of Engerix-B i.m.

   b. Infants and children <11 years, HbsAg-positive mother: 5 μg of recombivax HB i.m. or 10 μg of Engerix-B i.m.

   c. Children 11−19 years: 10 μg of recombivax HB i.m. or 20 μg of Engerix-B i.m.

   d. Adults: 10 μg of recombivax HB i.m. at months 0, 1, and 6, or 20 μg of Engerix-B i.m. at months 0, 1, and 6.

      • In immunosuppressed or dialysis patients, the

dose should be increased to 40 μg of either vaccine.
- Deltoid i.m. in children and adults.
- American Academy of Pediatrics recommends all infants be vaccinated for hepatitis B.
- Safe in pregnancy.
- 90%–95% effective.

Postexposure prophylaxis: HBIG, 0.06 mL/kg i.m. within 14 days of exposure to the hepatitis B patient.

Hepatitis vaccine should be administered prophylactically in the doses and regimens described to people who are not infected but who are at high risk for exposure, such as health care workers, close associates (family members) of i.v. drug abusers, noninfected i.v. drug abusers, and noninfected promiscuous people.

E. **Viral hepatitis C**
1. The **specific manifestations** of viral hepatitis C, in addition to those described in the section on acute manifestations are based on the biology, pathogenesis, and natural history of the virus itself.

   The **organism** that causes this form of hepatitis is an RNA virus that is transmitted in and by blood and body fluids. This had been the most common cause of transfusion-related hepatitis in the United States in the 1970s and 1980s and has decreased in incidence only over the past several years as the result of a somewhat effective screening test: IgG HCV antibodies. Specific **risk factors** for infection are as listed in viral hepatitis B.

   The **natural history** of this entity includes an incubation period of 2 weeks to 6 months after exposure. The patient has manifestations very similar to those of hepatitis B, see the preceding. There is virtually never any lymphadenopathy in hepatitis C, and the mortality of acute infections is 1%–2%. This form of viral hepatitis, like hepatitis B, can have several severe and potentially mortal sequalae. See section D for specifics.

2. The **specific evaluation** includes the fact that this is a diagnosis of exclusion, as there is no test to detect the hepatitis C antigen itself, although research continues on IgM HCV antibody and a direct measurement of HCV RNA. Past exposure to the virus can be demonstrated by the presence of IgG anti-HCV in the patient's plasma.

3. The **management** includes that listed in Box 2-10.

4. **Sequelae** are as listed in the previous discussion of hepatitis B. Several caveats germane to the discussion

of hepatitis C are appropriate here. Fulminant hepatitis with massive necrosis is decidely rare in hepatitis C, as opposed to hepatitis B; chronic sequelae are unfortunately not uncommon. Such sequelae of chronic hepatitis C have been treated with interferon alfa-2b, 3 million units thrice weekly.

5. **Prevention:** Only by primary risk-factor modification. There is no effective vaccine, nor is there any evidence that postexposure immunoglobulin prevents infection.

IV. Consultation

Problem	*Service*	*Time*
Any complication	GI	Urgent/emergent
Any viral hepatitis	Public Health	Required
Overdose in a suicide attempt	Psychiatry	Required

V. **Indications for admission:** Hypoglycemia, a coagulopathy, any suspicion of an ingestion or suicide attempt, or any evidence of intravascular volume depletion. The majority of patients can be treated as outpatients. Jaundice is not, in and of itself, an indication for admission.

Hernia

Hernias, colloquially referred to as "ruptures," are quite common. The vast majority are discovered and brought to the attention of the patient during a routine physical examination or are known by the patient, who has had it as a stable entity for years and has no specific complaints regarding it. The classic and most useful definition of a hernia is an abnormal protrusion through an abnormal anatomic defect, irrespective of the contents of the hernial sac. Hernias can be classified by severity and by location. Refer to Table 2-15.

Pyrosis and Gastroesophageal Reflux Disease

The esophagus, a long, relatively straight and narrow tube normally lined by stratified squamous epithelium, enters into the superior aspect of the stomach, a saclike structure normally lined by simple columnar epithelium. The transition between the mucosa of these two structures is marked by a discrete intraluminal mucosal line, the Z-line.

Both of these structures contribute differently to the overall goal of food digestion. The esophagus acts as a conduit for food and fluids to reach the stomach. It has a relatively neutral pH. The stomach has a major function in the direct digestion of food, and integral to this digestion is an acidic pH. In the normal state, the low-pH contents of the stomach rarely, if ever, enter the esophagus.

Certain physiologic mechanisms keep the low pH contents of

T A B L E 2-15
Hernias

Location	Pathogenesis	Manifestations	Treatment
Indirect inguinal hernia	*Congenital defect:* A defect in the internal ring such that the hernia sac passes through the internal ring alongside the spermatic cord through the external ring into the ipsilateral scrotum	Hernial sac in scrotum May also have hydrocele Males >>>> females Low risk of incarceration	Surgical referral
Direct hernia	*Acquired defect:* Through Hasselbach's triangle; increases with Valsalva (i.e., straining)	Hernial sac in scrotum Rare, if ever has a concurrent hydrocele Males >>>> females Low risk of incarceration	Surgical referral
Umbilical hernia	*Congenital:* Defect in the fascia deep to within umbilicus; usually closes by age 2 yr *Acquired:* Chronic increase in intraabdominal pressure, as the result of ascites, pregnancy, tumor in the abdomen; straining due to Valsalva or straining during urination	Hernial sac at umbilicus Examine for reason for straining (e.g., tumor, colon carcinoma, prostatic hypertrophy, occupation) Examine patient for ascites/signs of liver dysfunction High risk of incarceration	Surgical referral
Femoral hernia	Defect in the fascia deep to the inguinal ligament; sac passes through the femoral canal (i.e., medial to the femoral vein)	Hernial sac in medial thigh, medial to the femoral vein and deep to inguinal ligament Females >>>> males High risk of incarceration	Surgical referral
Incisional hernia	Defect in fascia at surgical site Increased risk in patients with poor wound healing (i.e., steroids/diabetes mellitus)	Hernial sac in a scar site	Surgical referral

Reducible, Sac easily put back through defect; *elective repair; Irreducible/incarcerated,* Sac cannot be put back through defect (i.e., "stuckout": urgent repair; *Strangulated,* Type of incarceration in which the hernia is ischemic: emergency repair.

the stomach from refluxing into the esophagus. The most important of these is the lower esophageal sphincter (LES), a collection of smooth muscle in the wall of the distal esophagus that constricts the luminal size of the distal esophagus in the immediate postprandial state. If the stomach contents do enter the esophagus, the mucosa of the esophagus will become damaged. The stratified squamous epithelium changes to a simple columnar epithelium in a process called metaplasia.

I. Pathophysiology

The underlying pathophysiology in the development of gastroesophageal reflux disease (GERD) and recurrent pyrosis may be an abnormal hypofunctioning of the LES sphincter or chronic increases in intraabdominal pressure.

A. Abnormal hypofunctioning of the LES

This occurs as the result of the use of nicotine, ethanol-based anticholinergic medications, estrogen agents, or chocolate ingestion. This is the most important factor in the development of GERD.

B. A chronic increase in intraabdominal pressure

This usually occurs as the result of a significant infradiaphragmatic process, such as ascites, abdominal masses, and pregnancy.

C. Hiatal hernia

It has long been postulated that a hiatal hernia (i.e., the abnormal slippage of the stomach through the diaphragm) plays a role in the pathogenesis of pyrosis. This is controversial, and presently a hiatal hernia is thought to play, at most, a minor role in its development.

II. Natural history and sequelae

The natural history of this disorder is one of chronic, recurrent symptomatic episodes that can lead to significant sequelae. Some of the most common sequelae are described subsequently.

A. Bronchospasm

A not infrequent but underrecognized complication of GERD is the development of reactive airway disease as a result of reflux and inhalation of gastric juices, especially when the patient is recumbent. The patient usually is seen with a cough or shortness of breath at night, and in the evaluation, no other cause is demonstrable. The pathogenesis of this sequela involves extrinsic bronchospasm. Pulmonary function tests are invariably quite normal. When the GERD is effectively managed, symptoms resolve completely.

B. Barrett's esophagus

This specific complication is usually quite asymptomatic. This process is one in which the chronic reflux of low-pH gastric fluids induces metaplasia of the distal esophageal mucosa from its normal stratified squamous epithelium

B O X 2-11

***Overall Evaluation and Management of Pyrosis
and Suspected GERD***

Evaluation

1. The history and physical examination are of paramount importance in this diagnosis. Salient features
   include:
   a. A burning sensation in the middle of the chest,
      which may mimic angina pectoris.
   b. Dyspnea at night, especially when the patient is ly-
      ing flat; probably a result of reflux-mediated bron-
      chospasm.
   c. Exacerbation of the pyrosis symptoms when the
      patient is lying flat and occasionally after inges-
      tion of spicy foods.
   d. Relief of symptoms with standing or use of ant-
      acids.
   e. Regurgitation of solid and liquid foodstuffs.
   f. Sour, acid taste in the mouth.
   g. Halitosis.
   h. "Water brash"—a significant, reflex increase in
      oral saliva usually precipitated by food or an epi-
      sode of pyrosis.
   i. It is quite rare to have significant odynophagia or
      dysphagia associated with GERD unless as a mani-
      festation of the underlying pathologic entity.
   j. Wheezes and evidence of bronchospasm during
      the attack.
2. Examine the patient for evidence of abdominal distention and, if present, for a fluid wave, tympany,
   and an enlarged uterus with heartbeats (a gravid
   uterus).
3. Perform radiographic imaging. An upper GI series
   can be of benefit in assessment, especially if real-
   time imaging under fluoroscopy demonstrates reflux.
   Other findings of note include any esophageal stricture, any associated PUD, and, potentially of import,
   a hiatal hernia.
4. If there is any suspicion of cardiac origin, perform a
   12-lead ECG.

(continued)

B O X 2-11 (continued)

Management

1. Educate the patient to dietary modifications (i.e., decrease fats in the diet, decrease weight if obese, and decrease ethanol and caffeine ingestion, either of which can decrease LES function).
2. Instruct the patient to keep the head of the bed >15° from horizontal (not just the pillow, but the entire bed head).
3. Discourage the oral intake of food or fluids within 1 hour of bedtime.
4. Prescribe use of antacids at bedtime (e.g., Mylanta II liquid, 15–30 mL p.o., q HS).
5. Prescribe H_2 blockers (e.g., cimetidine, 800 mg p.o., b.i.d., or ranitidine, 150 mg p.o., b.i.d., for 8 weeks).
6. If still symptomatic after 8 weeks of significant H_2 therapy, change to omeprazole, 20 mg p.o. q HS for 6–8 weeks; if still refractory, increase to 40 mg p.o. q HS, or lansoprazole, 15–30 mg p.o., q day.
7. If patient is receiving long-standing omeprazole, check for *H. pylori,* and treat with antibiotics if necessary.

to columnar cell epithelium, which is quite similar to gastric mucosa. This metaplasia has been indicated as a potential risk factor in the development of distal esophageal adenocarcinoma. Therefore, once Barrett's esophagus has been confirmed by EGD and biopsy, long-term follow-up is indicated.
C. **Erosive esophagitis** with a secondary stricture
D. **Dental erosions** and an increase in caries
The distal esophagus can become strictured as a result of the chronic recurrent inflammation and irritation of the mucosa and deeper tissues by GERD.

III. **Evaluation**
Evaluation of this disorder includes making the clinical diagnosis based on the features listed in Box 2-11. Often EGD is of clinical utility. Although EGD is not indicated in all cases, it should be performed in patients with symptoms that do not respond to 6 weeks of standard therapy, or if any abnormalities are demonstrated on an upper GI study, or if there are significant associated symptoms and signs (e.g., hematemesis or odynophagia), or if the process is recurrent. This direct

imaging technique allows the clinician to view the mucosa and to biopsy any affected areas. If there is any evidence of cough at night or of concurrent wheezing, pulmonary function tests should be performed. A final evaluative tool is the Bernstein test. A small-caliber NG tube is placed in the distal esophagus. Water and 0.1N HCl are instilled. If symptoms of pyrosis are reproduced with the acid instillation, the picture is consistent with GERD.

IV. **Management**

The **specific management,** in addition to that described in Box 2-11, includes the initiation of metoclopramide (Reglan), a dopamine agonist that aids in gastric emptying through the pylorus and increases LES pressure, resulting in a decrease in GERD symptoms. This medication should be reserved for patients for whom standard therapy has failed and thus usually who have undergone EGD to rule out other pathologic conditions.

V. **Consultation**

Problem	Service	Time
Recurrent GERD	GI	Elective
Chronic GERD (unresponsive)	GI	Elective
Associated symptoms	GI	Required
Abnormalities on upper GI series	GI	Required

VI. **Indications for admission:** None.

Bibliography

Abdominal Pain, General Approach

Adelman A: Abdominal pain in the primary care setting. J Fam Pract 1987;25:27–32.

Almy T, Howell DA: Diverticular disease of the colon. N Engl J Med 1980;302:324.

Brewer RJ, et al: Abdominal pain. Am J Surg 1976;131:219–223.

Dueholm S, et al: Laboratory aids in the diagnosis of acute appendicitis. Dis Colon Rectum 1989;32:855–859.

Edwards MW, et al: Audit of abdominal pain in general practice. J R Coll Gen Pract 1985;35:235–238.

Ernst CB: Abdominal aortic aneurysm. N Engl J Med 1993;328:1167–1172.

Roth J: Diagnosis and management of colonic diverticulitis. Contemp Gastroenterol 1988;1:7–16.

Staniland JR, et al: Clinical presentation of acute abdomen: study of 600 patients. Br Med J 1972;3:393–398.

Cholelithiasis

Glenn F: Acute acalculous cholecystitis. Ann Surg 1979;189:458–465.

Johnston DE, et al: Pathogenesis and treatment of gallstones. N Engl J Med 1993;328:412–421.

Marton KI, Doubilet P: How to image the gallbladder in suspected cholecystitis. Ann Intern Med 1988;109:722–729.

Welch CE, Malt RA: Surgery of the stomach, gallbladder, and bile ducts. N Engl J Med 1987;316:999–1008.

Wenckert A, Robertson B: The natural history of gallstone disease. Gastroenterology 1966;50:376–381.

Pancreatitis

Fan ST, et al: Early treatment of acute biliary pancreatitis by endoscopic papillotomy. N Engl J Med 1993;328:228–232.

Geokas MC, et al: Acute pancreatitis. Ann Intern Med 1985;103:86–100.

McPhee M: Treatment of acute pancreatitis. Hosp Pract 1985;1:83–90.

Ranson JHC, et al: Prognostic signs and the role of operative management in acute pancreatitis. Surg Gynecol Obstet 1974;139:69–80.

Steinberg W, et al: Acute pancreatitis. N Engl J Med 1994;330:1198–1210.

Willams KJ, et al: Pancreatic pseudocyst. Am Surg 1992;58:199–205.

Peptic Ulcer Disease

Agrawal NM, et al: Misoprostol compared with sucralfate in the prevention of nonsteroidal anti-inflammatory drug-induced gastric ulcer. Ann Intern Med 1991;115:195–200.

Cryer B, et al: Effects of NSAIDs on endogenous GI prostaglandins and therapeutic strategies for prevention and treatment of antiinflammatory drug-induced damage. Arch Intern Med 1992;152:1145–1155.

Feldman M, Burton ME: Histamine-2 receptor antagonists. N Engl J Med 1990;323:1749–1755.

Gough KR, et al: Ranitidine versus cimetidine in prevention of duodenal ulcer relapse. Lancet 1984;2:659–662.

Graham DY, et al: Duodenal and gastric ulcer prevention with misoprostol in arthritis patients taking NSAIDs. Ann Intern Med 1993;119:257–262.

Griffin MR, et al: Nonsteroidal anti-inflammatory drug use and increased risk for peptic ulcer disease in elderly persons. Ann Intern Med 1991;114:257–262.

Gugler R: Current diagnosis and selection of patients for treatment of peptic ulcer disease. Dig Dis Sci 1985;30:30–35.

Hentschel E, et al: Effect of ranitidine and amoxicillin plus metronidazole on the eradication of *Helicobacter pylori* and the recurrence of duodenal ulcer. N Engl J Med 1993;328:308–312.

Maton PN: Omeprazole. N Engl J Med 1991;324:965–975.

Ohning G, Soll A: Medical treatment of peptic ulcer disease. Am Fam Pract 1989;39:257–270.

Parsonnet J, et al: *Helicobacter pylori* infection and gastric lymphoma. N Engl J Med 1994;330:1267–1271.

Roth SH, Bennett RE: Nonsteroidal antiinflammatory drug gastropathy. Arch Intern Med 1987;147:2093–2100.

Schiller LR, Firdtran JS: Ulcer complications during short-term therapy of duodenal ulcer with active agents and placebo. Gastroenterology 1986;90:478–481.

Soll AH, et al: Nonsteroidal anti-inflammatory drugs and peptic ulcer disease. Ann Intern Med 1991;114:307–319.

Strum WB: Prevention of duodenal ulcer recurrence. Ann Intern Med 1986;105:757–761.

Taha AS, et al: Famotidine for the prevention of gastric and duodenal ulcers caused by nonsteroidal antiinflammatory drugs. N Engl J Med 1996;334:1435–1439.

Walsh JH, et al: The treatment of *Helicobacter pylori* infection in the managment of peptic ulcer disease. 1995;333:984–991.

Anorectal Disorders

Frisch M, et al: Benign anal lesions and the risk of anal cancer. N Engl J Med 1994;331:300–302.

Goldstein SD: Anal fissures and fistulas. Postgrad Med 1987;82:86–92.

Leff E: Hemorrhoids. Postgrad Med 1987;82:95–100.

Moore KT: The outpatient treatment of fissure-in-ano. Br J Clin Pract 1975;29:181–182.

Parks AG: Pathogenesis and treatment of fistula-in-ano. Br Med J 1961;1:463–469.

Smith LE, et al: Operative hemorrhoidectomy versus cryoreduction. Dis Colon Rectum 1979;22:10–16.

Thomson WH: The nature of hemorrhoids. Br J Surg 1975;62:542–552.

Dysphagia/Odynophagia

Bonacini M, et al: The causes of esophageal symptoms in human immunodeficiency virus infection. Arch Intern Med 1991;151:1567–1572.

Dabaghi R, Scott L: Evaluation of esophageal diseases. Am Fam Pract 1986;33:119–129.

Heit HA, et al: Palliative dilation for dysphagia in esophageal carcinoma. Ann Intern Med 1978;89:629–631.

Katz PO, et al: Esophageal testing of patients with noncardiac chest pain or dysphagia. Ann Intern Med 1987;106:593–597.

Ott DJ, et al: Radiological evaluation of dysphagia. JAMA 1986;256:2718–2721.

Pasricha P, et al: Botulinum toxin for achalasia. Gastroenterology 1996;110:1410–1415.

Diarrhea

Blacklow NR, Greenberg HB: Viral gastroenteritis. N Engl J Med 1991;325:252–264.

Cantey JR: Infectious diarrhea. Am J Med 1985;78:65–71.

Donowitz M, et al: Evaluation of patients with chronic diarrhea. N Engl J Med 1995;332:725–729.

DuPont HL: Nonfluid therapy and selected chemoprophylaxis of acute diarrhea. Am J Med 1985;78:81–90.

DuPont HL, et al: Prevention and treatment of traveler's diarrhea. N Engl J Med 1993;328:1821–1827.

DuPont HL, et al: Prevention of traveler's diarrhea by the tablet formulation of bismuth subsalicylate. JAMA 1987;257:1347–1350.

Fischer MC, Agger WA: Cryptosporidiosis. Am Fam Pract 1987;36:201–204.

George J, et al: The long term outcome of ulcerative colitis treated with 6-mercaptopurine. Am J Gastroenterol 1996;91:1711–1714.

Gerding DN, et al: *Clostridium difficile*-associated diarrhea and colitis in adults. Arch Intern Med 1986;146:95–100.

Gitnick G: Inflammatory bowel diseases: classification and cancer risk. Am Fam Pract 1989;39:216–220.

Goepp JG: Oral rehydration therapy. Am Fam Physician 1993;47:843–848.

Guerrant RL, Bobak DA: Bacterial and protozoal gastroenteritis. N Engl J Med 1991;325:327–340.

Juckett G: Intestinal protozoa. Am Fam Physician 1996;53:2507–2516.

Kelly CP, et al: *Clostridium difficle* colitis. N Engl J Med 1994;330:257–262.

Lichtiger S, et al: Cyclosporine in severe ulcerative colitis refractory to steroid therapy. N Engl J Med 1994;330:1841–1845.

Lynn RB, et al: Irritable bowel syndrome. N Engl J Med 1993;329:1940–1945.

Mekhjian HS, et al: Clinical features and natural history of Crohn's disease. Gastroenterology 1979;77:898–906.

Monson TP: Pediatric viral gastroenteritis. Am Fam Pract 1986;34:95–99.

Nelson JD: Etiology and epidemiology of diarrheal diseases in the United States. Am J Med 1985;78:76–80.

Peppercorn MA: Advances in drug therapy for inflammatory bowel disease. Ann Intern Med 1990;112:50–60.

Singleton JW, et al: A trial of sulfasalazine as adjunctive therapy in Crohn's disease. Gastroenterology 1979;77:887–897.

Steffen R, et al: Epidemiology of diarrhea in travelers. JAMA 1983;249:1176–1180.

Teasley DG, et al: Prospective randomized trial of metronidazole versus vancomycin for *Clostridium difficile*-associated diarrhea and colitis. Lancet 1983;2:1043–1046.

Vigneri S, et al: A comparison of five maintenance therapies for reflux esophagitis. N Engl J Med 1995;333:1106–1110.

End-Stage Liver Disease

Arroyo V, et al: Treatment of ascites in cirrhosis. Garoenterol Clin North Am 1992;21:237–256.

Basile AS, et al: The pathogenesis and treatment of hepatic encephalopathy. Pharm Rev 1991;27–57.

Bhuva M, et al: Spontaneous bacterial peritonitis: evaluation, management and prevention. Am J Med 1994;97:169–175.

Busuttil RW, et al: Liver transplantation today. Ann Intern Med 1986;104:377–389.

Christensen E, et al: Prognostic value of Child-Turcotte criteria in medically treated cirrhosis. Hepatology 1984;4:430–435.

Hoyumpa AM, et al: Hepatic encephalopathy. Gastroenterology 1979;76:184.

Laine L, et al: Endoscopic ligation compared with sclerotherapy for the treatment of bleeding esophageal varices. Ann Intern Med 1993;119:1–7.

Powell WJ, Klatskin G: Duration of survival in patients with Laënnec's cirrhosis. Am J Med 1968;44:406.

Rector WG: Drug therapy for portal hypertension. Ann Intern Med 1986;105:96–107.

Rossle M, et al: The TIPS procedure for variceal bleeding. N Engl J Med 1994;330:165–171.

Runyon BA: Care of patients with ascites. N Engl J Med 1994;330:337–342.

Runyon BA, et al: The serum-ascites albumin gradient is superior to exudate-transudate concept in the differential diagnosis of ascites. Ann Intern Med 1992;117:215–220.

Shear L, et al: Compartmentalization of ascites and edema in patients with hepatic cirrhosis. N Engl J Med 1970;282:1391.

Wong F, et al: TIPS in cirrhosis and refractory ascites. Ann Intern Med 1995;122:816–822.

Gastrointestinal Bleeding

Geelhoed GW: Gastrointestinal bleeding. Am Fam Pract 1984;29:115–125.

Graham DY, Schwartz JT: The spectrum of Mallory-Weiss tears. Medicine 1977;57:307–318.

Johnson RE, Velozzi CJ: Colonic angiodysplasia and blood loss. Am Fam Pract 1985;32:93–102.

Larson DE, Farnell MB: Upper gastrointestinal hemorrhage. Mayo Clin Proc 1983;58:371–387.

Pascal JP, et al: Propranolol in the prevention of first upper gastrointestinal tract hemorrhage in patients with cirrhosis of the liver and esophageal varices. N Engl J Med 1987;317:356–361.

Sauerbruch T, et al: Prophylactic sclerotherapy before the first episode of variceal hemorrhage in patients with cirrhosis. N Engl J Med 1988;319:8–15.

Sutton FM: Upper gastrointestinal bleeding in patients with esophageal varices. Am J Med 1987;83:273–275.

Wilcox CM, Truss CD: Gastrointestinal bleeding in patients receiving long-term anticoagulant therapy. Am J Med 1988;84:683–690.

Hepatitis

American Medical Association: Prevention, diagnosis, and management of viral hepatitis. Chicago: American Medical Association, 1995.

Centers for Disease Control: Update on hepatitis B prevention. Ann Intern Med 1987;107:353–357.

Chopra S, Griffin PH: Laboratory tests and diagnostic procedures in evaluation of liver disease. Am J Med 1985;79:221–230.

Corless JK, Middleton HM: Normal liver function. Arch Intern Med 1983;143:2291–2287.

Edwards CQ, et al: Screening for hemochromatosis. N Engl J Med 1993;328:1616–1620.

Farci P, et al: A long-term study of hepatitis C virus replication in non-A, non-B hepatitis. N Engl J Med 1991;325:98–104.

Kolts BE, Spindel E: Chronic active hepatitis. Am Fam Pract 1984;29:228–243.

Koretz RL: Chronic hepatitis. Am Fam Pract 1989;39:197–202.

Krugman S, et al: Viral hepatitis B: studies on natural history and prevention re-examined. N Engl J Med 1979;300:101.

Larsen LC, et al: Management of acetaminophen toxicity. Am Fam Pract 1996;53:185–190.

Little DR: Hemochromatosis: diagnosis and management. Am Fam Pract 1996;53:2623–2628.

McKenna JP, et al: Abnormal liver function tests in asymptomatic patients. Am Fam Pract 1989;39:117–126.

Maddrey WC: Hepatic effects of acetaminophen. J Clin Gastroenterol 1987;9:180–185.

Murray BJ: The hepatitis B carrier state. Am Fam Pract 1986;33:127–233.

Osmon DR, et al: Viral hepatitis. Arch Intern Med 1987;147:1235–1240.

Poynard T, et al: Meta-analysis of interferon randomized trials in the treatment of viral hepatitis C: effects of dose and duration. Hepatology 1996;24:778–789.

Ramond MJ, et al: A randomized trial of prednisolone in patients with severe alcoholic hepatitis. N Engl J Med 1992;326:507–512.

Rumack BH, Matthew H: Acetaminophen poisoning and toxicity. Pediatrics 1975;55:871–876.

Zarro VJ: Acetaminophen overdose. Am Fam Pract 1987;35:235–237.

Hernias

Dunphy JE, Botsford TW: Physical examination of the surgical patient. In: An introduction to clinical surgery, 4th ed. Philadelphia: WB Saunders, 1975:117.

Pyrosis/GERD

Adelman AM: Management of dyspepsia. Am Fam Pract 1987;35:222–230.

Barish CF, et al: Respiratory complications of gastroesophageal reflux. Arch Intern Med 1988;145:1882–1888.

Bozymski EM, et al: Barrett's esophagus. Ann Intern Med 1982;97:103–107.

Kitchin LI, Castell DO: Rationale and efficacy of conservative therapy for gastroesophageal reflux disease. Arch Intern Med 1991;151:448–454.

Klinkenberg-Knol EC, et al: Long term treatment with omeprazole for refractory reflux esophagitis. Ann Intern Med 1994;121:161–167.

Kuipers C, et al: Atrophic gastritis and *Helicobacter pylori* infection in patients with reflux esophagitis treated with omeprazole or fundoplication. N Engl J Med 1996;334:1018–1022

Lieberman DA: Medical therapy for chronic reflux esophagitis. Arch Intern Med 1987;147:1717–1720.

Lieberman DA, Keeffe EB: Treatment of severe reflux esophagitis with cimetidine and metoclopramide. Ann Intern Med 1986;104:21–26.

Pope CE: Acid-reflux disorders. N Engl J Med 1994;331:655–660.

Robinson M, et al: Effective maintenance treatment of reflux esophagitis with low dose lansoprazole. Ann Intern Med 1996;124:859-866.

Simpson WG: Gastresophageal reflux disease and asthma. Arch Intern Med 1995;155:798–803.

—D.D.B.

Chapter 3

Renal Disorders and Hypertension

Hematuria

The filtering efficiency of the kidneys is tremendous. The entire volume of blood is continuously and effectively filtered in the glomeruli. The effectiveness of the filter is matched only by its specificity. This is clearly demonstrated by the fact that only negligible amounts of albumin, plasma proteins, and cellular elements are lost in the urine. The specificity, however, is not 100%, even in the normal setting. It has been demonstrated that in the normal setting, <1,000 red blood cells (RBCs) are lost in the urine per minute, an essentially negligible loss. This loss is below the level of clinical detection by either the dipstick method or microscopic analysis.

Therefore, any blood loss greater than ~1,000 RBCs/min is, by definition, the pathologic problem hematuria. There are two categories of clinical hematuria, microscopic and gross.

1. **Microscopic hematuria.** This is an abnormal loss of RBCs in the urine that remains undetectable by visual examination of the urine. The loss of RBCs is >1,000 RBCs/min. The problem is detected by the dipstick analysis or by microscopic evaluation of the urine sample. The hematuria is unknown to the patient.
2. **Gross hematuria.** Red- or brown-colored urine, usually of acute onset. It may be the chief presenting complaint. Usually gross or macroscopic hematuria is >1,000,000 RBCs lost per minute.

Other conditions can cause significant brown or red discoloration to the urine. These conditions include bilirubinuria, myoglobinuria, and medication-induced discoloration, particularly that induced by rifampin. The dipstick test and microscopic urinalysis will differentiate these conditions from gross hematuria.

I. Differential diagnosis

The differential diagnosis of red- or brown-colored urine includes the following entities. The most common causes, especially of painful hematuria, are infections of the urinary tract and nephrolithiasis.

A. Coagulopathy

1. The **specific manifestations** include microscopic and/or macroscopic hematuria with the acute to sub-acute onset of nonpalpable purpura, multiple pete-chiae, gastrointestinal (GI) bleeding, easy bruising, menorrhagia, or recurrent epistaxis. Usually no urinary tract symptoms are present.

2. The **underlying pathogenesis** is a defect of coagulation. Thrombocytopenia, elevations in PT or PTT, and any consumptive or hypoproductive coagulopathy can manifest with microscopic or macroscopic hematuria. Usually the hematuria is a small component of the overall constellation of presenting signs and symptoms.

3. The **specific evaluation and management** of hematuria due to a coagulopathy include making the clinical diagnosis by using the evaluative tools described in Box 3-1 and managing the underlying coagulopathy. Expedient referral to hematology may be indicated. (See the section on excessive bleeding states in Chapter 5, page 268)

   Note: A coagulopathy will unmask any concurrent primary urinary tract lesion and therefore should not be accepted as the cause of hematuria until a complete evaluation has been performed.

B. Urinary tract infection (UTI), bacterial (See section on Pyuria Syndromes, page 172)

C. UTI, mycobacterial

1. **Manifestations**
   The patient is invariably asymptomatic, and thus, this is a true form of painless hematuria. Query the patient for any exposure to mycobacterial disease, any risk factors for development, and, if the patient has had a mycobacterial disease, what therapy was administered.

2. The **underlying pathogenesis** of this fairly rare cause of hematuria is of an infection of the kidney by *Myco-bacterium hominis.* Usually the infection is hema-togenously spread from another site, usually pulmonary.

3. The **specific evaluation and management** of hematuria due to a mycobacterial UTI include making the clinical diagnosis by using the evaluative tools de-

B O X 3-1

Overall Evaluation of Hematuria, Microscopic and Gross

Evaluation

1. Take a thorough history and perform a physical examination, including a prostate examination in males, looking for tenderness or enlargement, and a pelvic examination in females, looking for menstrual flow or cervical tenderness.
2. Obtain a urine specimen for urinalysis by dipstick and microscopic analysis. This test is mandatory.
3. If an infectious origin is suspected, as evidenced by prostate tenderness, pyuria concurrent with hematuria, or a positive nitrite or positive leukocyte esterase (LE) assay, send urine for culture and sensitivity testing and treat the patient with antibiotics. (See discussion in the text and in the section on Pyuria Syndromes, page 171.)
4. If nephritic sediment is present (i.e., hematuria, RBC casts, proteinuria, and fat oval bodies), the following laboratory tests are indicated to evaluate the patient for an underlying vasculitis, glomerulonephritis (GNP).
   a. Antinuclear antibody (ANA) assay.
   b. Anti-dsDNA assay.
   c. Antistreptolysin O (ASO) titer.
   d. CH_{50} of serum.
   e. C_3 and C_4 levels in serum.
5. If no specific cause of the problem is evident from these tests or if the problem is recurrent, perform the following studies:
   a. Urine culture and sensitivity tests.
   b. Urine myoglobin test. Myoglobin, a breakdown product of muscle, may produce a dark discoloration of urine.
   c. Complete blood cell (CBC) count with differential, looking for any concurrent anemia.
   d. Platelet count, prothrombin time (PT), and activated partial thromboplastin time (aPTT), looking for evidence of a concurrent or antecedent coagulopathy.
   e. Chest radiography, posteroanterior (PA) and lateral views, looking for any granulomatous disease suggestive of mycobacterial disease or Wegener's granulomatosis.

(continued)

B O X 3-1 (continued)

f. Purified protein derivative (PPD) test with controls applied to the skin, looking for exposure to mycobacterial disease (see Table 4-15).

g. Urine cytology. To optimize the sensitivity of this test, use the first urine sample of the morning.

h. Acid-fast bacilli (AFB) smear and culture of urine. To optimize the sensitivity of these tests, use the first urine sample of the morning.

i. Serum electrolytes, blood urea nitrogen (BUN), and creatinine, for baseline purposes.

j. Ultrasound (US) of the kidneys to demonstrate any renal parenchymal lesions, nephrolithiasis, or obstruction.

k. Computed tomography (CT) scan of the kidneys if any abnormality is present on the renal US study.

l. Referral to genitourinary (GU) surgeons for cystoscopy (i.e., the direct imaging) and, if needed, biopsy of the mucosa of the urinary tract.

scribed in Box 3-1 and treating the underlying infection. Obtain a morning urine specimen for AFB smear and culture. Perform PPD skin tests, unless the skin PPD was reactive in the past. Referral to GU and infectious disease experts is indicated. (See section on Mycobacterial Diseases in Chapter 4 for further details.)

D. Trauma

1. **Manifestations**

   Except for manifestations attributable to trauma to the back or flank, there are few associated manifestations. Trauma may cause painless hematuria.

2. The **underlying pathogenesis** is significant trauma to the kidneys or urinary bladder with resultant damage to these structures. The most dramatic event is trauma-induced rupture of the kidney.

3. The **specific evaluation and management** of hematuria due to trauma include making the clinical diagnosis by using the evaluative tools described in Box 3-1 and immediate referral to GU.

E. Transitional cell carcinoma of the bladder

1. **Manifestations**

   Transitional cell carcinoma of the bladder is invariably asymptomatic in its early, curable stage. This results in painless microscopic hematuria.

2. The **underlying pathogenesis** is a primary malignant neoplasm in the mucosa of the urinary bladder.
3. The **specific evaluation and management** of hematuria due to transitional cell carcinoma of the bladder include making the clinical diagnosis by using the evaluative tools described in Box 3-1 and immediate referral to GU. A morning urine specimen for cytology, looking for malignant cells shed in the urine, should be obtained at the outset. The first morning specimen has remained in the bladder overnight, which increases the sensitivity of the examination.

F. **Adenocarcinoma (clear cell carcinoma) of the kidney**
   1. **Manifestations**
      Adenocarcinoma of the kidney is invariably asymptomatic in its early, curable stage. This results in painless microscopic hematuria.
   2. **Pathogenesis**
      The **underlying pathogenesis** is a primary malignant neoplasm in the renal parenchyma.
   3. The **specific evaluation and management** of hematuria due to adenocarcinoma of the kidney include making the clinical diagnosis by using the evaluative tools described in Box 3-1 and immediate referral to GU. A morning urine specimen for cytology, looking for malignant cells shed in the urine, should be obtained at the outset.

G. **Berger's disease**
   1. **Manifestations**
      The **specific manifestations** of this not uncommon cause of microscopic painless hematuria in adults are few. In fact, it is invariably asymptomatic.
   2. **Pathogenesis**
      The **underlying pathogenesis** is an immunoglobulin A (IgA) nephropathy, which is quite benign and rarely progresses to any renal dysfunction.
   3. The **specific evaluation and management** of hematuria due to Berger's disease include making the clinical diagnosis by using the evaluative tools described in Box 3-1 and serum protein electrophoresis. The IgA titer will be elevated in Henoch–Schönlein purpura and Berger's disease, but Berger's disease will not have any of the extrarenal manifestations of Henoch–Schönlein purpura. Referral to nephrology is encouraged, but once the diagnosis is confirmed, reassurance and observation are the interventions required.

H. **Henoch–Schönlein syndrome**
   1. The **specific manifestations** include the development of nonpalpable purpura on the lower extremi-

ties with no evidence of concurrent or antecedent coagulopathy; arthralgias; painless microscopic or gross hematuria; and an increased risk of intussusception of the distal small bowel (ileum). The incidence is highest in children and young adults.

2. The **underlying pathogenesis** of this systemic disease is not completely known but probably is autoimmune in nature. **Natural history:** The disease is usually self-limited.

3. The **specific evaluation and management** of hematuria due to Henoch–Schönlein syndrome include making the clinical diagnosis by using the evaluative tools described in Box 3-1 and serum protein electrophoresis. The IgA titer will be elevated in Henoch–Schönlein purpura and Berger's disease, but Berger's disease will not have any of the extrarenal manifestations of Henoch–Schönlein purpura. **Referral** to nephrology, initiation of salicylates (aspirin, 325 g q.6hr), and observing for sequelae are indicated.

I. **Medications**

1. The **specific manifestations** can include massive hematuria with a decrease in hematocrit and the potential for hemodynamic instability. Although many different medications can cause a discoloration to the urine, few will result in true hematuria.

2. The **underlying pathogenesis** is direct irritation of the bladder mucosa by an agent or its catabolites. The medication most commonly described as causing microscopic or macroscopic hematuria is the chemotherapeutic and alkylating agent cyclophosphamide (Cytoxan).

3. The **evaluation and management** of medication-induced hematuria include making the clinical diagnosis by using the evaluative tools described in Box 3-1 and referral to nephrology. The best treatment method is prevention. **Specific modalities of prevention** of the cyclophosphamide-induced hemorrhagic cystis include maintaining a urine output of >100 mL/hr and the concurrent administration of the agent MESNA. MESNA is an agent that binds to and inactivates the active catabolites of cyclophosphamide in the urine, thereby preventing urinary bladder mucosal damage.

J. **Nephrolithiasis**
Nephrolithiasis causes painful hematuria and is discussed later in this chapter (page 158).

K. **Other glomerulonephritides;** see page 188 for systemic lupus erythematosus (SLE), Table 3-7, page 169 for lupus nephritis and page 188 for Wegener's.

II. **Consultation**

Problem	Service	Time
Nephritic sediment	Renal	Urgent
Acute renal failure	Renal	Emergent
Nephrolithiasis	Renal	Elective
Recurrent prostatitis	GU	Elective
Unexplained hematuria	GU	Required
Any positive cytology	GU	Required

III. **Indications for admission:** Massive hematuria, evidence of pyelonephritis, concurrent acute renal failure (ARF), or evidence of obstruction.

Hypertension

Hypertension is a disease process of significant import for health care in the United States and the industrial nations of the world. It is quite prevalent in the United States and is also virtually asymptomatic until it manifests with morbid, even mortal sequelae. Because it is prevalent and asymptomatic early in its course, because the sequelae of untreated hypertension are significant, and because early and chronic treatment has been demonstrated to prevent the morbid and mortal sequelae, hypertension is a disease for which screening is beneficial. Fortunately, effective screening techniques are available. The best is a blood pressure check at the physician's office or at a clinic or a health fair every 6 months.

I. **Overall manifestations**

The **overall manifestations** of hypertension are few early in the course of the disease. The patient may be seen by a primary care physician after having an elevated blood pressure reading at a screening location or in the physician's office. Table 3-1 lists diagnostic criteria published by the Joint National Commission on the Detection, Evaluation, and Treatment of High Blood Pressure. Unless the patient has a hypertensive urgency or emergency, the blood pressure must be measured at three different times over a period of 1–2 weeks to confirm the diagnosis.

II. **Pathogenesis**

The **underlying pathogenesis** is a chronic increase in systolic and diastolic arterial blood pressure. The arterial tree can be thought of as a plumbing system in which the heart is the pump, the blood is the water, and the arteries are the pipes. Blood pressure is the product of the cardiac output (i.e., the pump function) and the total peripheral resistance of the arterial bed (i.e., the overall decrease in caliber of the pipes). Therefore, blood pressure can be increased by an increase in cardiac output or by an increase in arterial resistance to flow. There is a high correlation between essential hypertension and mutations in the angiotensinogen gene on

T A B L E 3-1
Categories of Hypertension

Diastolic Pressure

<85 mm Hg	Normal
85–89 mm Hg	High normal
90–104 mm Hg	Mild hypertension
105–114 mm Hg	Moderate hypertension
>115 mm Hg	Severe hypertension

Systolic Pressure (when the diastolic pressure is <90 mm Hg)

<140 mm Hg	Normal
140–160 mm Hg	Isolated borderline systolic hypertension
>160 mm Hg	Isolated systolic hypertension

(Modified from the Joint National Committee on the Detection, Evaluation, and Treatment of High Blood Pressure. 1988 Report. Arch Intern Med 1988; 148:1023.)

chromosome 1q. Two different categories of mechanisms are known in the pathogenesis of hypertension, primary and secondary.

A. **Primary or essential arterial hypertension** is the result of either an increase in cardiac output or an increase in the total peripheral resistance. The exact mechanism is unknown. The vast majority of patients with hypertension have primary hypertension.

B. **Secondary arterial hypertension** occurs as a result of a known, definable, and potentially curable underlying cause. A mechanism of secondary hypertension can be demonstrated in a small but significant minority of patients, ~10%–15%. Secondary causes include disorders of the endocrine, renal, and vascular systems. Table 3-2 lists specific causes of secondary hypertension.

   1. The **endocrine lesions** that can result in hypertension include hypercortisolism, hyperaldosteronism, pheochromocytoma, and hypothyroidism.

      a. **Hypercortisolism,** either iatrogenic or as the result of adrenal hyperplasia or adrenal hyperfunction with increased levels of glucocorticoids, results in hypertension with concurrent hypokalemia. Other **specific manifestations** of this cause of secondary hypertension include truncal obesity, hyperglycemia, and an increased incidence of cutaneous fungal infections.

      b. **Hyperaldosteronism,** or Conn's disease, is hyperplasia or adenoma of the zona glomerulosa of the adrenal gland with increased levels of mineralo-

T A B L E 3-2
Some Causes of Secondary Hypertension

1. Hypercortisolism
   a. Cushing's disease
   b. Cushing's syndrome
   c. Iatrogenic
2. Primary hyperaldosteronism (Conn's syndrome)
3. Renal arterial stenosis
4. Pheochromocytoma
5. Coarctation of the aorta
6. Hypothyroidism
7. Renal failure
8. Mutation on angiotensinogen gene (chromosome 1q)

corticoids. This results in hypertension with concurrent hypokalemia.
  c. **Pheochromocytoma** is the hyperplasia or adenoma of the adrenal medulla or of a sympathetic
  ganglion with increased levels of the catecholamines, either epinephrine or norepinephrine.
  Other **specific manifestations** include supraventricular or ventricular tachycardia, hypertension,
  paradoxic orthostatic hypotension, and hypokalemia.
  d. **Hypothyroidism** is the decrease in thyroid hormone with resultant manifestations of thyroid
  hormone deficiency: cold, decreased energy, constipation, and hypertension (see section on thyroid dysfunctional states in Chapter 9, page 497).
2. The **renal lesions** that may result in hypertension
include any significant renal failure or renal arterial stenosis.
  a. **Renal failure** results in hypertension via multiple
  mechanisms, including chronic volume overload
  and the potential development of secondary hyperaldosteronism. Other specific manifestations
  include those described in the section on Renal
  Dysfunction, page 179.
  b. **Renal arterial stenosis** occurs as a result of either
  atherosclerosis or fibromuscular hyperplasia. In
  arterial stenosis, a decrease in perfusion of the
  kidneys results in an increase in aldosterone and
  renin, with resultant hypertension and hypokalemia. Specific manifestations include an abdominal bruit.
3. The **vascular cause** of hypertension is **coarctation
of the aorta.** This is a rare entity that manifests with
unilateral upper extremity hypertension with concurrent relative hypotension in other extremities.

III. **Natural history**

If untreated, hypertension will result in damage to any and potentially all areas of the arterial system. To continue the analogy with a closed plumbing system, the chronic elevation of fluid pressure (i.e., arterial pressure elevation) damages not only the pipes (the arteries) and the pump (the heart) but also any filter system (the kidneys). These sequelae, which usually occur only after a long history of uncontrolled hypertension and also referred to as "**target organ**" damage, include the following:

A. **Cardiac dysfunction.** There is abnormal hypertrophy of the left ventricle in patients with long-standing uncontrolled hypertension. The hypertrophy causes a problem with filling of the ventricle and thus causes diastolic heart failure. Over time, the ventricle evolves from hypertrophy to dilation and frank systolic heart failure.

B. **Renal failure,** invariably antedated by proteinuria.

C. **Cerebrovascular accidents** as a result of hemorrhage in the intracranial space or thrombotic infarctions.

D. **Damage to the thoracic and abdominal aorta,** with resultant dissection or aneurysm formation.

E. **Acceleration of atherosclerotic disease.** This acceleration of atherosclerotic disease is of tremendous import: along with cigarette smoking, diabetes mellitus, obesity, and hypercholesterolemia, it is a major risk factor in the development of atherosclerotic heart disease and cerebrovascular atherosclerotic disease.

IV. **Manifestations of late hypertension**

The **specific manifestations** of late, uncontrolled hypertension reflect the natural history of the disease and the known areas of target-organ damage.

A. **Cardiac manifestations** include cardiomegaly, a fourth heart sound, and, if heart failure is present, orthopnea, paroxysmal nocturnal dyspnea, bipedal edema, dyspnea on exertion, a third heart sound, and crackles in the lung fields. Furthermore, the entity can manifest with the findings of ischemic heart disease, either angina pectoris or an acute coronary syndrome such as a myocardial infarction (see section on Chest Pain in Chapter 1, page 3).

B. **Renal manifestations** include pedal edema, anasarca, and an exacerbation of symptoms of heart failure (see section on Renal Dysfunction, page 179).

C. Other manifestations include a cerebrovascular accident; a palpable, pulsatile abdominal mass, indicative of an abdominal aortic aneurysm; and retinopathy on funduscopy.

V. **Management**

The **overall management** of hypertension entails documenting its presence, documenting any sequelae, and screening for and evaluating any secondary cause (see Boxes 3-2 and

B O X 3-2

Overall Evaluation of Newly Diagnosed Hypertension

1. Make certain that the episode is not a hypertensive emergency or urgency (see page 150).
2. Take a thorough history and perform a physical examination, looking for a history of diabetes mellitus, the age of first elevated blood pressure, any concurrent medication use, the quantity of ethanol ingested, and any symptoms referable to target-organ damage. The physical examination includes determining the blood pressure in both arms to look for coarctation of the aorta; a cardiac examination for PMI displacement and a third or fourth heart sound; an extremity examination for edema; an abdominal examination for pulsatile or nonpulsatile masses or bruits; and a funduscopic examination to look for any microvascular disease. Funduscopy is mandatory.
3. Determine electrolyte, BUN, and creatinine levels for baseline purposes and to look for any concurrent hypokalemia, hyperglycemia, or renal dysfunction.
4. Perform urinalysis with microscopic examination to look for proteinuria or a nephritic sediment.
5. Determine calcium, phosphorus, and albumin levels as part of baseline evaluation.
6. Obtain a 12-lead ECG for baseline purposes and to look for any evidence of left ventricular hypertrophy.
7. Obtain chest radiographs in PA and lateral views to look for any left ventricular hypertrophy.
8. If there is any evidence of heart failure or of left ventricular (LV) hypertrophy on the ECG, obtain an echocardiogram to determine the size and wall-motion activity of the left ventricle.
9. If there is any evidence of a pulsatile mass in the abdomen, image the abdomen with CT or US to define the probable abdominal aortic aneurysm.
10. Evaluation for secondary hypertension should be performed only in patients who are at risk or who have specific markers that make a secondary origin more likely (see Box 3-3 for the evaluation of secondary hypertension). Patients in whom an evalua-

(continued)

B O X 3-2 *(continued)*

> tion for secondary hypertension should be performed include:
> a. Those with concurrent hypokalemia or hypomagnesemia.
> b. Those with a renal bruit.
> c. Those with an onset at age <25 years or >65 years.
> d. Those with orthostatic manifestations or concurrent tachydysrrhythmias.
> e. Those with disease difficult to control.

3-3; see Table 3-2). The **specific management** includes the following basic concepts:

A. Use nonpharmacologic management as first-line therapy for mild to moderate hypertension. This includes limiting salt intake, weight reduction if the patient is obese, and prescription of an exercise program.

B. If and when pharmacologic intervention is required, use agents that optimize compliance, such as those with minimal side effects; that can be taken in a once daily regimen; and that are effective as monotherapy.

C. Modify other risk factors for the development of atherosclerotic heart disease to minimize the risk-factor profile. This is even more important because some of the antihypertensive agents (listed in Table 3-3), while decreasing blood pressure, may worsen the risk factor of hypercholesterolemia by increasing low-density lipoprotein (LDL) or decreasing high-density lipoprotein (HDL) cholesterol levels.

B O X 3-3

Evaluation and Management of Suspected Secondary Hypertension

1. If **Cushing's syndrome or disease** is suspected:
   Tests:
   a. Perform a **24-hour urine collection for free cortisol** and creatinine. Normal free cortisol is <100 μg/day. If elevated, consistent with hypercortisolism.

(continued)

B O X 3-3 *(continued)*

    b. Obtain plasma adrenocorticotropic hormone **(ACTH) level**. If the ACTH is >20 pg/dL, consistent with ACTH-dependent Cushing's disease. If the ACTH is <20 pg/dL, consistent with ACTH-independent Cushing's syndrome.

    c. **Low-dose** overnight suppression test: At 2300, administer 1 mg dexamethasone p.o., and then measure the plasma cortisol at 0600 on the next day. If the plasma cortisol is <5 μg/dL, normal; if the plasma cortisol is >5 μg/dL, positive screen for hypercortisolism (many false positives).

    d. If hypercortisol and increased ACTH, perform CT scan of sella to look for tumor; refer to endocrinology.

    e. If hypercortisol and decreased ACTH, perform CT scan of adrenals; refer to endocrinology.
     Therapy: Refer to Endocrine; if syndrome, ketoconazole is the agent of choice medically to decrease the production of cortisol. Referral to surgery for resection of adrenal gland (syndrome) or pituitary adenoma (disease) is indicated.

2. If **renal arterial stenosis** is suspected:
   Tests:

    a. **Captopril test:** Patient with normal salt intake and off of all agents and diuretics, measure baseline plasma renin activity (PRA) and administer 25–50 mg p.o. captopril. Repeat the PRA 60 minutes later. Monitor the blood pressure over the course of the test period. If there is a marked decrease in blood pressure, consistent with renovascular hypertension; If the PRA increases by >150% of baseline, consistent with renovascular hypertension.

    b. **Renogram:** The diseased kidney will take up, accumulate, and excrete the [131I]iodohippurate agent more slowly than the normal kidney, consistent with renovascular hypertension. Sensitivity, 77%; specificity, 75%.

    c. **Digital subtraction angiography:** Sensitivity, 88%; specificity, 90%
   Therapy:

    a. Angiotensin-converting enzyme (ACE) inhibitors may be of benefit if used judiciously and if the K and creatinine are followed, i.e., closely on a q.2–4-week basis initially, as the patient may develop renal failure with or without hyperkalemia;

(continued)

surgery or angioplasty may be of benefit in delaying the progression to renal failure.

3. If **pheochromocytoma** is suspected:
   Tests:
   a. Perform a **24-hour urine collection for catecholamines**: If elevated, consistent with a pheochromocytoma. Sensitivity, 75%; specificity, 95%.
   b. Perform a 24-hour urine collection for **vanillylmandelic acid**: If >11 mg/24 hours, consistent with a pheochromocytoma. Sensitivity, 42%; specificity, 100%.
   c. Perform a 24-hour urine collection for **metanephrines**: If >1.8 mg/24 hours, consistent with a pheochromocytoma. Sensitivity, 79%; specificity, 93%.
   d. Perform **plasma catecholamines** (norepinephrine and epinephrine): If >950 pg/mL, consistent with pheochromocytoma. Sensitivity, 94%; specificity, 97%.
   e. **Clonidine suppression test:** Background: Clonidine will suppress catecholamines in normal patients as the result of central alpha blockade. Steps: Administer 0.3 mg clonidine p.o., repeat plasma catecholamines 3 hours later. If <500 pg/ml, normal; if >500 pg/ml, consistent with pheochromocytoma.
   Therapy:
   Labetolol is the drug of choice; localization with an MIBG scan and referral to surgery for resection are indicated.

4. If **Conn's syndrome** (i.e., primary hyperaldosteronism) is suspected:
   Tests:
   a. Determine **plasma aldosterone (ng/dL)/ plasma renin activity** (i.e., PRA (ng/ml/hr): If the ratio is >25: consistent with Conn's syndrome; if the ration is <25, consistent with normal or secondary causes.
   b. **Perform a captopril suppression test:** Administer 25 mg of captopril p.o., then perform the aldosterone/PRA ratio. If, from baseline, there is a decrease in aldosterone and an increase in PRA: normal; if there is no change (i.e., the aldosterone remains >15 ng/dL; or if the ratio remains high, very suggestive of Conn's syndrome.
   Therapy:
   a. Spironolactone and calcium channel blocker; localization with a ^{131}I-19-iodocholesterol (NP-59) scan is indicated and, if an adenoma, surgical intervention may be indicated.

D. If other disease processes are present, attempt to use agents that will treat that disease and the hypertension concurrently. Examples include:

1. Hypertension with **concurrent angina pectoris.** Treatment can include nitrates and/or β-blockers (if not contraindicated) and/or calcium channel blockers.

2. Hypertension with **concurrent LV failure.** An ACE inhibitor is strongly indicated to decrease afterload.

3. Hypertension with **concurrent diabetes mellitus.** An ACE inhibitor is strongly indicated, as recent data indicate that an ACE inhibitor may slow or even prevent the development of nephropathy in hypertensive diabetics.

4. The agents that fit the best profile today (i.e., have minimal side effects, have a long duration of action resulting in once daily dosing, and provide effective control of hypertension without exacerbating other risk factors for atherosclerotic disease) are calcium channel blockers or ACE inhibitors. An agent from either one of these categories should be initiated and titrated to establish a normal arterial blood pressure or to maximal dosage. If maximal dosage is reached without effective arterial pressure control, another agent can be added and increased, again titrated to the normal blood pressure range. Table 3-3 lists commonly used antihypertensive agents.

VI. **Hypertensive emergencies**

A hypertensive emergency is defined as an acute syndrome directly attributable to the hypertension that will, if the hypertension is not emergently treated, result in severe morbidity or mortality. The patient is hypertensive, usually but not always has a diastolic blood pressure >120 mm Hg, and has one or more of the syndromes listed under A.

A. **Specific syndromes** precipitated by hypertension, thus defining a hypertensive emergency, include:

1. Left ventricular heart failure.
2. Cerebrovascular accident.
3. Dissecting thoracic aortic aneurysm.
4. Eclampsia.
5. Acute renal failure.
6. Papilledema on funduscopic examination.
7. Hypertensive encephalopathy.

B. The **specific evaluation and management** of hypertensive emergencies include making the clinical diagnosis, performing the ACLS protocol as indicated, performing the overall evaluation as described in Box 3-2, and initiating emergent, therapeutic intervention. The agent of choice is sodium nitroprusside (see Table 3-4 for dosing). Place an arterial line, and strive for a blood pressure of 180–200/95–105 mm Hg in the first 4–6 hours. Then

slowly decrease the elevated blood pressure to normal
in 24–36 hours.

1. Once the patient has stabilized, add an oral agent
   that will be used on a long-term outpatient basis and
   gradually withdraw the nitroprusside. These steps
   are performed in the hospital, invariably in the ICU,
   and are included here for the reader's edification.
2. Eclampsia is managed differently, with admission,
   emergent referral to obstetrics, and the initiation of
   magnesium and/or hydralazine.

VII. Hypertensive urgencies

In hypertensive urgencies, the diastolic blood pressure is
significantly elevated, but no acute syndromes or findings
are directly attributable to or precipitated by the elevated
blood pressure. Thus an urgency is more an asymptomatic
severe hypertension (i.e., a numerical diagnosis). An urgency
is one in which the diastolic blood pressure is >115 mm Hg.

A. The **specific evaluation and management** of hypertensive urgencies include making the clinical diagnosis, performing the overall evaluation as described in Box 3-2,
   and making certain that there are no findings that would
   make the blood pressure elevation a hypertensive emergency.

   1. The short-term goal is to decrease the blood pressure
      to 180–190/95–105 mm Hg in the first several hours.
      Then give the patient an oral agent that will be con-
      tinued for the long-term control of the hypertension.
   2. In the acute setting, do not decrease the blood pres-
      sure to normal, as this can result in syncope or a
      cerebrovascular event.
   3. A model for therapy is to initiate therapy with the
      long-term agent to be used (e.g., atenolol, 25 mg; or
      felodipine, 5 mg, or lisinopril, 5 mg) administering
      one dose p.o. at outset of patient encounter. The
      blood pressure should be measured daily until stabi-
      lized, then weekly, and with the medication adjusted
      by following the principles discussed under V (Man-
      agement, page 145), until the patient is normotensive
      (see Table 3-3).
   4. A hypertensive urgency may be managed on an out-
      patient basis, especially if the blood pressure re-
      sponds to therapy and the patient is compliant with
      therapy and keeps appointments.

VIII. Consultation

Problem	Service	Time
Any renal failure	Renal	Urgent
Renal artery stenosis	Renal	Urgent
Conn's disease	Endocrine	Required
Hypercortisolism	Endocrine	Required
Pheochromocytoma	Endocrine	Urgent

T A B L E   3-3
Antihypertensive Agents

Class	Representative Agents and Doses	Side Effects/Contraindications	Special Uses
Diuretics	HCTZ, 25–50 mg p.o. q. day Dyazide (triamterene, 50 mg/HCTZ, 25 mg), one tablet p.o. q. day Maxide (triamterene, 75 mg/HCTZ, 50 mg), 1/2–1 tablet p.o. q. day Triamterene, 50 mg, one tablet p.o. q. day	Decreased intravascular volume Hypokalemia HypoMg Hyperuricemia Increased LDL Increased VLDL Special side effects of triamterene: hyperkalemia especially if patient has type IV RTA	Second- or third-line agent Excellent if in patients with calcium nephrolithiasis, hypoparathyroidism, or both
β-Blockers	Metoprolol (Lopressor), 50–100 mg p.o. b.i.d. Atenolol (Tenormin), 50–100 mg p.o. q. day	Decreases HDL Worsens systolic CHF Exacerbates the AV block Exacerbates asthma *Contraindications:* a) High-grade AV block b) Reversible airway disease c) Intermittent claudication d) Pheochromocytoma	Benefit in diastolic CHF Benefit in patients with ischemic heart disease, especially after MI, when it prolongs life and decreases reinfarction

Class	Drug/Dose	Side effects/Contraindications	Comments
	Labetolol 100 mg p.o. b.i.d.	As above, except it is the dose of choice for pheochromocytoma	Treatment of choice for pheochromocytoma or pre-eclampsia Benefit to hypertension in diabetics Benefit in diastolic hypertension
ACE inhibitors	Captopril, 6.25–25 mg p.o. q.8–12 hr Lisinopril, 2.5–40 mg p.o. q. day Quinapril, 2.5–10 mg p.o. q. day	Proteinuria Angioedema Lupus-like syndrome Bronchospasm Neutropenia Worsening of renal failure CONTRAINDICATED in pregnancy	
Calcium channel blockers	Verapamil SR, 120–240 mg q. day to b.i.d. Nifedipine XL, 30–60 mg p.o. q. day Amlodipine, 2.5–10 mg p.o. q. day Felodipine, 2.5–10 mg p.o. q. day	Peripheral edema Verapamil exacerbates AV block Exacerbation of systolic CHF Constipation with verapamil Short-acting calcium channel blockers (e.g., nifedipine t.i.d./q.i.d.) should not be used, as there may be an increased risk of myocardial infarction	Useful in control of supraventricular tachycardia, atrial fibrillation, or both Verapamil Diltiazem Effective, easy to use, with few side effects

T A B L E 3-4
Agents Used in the Management of Hypertensive Emergencies and Urgencies

Agent	Indications	Dosage	Side Effects
Sodium nitroprusside (Nipride)	All hypertensive emergencies except eclampsia	0.5 μg/kg/min IV initially, titrate dosage (increase/adjust) by increments of 0.5 μg/kg/min to target blood pressure (see text), maximum dosage is 8.0 μg/kg/min Concurrent use of intra-arterial catheter is recommended IV loop diuretics, 20 mg furosemide IV, usually needed at or soon after intiation of nitroprusside Advantage: Extremely short half-life, which allows clinician to rapidly titrate dose to target blood pressure; if overshoot, can rapidly adjust dosage down	Hypotension Hypotension Fluid retention Headache Thiocyanate toxicity if used >3–5 days

Drug	Indication	Dose	Complications
Hydralazine	Eclampsia/preeclampsia	**Loading dose:** 50 mg i.v. **Maintenance dose:** 5–20 mg i.v. q. 30 min, titrate to target blood pressure (see text) **Deliver fetus**	Hypotension Tachycardia See Chapter 11, Table: Pregnancy, page 558
Nifedipine (Procardia)	Urgency	10 mg p.o.; can repeat dose in 30–40 min; titrate to target blood pressure (see text) Can initiate chronic oral therapy with this agent as soon as target blood pressure is reached	Hypotension
Nitroglycerin ointment (Nitropaste)	Urgency	Apply 0.5–1 inch of paste to skin; titrate to target blood pressure (see text); can easily control if overshoot, just wipe off Best in emergency room (ER), especially in patients with concurrent atherosclerotic heart disease	Hypotension Headache
Labetalol (Normodyne)	Pheochromocytoma Preeclampsia/eclampsia	20 mg i.v. infusion over 2 min; repeat 20–80 mg doses q 5–10 min to a maximum of 300 mg	Bronchospasm Bradycardia

T A B L E 3-5
Incontinence: Types, Evaluation, and Management

Type	Manifestations	Etiologies	Management
Stress	Small amounts of urine released on events/episodes of acute intraabdominal pressure (i.e., Valsalva) Cough Sneeze Bowel movements Laughing If as the result of childbirth, concurrent rectal and cervical prolapses are possible	Weakness and laxity of pelvic floor muscles Weakness of the sphincter as the result of either a) Childbirth b) Surgery	Prevention Kegel exercises to strengthen musculature Surgery: repair of any prolapse with bladder neck suspension
Urge	Large amounts of urine released when sensation of full bladder perceived by the patient; unable to delay voiding If related to spinal cord damage, there is a decrease in the anal wink	Detrusor hyperactivity a) UTI, urethritis b) UTI, cystitis c) CVA d) Spinal cord injury e) Multiple sclerosis	Treat any infection Agents to decrease detrusor function (anticholinergic agents) a) Propantheline, 15–30 mg t.i.d./q.i.d. p.o. *or*

Overflow	Leakage of urine in small amounts from a distended (overdistended) bladder Postvoid residual of >100 mL Enlarged prostate Cystocele If as the result of spinal cord damage, there is a decrease in the anal wink	Prostate hypertrophy or carcinoma Cystocele Acontractile bladder secondary to lesion in the spinal cord, either trauma or dysmyelination	b) Oxybutynin, 2.5-5 mg b.i.d. to q.i.d. (side effects, dry mouth, dry eyes, decrease in cognitive skills) Prazosin 1-2 mg p.o. q.hs or other α agents Surgery (TURP) for BPH Surgery (prostatectomy) for prostate carcinoma Surgery/pessary of cystocele Bethanechol (cholinergic) 10-15 mg p.o. b.i.d. if a nonobstructive etiology Toilet-training techniques
Functional	Impaired cognition Psychologic changes Dementia	Immobility Dementia Physical restraints	

IX. **Indications for admission:** All hypertensive emergencies and all hypertensive urgencies that are refractory to short-term intervention.

Incontinence

This is a major problem, especially in the elderly. See Table 3-5 for types and overall management. Recent reports demonstrate that 41% of older women report daily urinary incontinence.

Nephrolithiasis

The presence of calculi (stones) in the urinary tract is a medical problem that is quite prevalent in the United States, affecting between 4% and 8% of the population at some time during life. The stones may be in the upper tract (nephrolithiasis) and/or in the lower urinary tract (cystolithiasis).

I. The **overall manifestations** of urinary tract stones include the acute onset of unilateral flank pain that is invariably quite severe. The pain originates in the flank and radiates into the ipsilateral labium majora or scrotum. There may be associated nausea, anorexia, vomiting, dysuria, and gross hematuria. The patient may have a history of UTIs or of crystal arthropathies, especially gout. Also, because there is a high recurrence rate for any type of urinary tract calculus, there often is a history of antecedent nephrolithiasis. Although the majority of patients have symptoms, many quite severe, the stones can be asymptomatic and thus found incidentally, during the workup for microscopic hematuria or recurrent pyuria.

II. **Types of stones**

Although virtually all urinary stones have the same manifestations and require the same overall short-term evaluation and management, there are several types of urinary stones, each with different physical properties, a unique pathogenesis, a unique natural history, and specific features in long-term management (Table 3-6).

A. **Calcium stones**

Calcium stones are by far the most common crystal stones that result in symptomatic nephrolithiasis. There are two subtypes of calcium stones—calcium oxalate, which causes 40% of all stones, and calcium phosphate-oxalate, which causes 40% of all stones in the renal system. Any of the calcium-containing stones are radiopaque and thus are easily visualized on standard radiographic imaging.

1. The **underlying pathogenesis** in virtually all cases is an increase in levels of calcium in the urine. The differential diagnosis and the unique pathogenetic

T A B L E 3-6
Nephrolithiasis

Stone Type	Urine pH	Radiographic Appearance	Sex Ratio
Calcium	Alkaline (>7)	Radiopaque	Men > women (most common type in both)
Calcium apatite			
Calcium oxalate			
Urate (purine)	Acidic (<7)	Radiolucent	Men > women
Struvite	Alkaline (>7)	Radiopaque	Women > men
Cystine	Variable	Radiopaque	Equal

features resulting in the development of calcium-based calculi include:

a. **Primary hyperparathyroidism.** This is hypersecretion of parathyroid hormone (PTH) from the parathyroid glands, either as a result of a parathyroid adenoma or of parathyroid hyperplasia. The mechanism is an elevated PTH level, causing a secondary hypercalciuria, which increases the risk of calcium stone development in the renal system.

b. **Increased GI load and/or absorption of calcium.** This is the chronic ingestion of large quantities of calcium, usually in the form of calcium carbonate antacids, with or without a concurrent increase in the amount of vitamin D ingested, by a patient with normally functioning kidneys. The normally functioning renal tubules handle the overall increased calcium load by excreting more, with resultant hypercalciuria. This increases the risk of calcium stone development in the renal system.

c. **Renal tubular dysfunction, usually type I** (distal), is an uncommon cause. The mechanism is one of tubular dysfunction, causing an inappropriate loss of calcium in the urine and a concurrent decrease in the normal amount of citrate within the urine. Citrate normally will chelate calcium in the urine, thus decreasing the risk of calculus formation. Thus a significant hypercalciuria results, which increases the risk of calcium stone development in the renal system.

d. **Hyperoxaluria.** This is most common in patients who frequent health-food stores and ingest large doses of water-soluble vitamin C. These patients may ingest 1–4 g of vitamin C per day. The mechanism is one in which there is an increase in oxalate in the urine. The presence of this anion in the urine results in an increased risk for the development of calcium oxalate calculi. Other causes of hyperoxaluria include inflammatory bowel disease, intestinal bypass surgery, and hereditary hyperoxaluria.

2. The **specific evaluation and management** of calcium stones in the urinary tract include making the clinical diagnosis and treating immediately as described in Box 3-4. Specific evaluative tools include:

a. Obtaining 24-hour urine collections to measure calcium. Normal is <300 mg/24 hr. If >300 mg/24 hr, the chance is greater that the stone is indeed calcium related.

b. If renal tubular acidosis is suspected (i.e., the

B O X 3-4

Overall Evaluation and Management of Nephrolithiasis

Evaluation

1. Take a thorough history directed toward uncovering past UTIs, arthritides, diet of the patient, medication and vitamin use, or a family history of renal calculi.
2. Perform a physical examination, looking especially for costovertebral angle tenderness and fever.
3. Perform urinalysis with microscopic analysis, looking especially for any crystals (Fig. 3-1).
4. Determine urine pH, as it can aid in predicting the type of stone present. An alkaline pH is associated with struvite calculi.
5. Determine serum electrolyte levels for baseline purposes.
6. Determine serum uric acid level, especially if the patient has gout or is at risk for uric acid nephrolithiasis.
7. Perform renal US. This is an important imaging technique to ascertain:
   a. The presence of a stone.
   b. The size of the stone.
   c. The size of the kidneys.
   d. The presence or absence of ureteral obstruction. The advantages of US over standard radiographic imaging are several: (a) there is no radiation exposure; therefore, the study can be safely performed in pregnant women; (b) one can directly image all stones, including radiolucent uric acid stones; and (c) one can directly image the size of the ureters and therefore detect early renal obstruction.
8. Determine serum calcium, PO_4, albumin, and magnesium levels for baseline purposes and to screen for hyperparathyroidism.
9. Determine CBC count with differential for baseline purposes.
10. Strain all urine; 80% of first stones will pass.
11. Send the stone for chemical-structure analysis.
12. Perform spot tests for urine calcium and creatinine, and calculate the ratio of calcium to creatinine:
    a. Normal: <0.1.
    b. Hypercalciuria: >0.3. Hypercalciuria is a risk factor for the development of calcium stones.

(continued)

B O X   3-4 (continued)

Management

1. If the patient is acutely ill and vomiting, place on NPO orders.
2. Replete any fluid deficit, and then maintain i.v. fluids with 0.9 normal saline.
3. Provide analgesics. For the short term, patients usually need narcotic analgesia. The following regimens can be used:
   a. Meperidine (Demerol), 50 mg, plus hydroxyzine (Vistaril), 25 mg i.m., q.3–4hr prn.
      -or-
   b. Morphine sulfate, 2–3 mg i.v., q.2–3hr. Occasionally a morphine sulfate drip, 1–3 mg/hr i.v., is necessary for short-term management.
4. Monitor fluid input and output closely. Maintain a urine output of ≥ 100 ml/hr to aid in flushing the stone out.
5. If pyuria is present and the urine is alkaline, treat the UTI with ampicillin and an aminoglycoside, covering for *Proteus mirabilis* (see section on Pyuria Syndromes, page 171).

Referral

1. Obtain a renal consultation.
2. If the stone is large (>5 mm in diameter) or if obstruction is present, consult urology urgently or emergently.

---

patient has a non–anion gap metabolic acidosis and an inappropriately alkaline urine), obtain a 24-hour urine collection to measure citrate. Normal urinary citrate is >250 mg/24 hr. Thus <250 mg is indirect evidence not only of calcium nephrolithiasis, but also of a concurrent distal renal tubular acidosis (RTA) (see page 489).
   c. If hyperparathyroidism is suspected, determine the serum PTH-N-terminal (intact).
3. **Long-term management**
   Long-term management and secondary prevention of calcium nephrolithiasis include:
   a. Initiation of a thiazide diuretic (e.g., hydrochlorothiazide, 25 mg/day p.o.), which acts on the renal tubules to decrease the calcium in the urine.

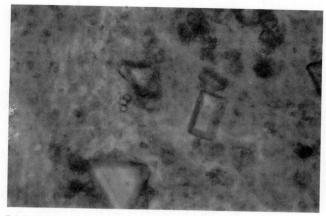

F I G U R E 3-1
Urine-microscopic: Struvite crystals in a patient with a *Proteus mirabilis* urinary tract infection.

    b. Attempting to discontinue or limit the administration of agents that can exacerbate the pathogenesis of these stones (e.g., loop diuretics and vitamin C).

    c. Recommending that the patient increase oral fluid intake to increase urine output and thus decrease the risk of stasis and crystal formation.

    d. If RTA is the underlying cause, referral to nephrology and the initiation of potassium citrate, 1 mEq/kg/day p.o., are indicated.

    e. If hyperparathyroidism is diagnosed, referral to an endocrinologist is indicated, as well as referral to nephrology for treatment of recurrent stones or any evidence of renal tubular dysfunction.

B. Uric acid stones

Uric acid stones are relatively uncommon. This crystal type makes up ~5%–10% of all urinary calculi. They are the only stones that are radiolucent and thus invisible on standard radiographic imaging techniques.

    1. The **underlying pathogenesis** in virtually all cases is increased uric acid in the urine. The differential diagnosis and unique pathogenetic features of uric acid–based calculi include:

        a. Tophaceous gout. This is a specific form of gout in which the patient has a long history of severe, recurrent, untreated gouty arthritis. The total body stores of uric acid are extremely increased.

The uric acid is deposited in the soft tissues, resulting in formation of indurated, nontender lesions (i.e., tophi). As an outcome of these elevated purine and urate stores in the body, there invariably is concurrent hyperuricosuria and therefore an increased risk of uric acid stone formation.

b. **Deficiency in hypoxanthine-guanine phosphoribosyl transferase** (HGPT). The partial or complete deficiency of this ubiquitous enzyme results in a decreased ability of the cells to catabolize purines, with resultant chronically extremely elevated uric acid levels in the serum and the urine and, therefore, an increased risk of uric acid stone formation. Complete deficiency may manifest as the Lesch–Nyhan syndrome.

c. **Medication side effect.** Several medications, including salicylates in high doses and probenicid, will effect a decrease in uric acid in the body and in the serum by increasing the tubular excretion of uric acid and increasing the risk of uric acid nephrolithiasis. Thus, when prescribing high-dose aspirin or probenicid, one must know of this potential side effect.

2. The **specific evaluation and management** of uric acid stones in the urinary tract include making the clinical diagnosis and treating in the short term as described in Box 3-4. Specific evaluative tools include:

a. Obtaining a 24-hour urine collection to determine uric acid. The normal value is <700 mg/24 hr. Thus >700 mg/24 hr increases the probability that the stone is indeed uric acid.

3. **Long-term management**
The specifics in the **long-term management** and prevention of uric acid nephrolithiasis, once the diagnosis is made, include initiating allopurinol, 300 mg p.o., once daily. This agent, which should be used over the long term, decreases the overall serum and urinary uric acid levels by inhibiting the enzyme, xanthine oxidase. Other steps include alkalinizing the urine with oral $NaHCO_3$, and discontinuing probenicid or high-dose aspirin.

C. **Struvite stones**
This crystal type, referred to as triple phosphate, with a chemical composition of $NH_4Mg(PO_3)3:(6\ H_2O)$, accounts for ~5%–10% of all urinary calculi. These calculi are uniformly radiopaque and thus are easily demonstrated by standard radiographic techniques. The stones are usually quite large and can cause ureteral obstruction.

1. The **underlying pathogenesis** is recurrent infection with urea-splitting organisms, most commonly *Proteus* or *Morganella* spp. These organisms contain the enzyme urease, which effectively breaks down urea and causes an alkaline urine and NH_4 in the urine. These two processes (i.e., alkalosis and increased urinary NH_4) increase the risk of formation of triple-phosphate crystals and thus of struvite, also known as "staghorn" calculi. These calculi are foreign bodies and, once present, increase the risk of future UTIs, which in turn leads to further growth of the calculi.

2. The **specific evaluation and management** of struvite stones in the urinary tract include making the clinical diagnosis and acutely treating as described in Box 3-4. Invariably, the diagnosis is clinically evident at the time of presentation. The crystals are "coffin" shaped on urinalysis (see Fig. 3-1). Specific acute management includes obtaining urine culture and sensitivity and the empiric initiation of antibiotics. Regimens can include amoxicillin, 500 mg p.o., q.i.d., for 7–10 days, or, if inpatient management is required, ampicillin and an aminoglycoside or ampicillin-sulbactam (Unasyn). Expedient referral to urology for stone removal, either surgically or by lithotripsy, is indicated.

3. **Long-term management**
   The specifics in the **long-term management** and prevention of struvite stones include effective removal of the stones and aggressive treatment of the underlying UTIs. Follow-up with urology is mandatory.

D. **Cystine stones**
   These stones are quite uncommon and usually occur as a result of a congenital process. Approximately 0.5% of all calculi are cystine stones. The stones are radiopaque and thus easily visualized on radiographic imaging.

   1. The **underlying pathogenesis** is an increase in the urinary levels of cystine. The most common cause is hereditary cystinuria, inherited as an autosomal recessive trait.

   2. The **specific evaluation and management** of cystine stones in the urinary tract include making the clinical diagnosis and treating in the short term as described in Box 3-4. The crystals are hexagonal on urinalysis. Further evaluation includes querying the patient regarding a family history of stones affecting both sexes and screening for it in the patient and family members by performing a nitroprusside test on the urine. **Specific management** includes referral to a nephrology consultant and is beyond the scope of this text.

III. Consultation

Problem	Service	Time
Obstruction	GU	Emergent/urgent
Large calculus (>5 mm)	GU	Urgent
Recurrent calculi	Renal	Elective
Hyperparathyroidism	Endocrinology	Elective

IV. Indications for admission: Any evidence of ureteral obstruction, pyelonephritis, septicemia, severe pain, or intravascular volume depletion.

Proteinuria

One of the most important and central functions of the kidneys is to filter the blood. The filtering activity is performed by the glomeruli. This filtration is efficient and quite specific in that only low-molecular-weight substances are filtered out of the blood. The specificity is such that medium- and large-molecular-weight molecules, such as albumin and plasma proteins and all cellular components, are uniformly not filtered out of the blood. Although the filter system is efficient and specific, there is, even in the normal setting, the potential for some loss of scant amounts of albumin and protein. Moreover, the cells of the urinary tract distal to the glomeruli can produce small amounts of protein, including the protective immunoglobulin IgA, which eventually is lost in the urine. Therefore in healthy people, a very small amount of protein may be lost in the urine. This protein loss does not exceed 150 mg/24 hr and is below the detection threshold of the test for proteinuria most commonly used, the urine dipstick analysis.

I. Definition

Proteinuria, by definition, is the loss of an excessive quantity of protein in the urine. The patient may have significant manifestations directly attributable to the loss of protein and albumin, as well as manifestations indirectly associated with the underlying disease process. Any quantity of protein greater than normal (i.e., 150 mg/day in the urine) is by definition proteinuria. Therefore even a trace of protein on the dipstick is considered proteinuria.

II. Nephrotic range proteinuria

This is a large amount of protein lost in the urine—by definition, >2 g/24 hr. The classic nephrotic syndrome is the quintessential but nonspecific example of this type of protein loss. This classic syndrome consists of hypoalbuminemia, hypercholesterolemia, and >2 g of protein lost in the urine per 24 hours.

A **spot urine protein/creatinine ratio >3.5** is quite sensitive and specific for nephrotic-range proteinuria, thus giving the clinician a simple and inexpensive evaluative tool with which to document proteinuria. This evaluative tool should replace the older, more expensive, and less convenient 24-hour urine collection for protein and creatinine determination.

A. The **specific manifestations** of nephrotic-range proteinuria include those related to the nephrosis itself and those related to the underlying cause of the nephrotic-range proteinuria. The manifestations specific to the nephrotic-range proteinuria include the development of edema, first dependent and then diffuse, leading to anasarca and biventricular heart failure. Further findings include the onset of frothy or foamy urine without other urinary symptoms, as a result of albumin in the urine, or xanthelasma as a result of the secondary hypercholesterolemia present.

B. The **differential diagnosis** includes membranous GNP; minimal-change GNP; SLE, especially if mesangial or membranous GNP is present; primary or secondary amyloidosis; diabetes mellitus; uncontrolled hypertension; exposure to heavy metals; and monoclonal gammopathies, including multiple myeloma. The pathogenesis of proteinuria in each of these entities is different but beyond the scope of this textbook.

   The most common causes of nephrotic-range proteinuria in the United States today are hypertension and diabetes mellitus.

C. The **specific evaluation and management** of this disorder include making the clinical diagnosis by using the evaluative tools described in Box 3-5, performing specific tests to determine the underlying cause and concurrent sequelae. These tests include US of the kidneys to reveal the size of the kidneys. If the disease process is acute, the kidney size is usually normal, whereas if the process is chronic, the kidney size is small.

   1. If a vasculitis or glomerulonephritis (GNP) is suspected, the erythrocyte sedimentation rate (ESR) and antinuclear antibody (ANA) titer should be determined; both would be abnormally elevated. Referral to nephrology to consider a renal biopsy and to consider the initiation of steroid or cytotoxic agent (e.g., cyclophosphamide for Wegener's) treatment is indicated. Refer to Table 3-7 (page 169) and section on Renal dysfunction (page 188), types and treatment of lupus nephritis.

   2. If the sulfosalicylic acid (SSA) assay is positive, urine protein electrophoresis on a 24-hour collection of urine should be performed. It will demonstrate what specifically the protein is, κ or λ light chains, or albumin. Furthermore, serum protein electrophoresis should be performed.

   3. A fasting glucose and examination of the retinas,

B O X 3-5

Overall Evaluation of Proteinuria

Evaluation

1. Take a thorough history and perform a physical examination, looking for any signs of chronic protein or albumin loss (e.g., peripheral edema, heart failure, ascites).
2. Repeat the dipstick analysis of the urine and perform a microscopic analysis of the urine, specifically looking for the concurrent findings of RBC casts, RBCs, WBCs, bacteria, and fat oval bodies, which are manifestations of a "nephritic" urinary sediment.
3. The sulfosalicylic acid (SSA) test should be performed on the urine specimen. This reagent is used to determine whether Bence Jones proteins (light chains in a gammopathy) are present in the urine. Two drops of the SSA reagent are added to a small sample of urine. If light chains are present, a white precipitate forms. Light chains (Bence Jones proteins) are not revealed by the standard dipstick method.
4. Obtain spot levels of protein and creatinine in the urine, both in mg/dL. If the ratio of protein to creatinine is >3.5, it is consistent with nephrotic-range proteinuria. This rapid test has virtually supplanted the 24-hour collection of urine for protein determination. Alternatively, the clinician can perform the traditional 24-hour urine collection for protein.
5. Determine serum electrolyte levels for baseline purposes.
6. Determine serum creatinine, BUN, and glucose levels for baseline purposes and to document the degree of renal impairment.
7. Determine the serum albumin, calcium, and phosphorus levels for baseline purposes and to document any hypoalbuminemia.
8. Determine the CBC count with differential for baseline purposes.
9. Categorize the proteinuria into nephrotic-range proteinuria (>2 g/24 hr or a spot protein/creatinine ratio of >3.5) or nonnephrotic-range proteinuria (<2 g/24 hr or a spot protein/creatinine ratio of <3.5).

TABLE 3-7
WHO Classification of Lupus Nephritis

Class	Renal Histology	Laboratory Evaluation	Prognosis/Treatment
I. (Normal)	Normal	Normal	Excellent/No need for treatment
II. (Mesangial lupus nephritis)	Mesangial hypertrophy	Minimal proteinuria (normal in 25%) Anti-DNA in minority	Good/No need for treatment
III. (Focal proliferative nephritis)	Mesangial and endothelial proliferation Immune deposition in capillaries with narrowing <50% of glomeruli are involved	Mild proteinuria Decreased C3 and C4 Anti-DNA in majority	Moderate/High-dose steroids *or* Cyclophosphamide
IV. (Diffuse proliferative nephritis)	As in III, except >50% of the glomeruli are involved Crescents are present Thrombi are present	Heavy proteinuria RBC casts Renal failure Hypertension Decreased C3 and C4 Anti-DNA in all	Poor/High-dose steroids *or* Cyclophosphamide
V. (Membranous GNP)	Subepithelial granular deposits	Heavy proteinuria Microhematuria Normal C3 and C4 levels Anti-DNA: negative	Good to moderate
VI. (Sclerosing GNP)	Sclerosis; crescents and fibrosis are present		Poor

looking for hypertensive or diabetic changes, should be performed. Furthermore, aggressive control of serum glucose and aggressive control of any hypertension must be done. If the patient has no renal failure yet, the drug classes of choice to control hypertension, especially in patients with concurrent diabetes mellitus, are ACE inhibitors and/or calcium channel blockers.

III. **Nonnephrotic-range proteinuria**

This is a modest but abnormal amount of protein lost in the urine—<2 g of protein lost in 24 hours. A spot urine protein/creatinine ratio <3.5 is quite sensitive and specific for nonnephrotic-range proteinuria, thus giving the clinician a simple and inexpensive evaluative tool with which to document proteinuria.

A. The **specific manifestations** of nonnephrotic-range proteinuria include the fact that it is virtually always asymptomatic unless it is due to a UTI, in which case the findings of dysuria, pyuria, and increased frequency are to be expected (see section on Pyuria Syndromes, page 171).

B. The **differential diagnosis** includes UTIs, fever, diabetes mellitus, hypertension, exercise (especially if strenuous), and benign positional proteinuria (mild proteinuria that occurs when the patient is in an upright position but resolves when the patient is recumbent). The pathogenesis of proteinuria in each of these entities is different and beyond the scope of this textbook.

The most common causes of nonnephrotic-range proteinuria in the United States today are hypertension and diabetes mellitus.

C. The **specific evaluation and management** of this disorder include making the clinical diagnosis by using the evaluative tools described in Box 3-5 and performing specific evaluative tests, listed subsequently.

1. If diabetes mellitus is suspected, determine the fasting blood glucose level. If it is >129 mg/dL, the diagnosis of diabetes is confirmed; then look for any proliferative retinal changes consistent with microvascular diabetic disease. Treat aggressively (see section on Diabetes Mellitus in Chapter 9, page 464).

2. If hypertension is thought to be poorly controlled, obtain a 12-lead ECG to look for evidence of hypertension-induced LV hypertrophy, and perform a retinal examination. Treat aggressively (see section on Hypertension, page 142).

3. If benign positional proteinuria is suspected, obtain two urine collections, one during the day (~12 hours) and the other at night while the patient is

recumbent (~12 hours). The mild proteinuria should resolve when the patient is recumbent.

4. If UTI is found, treat as such (see section on Pyuria Syndromes, below).

5. If no clear cause can be determined or if the proteinuria is thought to result from hypertension or diabetes mellitus, consultation with a nephrologist, performing urinalysis, and monitoring serum electrolyte, BUN, and creatinine levels every 4–6 months are all indicated. If the proteinuria progresses to the nephrotic range, perform the evaluations listed for that entity.

IV. **Consultation**

Problem	Service	Time
Nephrotic range	Nephrology	Urgent
Nonnephrotic range	Nephrology	Elective

V. **Indications for admission:** Any evidence of biventricular failure, especially if new onset, or of new-onset anasarca.

Pyuria Syndromes

Pyuria is the abnormal presence of leukocytes in the urine. The overall manifestations of pyuria include a diverse array of symptoms and signs, among them dysuria (pain or burning on urination), an increased frequency of urination, a clear or purulent discharge from the urethral orifice, and the onset of cloudy urine. Further manifestations include pruritus of the vulva or distal glans, hesitancy (inability to generate a forceful urinary stream), and dribbling of urine after the completion of voiding.

Associated manifestations may include nausea, vomiting, urinary incontinence, and pain and tenderness in the suprapubic area. If pyelonephritis develops, there invariably will be unilateral pain and tenderness in the flank or costovertebral angle area.

The intensity of the overall manifestations can range from very severe to virtually asymptomatic. In fact, many cases of pyuria are completely asymptomatic and are diagnosed only by urinalysis.

The sex of the patient plays a major role in the differential diagnosis and even in the evaluation and management of pyuria. Thus one should approach pyuria in female patients differently from pyuria in male patients. The distal urinary tracts and adjacent reproductive structures are significantly different in female and male subjects.

I. **Pyuria in female patients**

Pyuria, either asymptomatic or symptomatic, is quite common in females.

A. The **underlying pathogenesis** of many pyuria syndromes in females is an infection that initially infects the distal urethra and, if not treated, ascends the urinary tract to the kidneys. Certain procedures and activities predispose to UTIs. These **risk factors** include but are not limited to:

1. The presence of a Foley catheter.
2. Poor perineal hygiene or techniques of hygiene, such as wiping posterior to anterior, potentially infecting the urethra with fecal material.
3. Anal intercourse with subsequent vaginal intercourse.
4. Nephrolithiasis.
5. Diaphragm and spermicide use. Specific pathogen: *Escherichia coli.*

B. **Subcategories**

Two major subcategories are discussed, symptomatic pyuria without bacteriuria and symptomatic pyuria with bacteriuria.

1. **Symptomatic pyuria without bacteriuria**
   a. The **specific manifestations** include those listed in the introductory material of this section. They usually are mild to moderate in intensity and usually are referable to only the distal aspects of the urinary tract. Invariably, the number of WBCs/HPF is low, 5–10. On dipstick analysis, the LE in the urine is positive, whereas the nitrite in the urine is negative. This is a not uncommon form of pyuria, especially in females. No bacteria are demonstrated on urinalysis or urine culture. Urine culture will reveal <10,000 organisms/mL of a specific bacterium.
   b. The **differential diagnosis** includes cervicitis; vaginitis; or primary UTIs with atypical bacteria, including *Chlamydia trachomatis* or *Mycobacterium hominis* (i.e., tuberculosis). Chlamydial infections are the most common of these causes.
   c. The **specific evaluation and management** of this category of pyuria in females include performing those examinations described in Box 3-6. If an extraurinary source is found, such as cervicitis or vaginitis, treat that entity. If the source is the urinary tract (i.e., no extraurinary source is demonstrated), the clinician can initiate antibiotics to cover *Chlamydia*. The best regimen (which, however, is **contraindicated in pregnancy**) is that of doxycycline, 100 mg p.o., b.i.d., for 7–10 days (see section on STDs, chapter 6, page 341).

2. **Symptomatic pyuria with bacteriuria**
   a. The **specific manifestations** of this not uncommon form of pyuria include those described in the introductory material of this section. The manifestations may range from mild to moderate

B O X 3-6

Overall Evaluation and Management of Pyuria Syndromes

Evaluation

1. Take a thorough history and perform a physical examination. In the history, emphasis should be placed on the manifestations described at the beginning of this section (page 171). The physical examination in female patients includes a pelvic examination looking for any areas of inflammation, discharge, or tenderness. In male patients, the GU tract must be examined with emphasis on the testes, penis, and prostate gland, again looking for tenderness or discharge. The prostate must be examined by rectal examination.
2. Obtain a sample of urine for dipstick and microscopic urinalysis. The dipstick analysis is for nitrite and LE; the microscopic analysis is for leukocytes, WBC casts (Fig. 3-2), erythrocytes, and bacteria.
3. If pyelonephritis is suspected, send the urine for a Gram stain.
4. Send the urine for culture and sensitivity testing.
5. Further evaluation and management differ according to the sex of the patient, reflecting different anatomic organization.

to severe in intensity and may be referable to the distal and/or proximal aspects of the urinary tract. On microscopic analysis, the number of WBCs/HPF is variable from low (5–10) to "too numerous to count." Also, the microscopic analysis will reveal bacteria in the urine specimen. On dipstick analysis the LE in the urine is positive, and the nitrite in the urine is positive if the infection is with a gram-negative organism, but the nitrite is negative if the infection is with a gram-positive organism. Culture of the urine will yield the etiologic organism. Positive culture is one that has >100,000 organisms/mL.

b. The differential diagnosis includes extraurinary (cervicitis, vaginitis) and primary UTIs with gram-negative bacilli (i.e., the Enterobacteriaceae), and the gram-positive cocci (i.e., *Staphylo-*

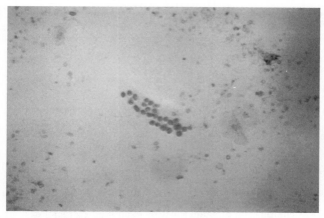

F I G U R E   3-2
Urine-microscopic: White blood cell cast in a patient with a urinary tract infection.

coccus saprophyticus and the group D streptococci).

The most common examples of gram-negative bacilli that result in UTIs are *Proteus, E. coli, Pseudomonas,* and *Morganella* spp.

  c. The **specific evaluation and management** of this category of pyuria in females include performing the evaluative examinations listed in Box 3-6. The urine pH is a useful tool, in that an alkaline pH indicates an infection with a urea-splitting organism and thus an increased risk for struvite nephrolithiasis. If an extraurinary source is found (e.g., cervicitis or vaginitis), treat that entity. If the source is the urinary tract, the clinician must initiate antibiotics. The Gram stain of the urine shows no specific organism unless pyelonephritis has developed.

The **specific antibiotic regimen** used should reflect the clinical picture of the patient. If the infection is limited to the lower tract and is without sequelae, a single-dose regimen can be used. If the patient is febrile and has flank pain, findings suggestive of pyelonephritis or impending sepsis, parenteral agents are mandatory. Typical regimens, categorized according to the clinical picture, are listed:

  i. If this is the first episode in the distal tract (i.e., the urethra or urinary bladder):

Trimethoprim (TMP)/sulfa (Bactrim DS), 1 tablet p.o., b.i.d. for 3 days
-or-
Ciprofloxacin, 250 mg p.o. q.12hr for 3 days
-or-
Amoxicillin, 250 mg p.o., t.i.d. for 3 days

ii. If the patient uses a diaphragm or if she has diabetes mellitus or if she is aged >65 years:

TMP/sulfa (Bactrim DS), 1 tablet p.o., b.i.d. for 7 days
-or-
Ciprofloxacin, 250 mg p.o., q.12hr for 7 days
-or-
Amoxicillin, 250 mg p.o., t.i.d. for 7 days

iii. If the patient is febrile and ill-appearing, parenteral antibiotics are required from the outset. This is pyelonephritis. The urine Gram stain will demonstrate polymorphonuclear leukocytes (PMNs) and often the organism itself. Regimens may include:

Ampicillin, 2 g i.v. q.4–6hr with or without an aminoglycoside
-or-
Piperacillin, 3 g i.v. q.4–6hr with or without an aminoglycoside

3. **Risks for recurrent UTIs in women:**
   a. Exogenous reinfection (e.g., after coitus)
   b. Use of diaphragm and a spermicide (increased risk of *E. coli*)
   c. Antigen nonsecretors (increased risk of *E. coli*).
   d. Rare to have an anomaly, therefore no exhaustive evaluation is mandated.
   e. Foley catheter
   f. Nephrolithiasis
   g. Poor perineal hygiene (wiping back to front, potentially contaminating the urethra with fecal material)
4. **Prevention of recurrent UTIs:**
   a. Teach hygiene techniques
   b. If nephrolithiasis is suspected, see page 158
   c. If there is a relation to coitus:

Bactrim SS, one tablet p.o. after intercourse
-or-
Cephalexin, 250 mg p.o. after intercourse

    d. If there is no relation to coitus:

        TMP, 100 mg p.o., 2–3 times/week for 1 month
        -or-
        Bactrim SS p.o., 2–3 times/week for 1 month

II. Pyuria in male patients

There are three different categories of pyuria in males: those of the urinary tract proper, the sexually transmitted purulent urethritides, and prostatitis. Each is discussed separately.

  A. Categories

    1. Symptomatic pyuria, not sexually transmitted

      a. The **specific manifestations** of this quite uncommon form of pyuria in males are described in the introductory material to this section. Symptoms are present in virtually all males who have pyuria. The intensity of the manifestations can be mild to moderate to severe, and the manifestations may be referable to both the lower and upper urinary tract. On microscopic analysis, the number of WBCs/HPF is variable from low (5–10) to "too numerous to count." Also, the microscopic analysis will reveal bacteria in the urine specimen. On dipstick analysis, the LE in the urine is positive, and the nitrite in the urine is positive if the infection is with a gram-negative organism, but the nitrite is negative if the infection is with a gram-positive organism. Culture of the urine will yield the etiologic organism.

      b. **Risk factors** that predispose to UTIs in males include but are not limited to prostatic hypertrophy, nephrolithiasis, anal intercourse, straight catheterization, and Foley catheter placement. In addition, individuals who are uncircumcised or have a partner with *E. coli* are at risk for infection.

      c. The **differential diagnosis** includes extraurinary (e.g., prostatitis or sexually transmitted purulent urethritis) and primary UTIs with gram-negative bacilli (i.e., the Enterobacteriaceae), and the gram-positive cocci (i.e., *Staphylococcus saprophyticus* and the group D streptococci). The most common gram-negative bacilli that result in UTIs are *Proteus*, *E. coli*, *Pseudomonas*, and *Morganella* spp.

      d. The **specific evaluation and management** of this category of pyuria in males include performing those examinations described in Box 3-6. The urine pH is a useful tool, in that an alkaline pH indicates an infection with a urea-splitting organism and thus an increased risk for struvite nephrolithiasis. If an extraurinary source is found (e.g.,

prostatitis or sexually transmitted purulent urethritis), treat that entity. If the source is the urinary tract, the clinician must initiate antibiotics.
The **specific antibiotic regimen** used should
reflect the clinical picture of the patient. If infection is limited to the lower tract and is without
sequelae, an oral regimen may be used. If the
patient is febrile and has flank pain, findings suggestive of pyelonephritis or impending sepsis,
parenteral agents are mandatory. Single-dose regimens for pyuria in males are contraindicated.
Several regimens, categorized according to the
clinical picture, are listed:

    i. If the patient has had acute or recurrent UTIs
in the past, regimens include:

> Amoxicillin, 500 mg p.o., t.i.d. for 10 days
>   -or-
> Bactrim DS, 1 tablet p.o., b.i.d. for 7–10 days
>   -or-
> Augmentin (ampicillin–clavulinic acid), 500
> mg p.o., b.i.d. for 7–10 days
>   -or-
> Ciprofloxacin, 250–500 mg p.o., b.i.d. for 7 days

    ii. If the patient is febrile and ill-appearing (i.e.,
a pyelonephritis), parenteral antibiotics are required from the outset. Regimens may include:

> Ampicillin, 2 g i.v., q.4–6hr with or without
> an aminoglycoside
>   -or-
> Piperacillin, 3 g i.v., q.4–6hr with or without
> an aminoglycoside

    Further evaluation is mandatory in all cases of
UTI in males. Expedient referral to GU and renal
US are indicated. All cases of nonsexually transmitted pyurias must be thoroughly evaluated by
a GU colleague.

2. **Sexually transmitted purulent urethritis.** This is the
most common form of pyuria in males and is usually
clinically evident (see the section on Sexually Transmitted Diseases in Chapter 6, page 340).

3. Prostatitis

    a. The **specific manifestations** of this fairly common
origin of pyuria in males are best described by
categorizing prostatitis as either acute or chronic
in duration. Chronic prostatitis is defined as
symptoms present for >2 weeks.

        i. Acute prostatitis. Manifestations include an
acute onset of perineal pain and, on examina-

tion, an enlarged, boggy feeling, and exquisitely tender prostate gland. Other manifestations include leukocytes, but rarely bacteria,
on microscopic analysis of the urine, and, on
dipstick analysis, a positive LE test but not
necessarily a positive nitrite.

    ii. **Chronic prostatitis.** There can be, but not necessarily is, an antecedent history of acute
prostatitis with recurrent pain and discomfort
in the groin and perineum. Often there are
some associated urinary obstructive symptoms, including hesitancy, dribbling, and frequency. On examination, the gland is, at
most, mildly tender and moderately enlarged.
Other manifestations include leukocytes, but
rarely bacteria, on microscopic analysis of the
urine, and, on dipstick analysis, a positive
LE test but not necessarily a positive nitrite.

b. The **underlying pathogenesis** is inflammation,
usually as the result of an infection, of the prostate
gland. The prostate gland is located at the base
of the penis and, in the pelvis, is immediately
anterior to the rectum. The gland completely surrounds the urethra as it enters the penis, and thus
causes manifestations of urinary tract obstruction
when inflamed or enlarged. Causative agents in
prostatitis, acute or chronic, include the gram-
negative bacillary organisms (i.e., the Enterobacteriaceae) and *Chlamydia trachomatis.* Very
rarely, Mycobacterium or *Blastomycetes* will result in chronic but never acute prostatitis.

c. The **specific evaluation and management** of this
category of pyuria in males include performing
those examinations described in Box 3-6. Antibiotic regimens include the following:

Acute prostatitis:
Bactrim DS, 1 tablet p.o., b.i.d. for 21 days,
   -or-
Amoxicillin, 500 mg p.o., t.i.d. for 21 days,
   -or-
Doxycycline, 100 mg p.o., b.i.d. for 21 days,
   -or-
Ciprofloxacin, 500 mg p.o., b.i.d. for 14–21
days.

Chronic prostatitis: The treatment is the same
as for acute prostatitis but is of longer duration
(i.e., 6 weeks). In addition, GU should be consulted.

III. Consultation

Problem	*Service*	*Time*
Recurrent infections	GU	Elective
First infection in males	GU	Required
Nephrolithiasis	GU	Elective
Chronic or recurrent prostatitis	GU	Elective
Benign prostatic hypertrophy	GU	Elective
Prostatic nodule	GU	Required

IV. Indications for admission: Pyelonephritis, inability to take adequate fluids by mouth, or any signs of impending sepsis.

Renal Dysfunction, Acute or Chronic

Acute renal failure (ARF) is the sudden onset of decreased renal function, which has significant manifestations and sequelae. It may be a new episode or an exacerbation of chronic renal dysfunction. Any acute decrease in renal function, even if asymptomatic, is by definition ARF and mandates an aggressive evaluation. Further underscoring the need for aggressive evaluation and management is the fact that although the differential diagnosis is quite large and diverse, many of the specific causes of ARF are, especially early in their course, quite reversible. ARF, when it develops in the presence of intercurrent disease, is a poor prognostic factor.

Chronic renal failure may be the result of an episode of irreversible ARF or of long-standing systemic disease (Table 3-8).

I. Physiologic functions of the normal kidneys
A. Excretion of nitrogenous wastes
The kidneys filter the entire volume of blood on a repetitive, continuous basis. The blood is filtered through one of the active sites of the kidneys, the glomeruli. It is in the glomeruli that low-molecular-weight nitrogenous

T A B L E 3-8
Clinical Differentiation of Acute from Chronic Renal Failure

Size of the kidneys on ultrasound	
Normal:	Acute
Small:	Chronic
Anemia	
Absent:	Acute
Present:	Chronic
Phosphorus	
Normal:	Acute
Elevated:	Chronic
Calcium	
Normal:	Acute
Low:	Chronic

wastes, such as the catabolites of respiration, are filtered from the plasma to be excreted in the urine. Although this effective filter removes the low-molecular-weight wastes from the blood, it does not filter out the formed cellular elements of the blood, the plasma proteins, or albumin. A physiologic measurement of kidney function is therefore the **glomerular filtration rate (GFR),** or the amount of blood filtered through the entire set of glomeruli in the renal cortices.

B. **Intravascular volume homeostasis**

Because the kidneys filter the blood continuously, a basic physiologic function of the kidneys is to maintain volume status. This is maintained by using the other active portion of the kidneys, the renal tubules, and is mainly under the direction of antidiuretic hormone (ADH) from the neurohypophysis and of mineralocorticoids from the adrenal cortices.

1. If the patient is **intravascularly volume depleted,** the neuroendocrine cells of the thirst center of the hypothalamus will secrete **ADH** through the neurohypophysis. ADH acts on and stimulates the collecting tubules of the kidneys actively to resorb free water from the urine. Furthermore, the glomeruli sense the decrease in volume being filtered and produce the hormone **angiotensin.** This hormone, produced by the juxtaglomerular (JG) cells of the kidneys, is activated in the lung parenchyma and stimulates the release of the mineralocorticoid, aldosterone, from the adrenal cortices. **Aldosterone** acts on the renal tubules to increase the resorption of water and sodium from the urine. All of these activities lead to appropriate retention of free water by the blood and concentration of the urine.

2. If the patient is **intravascularly volume overloaded,** the converse of these processes occurs, with the secretion of ADH and aldosterone being minimal. Furthermore, as the result of more volume, quite often the GFR increases. All of these steps lead to an appropriate loss of free water from the blood and dilution of the urine.

C. **Endocrine function**

The kidneys can, through the hormone **erythropoietin,** stimulate erythropoiesis and thus act to maintain a normal level of hemoglobin and therefore oxygen-carrying capacity of the blood.

D. **Calcium homeostasis**

The kidneys are integral to calcium homeostasis. Under the direction and influence of PTH, the renal tubules adjust the level of calcium in the urine and therefore in the serum. An increase in PTH results in decreased tubular secretion of calcium (i.e., retention of calcium in the serum), whereas a decrease in PTH results in increased excretion of calcium into the urine. Furthermore, the kidneys are the site of hydroxylation of 25-hydroxyvitamin D into its active component, 1,25-OH vitamin D. 1,25-OH vitamin D is required for effective absorption of calcium from the GI tract.

  E. **Phosphorus homeostasis**

The kidneys are integral to the homeostasis of phosphorus. Under the direction and influence of PTH, the renal tubules control the loss of phosphorus. An increase in PTH results in increased excretion of phosphorus, whereas a decrease in PTH results in decreased phosphorus excretion.

  F. **Acid–base homeostasis**

The renal tubules play a major role in maintaining the serum pH at a constant level of 7.4. The tubules control pH by adjusting the loss of hydrogen ions and HCO_3 ions. If there is an increase in fixed acids within the body, the tubules compensate by retaining HCO_3 and excreting H^+.

  G. **Potassium homeostasis**

The kidneys, under the direct influence of aldosterone, maintain serum potassium levels at a constant physiologic level. The normal range of serum potassium is 3.8–5.0 mEq/dL. When the serum potassium level increases, there is an increase in aldosterone secretion by the zona glomerulosa of the adrenal cortices, which acts on the renal tubules to increase the excretion of potassium.

II. **Overall manifestations of renal failure** (see Table 3-8)

  A. **Edema**

Both pulmonary and peripheral edema are common. Clinically, edema manifests with a subacute to insidious onset of orthopnea, paroxysmal nocturnal dyspnea (PND), a third heart sound, dependent pitting edema (especially of the lower extremities), and pleural effusions. The **underlying pathogenesis** is based on:

   1. An **overall decrease in GFR.** If the blood is not filtered, the excess volume cannot be removed by the kidneys. This is central to the pathogenesis.

   2. An **abnormal loss of albumin into the urine.** Albumin is an osmotically active substance—that is, it takes water with it—and thus is a major factor in maintaining water in the intravascular tree. If albumin is lost and the patient develops hypoalbuminemia, water, which as a result of the decreased GFR cannot be efficiently excreted, transudes (is lost) into the extracellular tissues, with resulting edema.

  B. **Oliguria**

Oliguria clinically manifests with the decrease in urine output to <30 mL/hr. This manifestation usually is not present until late in the course of disease. The **underlying pathogenesis** is a decrease in urine production due to an overall decrease in the normal GFR.

Even in relatively marked chronic renal failure, if the damage is predominantly to the tubules and relatively spares the glomeruli, the patient may be nonoliguric (i.e., with a normal urine output) or even polyuric (i.e., with an increased urine output).

C. **Anemia, normochromic normocytic**

The anemia is usually mild to moderate, but it can result in increased fatigability and a pale color to the nail beds and mucous membranes. Moreover, it can exacerbate any concurrent angina pectoris or heart failure. The **underlying pathogenesis** is a deficiency in the hormone erythropoietin, and therefore the reticulocyte count is low. An anemia usually is a manifestation of chronic rather than ARF.

D. **Hypocalcemia**

Usually this will be quite asymptomatic as it rarely will be of a magnitude as to cause the classic findings of hypocalcemia (i.e., tetany, Trousseau's sign, Chvostek's sign, and/or seizures). The **underlying pathogenesis** is twofold, involving first, the loss of renal tubular function and therefore response to PTH, and second, a decrease in the hydroxylation of the inactive 25-OH vitamin D to the active 1,25-OH vitamin D. Through these mechanisms, the serum calcium levels slowly but steadily decrease.

E. **Osteodystrophy**

This disorder closely resembles rickets. The patient develops an asymptomatic decrease in the mineral component of bone and bony structures. There is an increased risk for vertebral-compression fractures and fractures of the long bones; quite often, a fracture is the sentinel manifestation of this disorder. The **underlying pathogenesis** is essentially twofold, involving first, a decrease in the hydroxylation of 25-OH vitamin D with a resultant decrease in calcium absorption from the GI tract, and second, the development of secondary hyperparathyroidism caused by the chronic hypocalcemia, which results in increased resorption of calcium from bone, with a resultant osteodystrophy. This entity has been termed "vitamin D−resistant rickets," but actually it responds to **high doses** of oral 1,25-OH vitamin D.

F. **Hyperphosphatemia**

Although it is usually asymptomatic until markedly increased, the manifestations can include lethargy and increased fatigability. The **underlying pathogenesis** is a significant decrease in the GFR as the kidneys fail and a decrease in the ability of the kidney tubules to excrete phosphorus.

G. **Metabolic acidosis**

As the kidneys fail, there is a decreased ability of the renal tubules to excrete H^+ and fixed acids, resulting in a chronic, usually high anion gap, metabolic acidosis.

H. **Hyperkalemia**

Hyperkalemia usually is not a major problem until late in renal failure, when the patient becomes **oliguric** because the GFR has been markedly compromised. The **underlying mechanism** is a decrease in GFR and, concurrently, a decrease in tubular function and therefore ability to excrete potassium, even if aldosterone is markedly elevated. The hyperkalemia is further exacerbated by the metabolic acidosis that is usually concurrently present. (See the section on Hyperkalemia in Chapter 9, page 491.)

I. **Encephalopathy**

Encephalopathy manifests clinically with a diverse set of findings ranging from an insidious onset of lethargy to an acute onset of delirium. There often is asterixis, or "flap," present on examination. A harbinger is the development of intractable hiccups, myoclonic jerks, i.e., of the diaphragm. The **underlying pathogenesis** is an accumulation of nitrogen and other wastes of respiration and catabolism, which, over a given threshold, will result in decreased function of the brain. Encephalopathy is more common in chronic than in ARF. The **natural history** of uremic encephalopathy is grave; if no intervention is implemented, the mean survival time is <100 days.

J. **Coagulopathy**

Coagulopathy manifests clinically with the acute, subacute, and/or chronic onset of epistaxis, menorrhagia, easy bruisability, petechiae, and/or nonpalpable purpura. The **underlying pathogenesis** is an abnormal elevation in nitrogenous wastes, which, over a certain threshold, causes significant dysfunction of the platelets. Coagulopathy is more common in chronic than in ARF.

K. **Hypertension**

Hypertension is one of the most common manifestations of chronic renal failure. It results from and is exacerbated by the secondary hyperaldosteronism that develops in chronic renal failure. Hypertension is a risk factor for the development of other significant cardiovascular diseases and independently exacerbates and accelerates renal failure (see the section on Hypertension, page 142).

III. **Acute renal failure**

The causes of ARF are quite diverse but relatively easy to recall if they are divided into prerenal, renal, and postrenal subsets. This classification is somewhat artificial, as there is some overlap between the subsets, and acute renal dysfunction often is multifactorial.

A. **Prerenal**

1. The **specific manifestations** include orthostatic blood pressure and volume changes (see Box 3-7), an overall decrease in urine output, and an increase in concentration of the urine. Also seen are dry mu-

B O X 3-7

Overall Evaluation and Management of Renal Dysfunction

Evaluation

1. Take a thorough history and perform a physical examination with emphasis on the manifestations of acute renal dysfunction (see page 181). In addition, the history should focus on medication use, illicit drug use, and a history of renal or hepatic dysfunction. A rectal examination to determine prostate size is mandatory.
2. Assessment of the volume status clinically is of utmost importance. This is best done by determining blood pressure and pulse parameters with the patient supine and standing (i.e., orthostatic parameters), by examining the cardiopulmonary system, and by weighing the patient. By using the results of these examinations, the clinician assesses the patient's volume status and places the patient in one of three intravascular volume groups: hypovolemic, euvolemic, and hypervolemic.
    a. Hypovolemic—Characterized by a decrease in blood pressure and/or an increased heart rate when the patient stands up and a decrease in the patient's weight from a pre-illness baseline weight.
    b. Hypervolemic—Examination of the cardiopulmonary system discloses rales, a third heart sound, increased jugular venous pulsations, and dependent pitting edema. The weight is invariably increased from a pre-illness baseline weight.
3. Straight catheterization of the urinary bladder to determine volume, to relieve any retention or obstruction, and to obtain a specimen of urine for analysis. If the specimen is obtained in the postvoid state (i.e., immediately after the urinary bladder has been voluntarily emptied), any quantity >50 mL is abnormal.
4. US of the kidneys and bladder is indicated in all cases to ascertain the size of the kidneys and if obstruction (i.e., hydronephrosis) is present. Normally, the kidneys are ~12 cm long. If the kidneys are small, the failure is essentially irreversible; if the

(continued)

kidneys are normal sized, the failure is more likely reversible.

5. Perform urinalysis with microscopic examination. Many clues to the cause of renal dysfunction are gleaned from the urinalysis. Urinalysis should be done by the primary care physician and, if needed, with the direct assistance of a nephrology consultant. The importance of this examination cannot be overstressed. Clinical clues include the following:

 a. Pyuria (>5 WBCs/HPF) indicates infection of the urinary tract (see section on Pyuria Syndromes, page 171).
 b. Muddy brown casts (i.e., broad-based casts with pigment within) indicate acute tubular necrosis.
 c. Eosinophils on urinalysis, specifically demonstrated on Wright's stain, indicate interstitial nephritis.
 d. Red cell casts (i.e., smaller casts composed of RBCs) indicate a glomerular origin.
 e. Fat oval bodies (i.e., oval-shaped collections of fat) indicate a glomerular origin.
 f. Granular casts (i.e., clear narrow casts). These are nonspecific findings and not necessarily pathologic.
 g. White cell casts (i.e., casts composed of PMNs) indicate an infection of the urinary tract (Fig. 3-2).

6. Wright's stain of urine for eosinophils. If eosinophils are present, it is consistent with interstitial nephritis.

7. Spot urine for protein, creatinine, and sodium.

 a. The spot urine protein/creatinine ratio indicates whether significant proteinuria is present. A value >3.5 indicates nephrotic-range proteinuria (see section on Proteinuria, page 166).
 b. Spot Na can help differentiate certain forms of ARF. The subsets include:
  Urine Na <10 mEq/L:
   Prerenal ARF
   Hepatorenal syndrome
   Acute GNP
  Urine Na >10 mEq/L:
   Oliguric phase of acute tubular necrosis (ATN)
   Obstructive nephropathy

(continued)

B O X 3-7 *(continued)*

8. Send urine for culture and sensitivity testing if any pyuria is demonstrated.
9. Determine serum electrolytes for baseline purposes.
10. Determine serum creatinine and BUN levels for baseline purposes.
11. Determine albumin, PO_4, Ca, and creatine phosphokinase (CPK) levels, determine ESR, and perform a drug screen at the time of presentation.
12. If possible, discontinue all nephrotoxic agents. Adjust dosages of all agents that are excreted through the renal system, and if possible, follow up the serum levels of these drugs. Examples of this category of agents are digoxin, aminoglycoside antibiotics, and penicillin antibiotics.
13. Differentiate acute from chronic renal failure: see Table 3-8.

cous membranes, dry axillae, and skin "tenting." The patient is assessed to be hypovolemic. Finally, there invariably are manifestations of the underlying cause of the loss of intravascular volume. Both serum BUN and serum creatinine are increased; however, the elevation in serum BUN is relatively greater than the elevation in serum creatinine.

2. The **underlying pathogenesis** of this very common cause of renal dysfunction is an overall decrease in fluid in the intravascular tree, a decrease in blood flow to the kidneys, and therefore a decrease in GFR. In other words, there is an effective decrease in the intravascular volume of the patient. Specific states that result in a significant decrease in renal perfusion include intravascular volume depletion, acute hemorrhage from any source, low-output left ventricular failure, and inappropriate third spacing of fluids. Third spacing of fluids is a unique mechanism in that the patient has an overall increase in total body water, but the increase is mainly in third spaces (e.g., producing ascites or pleural effusions) and paradoxically results in a decrease in effective intravascular volume.

3. **Evaluation** includes making the clinical diagnosis by performing the evaluations listed in Box 3-7 and looking for any evidence of concurrent GI hemorrhage by performing stool guaiac measurements.

4. **Specific management** includes administering fluids to the patient. The fluid of choice is 0.9 normal saline first and a repletion rate of >250–300 mL/hr for several hours. The **goal** is to replete half of the total volume deficit in the first 12–18 hours and complete repletion in 24–30 hours. Use the baseline, pre-illness weight of the patient as a target for volume repletion and therefore euvolemia. Once euvolemia is achieved, administer maintenance fluids at 100–150 mL/hr until the underlying cause of the volume depletion has been effectively treated.

   a. One must always follow up weight, orthostatic parameters, creatinine, urine output, K, PO_4, Mg, and BUN levels on a frequent basis. Observe the patient for any signs of volume overload or heart failure. If these signs appear, decrease the rate of fluid input.

   b. In the short term, a consultation with nephrology is strongly recommended for all patients unless the renal dysfunction is mild, is due to a known and documented cause, and rapidly reverses.

B. **Renal**

1. The **specific manifestations** include those described in the section on overall manifestations (page 181), but the patient is clinically euvolemic. Furthermore, there are manifestations specific to the underlying condition causing the renal failure, such as arthralgias, serositis in SLE, and hemoptysis in Wegener's granulomatosis.

2. The **underlying pathogenesis** of this category of renal failure is direct damage to the kidneys themselves. Specific conditions that can result in renal damage may be subgrouped into tubular or glomerular types.

   a. **Tubular damage** or dysfunction results from one of two mechanisms:

      i. An episode of renal ischemia due to profound **hypotension,** or

      ii. **Direct damage** to the tubules by nephrotoxic agents, including i.v. contrast agents, acetaminophen, aminoglycoside antibiotics, *cis*-platinum chemotherapy, nonsteroidal antiinflammatory drugs (NSAIDs), and a vast array of other agents.

   b. *Glomerular damage* or dysfunction results from many discrete entities. Classic or common entities are described subsequently.

      i. *Poststreptococcal GNP,* or GNP that closely follows a suspected or documented streptococcal infection, usually a pharyngitis. This is a complement-fixing proliferative type of

GNP that is invariably reversible with supportive care.

  ii. **Vasculitides,** including SLE, polyarteritis nodosum, and Wegener's granulomatosis (see
the section on Polyarticular Arthritis in Chapter 7, page 406, for a discussion of SLE). SLE
is a systemic autoimmune process that results
in significant GNP (Table 3-7). Wegener's
granulomatosis is a necrotizing vasculitis that
manifests with rapidly progressive GNP, sinusitis with nasal and sinus mucosal lesions,
and hemoptysis due to necrotizing pulmonary lesions. Polyarteritis nodosum is a vasculitis of medium-sized arteries that may rapidly develop into progressive GNP.

 iii. **Thrombotic thrombocytopenic purpura**/he-
molytic uremic syndrome (TTP/HUS). This
syndrome consists of the pentad of microangiopathic hemolytic anemia, thrombocytopenia, fever, mental-status changes, and ARF.

  iv. The **hepatorenal syndrome** [i.e., the development of acute renal dysfunction in the face
of severe (Child's C) hepatic failure]. This is
a grave and irreversible form of ARF.

   v. **Hypertension**—Uncontrolled hypertension
can cause acute, subacute, or chronic renal
failure as a result of significant glomerular
damage.

  c. **Mixed:** Many etiologies, including HIV and diabetes mellitus, may result in tubular and glomerular damage.

3. **Evaluation** includes making the clinical diagnosis
by performing the evaluations listed in Box 3-7 and
looking for the underlying cause. The patient is usually euvolemic. Specific evaluative tools should include, if a vasculitis or GNP is suspected, serum
levels of ANA, RF, ESR, CH_{50}, C_3, C_4, and anticy-
toplasmic antibody. The ANA, RF, and ESR often
will be, in general, increased, whereas often the complement levels will be decreased. The anticytoplas-
mic antibody may be quite specific for Wegener's
granulomatosis. If there is any evidence of concurrent hepatic dysfunction, obtain LFTs, including total bilirubin, AST, ALT, GGT, alkaline phosphatase,
PT, and albumin (see the section on Polyarticular
Arthritis in Chapter 7 for specifics on ANA assays,
page 403).

4. **Specific management** includes making the clinical
diagnosis and monitoring the parameters of weight,
creatinine, urine output, K, PO_4, Mg, and BUN on a
frequent basis. In the short term, a nephrology con-

T A B L E 3-9
Indications for Emergency Dialysis

1. Volume overload that is resistant to aggressive diuretic therapy and is symptomatic
2. Hyperkalemia that is resistant to aggressive standard treatment (see the section on Hyperkalemia in Chapter 9, page 491)
3. Severe, refractory acidosis
4. Uremic encephalopathy
5. Uremia-induced pericardial friction rub
6. Uncontrollable bleeding due to uremia, causing platelet dysfunction
7. Severe rhabdomyolysis
8. Dialyzable toxin or an overdose of agent that is dialyzable (e.g., theophylline)

sult is strongly recommended for all patients. Hemodialysis or peritoneal dialysis should be initiated if severe (Table 3-9). Consultation with a dietitian to modify diet to decrease potassium, sodium, and fixed acids (i.e., proteins) is also clearly indicated. Specifics in management are beyond the scope of this text.

C. **Postrenal**
1. The **specific manifestations** include, in addition to those described in the overall manifestations section, a recent onset of a UTI and manifestations of urinary obstruction. These associated manifestations can include hesitancy, dribbling, urgency, and frequent small-quantity urination episodes.
2. The **underlying pathogenesis** is obstruction to the flow of urine between the kidneys and the external environment. The kidneys are functioning appropriately. The **differential diagnosis** includes multiple renal calculi (see the section on Nephrolithiasis, page 158). A second cause is urinary bladder obstruction with retention of urine as a result of benign prostatic hypertrophy (BPH), prostate adenocarcinoma, or the use of anticholinergic agents. A third cause is retroperitoneal lesions, including lymphoproliferative disorders, fibrosis, or sarcomas, causing bilateral ureteral obstruction. A final, uncommon cause of obstruction is iatrogenic, such as an obstructed Foley catheter.
3. **Evaluation** includes making the clinical diagnosis by performing the overall evaluation listed in Box 3-7 and looking for the underlying cause. The patient is usually euvolemic but may be hypervolemic.
4. **Specific management** includes the placement (or re-

placement) of a Foley catheter and emergent referral to a urologist for evaluation and potential placement of internal or external drainage stents. A nephrology consult is strongly recommended for all patients, as significant electrolyte disturbances and polyuria may develop after immediate relief of the obstruction. This polyuric phase occurs as a result of nephrogenic diabetes insipidus after the immediate relief of obstruction. The polyuric phase is treated supportively with repletion of the excessive urine output with 0.45 normal saline.

IV. **Chronic renal failure**

The causes of chronic renal failure include irreversible or recurrent ARF and systemic diseases.

A. **Etiologies: renal subgroup**

The most common conditions giving rise to ARF that progresses to chronic renal failure are in the "renal" subgroup, that is, the vasculitides and many of the glomerulonephritides. Most prerenal, postrenal, and drug-related causes of ARF will not progress to chronic renal failure if they are effectively treated.

B. **Etiologies: systemic diseases**

Systemic diseases are the most common conditions leading to chronic renal dysfunction in the United States today. These diseases include diabetes mellitus and hypertension.

1. **Diabetes mellitus.** Uncontrolled diabetes mellitus, especially with concurrent hypertension, will result in glomerular damage. This is more commonly subacute to chronic renal failure.

2. **Hypertension.** Uncontrolled hypertension may cause acute, subacute, or chronic renal failure as a result of significant glomerular damage.

C. **Evaluation and management**

The specific evaluation and management of chronic renal failure include making the clinical diagnosis and performing the tests described in Box 3-7. Other tools are described subsequently.

1. **Reciprocal creatinine line.** To determine whether any component of ARF is exacerbating the chronic dysfunction, the clinician should attempt to obtain several creatinine levels from the past and plot the reciprocals of the serum creatinine values against time. One can then easily determine the slope of the line. The clinician then plots the most recent 1/creatinine value. If the most recent reciprocal creatinine value is in the same line—that is, if the slope of the line is unchanged—the creatinine elevation is due to a natural progression of the chronic

failure, whereas if the value changes the slope of the line, a concurrent acute process is occurring.

2. **Long-term monitoring** of the patient's vital signs, K, BUN, creatinine, general urine output, PO_4, and CO_2 every 2–4 weeks. Monitor drug levels, Ca, and hemoglobin every 8–12 weeks.

3. **Define and treat any concurrent cause of ARF.**

4. Administer the pneumococcal vaccine (Pneumovax) and *Haemophilus influenzae* vaccine at the time of presentation and provide yearly influenza vaccinations.

5. **Aggressively control hypertension.** The goal is completely to normalize the blood pressure. An effective regimen includes a calcium channel blocker with a loop diuretic. The loop diuretic is especially useful to treat any evidence of fluid retention, either due to the renal failure or as a result of a calcium channel blocker. The dose of loop diuretic often is very large. A rule of thumb is to start with furosemide (Lasix), 20 mg p.o., and double the dose every 5–7 days until an effective diuretic dose is found. It is not uncommon to require 160–200 mg of Lasix p.o. or 4–5 mg of bumetanide (Bumex) p.o. every day.

6. **Dietary modifications.** The diet that should be recommended and described to the patient is 1 g of salt (NaCl), 1,500-mL fluid restriction, and low protein (0.5 g/kg/day). This diet is required in patients with oliguric renal failure who are not receiving dialysis. If the patient is nonoliguric, sodium and fluid restrictions can be liberalized significantly. Evidence is extant that the prescription of a low-protein diet (0.5 g/kg/day) delays progression of moderate renal insufficiency in chronic renal failure.

7. Administer calcitriol 0.25 μg/day p.o.; $CaCO_3$, 1–2 g p.o., b.i.d., and $NaHCO_3$, dosed to keep the serum CO_2 >15 mEq/dL. The usual dose is 500 mg p.o., once or twice a day.

8. If hiccups are bothersome or recurrent, administer thorazine, 25 mg p.o., q.6–8hr prn.

9. If recurrent bleeding due to uremia-induced platelet dysfunction is present, 1-deamino-8-D-arginine vasopressin (DDAVP) can be used (see previous discussion and page 268, Bleeding tendency).

10. Kayexalate, 15–30 g p.o., b.i.d., is effective in the long-term management of hyperkalemia in patients not yet receiving hemodialysis or continuous ambulatory peritoneal dialysis (CAPD). If there is an acute increase in serum potassium, one must treat emergently (see page 491).

11. Erythropoietin is now available as a therapeutic

agent. It is effective in increasing the hemoglobin in patients with renal failure–induced anemia. The target is to keep hematocrit in the mid-30s.

12. $Al(OH)_3$ antacids (e.g., Amphogel, 15–30 mL p.o., t.i.d. to q.i.d. with meals) bind the phosphorus in food. Aluminum-containing antacids should not be used on a long-term basis as they can exacerbate metabolic bone disease.

13. **CAPD/HD:** The patient must be prepared for the need for dialysis, either hemodialysis by using a surgically constructed arteriovenous fistula or peritoneal dialysis by using a peritoneal catheter (see Table 3-9). The patient should have dialysis initiated when the creatinine time is <10 mL/min. Specifics are beyond text.

14. Consider the patient for **renal transplantation.** The primary care physician should discuss this issue with the patient. The patient should be informed that renal transplants are effective and that none of these treatments including dialysis is a contraindication to transplant. The patient should discuss this with family members, and any first-degree relatives should be typed for blood and human leukocyte antigen (HLA) tissue as potential donors. Cytomegalovirus (CMV) titers of the patient should be obtained at baseline. If CMV-negative, the patient should receive, if transfusions are ever required, CMV-negative blood.

V. **Prevention**

This is one of the most critical areas in which the primary care physician or ambulatory care physician can have a major impact. Because many cases of ARF are iatrogenic, it is of great importance to monitor the renal function of patients given potentially nephrotoxic agents, such as NSAIDs or ACE inhibitors. Levels of agents that can be nephrotoxic, such as aminoglycoside antibiotics or lithium, should be determined regularly. Finally, when i.v. contrast media are used for radiographic imaging studies in patients at high risk for contrast-induced tubular damage (i.e., the elderly, any patient with diabetes mellitus, and any patient with a monoclonal gammopathy), the following preventive measures should be undertaken.

• Minimize the dose of contrast agent.
• Make certain the patient is euvolemic at the time of contrast-enhanced imaging.
• After injection of the contrast agent, one might administer mannitol, 12.5–25 g i.v., to cause a forced diuresis and aid in excreting the agent, thereby minimizing potential tubular damage.

VI. Consultation

Problem	Service	Time
All	Dietary	Elective
If dialysis is indicated	Renal	Emergent
All	Renal	Urgent/emergent
Complete obstruction	GU	Emergent
BPH with partial obstruction	GU	Urgent
Chronic renal failure	Transplant	Elective

VII. Indications for admission: Urgent or emergent need for dialysis, significant hyperkalemia, significant volume overload, hemodynamic instability, or acute tubular necrosis.

Bibliography

Hematuria

Mohr DN, et al: Asymptomatic microhematuria and urologic disease. JAMA 1986;256:224–229.

Restrepo NC, Carey PO: Evaluating hematuria in adults. Am Fam Pract 1989;40:149–156.

Sutton JM: Evaluation of hematuria in adults. JAMA 1990;263:2475-2480.

Thompson C: Hematuria: A clinical approach. Am Fam Pract 1986; 33:194–200.

Hypertension

Avgerinos PC, et al: The metyrapone and dexamethasone suppression tests for the differential diagnosis of the ACTH-dependent Cushing's syndrome: a comparison. Ann Intern Med 1994;121:318–327.

Blumenfeld JD, et al: Diagnosis and treatment of primary hypoaldosteronism. Ann Intern Med 1994;121:877–885.

Buck C, et al: The prognosis of hypertension according to age at onset. Hypertension 1987;147:820.

Caulfield M, et al: Linkage of the angiotensinogen gene to essential hypertension. N Engl J Med 1994;330:1629–1633.

Croog SH, et al: Sexual symptoms in hypertensive patients. Arch Intern Med 1988;148:788–794.

Ferguson RK, Vlasses PH: Hypertensive emergencies and urgencies. JAMA 1986;255:1607–1613.

Frolich ED, et al: Recommendations for human blood pressure determinations by sphygmomanometers. Hypertension 1988;11:209A.

Grossman E, et al: Should a moratorium be placed on sublingual nifedipine capsules given in hypertensive emergencies and pseudoemergencies? JAMA 1996;276:1320–1331.

Hommel E, et al: Effect of captopril on kidney function in insulin-dependent diabetic patients with nephropathy. Br Med J 1986;293:467–470.

Joint National Committee on Detection, Evaluation, and Treatment of High Blood Pressure. Arch Intern Med 1997;157:2413–2446.

Kaplan NM: Non-drug treatment of hypertension. Ann Intern Med 1985; 102:359–373.

Kaplan NM, et al: A differing view of treatment of hypertension in patients with diabetes mellitus. Arch Intern Med 1987;147:1160–1162.

Mann SJ: Systolic hypertension in the elderly: Arch Intern Med 1992; 152:1977–1984.

Mann SJ, et al: Detection of renovascular hypertension: state of the art. Ann Intern Med 1992;117:845–853.

Orth DN: Cushing's syndrome. N Engl J Med 1995:332:791–803.

Pacheco JP, et al: Monotherapy of mild hypertension with nifedipine. Am J Med 1986;81(suppl 6A):20–24.

Ruggenenti ML, et al: Nitrendipine and enalapril improve albuminuria and glomerular filtration rate in non-insulin dependent diabetes. Kidney Int 1996;49(suppl 55):S–91.

Sinclair AM, et al: Secondary hypertension in a blood pressure clinic. Arch Intern Med 1987;147:1289–1293.

Wikstrand J: Primary prevention with metoprolol in patients with hypertension. JAMA 1988;259:1976–1982.

Williams GH: Converting-enzyme inhibitors in the treatment of hypertension. N Engl J Med 1988;319:1517.

Incontinence

Ouslander JG, et al: Incontinence in the nursing home. Ann Intern Med 1995;122:438–449.

Nephrolithiasis

Jacobson EJ, Fuchs G: Nephrolithiasis. Am Fam Pract 1989;39:233–244.

Levy FL: Ambulatory evaluation of nephrolithiasis: an update of a 1980 protocol. Am J Med 1995;98:50–58.

O'Brien WM, et al: New approaches to the treatment of renal calculi. Am Fam Pract 1987;36:181–194.

Pak CY, et al: Ambulatory evaluation of nephrolithiasis. Am J Med 1980; 69:19–29.

Uribarri J, et al: The first kidney stone. Ann Intern Med 1989;111:1006–1009.

Proteinuria

Bernard DB, et al: Extrarenal complications of the nephrotic syndrome. Kidney Int 1988;33:1184–1202.

Levey AS, et al: Idiopathic nephrotic syndrome. Ann Intern Med 1987; 107:697–713.

Schwab SJ, et al: Quantitation of proteinuria by use of protein-to-creatinine ratios in single urine samples. Arch Intern Med 1987;147:943–944.

Stewart DW, et al: Evaluation of proteinuria. Am Fam Pract 1984; 29:218–225.

Pyuria Syndromes

Fihn SD, et al: Trimethoprim-sulfamethoxazole for acute dysuria in women: a single dose or ten day course. Ann Intern Med 1988;108:350–357.

Hoffman SA, Moellering RC: The enterococcus: putting the bug into our ears. Ann Intern Med 1987;106:757–761.

Hooten TM, et al: Erythromycin for persistent or recurrent nongonococcal urethritis. Ann Intern Med 1990;113:21–26.

Komaroff AL: Urinalysis and urine culture in women with dysuria. Ann Intern Med 1986;104:212–218.

Pels, et al: Dipstick urinalysis screening of asymptomatic adults for urinary tract disorders II. Bacteriuria. JAMA 1989;262:1221–1224.

Stamm WE, et al: Management of UTIs in adults. N Engl J Med 1993; 329:1328–1334.

Stamm WE, et al: Acute renal infection in women: treatment with trimetho-prim-sulfamethoxazole or ampicillin for two or six weeks. Ann Intern Med 1987;106:341–345.

Zweig S: Urinary tract infections in the elderly. Am Fam Pract 1987; 35:123–130.

Renal Dysfunction, Acute or Chronic

Clive DM, Stoff JS: Renal syndromes associated with nonsteroidal antiin-flammatory drugs. N Engl J Med 1984;310:563–572.

Eschbach JW, et al: Recombinant human erythropoietin in anemic patients with end-stage renal disease. Ann Intern Med 1989;111:992–1000.

Fine RN, et al: Renal transplantation update. Ann Intern Med 1984;100:246.

Fraser CL, Arieff AI: Nervous system complications in uremia. Ann Intern Med 1988;109:143–153.

Goldstein MB: Acute renal failure. Med Clin North Am 1983;67:1325–1341.

Klahr S, et al: The effects of dietary protein restriction and blood pressure control on the progression of chronic renal failure. N Engl J Med 1994;330:877–884.

Madaio MP, Harrington JT: The diagnosis of acute glomerulonephritis. N Engl J Med 1983;309:1299–1302.

Mooradian AD, Morley JE: Endocrine dysfunction in chronic renal failure. Arch Intern Med 1984;144:351–353.

Moore J, Maher JF: Management of chronic renal failure. Am Fam Pract 1984;30:204–213.

Myers BD, Moran SM: Hemodynamically mediated acute renal failure. N Engl J Med 1986;314:97–105.

Porush JG: New concepts in acute renal failure. Am Fam Pract 1986; 33:109–118.

Suthanthiran M, et al; Renal transplantation. N Engl J Med 1995; 331:365–376.

—D.D.B.

Chapter 4

Pulmonary Diseases

Asthma

Asthma is a common disease that affects all age groups. It has its greatest incidence in the younger population, but it can begin in patients in their eighth and ninth decades. Furthermore, it can be concurrent with, but independent of, chronic obstructive pulmonary disease (COPD) and other cardiopulmonary problems. Asthma is similar to COPD in that it is a chronic recurrent pulmonary disease with bronchoconstriction and leads to morbid, even mortal events, but it is quite different from COPD in that it involves a pathogenic mechanism in which the bronchoconstriction is reversible.

I. **Pathogenesis of asthma**

The **pathogenesis** of asthma is based on reversible bronchoconstriction that occurs as a result of the release of histamine and other short- and intermediate-acting mediators (leukotrienes) from mast cells and other inflammatory cells that have been activated by an allergen–immunoglobulin E (IgE) complex. This results in the acute and significant contraction of smooth-muscle fibers within the airways, with resultant markedly increased airway resistance. Among the large number of allergens that can precipitate such a pathogenic response are pollens, dusts, and, by an analogous mechanism with the same reversible results, exercise. Exercise is as the result of the need to humidify and warm large quantities of cold dry air, so bronchospasm from exercise is most common when exercising outside in the cold, dry air of winter.

A. **Anaphylaxis**

Asthma and other processes that are mediated by IgE result not only in acute bronchoconstriction but also in other acute and life-threatening states, such as anaphylaxis, hypotension, urticaria, angioedema of the face and pharyngeal tissues, and even death. Therefore, in addition to the bronchoconstriction, the clinician must watch for

T A B L E 4-1
Acute Emergent Management of Anaphylaxis

1. Evaluate and maintain ABCs by using the techniques of basic and advanced life support
2. Administer epinephrine aqueous, 1:1000, 0.3 mL i.v. or s.c. May repeat the dose q 10 minutes prn
3. Establish i.v. access; if patient is hypotensive, give a 500-mL bolus of 0.9 normal saline
4. If the anaphylaxis is due to a skin test or an insect bite on an extremity, apply a tourniquet to an area 2–4 cm proximal to the bite or test site
5. Administer diphenhydramine (Benadryl), 50–75 mg i.m. or i.v. or p.o. q.6–8 hr. This should be continued for 48–72 hours after the acute event to prevent another anaphylactic event from the same allergen
6. Administer methylprednisolone (Solu-Medrol), 80 mg, by i.v. bolus
7. Administer cimetidine, 400 mg, by i.v. bolus
8. Clean the site of the bite
9. Prescribe a topical β_2-agonist (e.g., albuterol) by hand-held nebulizer for any bronchospasm

and be able to manage effectively any episode of anaphylaxis in any patient with asthma. The short-term management of anaphylaxis is described in Table 4-1.

II. **Overall manifestations**

The **overall manifestations** of asthma are quite diverse in terms of type and severity of symptoms and signs. Patients often are seen with symptoms of an acute attack; at other times, the problem of wheezing, shortness of breath, and cough at various times during the year or associated with certain activities becomes evident only after a thorough review of systems.

   A. If the patient is having an acute attack, the symptoms and signs include tachypnea, tachycardia, dyspnea, cough, diffuse wheezing in inspiration and expiration, and, in severely symptomatic patients, cyanosis, stridor, and hypotension. The patient invariably has had similar episodes in the past.

   B. In patients who are not acutely symptomatic, there is usually a paucity of clinical findings; however, one can increase the sensitivity of the auscultatory pulmonary examination by auscultating the lungs during maximal and forced expiration.

   C. The patient should be queried for specific precipitating factors, including seasonal occurrence, exposure to pet hair, and exercise. This information will indicate what specific allergens are involved. If the condition is sea-

B O X 4-1

Overall Evaluation and Management of Asthma

Evaluation

1. Evaluate and maintain ABCs—airway, breathing, and cardiac maintenance—by using basic and advanced life support protocols, as needed.
2. Consider chest radiography in posteroanterior (PA) and lateral views to look for any infiltrate.
3. Obtain a sputum specimen for Gram stain to look for polymorphonuclear leukocytes (PMNs) or organisms indicative of an infectious precipitating event.
4. Consider determining the complete blood cell count with differential, looking for a leukocytosis. If an eosinophilia is present, it is quite consistent with atopic-related bronchospasm.
5. Determine oxygen saturation by using a noninvasive finger monitor. If the oxygen saturation is <92% on room air, determine arterial blood gas (ABG) values while the patient is breathing room air. ABG values are sought to document any hypoxemia or hypoventilation, which manifest with a decreased P_aO_2 and an elevated P_aCO_2. An elevated P_aCO_2 is a risk marker for respiratory decompensation.
6. Take a thorough history and perform a physical examination.

Management

1. The immediate emergency management of anaphylaxis is described in Table 4-1.
2. If severe acute asthma (status asthmaticus), administer epinephrine 1:1,000, 0.3 mL subcutaneously. This agent is a potent β_2-receptor agonist that bronchodilates optimally and effectively.
3. β_2-Receptor agonists are excellent first-line modalities in the treatment of asthma. Specific agents include albuterol (Proventil), 2.5 mL in 3 mL normal saline, administered by hand-held nebulizer, or metoproterenol (Alupent), 0.3 mL in 3 mL normal saline, administered by hand-held nebulizer. Either is very effective.
4. Provide oxygen by nasal cannula, face mask, or, if necessary, mechanical ventilation to maintain P_aO_2 >60 mm Hg or O_2 saturation >90%.
5. Steroids are effective and indicated in the manage-

(continued)

B O X 4-1 *(continued)*

ment of bronchospastic disease. For immediate treatments, agents include methylprednisolone (Solumedrol), 80 mg i.v., q.8hr, or prednisone, 60 mg p.o., once daily. The steroids, once initiated, should have a dose taper. A specific model for tapering steroids is given in Table 4-2.

6. If exercise related, instruct the patient to perform adequate warm-ups, limit the amount of exercise in cold air; use two puffs of β_2 agonists (albuterol MDI) 10 minutes before exercise.

sonal, pollen or mold are the probable allergens; if pet-related, animal dander is the most likely allergen; if associated with exercise, the underlying cause is that of breathing in large quantities of cold, dry air; wheezing is maximal 5–10 minutes after the termination of exercise. Moreover, a history of other allergies, including "hay fever" and atopic dermatitis, is not uncommon.

III. **Evaluation and management** (see Box 4-1)

The long-term **evaluation and management** of reversible airways disease consist in first, preventing or minimizing the periods of asthma, and second, minimizing, treating, and preventing any concurrent exacerbating cardiopulmonary

T A B L E 4-2
Model for Tapering Steroids

Treat acutely: methylprednisolone, 80 mg i.v. q.8hr, or prednisone, 60 mg p.o. q.A.M. Continue until the desired effect has been achieved, and then the protocol for tapering is begun.
Weaning days 1–3: 60 mg prednisone
Weaning days 4–6: 50 mg prednisone
Weaning days 7–9: 40 mg prednisone
Weaning days 10–12: 30 mg prednosine
Weaning days 13–15: 20 mg prednisone
Weaning days 16–18: 10 mg prednisone
Discontinue
Notes:
1. Titrate to the symptoms and signs. If symptoms increase, slow the taper or increase the dose and start again
2. Invariably in severe cases, a slower taper is required
3. If unable to wean, document the symptoms that occur at that level and attempt to minimize dose to lowest level
4. Dosing of steroids for asthma should be on a daily basis

problems. Efforts to meet these long-term goals can be initiated during and immediately after the acute asthmatic or anaphylactic event has been reversed.

A. **Pulmonary-function tests** (PFTs) aid in defining the specific type of obstructive airway disease. Pulmonary function tests are described in Table 4-3; typical findings in various disease categories are summarized in Table 4-4.

T A B L E   4-3
Pulmonary-Function Tests

Pulmonary-function tests (PFTs) are routinely performed to aid in the diagnosis of pulmonary dysfunction. These tests should be performed after the clinician has formulated a clinical opinion of what the patient has and should be performed when the patient is at her baseline performance status.

FEV_1 (forced expiratory volume in 1 second): The patient is instructed to inspire maximally, and then maximally to exhale. The volume in the first second of expiration is measured. If this is decreased from normal for that age group, the finding is consistent with airway obstruction.

FVC (forced vital capacity): The patient is instructed to inspire maximally, and then, using maximal force in minimal time, to exhale all of the air. The entire volume of air is measured. If this is decreased from normal for the patient's age group, the finding is consistent with a restrictive disease process

FEV_1/FVC: This calculated ratio is normally 0.80. If it is <0.80, the finding is consistent with airway obstruction

Residual volume: The volume of air remaining in the lungs after the completion of maximal expiration. It is the dead-space air. The value cannot be directly measured, but it is calculated by using the following equation:

$$RV = FRC \backslash -\backslash ERV,$$

where FRC is forced respiratory capacity and ERV is expiratory residual volume. Normal is 1,200 mL. A decrease in residual volume is consistent with restrictive disease. An increase in residual volume is consistent with obstructive disease

DLco (diffusing capacity): This is a measurement of the ability of the alveolar membrane unit to perform gas exchange. It is measured by using carbon monoxide. If decreased, it is indicative of either a decrease in the number of alveoli (e.g., emphysema) or an increased alveolar–arterial gradient ($A-ao_2$) as a result of left ventricular failure, pulmonary thromboembolic disease, or interstitial lung disease

Arterial blood gas values

T A B L E 4-4
Classic PFT Findings in Various Diseases

Disease Type	FEV$_1$	FVC	FEV$_1$/FVC	DLco	RV
Chronic bronchitis	Decreased	Normal to increased	Decreased	Normal	Normal
Emphysema	Decreased	Normal to increased	Decreased	Decreased	Increased
Asthma	Decreased	Normal to increased	Decreased	Normal	Normal
Interstitial diseases	Normal	Decreased to normal	Decreased to normal	Decreased	Normal

1. If the test reveals obstructive disease, it must be immediately repeated after a topical β_2 agonist is administered. If the obstruction resolves, it is reversible and thus essentially diagnostic of asthma.

2. If the PFT results are equivocal, the patient is undiagnosed and asymptomatic, and the clinical suspicion is moderate to high, a **challenge** with the cholinergic agent **methacholine** can be performed to increase the sensitivity of PFTs for asthma.

B. Determine the precipitating agents or events, and then advise the patient to avoid them. This should be done with a meticulous history and skin tests performed under the direction of an allergist (see the section on Rhinitis, Chapter 12, page 583, for specifics).

C. Patient and family must discontinue smoking.

D. Chronic pharmacologic intervention is best divided into two groups of patients, mildly symptomatic and significantly symptomatic.

1. If the attacks are mild and infrequent, **β_2-receptor agonist inhaler** (Alupent or Proventil) can be prescribed, to be administered through a metered-dose inhaler, two puffs q.i.d. on a prn basis.

2. If the symptoms are recurrent or severe, the patient should be given scheduled β_2 agonists delivered by metered-dose inhaler, two puffs q.i.d., and topical steroid inhalers, e.g. beclomethasone, delivered by metered-dose inhaler, two puffs q.i.d. As described in the section on Chronic Obstructive Lung Disease, the β_2 agent should be taken 3–5 minutes before the topical steroid.

a. If the patient is still symptomatic, systemic steroids are indicated. The goal is to use the lowest possible daily oral dose and to wean when indicated. The topical steroid will usually aid in the weaning process.

E. Topical anticholinergic agents, oral methylxanthines, and oral β_2 agents are of little use in the management of reversible airway disorders; at most they are adjuvants. A qualification to this statement comes from a National Institutes of Health (NIH) consensus group, which recommends adjuvant theophylline therapy in patients with severe asthma.

F. If the symptoms are **exercise-induced,** the patient should be instructed to exercise in an environment with a warm ambient temperature. The patient also should be instructed not to go from a warm ambient temperature to exercise in the cold. The use of either a β_2 agonist delivered by metered-dose inhaler or cromolyn sodium, two puffs inhaled, at the initiation of exercise, is effective in preventing the development of this form of bronchospastic disease.

IV. **Consultation**

Problem	Service	Time
All atopic-related asthma	Allergy	Elective
Severe asthma	Pulmonary	Urgent

V. **Indications for admission:** Any evidence of anaphylaxis, or any concurrent angina pectoris, left ventricular failure, or pneumonia; the patient is not improving or is deteriorating after initial therapy.

Chronic Obstructive Lung Disease

Chronic obstructive pulmonary disease (COPD) comprises a large group of chronic disorders in which a major pathophysiologic component is nonreversible or minimally reversible airways disease. This is a chronic, often progressive disorder in which obstruction develops within the bronchi and bronchioles, with or without associated destruction of alveolar tissue itself. The result is an increase in resistance to air flow during both inspiration and expiration, but to a greater degree during expiration.

I. **Pathogenesis**

The **underlying pathogenesis** of COPD is damage, thickening, or destruction of airway tissue that results in the chronic disease process. If the underlying pathogenetic mechanism is corrected, the disease stabilizes: there is no further deterioration but also no improvement. However, if the underlying pathogenetic mechanism is not reversed, there will be continuation of the damage. Thus it is of great importance to attempt to determine and modify the underlying causes early in the course of the disease to prevent further damage.

Although there is considerable overlap, the group of disorders can be divided into two large subsets, **emphysema** and **chronic bronchitis.**

A. **Emphysema** is predominantly the destruction of pulmonary tissue, predominantly alveoli, with resultant irreversible loss of gas-exchange surface and the formation of bullae, but only a mild to modest increase in airway resistance.

B. **Chronic bronchitis** is mainly a minimally reversible airways disease with resultant increased resistance to air flow and, due to dysfunction of cilia within the airways, a decrease in the ability of the lungs to mobilize secretions. This decrease in sputum clearance results in the development of tenacious sputum and an increased risk of pulmonary infections.

II. **Prevalence**

The **prevalence of COPD** in the United States is quite high, particularly in middle-aged and elderly people. Smoking tobacco or marijuana is a major risk factor in the development of COPD and a major reason for its high prevalence. Even with

B O X 4-2

Overall Evaluation and Management of an Acute Exacerbation of COPD

Evaluation

1. Evaluate and maintain ABCs—airway, breathing, and cardiac maintenance—by basic and advanced life support protocols, as indicated.
2. Determine the underlying precipitating event and the basic underlying major pathologic group (see Table 4-5).
3. Take a thorough history, including tobacco use in the past or present, and perform a physical examination.
4. Determine ABG values on room air if possible, looking for hypoxemia or any evidence of hypoventilation, as manifested by a respiratory acidosis (i.e., an increased P_aco_2). The new onset of an elevated P_aco_2 is a marker for impending respiratory failure.
5. Perform laboratory examinations, including levels of theophylline, electrolytes, blood urea nitrogen (BUN), creatinine, and glucose, and a complete blood cell (CBC) count with differential for baseline purposes.
6. Obtain chest radiographs in PA and lateral views and a 12-lead electrocardiogram (ECG) at the time of presentation to look for any evidence of an infiltrate, indicative of a pneumonitis, or any ischemic cardiac changes, respectively.
7. Perform baseline spirometry at the bedside or in the examination room. Peak expiratory flow is a baseline marker and is repeated as an objective marker for therapeutic improvement in the acute setting. The normal value of this marker of airway resistance, in which the number measured is inversely related to airway resistance, is >300 mL. It is a crude objective measurement that is best used when interpreted in the clinical setting and for immediate follow-up of therapeutic interventions.
8. Obtain a sputum specimen of any productive cough for gross observation and Gram stain. The presence of PMNs and organisms strongly suggests an infection as the precipitating event.

(continued)

B O X   4-2 (continued)

Management

1. Administer oxygen by nasal cannula, face mask, or other methods (including mechanical ventilation) to maintain arterial oxygen pressure >60 mm Hg or O_2 saturation ≥90%. Monitor P_aCO_2 closely after initiating oxygen therapy as O_2 can, in some cases, decrease the patient's ventilatory drive and result in respiratory failure.

2. The short-term management of an acute exacerbation is tailored to the underlying specific precipitating cause (i.e., heart failure, pulmonary thromboembolic disease, bronchitis, or pneumonitis).
   a. If due to left ventricular failure, treat as such.
   b. If due to pulmonary thromboembolic disease, treat as such (see section on Pleuritic Chest Pain, Pulmonary Thromboembolic Disease, page 221).
   c. If an infectious origin is suspected, either bronchitis or pneumonitis, and especially if purulent sputum is present, antibiotics are clearly indicated.

---

public health education and legislative efforts to decrease the use of tobacco, 30% of the population still uses tobacco on a regular basis. Furthermore, there is a disconcerting increase in the use of such products by young people. Another risk factor for the development of COPD, especially emphysema, is a deficiency in the enzyme α_1-antitrypsin.

III. **Overall manifestations** (see Box 4-2)

The **overall manifestations** of COPD often will not occur until quite late in the disease course or during an acute exacerbation of the chronic process. Although there are some overlapping features, the symptoms and signs will be divided into those related to emphysema, chronic bronchitis, or acute exacerbations of COPD. A particularly useful test is that of the **forced expiration time (FET)**, which is measured by auscultation over the trachea and measuring the time it takes completely to exhale a maximal breath; if the FET is >6 seconds, it is consistent with significant COPD, with a sensitivity of 74% and specificity of 75%.

A. **Emphysema** in the chronic state manifests with diffuse hyperresonance, increased AP diameter of the chest wall, decreased exercise tolerance, nonproductive cough, and peripheral cyanosis.

B. **Chronic bronchitis** in the chronic state manifests with cough productive of purulent sputum. By definition, the

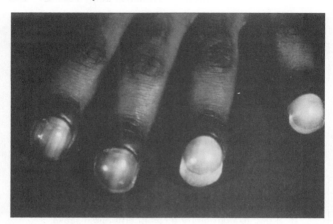

F I G U R E   4-1
Clubbing.

cough must be one that occurs daily and is productive of purulent sputum for >3 months per year for 3 consecutive years. In addition to the cough, other common findings include an increased AP diameter of the chest wall, significant wheezes, especially at the end of expiration, and potentially cyanosis.

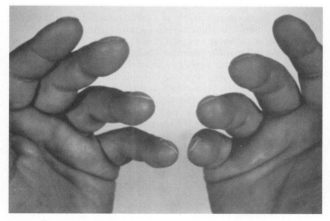

F I G U R E   4-2
Clubbing.

C. An acute exacerbation of any of the chronic processes includes an increase in cough from baseline, an increase in the quantity of sputum, and/or a change in sputum from white to yellow; fevers; chills; an increase in shortness of breath; an increase in wheezing; chest tightness; and any symptoms and signs associated with the precipitating factor. Table 4-5 describes the various precipitating factors and their specific manifestations.

IV. Pharmacologic agents

Agents of use in the management of an acute exacerbation of COPD include the following:

A. β_2-**Agonist inhalers** administered by hand-held nebulizer. Either albuterol (Proventil) or metoproterenol (Alupent) is quite effective.

    1. The **mechanism of action** is to increase cyclic adenosine monophosphate (cAMP) in the smooth-muscle

T A B L E 4-5
Precipitating Factors in Acute Exacerbations of COPD

Process	Features
Left ventricular failure	Orthopnea
	Paroxysmal nocturnal dyspnea
	Dyspnea on exertion
	Third heart sound
	Crackles, bibasilar
	Pulmonary vasculature redistribution and cardiomegaly on chest radiograph
Pulmonary thromboembolic disease	Pleuritic chest pain
	Dyspnea
	Asymmetric lower extremity swelling
	Tachypnea
	No acute change on chest radiograph
Acute bronchitis	Purulent sputum
	Low-grade fever
	Rhonchorous breath sounds
	Wheezing, diffuse
	Dyspnea
	No acute change on chest radiograph
Pneumonitis	Purulent sputum
	Fevers, often spiking to >102°F
	Lobar consolidation with bronchial breath sounds
	Infiltrate on chest radiograph

cells of the bronchial tree via the stimulation of β-adrenergic receptors on those cells. The increase in cAMP results in relaxation of these bronchi and therefore a decrease in the airway resistance.

2. **Side effects** include the development of supraventricular tachycardias and muscle tremulousness.
3. **Recommended regimens:**

> Albuterol (Proventil), 2.5 mL in 3 mL of normal saline by hand-held nebulizer,
> or
> Metoproterenol (Alupent), 0.3 mL in 3 mL of normal saline by hand-held nebulizer.

> These treatments can be repeated in 30–60 minutes.

B. **Antibiotics** are of use in the management of acute exacerbations of COPD, even when given empirically.
1. The **mechanism of action** of these agents is to kill any bacteria acutely infecting the bronchial airways, thus decreasing secretion production in general and purulent sputum production in specific.
2. **Side effects** include diarrhea and the risk of anaphylaxis.
3. The **doses and regimens** depend on the suspected infection.
   a. If pneumonitis, refer to the section on Community-Acquired Pneumonitis, page 231.
   b. If bronchitis or for empirical therapy, initiate therapy with:

   > Trimethoprim (TMP)-sulfa (Bactrim DS) p.o., b.i.d. for 7 days
   > or
   > Amoxicillin, 500 mg p.o., t.i.d. for 7 days
   > or
   > Ciprofloxacin, 500 mg p.o., b.i.d. for 7 days

   > Any of these regimens is effective against the most common bacterial pathogens in acute bronchitis, the gram-negative coccobacillus *Haemophilus influenzae* and the gram-positive coccus *Streptococcus pneumoniae*.

C. Topical anticholinergic agents are of benefit in the acute setting. These agents have been conclusively demonstrated to be the cornerstone in the treatment of COPD, specifically that of chronic bronchitis.
1. The **mechanism of action** of these agents, which include ipratropium bromide (Atrovent), is to relax smooth muscle and to decrease the quantity of secretions within the airways.
2. **Side effects** are rare but can include dry mouth and tachycardia.

3. **Dosage:**

Atrovent, two puffs q.i.d. by metered-dose inhaler, given 5 minutes after β-agonist inhalation therapy.

D. **Steroids** are indicated if the patient remains symptomatic or has signs of obstruction after initiation of this therapy, or if there is any component of atopic disease to the underlying process.

1. The **mechanism of action** of steroids is not completely clear but is probably multifactorial and includes inhibition of the release of inflammatory mediators (leukotrienes, histamines) that mediate the reversible component of the bronchoconstriction. These agents often take a longer time to be effective, and thus benefit from them is not immediate but occurs 12–24 hours after initiation.

2. **Side effects** include delirium and psychotic behavior, and, in the long term, immunosuppression, osteoporosis, and decreased wound healing.

3. The **dosing of steroids** in the acute setting is:

Solumedrol, 80 mg i.v., q.8hr,
or
Prednisone, 40–60 mg p.o., q.d.

Either regimen is continued for several (3–5) days and then tapered (see Table 4-2).

E. **Theophylline.** Before the development of other, more effective modalities, this agent was a mainstay of acute management of an exacerbation of COPD; this is no longer the case.

1. The **mechanism of action** of this agent is to increase cAMP by completely inhibiting the enzyme that degrades cAMP, phosphodiesterase, and, with the increased cAMP, to relax bronchiolar smooth muscle; furthermore, it has a mild diuretic effect.

2. **Side effects** include nausea, vomiting, tremor, restlessness, and tachycardia.

3. The **loading dose** is 5 mg/kg i.v., given over 15 minutes, followed by a **maintenance dose** of 0.5 mg/kg/hr i.v. The loading dose should be administered only after the baseline theophylline level has been checked and documented to be <4 mg/dL. If the patient has at presentation a theophylline level in the therapeutic range, give the patient the maintenance dose only. The therapeutic range is 10–20 mg/dL.

V. **Evaluation and management**

The intermediate and long-term evaluation and management of these disorders, whether emphysema or chronic bronchitis predominates, include the following points. The major goals of management are prevention, patient education, and providing pharmacologic palliation on a long-term basis.

A. Define the extent of the COPD and determine whether there is any underlying reversible component to the process. This is best done through the history and physical examination and PFTs after the patient is at baseline (i.e., not during an acute exacerbation of the process; see Tables 4-3 and 4-4 for PFT diagnostic criteria).

B. Instruct the patient and all family members to discontinue smoking, which will decrease the patient's exposure to direct and second-hand smoke.

C. Vaccinations include a one-time dose of Pneumovax (pneumococcal vaccine), *Hemophilus influenzae* vaccine, and a yearly influenza immunization.

D. **Pharmacologic interventions** for the long-term management of COPD include the same types of agents as are used for immediate exacerbations of COPD. Because this is not a reversible process, the agents used must assist the normally functioning pulmonary tissue, reverse any and all concurrent reversible bronchospastic disease, and minimize secretions.

   1. **Inhalation agents** include the β_2 agonists albuterol (Proventil) or metoproterenol (Alupent) delivered by metered-dose inhaler, two puffs q.i.d.; the topical anticholinergic ipratropium sulfate (Atrovent) delivered by metered-dose inhaler, two puffs q.i.d.; and the topical steroid beclomethasone delivered by metered-dose inhaler, two puffs q.i.d. These topical/inhalation modalities are the foundation of long-term pharmacologic therapy.

      a. The agents should be initiated and used in the order in which they are listed here. The β_2 agonist should be started first, and then, if the patient remains symptomatic, the topical anticholinergic agent should be added, followed by the topical steroid. If two or all three of the agents are being used, the patient should be instructed to use the β_2 agonist by metered-dose inhaler first, wait 3–5 minutes, use the topical anticholinergic agent, wait 3–5 minutes, and then use the topical steroid.

      b. Because all of the agents are delivered through a metered-dose inhaler, be sure the patient knows how to use this device.

   2. Long-term oral steroid use should be reserved for patients with severely symptomatic disease that remains clinically significant even with optimal and maximal therapy. The daily dose should be as small as possible and titrated to the symptoms of dyspnea and wheezing.

   3. Long-term oral methylxanthines such as theophylline can be of some adjuvant use, especially in patients who remain symptomatic on maximal topical therapy.

T A B L E 4-6
Indications for Low-Flow Home Oxygen Therapy (American Thoracic Society)

1. P_aO_2 <55 mm Hg on room air
2. O_2 saturation <90% on room air
3. Exercise-induced or sleep-induced decrease in P_aO_2 to <55 mm Hg
4. Primary pulmonary hypertension
5. Cor pulmonale

The oral maintenance dose is usually 200–300 mg p.o., q.12hr of the long-acting theophylline preparation (e.g., Theodur). The therapeutic range is 10–20 mg/dL.

4. The use of oral β_2 agents in addition to or instead of topical β_2 agents results in more side effects than does inhalation treatment alone and is of no clear advantage. Therefore, it is of little or no benefit even as an adjuvant modality.

5. **Low-flow long-term oxygen therapy** is a relatively high-cost modality that benefits only a subset of patients with COPD. These patients include patients with cor pulmonale (right ventricular failure), patients who have a P_aO_2 <55 mm Hg, and patients with sleep apnea. (The evaluation and management of sleep apnea is quite complex, requires the consultation of a pulmonary colleague, and is beyond the scope of this textbook). Table 4-6 lists specific indications for the home use of long-term oxygen therapy.

6. Phlebotomy to keep the hematocrit ≤52%, if secondary erythrocytosis is present, is of short- and long-term benefit.

7. Instruct the patient to initiate an oral antibiotic, e.g., Bacterim or Amotoxicillin, for which he or she has as a prewritten prescription, for 5–7 days at the onset of any purulent sputum changes.

VI. **Consultation**

Problem	Service	Time
Severe COPD	Pulmonary	Elective
Any atopic component	Allergy	Elective
If heart failure is present	Cardiology	Urgent

VII. **Indications for admission:** Any patient who requires steroids in the acute setting; any patient who does not improve after two β_2-agonist treatments; or any patient with concurrent or concomitant unstable angina pectoris, pulmonary thromboembolic disease, left ventricular failure, or pneumonitis.

Hemoptysis (see Box 4-3)

The anatomy of the airway system is quite simple. It is essentially an inverted hollow tree in which the trunk is the upper airway system, consisting of the nasopharynx, mouth, oropharynx, hypopharynx, larynx, and trachea; and the branches compose the lower airway system, consisting of the bronchi, bronchioles, and alveoli. Although the anatomy is simple to describe, the component structures are quite diverse, and any part of it can bleed, resulting in hemoptysis, the coughing up of blood. Because the blood can come from any part of the respiratory tract, because the gastrointestinal tract (GI) is contiguous with the respiratory tract, and because patients themselves define hemoptysis in different ways, the problem of hemoptysis is quite diverse.

I. **Overall manifestations**

The **overall manifestations** of hemoptysis include the features of the hemoptysis itself and associated manifestations. Hemoptysis is best described in terms of quantity. If there is a scant amount of blood or whitish yellow sputum streaked with blood, it is called mild hemoptysis, whereas if there is a large quantity of gross blood (i.e., >200 mL (~1/2 cup) in a 24-hour period), it is called massive hemoptysis.

The **associated manifestations** can include a change in the quantity or quality of sputum, tachypnea, dyspnea, chest

---

B O X 4-3

Overall Evaluation and Management of Hemoptysis

Evaluation

1. Evaluate ABCs and institute basic and advanced life-support modalities, as airway maintenance and ventilation are major concerns in patients with hemoptysis.
2. Take a thorough history and perform a physical examination, looking for features described under I. Overall manifestations. Query the patient regarding the source of the bleeding. Often the patient can localize the site of bleeding to the right or left lung, the upper airways, or the lower airways.
3. Examine the mouth for bleeding sites and the nose for epistaxis.
4. Obtain chest radiographs in PA and lateral views to look for infiltrates, nodules, and lesions.
5. Determine prothrombin time (PT), activated par-

(continued)

tial thromboplastin time (aPTT), and platelet count, looking for any evidence of coagulopathy such as an increased PT, an increased aPTT, or a decreased platelet count.

6. Determine the CBC count with differential for baseline purposes.
7. Determine ABG values for baseline purposes and to diagnose any hypoxemia, which would be indicative of significant blood in the pulmonary tree.
8. Examine the sputum directly visually to ascertain what specifically the patient is expectorating.
9. Obtain a Gram stain of the sputum, looking for any PMNs and bacteria indicative of an infectious bronchitis or pneumonitis.
10. Send a sputum sample for acid-fast bacillus (AFB) smear and culture. The presence of AFB is indicative of active mycobacterial disease. This procedure is unnecessary if the chest radiograph is normal.
11. Place the patient on respiratory isolation if mycobacterial disease is suspected.
12. Send a sputum sample for cytologic examination to look for malignant cells, diagnostic of a malignant lesion in the respiratory tree.
13. Provide oxygen supplementation to keep P_aO_2 >60 mm Hg.

Management

If the bleeding is mild, determine its source and cause, and treat the underlying condition. If the bleeding is massive, the patient's condition can rapidly deteriorate, and thus emergent management is clearly indicated. A basic approach to massive hemoptysis includes the following steps.

1. Admit the patient to a monitored bed, preferably in an intensive care unit (ICU).
2. If the lesion is localized on the chest radiograph, the patient should keep the ipsilateral side inferior.
3. Correct any coagulopathy.
4. Provide cough suppression with codeine, 30 mg p.o., q.4–6hr.
5. Obtain emergent consultation with cardiothoracic surgeons and pulmonologists for rigid bronchoscopy.

Further management is beyond the scope of this text.

T A B L E 4-7
Hemoptysis: Differential Diagnosis and Features

Etiology	Mild/Massive	Associated Features	Chest Radiograph	Evaluation and Management
Acute Bronchitis	Mild	Cough, worse at night Purulent sputum Low-grade fever	Normal, or no change from baseline	Box 4-3, sputa examination and Gram stain Organism: *H. influenzae* *Branhamella catrrhalis* *Streptococci sps* Cough suppression Bactrim DS b.i.d. p.o. or amoxicillin 500 mg p.o. t.i.d. for 7 days
Neoplastic lesion	Mild to massive	Weight loss Clubbing (Figs. 4-1 and 4-2) Smoking history Cough	Solitary nodule Can have cavity and/or an infiltrate	Box 4-3, and sputum cytology; sensitivity <50% for sputum cytology

Pulmonary infarction	Mild to massive	Pleuritic chest pain, asymmetric lower extremity swelling	Normal, or pleural-based infiltrate with effusion	Box 4-3 and see section on Pleuritic Chest Pain, page 221; V/Q, venous Doppler studies of lower extremities; Anticoagulate with heparin
Myobacterial infections	Mild to massive	Reactive PPD, weight loss	Simon foci; Ghon focus/complex; Cavitary apical lesion	Box 4-3 and respiratory isolation; INH/rifampin/ethambutol/PZA see page 9
Left ventricular failure	Mild	Orthopnea; PND; Dyspnea; Third heart sound	Cardiomegaly; Increased pulmonary vascular distribution	Box 4-3; see chapter 1, page 9
Aspergillosis	Massive	History of COPD/emphysema with bullae	Mass in cavity or bulla in one apex	Resection/CT surgery consult
Bronchiectasis	Mild	Cystic fibrosis; Intermittent purulent and bloody sputa; Severe chronic cough; Clubbing (Figs. 4-1 and 4-2)	Chronic infiltrate; dilated bronchi	Penicillin VK 500 mg p.o. q.i.d.; Pulmonary consultation

pain, pleuritic chest pain, nausea, vomiting, hematemesis, and fevers. Because the GI tract is contiguous with the respiratory tract, the clinician must differentiate hematemesis from hemoptysis.

II. **Differential diagnosis**

The **differential diagnosis** of hemoptysis, the pathogenesis, the unique characteristics of each underlying state, and a brief summary of evaluation and management are given subsequently and in Table 4-7.

III. **Consultation**

Problem	Service	Time
Any suspicion of neoplasia	Pulmonary	Urgent
Massive hemoptysis	Pulmonary	Emergent
Bronchiectasis	Pulmonary	Urgent
Massive hemoptysis	Cardiothoracic surgery	Emergent
Left ventricular failure	Cardiology	Urgent

IV. **Indications for admission:** Massive hemoptysis, heart failure, hemodynamic instability, or any evidence of respiratory compromise.

Pleural Effusions (see Box 4-4)

The pleural space is normally a potential space. It is, by definition, the area between the visceral pleura—a simple squamous epithelial lining directly applied to the lung—and the parietal pleura—a simple squamous epithelial lining applied to the inner surface of the chest wall. The pleural space in each hemithorax is essentially independent of the other in the normal state. The pleural space in the healthy, normal adult has <50 mL of transudative fluid in each hemithorax. Any quantity of fluid in excess of that amount in either hemithorax is termed a **pleural effusion.**

I. **Overall manifestations**

The **overall manifestations** of pleural effusions include orthopnea, especially if the effusions are bilateral; trepopnea, if the effusion is unilateral (the patient preferentially sleeps with the side ipsilateral to the effusion down); dyspnea on exertion; nonproductive cough; and baseline dyspnea. Further signs over the area of effusion include localized dullness to percussion with concurrent decreased breath sounds and decreased tactile fremitus in the same area. There is often an area of bronchial breath sounds at the superior border of the area of decreased breath sounds. The bronchial breath sounds occur as a result of adjacent atelectasis of the lung tissue.

II. **Additional evaluation**

Further evaluation entails categorizing the pleural effusion as transudative, exudative, or bloody. Each category of pleural effusion has differentiating features, a specific differential

B O X 4-4

Overall Evaluation of Pleural Effusions

Evaluation

1. Take a thorough history and perform a physical examination, looking for overall manifestations.
2. Obtain chest radiographs in PA, lateral, and decubitus views (Fig. 4-3). The decubitus radiograph is best obtained with the affected side down and is used to determine what quantity of fluid moves, or "layers out" with gravity. If >1 cm fluid layers out, then it is quite safe to perform thoracentesis. Any effusion that does not layer out or is <1 cm should be further localized by ultrasonography (US) and thoracentesis performed under US guidance.
3. Perform thoracentesis. The tests used to evaluate all pleural effusions include the following:
   a. Gross appearance: clear, bloody, or purulent.
   b. Pleural fluid lactate dehydrogenase (LDH).
   c. Plasma LDH (obtained within 24 hours of thoracentesis).
   d. Total protein content of pleural fluid.
   e. Total protein content of plasma (obtained within 24 hours of thoracentesis).
4. Categorize the fluid as transudative or exudative, based on these parameters; see discussion in this section and Table 4-8.
5. Save some fluids in case the fluid is exudative. If it is, further tests are indicated.
6. Obtain a postthoracentesis chest radiograph to rule out any postprocedure pneumothorax.
7. Specific tests to be performed on pleural effusions that are exudates:
   a. Glucose: Decreased in rheumatoid-related and in a complicated parapneumonic effusion.
   b. Antinuclear antibody (ANA): If >1:160, consistent with lupus pleuritis.
   c. ANA ratio (pleural fluid/plasma): If >1, consistent with lupus pleuritis.
   d. Lupus erythematosus (LE) cell prep: If present, consistent with lupus pleuritis.
   e. Amylase: If elevated, consistent with pancreatitis or esophageal rupture.
   f. Triglycerides: If >110 mg/dL, consistent with a chylothorax.

(continued)

B O X   4-4 (continued)

g. Chylomicrons: If present, consistent with a chylo-thorax.
h. Hematocrit: If >1%, consistent with pulmonary in-farction, malignant neoplastic or trauma related.
   (N.B. an RBC count of 100,000/mm³ is equiva-lent to an HCT of 1%)
i. White blood count: If >10,000/mm³, consistent with an inflammatory origin.
j. Differential count:
   If lymphocytosis: Malignancy or mycobacterial disease.
   If eosinophilia (i.e., >10%): Mycobacterial or drug-induced lupus; marked decrease in risk that it is malignant.
k. pH: If <6.0: rupture of the esophagus.
   If parapneumonic and <7.1, complicated para-pneumonic effusion.

diagnosis, and thus a different scheme of evaluation and man-agement (see Tables 4-8 and 4-9).

A. **Transudative effusions:** LDH of pleural fluid, <200 IU; protein of pleural fluid, <3.0 g; ratio of LDH in pleural fluid to LDH in plasma, <0.6; ratio of total protein in pleural fluid to total protein in plasma, <0.5.

   1. The **pathogenesis** of transudative effusions results from changes in the Starling forces that maintain fluid in the intravascular spaces, either an increase in the hydrostatic pressure (as in heart failure) and/or a de-creased albumin (e.g., as a result of cirrhosis or ne-phrotic syndrome; see Table 4-9).

   2. The **evaluation and management** of transudative effu-sions entail treating the underlying pathologic process, which is virtually always clinically evident. No other

T A B L E   4-8
Light's Criteria for Transudative versus Exudative Effusions

Parameter Evaluated	Transudative	Exudative
LDH	<200 IU	>200 IU
Pleural fluid/plasma LDH ratio	<0.6	>0.6
Total protein	<3 g	>3 g
Pleural fluid/plasma protein ratio	<0.5	>0.5

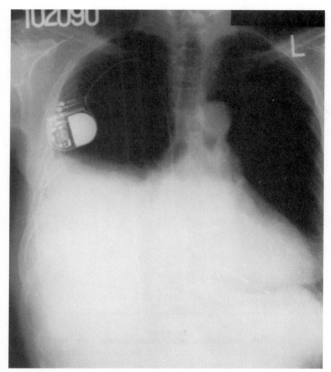

FIGURE 4-3
Posteroanterior chest radiograph showing massive right pleural
effusion.

evaluation of the fluid itself is necessary. **Therapeutic
thoracentesis** of 500–1,000 mL of fluid is indicated
only if the effusion is massive and the patient is quite
symptomatic due to its size. **Management** of left ventricular failure, cirrhosis, and nephrotic syndrome are
described elsewhere in the book.
  B. **Exudative effusions:** LDH of pleural fluid, >200 IU; protein of pleural fluid, >3 g; ratio of LDH in pleural fluid
to LDH in plasma, >0.6; ratio of total protein in pleural
fluid to total protein in plasma, >0.5.
    1. The **pathogenesis** of exudative effusions is more di-
verse and portends a more malignant course. The differential diagnosis is outlined in Table 4-9.

T A B L E 4-9
Differential Diagnosis of Pleural Effusions

Transudative

Left ventricular failure
Cirrhosis
Nephrotic syndrome

Exudative

Parapneumonic
Viral
Bacterial
Pulmonary infarction
Mycobacterial
Rheumatoid
SLE
Lymphoproliferative
Malignant neoplastic
Pancratitis

Bloody

Trauma
Malignant neoplasia
Mesothelioma
Pulmonary infarction

2. The **evaluation and management** are significantly more extensive than for transudative effusions. Laboratory tests on the pleural fluid itself include pH, Gram stain, cultures, cytology, AFB smear, glucose, amylase, cell count, and rheumatoid factor assay. Further evaluation and management depend on the results of these tests and are beyond the scope of this text.

a. If there is gross pus, if Gram stain demonstrates bacteria (i.e., empyema), or if the pleural fluid glucose is <20 mg/dL and pH is <7.0 (i.e., a complicated parapneumonic effusion as a result of a bacterial pneumonia), the clinician must involve pulmonologists or cardiothoracic surgeons for chest-tube drainage procedures.

b. If the effusion is parapneumonic but the glucose level is >20 mg/dL and the pH is >7.0 (i.e., an uncomplicated parapneumonic effusion), the clinician must watch closely and repeat the thoracentesis on alternate days until it has resolved, looking for a decrease in the pleural fluid glucose or pH, or the development of an empyema, any of which would necessitate the placement of a chest tube.

       c. If malignant cytology is present (i.e., malignant neo-plastic effusion), consultations with oncologists and pulmonologists should be sought. Chest-tube drainage is indicated if the effusion is massive and symptomatic.

  C. Bloody pleural effusions are not uncommon and are virtually always exudative in nature.

    1. The **pathogenesis** of bloody effusions is diverse and portends a more malignant course. The differential diagnosis is outlined in Table 4-9.

    2. The **evaluation and management** of bloody effusions are significantly more extensive than for transudative effusions. Laboratory studies of the pleural fluid itself include pH, Gram stain, cultures, cytology, AFB smear, glucose, amylase, cell count, hematocrit, and rheumatoid factor assay. As with other pleural effusions, therapy must be tailored to the underlying process. Consultation with pulmonologists should be sought.

III. Consultation

Problem	Service	Time
Exudative effusion	Pulmonary	Urgent
Bloody effusion	Pulmonary	Urgent
Empyema	Cardiothoracic surgery	Emergent
Nephrotic syndrome	Renal	Urgent
Malignant effusion	Oncology	Urgent

IV. Indications for admission: Any evidence of respiratory compromise due to the effusion, or any evidence of an empyema or a complicated parapneumonic effusion.

Pleuritic Chest Pain

Pleuritic chest pain is defined as pain that is exacerbated by inspiration or expiration. It is often pain that is invariably referable or attributable to irritation of the pleura. The pleura is a simple squamous epithelium that is derived from mesoderm and lines the lungs and chest wall. The visceral pleura lines the lungs, whereas the parietal pleura lines the inside of the chest wall. Inflammation, disruption, or dysfunction of either the parietal or visceral pleura manifests with pleuritic-type chest pain. Although many processes can manifest with pleuritic-type chest pain, four of the most common or reversible specific syndromes are discussed here: pneumothorax, musculoskeletal chest pain, pneumonitis, and pulmonary thromboembolic disease.

  I. Pneumothorax

    Pneumothorax may cause pleuritic chest pain. There is the acquired disruption of the parietal or visceral pleural membrane with resultant leakage of atmospheric air into the pleural space. The pleuritic chest pain is always on the same side as the pneumothorax. There are two types of pneumothoraces, simple and tension.

A. A **simple pneumothorax** remains the same size immediately, and then resolves with time. Simple pneumothoraces can be dangerous in and of themselves because they result in restriction of respiratory volume and may lead to significant respiratory compromise or develop into tension pneumothoraces. The **specific manifestations** include pleuritic-type chest pain, mild tachypnea, and decreased breath sounds in the lung ipsilateral to the pneumothorax. Precipitating causes of simple and tension pneumothoraces may be iatrogenic (e.g., thoracentesis or central-line placement), traumatic (e.g., rib fracture or a penetrating wound to the chest), or spontaneous, usually in patients with risk factors (e.g., coughing fits, bullous disease, a history of pneumothoraces). **Evaluation and management** include that described in Box 4-5 and watching for the development of a tension pneumothorax.

B. A **tension pneumothorax** is one in which the process is severe and unchecked, with a significant and progressive inflow of air into the pleural space. The process invariably results in collapse of the ipsilateral lung and displacement of all thoracic structures to the contralateral hemithorax.

B O X 4-5

Overall Evaluation and Management of Pneumothorax

Evaluation

1. Evaluate and maintain ABCs by using basic and advanced life-support protocols.
2. Obtain chest radiographs in PA and lateral views to look for, diagnose, or confirm the presence of a pneumothorax (Fig. 4-4).
3. Determine ABG values, preferably with the patient breathing room air, as baseline. Any hypoxemia is of significant import.
4. Provide supplemental oxygen via nasal cannula or face mask to maintain Pao_2 >60 mm Hg.
5. A tension pneumothorax or a simple pneumothorax that occupies >20% of the ipsilateral hemithorax requires immediate chest-tube placement.
6. If the patient has a simple pneumothorax and it is asymptomatic and <20% of the hemithorax is affected, conservative treatment is indicated. Follow up with examinations and chest radiographs every 12–24 hours until the process has resolved.

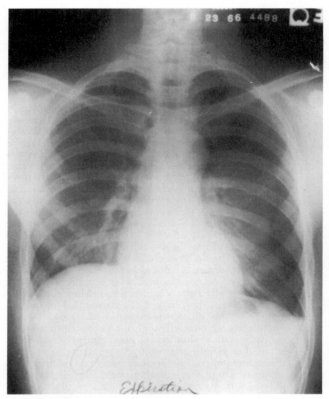

FIGURE 4-4
Anteroposterior chest radiograph taken in expiration and showing a
large left pneumothorax.

A tension pneumothorax can be rapidly fatal if not diagnosed and treated immediately. The **specific manifestations** of a tension pneumothorax include pleuritic-type
chest pain, decreased breath sounds, and hyperresonance,
all ipsilateral to the pneumothorax. Additional manifestations include tachycardia, tachypnea, and a shift of the
trachea and other mediastinal structures to the contralateral side. **Evaluation and management** of a tension pneumothorax include that described in Box 4-5 and emergency intervention. Intervention entails the insertion of
a 14-gauge needle into the affected hemithorax, or, better,
emergency chest-tube placement either laterally or, for
time efficiency, anteriorly. All tension pneumothoraces

require chest-tube placement with consultation with cardiothoracic surgeons. The pleuritic chest pain will resolve with resolution of the pneumothorax.

II. **Musculoskeletal chest pain**

This is the most common reason for pleuritic-type chest pain. In the vast majority of cases, it is self-limited and benign, but it may be a harbinger of a more significant problem.

A. **Trauma** is the most common cause of musculoskeletal chest pain. The **specific manifestations** include antecedent blunt trauma with associated bruising, ecchymosis, splinting, and potentially one or more rib fractures. **Evaluation and management,** especially if the pain is significant, include rib films and chest radiographs in PA and lateral views. The chest radiographs are required to rule out any concurrent pneumothorax or hemothorax. If there are no associated or evident complications, nonsteroidal antiinflammatory drugs (NSAIDs; e.g., ibuprofen, 600–800 mg p.o., q.6hr prn) or even a short course of a narcotic agent (e.g., Tylenol 3, one tablet p.o., q.4–6hr prn) can be prescribed and are effective in affording analgesia. The application of tape to the chest wall is of little value. Follow-up should be as clinically needed.

B. **Tietze's syndrome** is a not uncommon cause of pleuritic musculoskeletal chest pain. This is nonspecific, usually trauma-related, costochondritis (i.e., inflammation of the joints between the ribs and the sternum). The **specific manifestations** include pain that is demonstrable and completely reproduced by palpation of the costochondral joints. **Specific evaluation and management** include initiation of an NSAID or a narcotic-type agent.

C. **Nontraumatic rib fracture** can occur in a patient with severe recurrent cough or with lytic rib lesions; therefore, if a rib fracture occurs and there is no history of antecedent trauma, one must ask why it occurred. If a lytic lesion is present, evaluation and management with serum protein electrophoresis (SPEP), erythrocyte sedimentation rate (ESR), urine protein electrophoresis (UPEP), and bone biopsy are indicated, as the most likely diagnosis is a monoclonal gammopathy (See page 266.).

III. **Pneumonitis**

This is a not uncommon cause of pleuritic chest pain. Inflammation of the lung parenchyma invariably leads to inflammation of the adjacent pleura, causing pleuritic-type chest pain. This is most evident in *Streptococcus pneumoniae* pneumonitis. (See section on Community-Acquired Pneumonitis for further discussion, page 231.)

IV. **Pulmonary thromboembolic disease** (PTE; Box 4-6)

This is perhaps, with the exception of a tension pneumothorax, the most immediately ominous diagnosis that manifests

B O X 4-6

Overall Evaluation and Management of Potential Pulmonary Thromboembolic Disease

Evaluation

1. Take a thorough history and perform a physical examination, documenting any history of venous thromboembolic disease and the items described under IV, C (overall manifestations) in the text.
2. Assess the patient for risk factors.
3. Perform a guaiac test on the stool to document that the patient is not concurrently bleeding from a GI site, a contraindication to anticoagulation.
4. Determine ABG values for baseline purposes. Values suggestive of mild hyperventilation (i.e., a decreased P_aCO_2) and hypoxemia (i.e., a decreased P_aO_2) are consistent with pulmonary thromboembolic disease. A normal arterial oxygen level, however, does not rule out PTE, as evidenced by the fact that 20% of patients with PTE have arterial oxygen levels >80 mm Hg.
5. Obtain chest radiographs in PA and lateral views, looking for any infiltrates. The vast majority of patients with PTE disease will have normal chest radiographs.
6. Consider obtaining a 12-lead ECG for baseline purposes. The vast majority of patients with PTE disease will have sinus tachycardia as the sole ECG manifestation.
7. Determine aPTT and PT for baseline purposes in the event that anticoagulation is indicated.
8. Determine the CBC count with differential for baseline purposes in the event that anticoagulation is indicated.
9. Determine the platelet count for baseline purposes in the event that anticoagulation is indicated.
10. Further evaluation and management are based on the clinical suspicion for PTE as determined by the evaluation described (i.e. stratify the suspicion as to high, intermediate, or low clinical suspicion). Further evaluation and management is as in text (high suspicion: E.1, low suspicion: E.2, intermediate suspicion, E.3)
11. Consider hypercoagulable-state evaluation, especially for antithrombin III and factor V Leiden levels.

with pleuritic-type chest pain. It is a relatively common disease process, especially in patients at high risk for the development of deep venous thrombosis (DVT).

A. The **pathogenesis** and **natural history** of this disorder are
integral to its evaluation and management. This will be
divided into two areas of discussion, the sites where emboli originate and the risk factors for their development.

   1. Emboli that reach the pulmonary arteries originate
   from some specific site.

      a. The **deep venous systems** of the thighs and pelvis
      are the most common sites of formation of thrombi
      that embolize to the pulmonary arteries. In fact, the
      vast majority (>95%) of emboli come from these
      sites.

      b. Another site of potential thrombus formation is the
      deep system of the upper arm. Although it is quite
      uncommon for an arm DVT to develop, once pres-
      ent, it may embolize to the pulmonary arteries.

      c. Another potential but quite rare site of venous
      thromboembolism is the right ventricle.

   2. It is exceedingly rare for a thrombus isolated to the
   calf (i.e., distal to the popliteal fossa) to embolize to
   the pulmonary artery unless it has already propagated
   (extended) into the popliteal fossa or even further proximally into the thigh.

B. **Risk factors** for the development of thrombi and therefore
of thromboembolic events include, but are not limited to,
immobilization, concurrent carcinoma, the recent dona-
tion of plasma, a history of thromboembolism, a family
history of PTE events, the use of estrogens, and a congenital or acquired hypercoagulable state. **Defined hypercoagulable states** include deficiencies in natural anticoagulation factors such as antithrombin III, protein C, and
protein S. In addition, a quite common risk factor for the
development of DVT is **factor V Leiden.** This mutation
results in resistance to activated protein C and a change
in the primary polypeptide structure of Ara 506 Gln and
is found in 20% of patients with DVT/PTE.

C. The **overall manifestations** of PTE disease include pleuritic-type chest pain, but this is a far from universal finding. Other symptoms and signs include tachypnea, dyspnea, hemoptysis, pleural friction rub, low-grade fever,
and asymmetric swelling of the lower extremities. P_aO_2 is
decreased, as is P_aCO_2, all leading to an increased $A-aO_2$
gradient. Chest radiographs are usually at baseline or normal; however, a pleural-based infiltrate can be present in
severe pulmonary thromboembolism (Hampton's hump
sign). Finally, the ECG usually shows sinus tachycardia;
again, however, the classic pattern of a right-axis deviation, S_1, Q_3, T_3 pattern may be present.

D. Further evaluation and management are based on the **clinical suspicion for PTE** at the time of the initial assessment. This clinical suspicion is the cornerstone in the diagnosis and therapy of this condition. The three subsets are identified:

1. **High clinical suspicion.** Risk factors and baseline clinical evidence make PTE the likely cause of the pleuritic chest pain.

2. **Low clinical suspicion.** A condition other than PTE is known or is likely to be the cause of the pleuritic chest pain (e.g., angina pectoris, pneumothorax, pneumonitis, or musculoskeletal origins).

3. **Intermediate clinical suspicion.** Some features of PTE are present, but other diagnoses may be possible; thus no clear-cut diagnosis emerges from the initial assessment. This occurs in the majority of cases. Further diagnostic tests are necessary to aid the clinician in making the diagnosis of PTE.

E. The **evaluation and management** for each subgroup are described subsequently.

1. **High clinical suspicion.** Essentially the diagnosis is made. Treatment should not be postponed for any evaluative tools unless there is a relative or absolute contraindication to first-line, standard therapy, anticoagulation. (See Table 4-10 for contraindications to anticoagulation.)

   a. The patient should be **anticoagulated with heparin,** 5,000–10,000 units by i.v. bolus, followed by a maintenance dose of 1,300 units/hr i.v. The aPTT should be checked 6 hours after the initiation of therapy. The therapeutic goal is an aPTT of 60–80 seconds. The bolus can be given in the clinician's office as arrangements are made for inpatient admission. The heparin is continued for a total of 5–7 days. Early in the course, it is best to err on the high side, as the risk for PTE is greatest early in the course.

T A B L E *4-10*
Contraindications to Anticoagulation

1. Heparin-induced thrombocytopenia (only heparin is contraindicated)
2. Intracranial hemorrhage within the preceding 6 weeks
3. Major GI or GU bleeding within the preceding 6 weeks
4. Major surgery in an area that is not compressible (e.g., a neurosurgical or intraabdominal surgical procedure) within the preceding 6 weeks

Mechanism of action of heparin: Heparin acts on the naturally occurring inhibitor of thrombin formation, antithrombin III. Heparin prevents further propagation and embolization of the thrombus and allows the intrinsic fibrinolytic pathway to lyse some of the thrombus.

b. **Emergent systemic thrombolysis** with systemic streptokinase is indicated if:
   - Massive PTE with hypotension,
   - PTE with significant hypoxemia, or
   - PTE with right heart strain on ECG

c. After initiation of heparin and admission, a V/Q scan, venous duplex study of lower extremities, or a helical computed tomography (CT) scan of the chest, can be performed to confirm the diagnosis (see discussion under 3. Intermediate clinical suspicion).

d. The initiation of warfarin therapy is indicated, to begin the day after heparin is started (see Table 1-16). The starting dose of warfarin is 5–10 mg p.o., q.d., with a target of therapy being the PT-based international normalized ratio (INR). The **target INR should be 2.0–3.0.** The warfarin is continued for a total of 3 months.

   Mechanism of action of warfarin: Warfarin inhibits the activity of vitamin K–dependent coagulation factors, with a resultant anticoagulant effect.

e. If there is any contraindication to anticoagulation, a definitive diagnosis is required by pulmonary angiography and then inferior vena caval interruption/filter placement. Therefore, consultation with interventional radiologists for the pulmonary angiography and/or IVC placement is indicated.

2. **Low clinical suspicion.** Evaluation and management are directed toward the underlying suspected cause. The indications for admission and for consultations depend on the underlying clinical diagnosis and the stability of the patient. No further PTE-directed evaluation is necessary.

3. **Intermediate clinical suspicion.** The patient can be evaluated immediately (within 1–3 hours as an outpatient, or if logistically impossible or if the patient is not stable, admitted for the same evaluation as an inpatient). If the patient is stable, efficient, effective, immediate outpatient evaluation is optimal. This evaluation includes the following evaluative tools, which should be performed in the order listed.

   a. **Ventilation/perfusion scan.** This radionuclide imaging study is performed in two distinct parts. In one part, radiolabeled xenon gas is used to assess ventilation (V). In the other part, technetium 99m-labeled albumin microaggregates are used to assess pulmonary arterial perfusion (Q). To increase the sensitivity and specificity of this test, a chest radiograph should be obtained at the time of the V/Q scan. These scans are read as (or should be interpreted by the clinician to be) one of the following:

i. **High probability.** This scan has one or more subsegmental or larger V/Q mismatches. PTE is the diagnosis. Treat as such. No further PTE evaluation is necessary immediately. See Figs. 4-5 and 4-6.

ii. **Normal.** PTE is essentially ruled out as the cause of symptoms. No further PTE evaluation is necessary immediately.

iii. **Intermediate/indeterminate probability.** The scans are interpreted as "low probability." Most scans are in this group. **Low does not mean no probability.** An intermediate or indeterminate scan necessitates further evaluation. This further evaluation includes:

b. **Look for the site source of emboli,** specifically in the lower extremity system. If thrombus is demonstrated in the deep system, especially in the proximal deep lower extremity venous system (that is, in the area including and proximal to the popliteal fossa), the treatment is essentially the same as for PTE, and the diagnosis of PTE is strongly inferred. Modalities to image the lower extremity venous system, along with their clinical utility, include the following.

i. **Impedance plethysmography (IPG).** Sensitive for proximal DVT, and one of the best tools for evaluating the venous system proximal to the popliteal fossa for thrombus.

ii. **Venous duplex Doppler study.** A sensitive test for proximal DVT, and one of the best tools for evaluating the venous channels proximal to the popliteal fossa for thrombus.

iii. **Venography.** Entails injection of contrast material into the venous system of the lower extremity. The test is good for diagnosing the relatively benign distal thrombus, but it has only a fair sensitivity for the much more dangerous proximal thrombus. (See also the section on Peripheral Vascular Disease in Chapter 1, Table 1-15, page 31.)

c. If the V/Q scan is of little assistance and there is no evidence of thrombus in the lower extremities, the next step in the patient with an intermediate

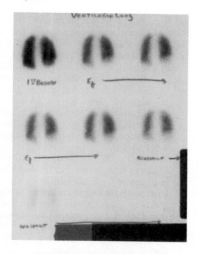

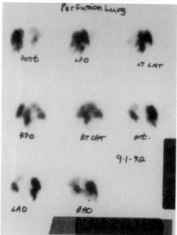

F I G U R E S   4-5 and 4-6
Ventilation–perfusion lung scans. The ventilation portion is completely
unremarkable, with normal ventilation to all areas of the lungs. The
perfusion portion is grossly abnormal, with several large perfusion
defects, predominantly in the right lung.

clinical suspicion is performing a contrast-enhanced helical CT scan. The helical CT scan will demonstrate pulmonary thrombus. The overall sensitivity of this test is 63% but increases to 86% if the thrombus is in a central pulmonary artery.

   d. If results on the lower extremity—imaging examination and helical CT scan are equivocal, perform pulmonary angiography to clarify the diagnosis. Consultation with pulmonologists and interventional radiologists is indicated at this time. If the angiogram is normal, PTE is ruled out; if the angiogram is positive, PTE is ruled in and therapy as discussed should be initiated.

F. The **long-term follow-up and management** of patients with PTE include the following steps:

   1. The duration of warfarin for the first episode of DVT or PTE is 3 months, and then warfarin is discontinued.

   2. If a DVT or PTE recurs, use the same regimen as for immediate therapy, but warfarin is continued for 1–2 years and may need to be continued indefinitely. A hematologist with specialty training in hypercoagulable states should evaluate the patient for a hypercoagulable state.

   3. If PTE or DVT recurs even though adequate anticoagulation has been provided, IVC interruption is indicated.

   4. The patient should never use aspirin concurrent with warfarin or heparin; other NSAIDs are relatively contraindicated for use concurrent with warfarin.

   5. Follow-up should be on a frequent and regular basis, usually every 2–4 weeks with a PT measurement.

   6. All estrogens, including oral contraceptive pills, are contraindicated for the remainder of the patient's life.

Community-Acquired Pneumonitis (see Box 4-7)

In the broadest sense, pneumonitis is the nonspecific inflammation of pulmonary parenchymal tissue. It is synonymous with the term pneumonia. Although a diverse set of pathogenetic mechanisms and causes exists for the development of inflammation of the pulmonary parenchymal tissue, only infectious agents (bacteria and viruses) in the local community are discussed here.

I. **Spectrum and pathogenesis**
   The spectrum and pathogenesis of infection-mediated lung disease can be generally overviewed by using the models of bronchitis, pneumonitis, and abscess formation.

   A. **Bronchitis** is an infection-related inflammation limited to the trachea and bronchial airways.

   B. **Pneumonitis** is an infection-mediated inflammation of the pulmonary parenchyma with exudative material, includ-

B O X 4-7

Overall Evaluation and Management of Pneumonias

Evaluation

1. Take a thorough history and perform a physical examination, with attention to the overall manifestations described in the text.
2. Determine the CBC count with differential to look for any leukocytosis or a left shift, indicative of an infectious process.
3. Determine basic serum chemistry for baseline purposes.
4. Determine ABG values for baseline purposes. Any evidence of hypoxemia is indicative of a significant process.
5. Obtain blood samples for culture in all patients with pneumonia and fever. Culture results will indicate the bacterial pathogen in a significant minority of cases. Blood cultures yield the pathogen in 30%–40% of cases of *Streptococcus pneumoniae*.
6. Obtain chest radiographs in PA and lateral views as an integral component of the evaluation. Chest radiography complements the physical examination in localizing any infiltrate present (Fig. 4-7).
   a. Lobar, consolidative infiltrates are associated with *Streptococcus pneumoniae*.
   b. Lobular, patchy infiltrates are associated with *Haemophilus influenzae*.
   c. Diffuse interstitial infiltrates are associated with *Mycoplasma pneumoniae*, *Legionella*, or viruses.
7. Sputum examination, both gross and with Gram stain, is mandatory. Gross inspection will reveal any purulence; Gram stain will reveal any PMNs and the predominant organism present.
8. Sputum cultures should be done only on samples representative of the pulmonary infectious process (i.e., those with PMNs and organisms). If the specimen is saliva only (i.e., contains no PMNs and only squamous epithelial cells), do not send it for culture as the data obtained will be misleading.
9. Initiate antibiotics based on the Gram stain results, chest radiograph, and the clinical picture.

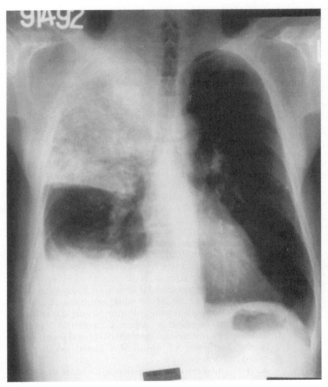

FIGURE 4-7
Chest radiograph in PA view showing right upper lobe consolidation with a concurrent parapneumonic effusion.

ing but not limited to PMNs and the pathogen itself, in the tissue itself, resulting in alveolar pneumonitis (i.e., material in the alveoli with resultant patchy or lobar infiltrates) or interstitial pneumonitis (i.e., material in the interstitium with resultant diffuse reticular or reticulonodular infiltrates).

   C. Abscess formation—any area of necrosis of lung tissue in an area of pneumonitis. This usually occurs in specific types of pneumonias. The most common organism types include gram-negative bacillary pneumonitis, in which necrosis of the tissue occurs acutely with the development of multiple small cavities; anaerobic pneumonias, in which the necrosis is insidious and a single large cavity forms; and reactive typical mycobacterial disease, which is insidious and forms a single large cavity.

II. **Manifestations, differential diagnosis, evaluation, and management**

The **manifestations,** differential diagnosis, evaluation, and management of community-acquired pneumonias are best approached by dividing the entities into two overall groups, typical pneumonias and atypical pneumonias (see Table 4-11).

A. The **classic or typical forms** of community-acquired pneumonia manifest with cough productive of yellow-green, even blood-streaked sputum; dyspnea; pleuritic chest pain, often in the site adjacent to the pneumonia; fevers, often spiking to 104°F; chills; and shaking rigors. The chest examination reveals signs of consolidation, including an area of dullness to percussion with concurrent increased tactile fremitus, and increased breath sounds, which are bronchial in nature.

1. The **organisms** that cause classic or typical pneumonias are the bacterial pathogens *Streptococcus pneumoniae* and *Haemophilus influenzae*.

2. **Sputum examination,** which is mandatory in all cases, will add significantly to the evaluation and management. A sputum from an *S. pneumoniae* infection will reveal polymorphonuclear cells and many gram-positive diplococci (positive = blue), whereas *H. influenzae* infection will reveal polymorphonuclear cells and many gram-negative coccobacilli (negative = pink).

3. The cornerstone in management of typical pneumonias is the initiation of antibiotics based on the suspected organism.

a. If *S. pneumoniae* is suspected, one of three regimens can be used:
   i. Penicillin G, 600,000 units q.4hr i.v., for 3–5 days, followed by penicillin VK, 500 mg p.o., q.i.d. for 5 days, or
   ii. Penicillin VK, 500 p.o., q.i.d., for 10 days, or
   iii. Erythromycin, 500 mg p.o. or i.v., q.6hr, for 10 days.

b. If *H. influenzae* is suspected, one of the following regimens can be used:
   i. A second-generation cephalosporin [e.g., cefuroxime (Zinacef), 750–1,500 mg i.v., q.8hr, for 5 days, followed by cefuroxime (Ceftin), 500 mg p.o., q.d., for 5 days, or
   ii. Cefuroxime (Ceftin), 500 mg p.o., b.i.d. for 10 days, or
   iii. Augmentin (amoxicillin–clavulanate), 500 mg p.o., b.i.d., for 10 days, or

T A B L E 4-11
Community-Acquired Pneumonias

Organism	History	Gram Stain	Chest Radiograph	Treatment
Streptococcus pneumoniae	Spiking fevers Rigors Pleuritic chest pain Cough Red-tinged sputum	Many PMNs Gram-positive diplococci	Lobar infiltrate	Penicillin Erythromycin
Haemophilus influenzae	Spiking fevers Cough Yellow-green sputum	Many PMNs Gram-negative coccobacilli	Lobar infiltrate or, more commonly, a patchy infiltrate	Ampicillin Second-generation cephalosporin
Legionella spp.	Low-grade fevers Cough Scant sputum Diarrhea	Many PMNs No organisms	Diffuse, interstitial	Erythromycin
Mycoplasma spp.	Low-grade fevers Cough Scant sputum Otalgia, ear popping	Many PMNs No organisms	Diffuse, interstitial	Erythromycin
Viral agents	Low-grade fevers Cough Myalgias Arthralgias Scant sputum Nausea, vomiting Diarrhea Rhinorrhea	Occasional PMNs No organisms	Diffuse, interstitial	Amantadine if influenza A is suspected Supportive; monitor for complication (e.g., superinfection with *Staphylococcus aureus*)

        iv. Ciprofloxacin, 500 mg p.o., b.i.d., for 7–10 days, (contraindicated in pregnancy).

B. The **nonclassic or atypical forms** of community-acquired pneumonias manifest with a low-grade fever; a hacking, nonproductive cough; dyspnea; rhinorrhea; and malaise. The chest examination usually reveals a slight tachypnea with diffuse crackles but rarely any signs of consolidation.

  1. The organisms that cause these classic or typical pneumonias are the bacterial and viral pathogens *Mycoplasma pneumoniae*, *Legionella pneumophila*, *Chlamydia psittaci* (psittacosis or "bird lover's pneumonia"), TWAR agent, and viruses, especially influenza A and B.

  2. The sputum examination is very important, but, because the cough is often nonproductive, sputum can be difficult to obtain. Gram stain will reveal PMNs but no organisms, for these pathogens do not stain with Gram stain.

  3. The cornerstone of management of atypical pneumonias is the initiation of antibiotics based on the suspected organism.

    a. Erythromycin, 500–1,000 mg i.v., q.6hr, for 5 days, followed by erythromycin, 500 mg p.o., for 5 days, or

    b. Erythromycin, 500 mg p.o., q.i.d., for 10 days.

  4. These pathogens, especially the RNA virus causing influenza A, cause a systemic infection that predisposes to bacterial superinfection, especially with *Staphylococcus aureus*. The physician in the ambulatory care setting must remain current with the specific pathogens in the community. The incidences of these pathogens change between different seasons (influenza A rarely occurs in summer but can be in epidemic proportions in late winter) and between communities (psittacosis is uncommon in the United States but quite common in Great Britain owing to the increased prevalence of birds as pets in the United Kingdom).

C. If the process cannot be defined as **typical or atypical** or if the process has components of both, initiate empiric therapy.

  1. A second-generation cephalosporin (cefuroxime, 750 mg i.v., q.8hr) and erythromycin (500 mg i.v. or p.o., for 10 days) are indicated; or

  2. Azithromycin (Z-Pac), 500 mg p.o., on day 1, and then 250 mg p.o., q. a.m. for 4 subsequent days. This novel macrolide antibiotic is effective against *S. pneumoniae*, *H. influenzae*, and the atypical pathogens. It must be taken on an empty stomach for optimal effectiveness; or

3. Clarithromycin (Biaxin), 500 mg p.o., b.i.d. for 10 days. Similar to azithromycin, refer to previous discussion.
4. If influenza A is in the community and is a potential diagnosis, amantadine, 100 mg p.o., b.i.d., for 7 days, can be added empirically to the regimen.

III. Follow-up

Follow-up is discussed in the acute, intermediate, and chronic settings.

A. **Acute follow-up** includes monitoring the symptoms and signs and temperature curve, whether the patient is an inpatient or an outpatient. It is not uncommon for the patient to have a febrile spike within the first 24–36 hours after initiation of therapy, and unless other factors indicate a deteriorating condition, this single spike should not affect the overall management scheme.

B. **Intermediate-duration follow-up** should include, if the patient clinically improves and has no clinical complications, chest radiography repeated ~4–6 weeks after treatment. Pneumonias take 3–6 weeks to resolve radiographically. If there is any evidence of complications or recurrence of symptoms earlier, chest radiography is repeated at that time, with closer radiographic follow-up as necessary.

C. Principles in **long-term follow-up:** If this is the second pneumonia, or if another pneumonia occurs, the clinician needs to ascertain whether there are any underlying systemic risk factors for recurrent pneumonias, such as immunodeficiency, hypogammaglobulinemia, or splenic dysfunction (e.g., splenectomy). If the patient is quite young and has had several pneumonias with gram-negative bacilli, cystic fibrosis must be entertained as an underlying process. If the recurrence is in same lobe, the clinician must evaluate for an anatomic lesion in that area, such as a neoplastic lesion with bronchial obstruction.

IV. Consultation

Problem	Service	Time
Recurrent pneumonia	Pulmonary	Required

V. **Indications for admission:** Most patients with active pneumonia need to be admitted for a short period for parenteral antibiotics. This is particularly true for the elderly population. Overall indications for admission include hypoxemia; a pneumonia that immediately exacerbates a chronic condition that itself is now symptomatic and requires therapy (e.g., COPD or left ventricular failure); a patient who is malnourished and needs nutritional supplementation to fight infection; a patient who is noncompliant; or any patient who is clinically ill with impending septicemia and cardiovascular or respiratory compromise.

Solitary Pulmonary Nodule

A solitary pulmonary nodule is usually discovered incidentally on a chest radiograph obtained for other reasons.

By definition, a nodule is a lesion <6 cm in diameter, whereas a mass is a lesion >6 cm in diameter. The definition of a solitary pulmonary nodule is quite specific and involves, in addition to size, the following qualifications, all of which must be met to make the diagnosis. The lesion is single, round, has distinct margins, is not based on pleura, and is without any concurrent mediastinal enlargement. The lesion may or may not have intralesional calcifications.

I. **Overall manifestations**

   Overall manifestations are minimal and, if present, are non-specific. This is true even on retrospective questioning of the patient after the nodule is discovered. Although there is a paucity of manifestations at the time of presentation, the patient's medical and personal history should be obtained, as certain features in the history will aid the clinician in establishing a ranked differential diagnosis and, more important, will aid the clinician in overall evaluation and management.

   A. **Smoking** of tobacco or marijuana as a habit is an important feature. There is clear and irrefutable evidence that smoking is a risk factor for the development of bronchogenic carcinoma.

   B. The patient's **geographic area** of residence, past and present, is important. Certain chronic infections that may manifest with a solitary pulmonary nodule are endemic to specific parts of the United States. As examples, histoplasmosis is endemic to the Ohio River valley, and blastomycosis is endemic to the upper Midwest.

   C. A history of exposure to mycobacterial disease must be sought. Mycobacterial lesions may rarely manifest as solitary pulmonary nodules.

   D. **Old chest radiographs** are important and, if available, are mandatory and integral to the evaluation and management.

II. **Diagnosis**

   The **differential diagnosis** includes bronchogenic carcinoma, which usually is noncalcified; the residua of primary mycobacterial disease, which usually is calcified and called a Ghon focus; histoplasmosis, which usually is calcified and associated with other calcified lesions, especially in the spleen; metastatic neoplastic disease, which is invariably non-calcified and multiple; and benign hamartoma, which invariably is calcified. Other specific differentiating features of these entities are listed in Table 4-12.

T A B L E 4-12
Differentiating Features of Solitary Pulmonary Nodules

Lesion Type	Patient Age	Lesion Rate of Growth	Smoking History	Calcification
Carcinoma: non–small cell	>30 yr	Doubling time >1 mo.	Present	Absent
Carcinoma: small cell	>30 yr	Doubling time <1 mo.	Present	Absent
Metastatic neoplasia	>30 yr	Doubling time <1 mo.	Present or absent	Absent
Hamartoma	Irrelevant	No change	Absent	Present, popcorn distribution
Mycobacterial	Irrelevant	No change	Absent	Present throughout the lesion
Histoplasmosis	Irrelevant	No change	Absent	Present; ringed calcifications in the lesion

T A B L E   4-13
Factors in Assessing the Risk of Malignancy of a Solitary Pulmonary Nodule

1. Age (<30 years or >30 years)
2. Rate of growth of lesion (no growth, doubling time <1 month, doubling time >1 month)
3. Presence or absence of calcifications in the nodule
4. Patient smokes or has ever habitually smoked tobacco products or marijuana

III. Evaluation and management

The **evaluation and management** of a solitary pulmonary nodule depend on the clinical suspicion of malignancy (Table 4-13). The clinician uses data gleaned from the history and physical examination and reviews, if at all possible, all old chest radiographs for comparison. If no old chest radiograph is available, one must assume the lesion is new.

A. If the patient is at **low risk for malignant neoplasm**—that is, the patient is <30 years old, the lesion shows no growth or rapid growth (i.e., doubling time <1 month) from baseline, the nodule contains calcifications, and the patient is a nonsmoker—management can be conservative. A conservative approach includes the following steps.

1. Perform a purified protein derivative (PPD) skin test (see Table 4-15).

2. Repeat the chest radiograph in 1–2 months. If there is no change in the lesion at that time, repeat the chest radiograph 2–4 months for two visits, to document the lack of change.

B. If the patient is at **moderate to high risk**—that is, the patient is >30 years old, the lesion shows slow, steady growth, the nodule contains no calcifications, and the patient is a past or current smoker (several or all factors present)—aggressive therapy is indicated. Furthermore, if the patient was at low risk but follow-up chest radiographs show that the nodule is slowly increasing in size, aggressive therapy is indicated. An aggressive approach includes the following measures.

1. CT of the thorax to look for concurrent lesions in the lungs or mediastinum.

2. Pulmonary function tests. These tests are indicated in all patients, because if forced expiratory volume (FEV_1) is <1.5 L, the patient is virtually never a candidate for thoracic surgery, as removal of a lobe or entire lung would be fatal to the patient.

3. If there is no evidence of metastatic disease and FEV_1 is >1.5 L, obtain a consultation with cardiothoracic surgery to resect the pulmonary lobe for diagnosis and,

in all likelihood, curative therapy. Preoperative bronchoscopy or needle biopsy would add little benefit if
surgery is to be performed.
4. If complete resection is performed and the tumor is
a non–small-cell carcinoma, expectant management
with repeated chest radiographs is indicated. If the
lesion is a small-cell carcinoma, adjuvant chemotherapy is indicated.

C. **Education of the patient** is of paramount importance. This
is especially true if the patient has an FEV_1 preoperatively
of <1.5 L. The primary care physician must inform the
patient of the likely outcome of the disease with and
without surgery and that, if the lesion is neoplastic, therapy will be palliative. The patient must be educated as
to the outcomes, response rates, and potential side effects
of various therapeutic modalities in the nonsurgical treatment of a solitary pulmonary nodule that is a malignant
neoplastic lesion.
1. If the **patient desires no therapy,** diagnosis by bronchoscopy or invasive needle biopsy is not indicated
until the patient becomes symptomatic. The reasoning
is as follows: palliative treatment, invariably local irradiation, would start only when and if symptoms begin;
moreover, the diagnosis may be made by sputum cytologic examination during subsequent follow-up, obviating the need for invasive testing.
2. If the **patient requests treatment,** the clinician should
obtain sputum for cytologic examination and then refer
to either an invasive radiologist for fine-needle biopsy
of the lesion or a pulmonologist for bronchoscopic
examination of the lesion. If and when the diagnosis
of a malignant neoplastic disease is made, referral to
an oncologist or radiation oncologist for therapy is
indicated. The response rates of non–small-cell carcinoma to the chemotherapeutic agents used today is
dishearteningly low. (For further discussion see the
section on Bronchogenic Carcinoma in Chapter 5,
page 280.)

IV. **Consultation**

Problem	Service	Time
If bronchoscopy is considered	Pulmonary	Elective
If needle biopsy is considered	Radiology	Elective
If SPN in high-risk patient	Cardiothoracic surgery	Urgent

V. **Indications for admission:** Admission is indicated on a
scheduled basis only for a specific procedure that has been
orchestrated by the primary care physician, or if the lesion
causes a secondary postobstructive pneumonitis requiring
palliative therapy.

Mycobacterial Diseases (see Box 4-8)

Typical mycobacterial disease, because of the AFB, *Mycobacterium hominis*, has become significantly less common in the United States after the availability of effective antimycobacterial chemotherapeutic modalities and the initiation of preventive health strategies in the 1940s and 1950s. There has been, however, a significant and disconcerting increase in the incidence of this disease in the recent past. Several potential reasons for this increased incidence can be postulated.

1. A decreased sensitivity of primary care and all physicians to this specific diagnosis, because it was uncommon during their training.

B O X   4-8

Overall Evaluation and Management of Mycobacterial Disease

The following discussion pertains to **typical** mycobacterial disease.

Evaluation

1. Take a thorough history and perform a physical examination. The history focuses on any history of PPD reactivity, any history of exposure to mycobacterial disease, inoculation with bacille Calmette-Guérin (BCG) vaccine, and any history of or risk factors for immunocompromise (see Table 4-14).
2. Obtain chest radiographs in PA and lateral views. Obtain and review any old chest radiographs and use these data, along with PPD results and the history, clinically to assess whether the patient has typical or atypical disease and whether the disease is primary, quiescent, or reactivation disease.
3. Respiratory isolation of the patient is strongly indicated, especially if there is any sputum production or any cavitary lesion on the chest radiographs. Respiratory isolation is relatively simple: a mask must be worn either by patient or by people who come in contact with the patient.
4. Obtain sputum for examination on three consecutive mornings for Gram stain, AFB smear, and culture.

(continued)

B O X *4-8 (continued)*

5. Perform a PPD test with controls unless there is a history of reactivity or BCG inoculation. This is because once a patient is reactive, the PPD should not again be applied. The PPD test is described in Table 4-15.

Management

1. If the sputum contains AFB or the suspicion of disease is high, initiate therapy with triple or dual chemotherapy (see Table 4-16). Regimens require more than one agent because the mycobacterial agents will develop resistance to one agent alone. One of the best regimens includes:
   a. Two-month course of isoniazid (INH), 300 mg p.o., q A.M., rifampin, 600 mg p.o., q A.M., pyrazinamide (PZA), 25–35 mg/kg/day p.o., and ethambutol, 15–25 mg/kg/day p.o., for 2 months, followed by 4 months of INH, 300 mg p.o., q A.M., and rifampin, 600 mg p.o., q A.M.;
      Or, if the patient is pyrazinamide intolerant,
   b. Two-month course of INH, 300 mg p.o., q A.M., rifampin, 600 mg p.o., q A.M., and ethambutol, 15–25 mg/kg/day p.o., for 2 months, followed by 4 months of INH, 300 mg p.o, q A.M., and rifampin, 600 mg p.o., q A.M.
2. If patient compliance is an issue, a modified regimen administered under **direct medical supervision** is indicated. This regimen consists of:
   a. Two-month course of INH, 300 mg p.o., q A.M., rifampin, 600 mg p.o., q A.M., and PZA, 25–35 mg/kg/day p.o., for 2 months, followed by 4 months of high-dose INH, 900 mg p.o., twice weekly, and rifampin, 600 mg p.o., twice weekly;
3. Obtain consultations with pulmonologists or infectious disease experts.
4. Report the case to the Public Health Service.
5. Screen other family members for disease. Screening includes a baseline PPD test, and, if the test is reactive, a chest radiograph. If exposed, INH chemoprophylaxis is indicated; if a family member has evidence of infection, treat as listed (see Table 4-17).
6. Administer pyridoxine (vitamin B_6), 50 mg p.o., q. A.M., to prevent the side effects of INH.

T A B L E 4-14
Groups at High Risk for the Development
of Mycobacterial Diseases

1. Immunocompromised hosts, especially in HIV
2. Recent immigrants to the United States from the tropics, especially from Southeast Asia
3. Untreated patients with reactive PPD skin tests (not including patients who received BCG in the past)
4. Patients with recent exposure to mycobacterial disease

2. Syndromes of immunodeficiency with predominantly cell-mediated deficiency (e.g., AIDS) increase the risk of mycobacterial disease development. Of interest is the relative risk (RR) for the development of mycobacterial disease in AIDS is 170, the RR in patients who are HIV reactive is 113!
3. The inherent immunosuppression of anticancer chemotherapeutic agents increases the risk of mycobacterial disease development.
4. Immunosuppression or immunocompromise is causing a significant increase in the incidence of the atypical mycobacterial diseases, especially those caused by *M. kansasii* and *M. avium-intracellulare* also known as MAC (*Mycobacterium avium-intracellulare complex*), agents with which a "normal" immune system adequately deals.
5. The fact that worldwide the prevalence of infection with mycobacterial organisms is 1.7 billion!

I. **Natural history of typical mycobacterial disease**
   The **natural history** of mycobacterial disease can be described by using infection by *M. hominis* as a model. The agent is transmitted by air, invariably by aerosolized sputum from an infected patient. Once the mycobacterial agent is transmitted into the pulmonary tree of a new host individual, its natural history belongs in three major and quite distinct temporal phases: primary disease, a quiescent period, and finally, reactivation disease.
   A. **Primary infection** is usually quite mild. Once the organism reaches the pulmonary airways, infection of the pulmonary tissue occurs. In the vast majority of cases, this is immediately followed by cell-mediated responses forming granulomas, usually of the caseating type. In the immunocompetent host, this stage of the infection is virtually always asymptomatic.
   B. The **quiescent period** begins after the cell-mediated responses have controlled and neutralized the original infection. These cell-mediated responses will, over months, result in granulomas in the pulmonary tissue and the

T A B L E 4-15
Skin Tests for Mycobacterial Diseases

Type	Indications	Contraindications	Mechanism	Reactive[a]
Purified protein derivative (PPD, intermediate strength, 5-TU	Demonstrate exposure to mycobacterial disease	Tested reactive in the past	Derivative of *M. hominis*	Immunocompromised: 5-mm induration[b] High-risk group, non-immunocompromised: 10 mm Nonimmunocompromised, nonhigh risk group: 15 mm
Trichophyton	Control, used to demonstrate active cell-mediated immunity	Tested reactive in the past	Derivative of this ubiquitous dermatophyte	10-mm induration
Mumps	Control, used to demonstrate active cell-mediated immunity	Tested reactive in the past	Derivative of this ubiquitous viral infection	10-mm induration

[a] Outcome of test measured at 48 hr.
[b] Immunocompromised: HIV, 15 mg prednisone/day, or lymphoproliferative disease.

TABLE 4-16
Antimycobacterial Agents

Agent	Mechanism of Action	Dose	Side Effects
Isoniazid (INH)	Bactericidal	300 mg p.o. q.d.	Hepatitis Peripheral neuritis, which can be prevented with vitamin B6, 50 mg p.o. q.d. Decreased seizure threshold
Rifampin	Bactericidal	600 mg p.o. q.d.	Hepatitis Thrombocytopenia Discoloration of all secretions to orange
Ethambutol	Bacteriostatic	25 mg/kg/day p.o. for 2 mo., then 15 mg/kg/day p.o. for 7–10 mo.	Optic neuritis; affects green-red vision
Streptomycin	Bactericidal	1 g i.m. for 60 days, then 1 g i.m. 2 times per week for 6 mo.	Vertigo Paresthesias Ototoxocity Nephrotoxicity

Drug	Action	Dose	Side effects
Pyrazinamide	Bactericidal	25 mg/kg/day p.o. in q.8h. dosing for 6–8 mo.	Arthralgias Hepatitis Hyperuricemia
Ciprofloxacin	Bactericidal	750 mg p.o. b.i.d.	Headache Gastrointestinal disturbances
Clarithromycin	Bactericidal	500 mg p.o. b.i.d.	Dysguesia Diarrhea
Amikacin	Bactericidal	7.5 mg/kg/day i.m.	Vertigo Ataxia Ototoxicity Nephrotoxicity
Rifabutin	Bactericidal	300 mg p.o. q. d.	Multiple drug interactions Discoloration of body secretions

T A B L E   4-17
Indications for Isoniazid (INH) Chemoprophylaxis for
Mycobacterial Diseases (American Thoracic Society)

Dose: INH, 300 mg p.o., q.a.m. for 12 mo.
Administer to:
1. Household contacts of patients with typical mycobacterial disease, even if contacts are PPD negative. If the contact remains PPD negative with reactive controls at 3 mo, can discontinue chemoprophylaxis
2. Untreated PPD-reactive patients >35 years old who have evidence of disease on old chest radiographs (Ghon foci, Simon foci)
3. PPD converters within the past 2 years of any age
4. All untreated PPD-reactive patients <35 years old
5. Any untreated PPD-reactive patients who develop any immunocompromise
Indications for Rifabutin chemoprophylaxis for MAC in HIV:
Dose: Rifabutin, 300 mg p.o., q day
1. When CD4 is <100/mm^3

adjacent draining mediastinal lymph nodes. Virtually all of these granulomas calcify over a relatively short period. These calcified lesions manifest as Ghon complexes or a Ghon focus on chest radiographs.

1. A **Ghon focus** is a calcified granuloma in the lung adjacent to the mediastinum.
2. A **Ghon complex** is a calcified granuloma and adjacent calcified mediastinal lymph nodes.

   Either or both of these findings are evidence and thus manifestations of past primary infection with *M. hominis* (i.e., the shadows of past, now quiescent mycobacterial infection). These lesions remain stable, asymptomatic, and quiescent for months, years, or even for the remainder of the lifetime of the patient. It is during the quiescent period that the majority of patients are first seen, usually discovered by the primary care physician from a chest radiograph that was obtained for other reasons.

C. **Reactivation** occurs after a period of dormancy or quiescence. If the patient did not receive therapy or chemoprophylaxis during the primary or quiescent period, the infection may reactivate. Reactivation occurs in both lung apices and manifests on chest radiographs as nodular infiltrates in the apices adjacent to the pleural surfaces (Simon foci) and the development of cavitary lesion(s) in the upper lobe(s). Invariably the reactivation begins in the posterior segment of the upper lobe(s). The **clinical manifestations** include cough, sputum production, hemoptysis, fevers, and night sweats. This phase, especially when cavitary lesions are present, is a phase in which the disease is highly transmissible to other people. If the disease in this phase is left unchecked, it will progress over variable periods to cause necrosis of the lung tissue, pleural diseases, systemic mycobacterial disease, and eventually death.

II. **Natural history of atypical mycobacterial disease**

The **natural history** of atypical mycobacterial disease is quite different from that of the typical disease. Although a comprehensive discussion is beyond the scope of this text, because the incidence of this disorder is markedly increasing, a brief discussion of the features of this infectious process is included.

A. The most common causative organisms are *M. kansasii* and *M. avium-intracellulare* (i.e., MAC). Neither of these organisms results in infection in an immunocompetent host with normal lung tissue.

B. The hosts are patients who invariably are immunosuppressed, especially that of cell-mediated immunity, or who have significant pulmonary disease.

C. The **primary disease** may be miliary or indolent.

1. **Miliary disease** is an intense and severe process in which there is an acute dissemination of the mycobacterial infection throughout the lungs and potentially the body. The **acute manifestations** of miliary tuberculosis include chest pain, dyspnea, low-grade or spiking fevers, hypoxemia, respiratory compromise, and even death.

2. **Indolent disease** is the other side of the spectrum. Infection with an atypical mycobacterial agent causes a slow, progressive disease with the development of diffuse nodular infiltrates in the middle and upper lung fields. The **pathophysiology** of the indolent form, which is the most common form of atypical mycobacterial disease, results in destruction of lung tissue and decreased pulmonary function. The clinical manifestations of this type are minimal until late in the process; they include dyspnea, especially on exertion, a nonproductive cough, and hypoxemia. The **evaluation and management** of atypical mycobacterial disease are beyond the scope of this text; however, early consultation with pulmonary and infectious disease colleagues for bronchoscopy and antimycobacterial chemotherapeutic initiation is clearly indicated. Often regimens will include four or five specific agents (see Table 4-16 for representative agents).

Bibliography

Asthma

American Thoracic Society. Diagnosis and care of patients with chronic obstructive pulmonary disease (COPD) and asthma. Am Rev Respir Dis 1987;136:225–246.

Bochner B, Lichtenstein L: Anaphylaxis. N Engl J Med 1991;324:1785–1790.

Fiel B, et al: Efficacy of short-term corticosteroid therapy in outpatient treatment of acute bronchial asthma. Am Med J 1983;75:259.

Gilbert R, Auchincloss H: The interpretation of the spirogram: how accurate is it for "obstruction"? Arch Intern Med 1985;145:1635–1639.

Kaliner MA: Inhaled corticosteroids for chronic asthma. Am Fam Pract 1990;42:1609–1616.

Littenberg B, Gluck E: A controlled trial of methylprednisolone in the emergency treatment of acute asthma. N Engl J Med 1986;314:150–152.

McFadden ER Jr: Clinical appraisal of the therapy of asthma: an idea whose time has come. Am Rev Respir Dis 1986;133:723.

McFadden ER, et al; Exercise-induced asthma. N Engl J Med 1994;330:1362–1366.

Mellion MB, et al: Exercise-induced asthma. Am Fam Pract 1992;45:2671–2677.

Stein L, Cole R: Early administration of corticosteroids in emergency room treatment of acute asthma. Ann Intern Med 1990;112:822–827.

Williams MH: Beclomethasone dipropionate. Ann Intern Med 1981;95:464.

Chronic Obstructive Lung Disease

American Thoracic Society. Standards for the diagnosis and care of patients with chronic obstructive pulmonary disease (COPD) and asthma. Am Rev Respir Dis 1987;136:225–246.

Anthonisen N, et al: Antibiotic therapy in exacerbations of chronic obstructive pulmonary disease. Ann Intern Med 1987;106:196–207.

Anthonisen NR: Long-term oxygen therapy. Ann Intern Med 1983;99:519.

Bertka K, Wunderink R: Outpatient management of COPD. Am Fam Pract 1988;37:265–280.

Crapo RO: Pulmonary function testing. N Engl J Med 1994;331:25–30.

Fulmer J, et al: American College of Chest Physicians–National Heart, Lung and Blood Institute Conference on Oxygen Therapy. Arch Intern Med 1984;144:1645–1655.

Gilbert R, Auchincloss H: The interpretation of the spirogram: how accurate is it for "obstruction"? Arch Intern Med 1985;145:1635–1639.

Kanner RE, et al: Predictors of survival in subjects with airflow limitation. Am J Med 1983;74:249.

Lakshminarayan S: Ipratropium bromide in chronic bronchitis/emphysema. Am J Med 1986;81(S):76–80.

Pennock B, et al: Pulmonary function testing: what is normal? Arch Intern Med 1983;143:2123–2127.

Rice K, et al: Aminophylline for acute exacerbations of chronic obstructive pulmonary disease. Ann Intern Med 1987;107:305–309.

Shapira R, et al: The outpatient diagnosis and management of COPD. J Gen Intern Med 1995;10:40–55.

Tobin M: The use of bronchodilator aerosols. Arch Intern Med 1985;145:1659–1663.

Hemoptysis

Jackson C, et al: Role of fiberoptic bronchoscopy in patients with hemoptysis and a normal chest roentgenogram. Chest 1985;87:142–144.

Johnston H, Reisz G: Changing spectrum of hemoptysis. Arch Intern Med 1989;149:1666–1668.

Morrissey JD, et al: The causes and management of hemoptysis. Cont Int Med 1994;6:10–26.

O'Neil K, Lazarus A: Hemoptysis: indications for bronchoscopy. Arch Intern Med 1991;151:171–174.

Pleural Effusions

Light R, et al: Pleural effusions: the diagnostic separation of transudates and exudates. Ann Intern Med 1972;77:507–513.

Light RW, Ball WC: Glucose and amylase in pleural effusion. JAMA 1973;225:259.

Light RW, et al: Cells and pleural fluid. Arch Intern Med 1973;132:854.

Peterman TA, Speicher CE: Evaluating pleural effusions. JAMA 1984;252:1051.

Pleuritic Chest Pain

Becker RC, et al: Antithrombotic therapy. Arch Intern Med 1995;155:149–161.

Fulkerson WJ, et al: Diagnosis of pulmonary embolism. Arch Intern Med 1986;146:961–967.

Ginsberg JS: Management of venous thromboembolism. N Engl J Med 1996;335:1816–1828.

Goodman LR, et al: Detection of PTE: helical CT versus angiography. AJR Am J Roentgenol 1995;164:1369–1374.

Hirsh J: Heparin. N Engl J Med 1991;324:1565–1574.

Hirsh J: Oral anticoagulant drugs. N Engl J Med 1991;324:1865–1875.

Hirsh J, et al: Oral anticoagulants: mechanism of action, clinical effectiveness and optimal therapeutic range. Chest 1995;(suppl 108):231S–246S.

Hull RD, et al: Diagnostic value of ventilation-perfusion lung scanning in patients with suspected pulmonary embolism. Chest 1985;88:819–828.

Hull RD, et al: Optimal therapeutic level of heparin therapy in patients with venous thrombosis. Arch Intern Med 1992;152:1589–1595.

Hull RD, et al: Pulmonary embolism in outpatients with pleuritic chest pain. Arch Int Med 1988;148:838–844.

Moser K: Venous thromboembolism. Am Rev Respir Dis 1990;141:235–249.

PIOPED Investigators: Value of the ventilation/perfusion scan in acute pulmonary embolism. JAMA 1990;263:2753–2759.

Simioni P, et al: The risk of recurrent venous thromboembolism in patients with an ARG 506 GLN mutation in the gene for factor V (factor V Leiden). N Engl J Med 1997;336:399–403.

Witty LA, et al: Thrombolytic therapy for venous thromboembolism, Arch Intern Med 1994;154:1601–1604.

Pneumonitis

American Thoracic Society. Prevention of influenza and pneumonia. Am Rev Respir Dis 1990;142:487–488.

Bartlett JG, et al: Community-acquired pneumonia. N Engl J Med 1995;333:1618–1623.

Chokshi S, et al: Aspiration pneumonia: a review. Am Fam Pract 1986;33:195–202.

Garibaldi RA: Epidemiology of community-acquired respiratory tract infections in adults. Am J Med 1985;78:32.

Gudiol F, et al: Clindamycin vs penicillin for anaerobic lung infections. Arch Intern Med 1990;150:2525–2529.

Levy M, et al: Community acquired pneumonias. Chest 1988;92:43–48.

Mayer RD: Legionella infections: a review of five years of research. Rev Infect Dis 1983;5:258.

McKellar P: Treatment of community acquired pneumonias. Am J Med 1985;79(S):25–31.

Schmitt SK, et al: Current guidelines for managing pneumonia in older patients. Contemp Intern Med 1993;12:15–24.

Stott GA: New macrolide antibiotics: clarithromycin and azithromycin. Am Fam Pract 1992;46:863–869.

Solitary Pulmonary Nodule

Lillington GA: Pulmonary nodules: solitary and multiple. Clin Chest Med 1982;3:361.

Stoller J, et al: Solitary pulmonary nodule. Cleve Clin J Med 1988;55:68–74.

Toomes H, et al: The coin lesion of the lung: a review of 955 resected coin lesions. Cancer 1983;51:534.

Trunk G, et al: The management and evaluation of the solitary pulmonary nodule. Chest 1974;66:236–239.

Mycobacterial Diseases

American Thoracic Society: Treatment of tuberculosis and tuberculosis infection in adults and children. Am J Respir Crit Care Med 1994;149:1359–1374.

Barnes PF, et al: Tuberculosis in the 1990s. Ann Intern Med 1993;119:400–410.

Centers for Disease Control: The use of preventive therapy for tuberculosis infection in the United States. MMWR 1990;39:153.

Dowling P: Return of tuberculosis: screening and preventive therapy. Am Fam Pract 1991;43:457–467.

Dutt A, et al: Short-course chemotherapy for tuberculosis with mainly twice-weekly isoniazid and rifampin. Am J Med 1984;77:233–241.

—D.D.B.

Chapter 5

Hematology/Oncology

Anemia

Erythrocytes are nonnucleated cells that contain a unique protein called hemoglobin. Hemoglobin allows the erythrocyte to perform with alacrity its main function, the delivery of oxygen to the tissues, and is also the basis for the unique red color of these cells. All normal erythrocytes are produced in the bone marrow by normoblasts. The life span of a normal erythrocyte is ~120 days.

I. Normal counts

The number of erythrocytes can be measured with various tests, but the two most common and reproducible measures are the hematocrit and the hemoglobin. The **hematocrit** is the percentage volume of cells in a given volume of blood; the hemoglobin is a direct measurement of this constituent and of the functional protein of erythrocytes. The normal ranges include:

Hematocrit
  Men: 42%–52%
  Women: 40%–50%
Hemoglobin
  Men: 14–18 g/dL
  Women: 13–16 g/dL

II. Overall manifestations

The **overall manifestations** of anemia include, but are not limited to, increased fatigability, a decrease in exercise tolerance, pale mucous membranes, pale conjunctivae, and high-output heart failure with a hyperdynamic heart; related findings include systolic murmurs, a fourth heart sound, and even unstable angina pectoris. Additional symptoms and signs that are directly attributable to the underlying anemia are described in the discussion of various entities that can give rise to anemia.

Compensatory mechanisms. Patients with mild to moderate degrees of chronic anemia may be asymptomatic as a result of adaptation to the anemia. Adaptive mechanisms

B O X 5-1

Overall Evaluation of Anemia

Evaluation

1. Take a thorough history, including the medication history, and perform a physical examination.
2. Perform laboratory studies to determine the characteristics of blood listed in Table 5-1.
3. Take a female patient's menstrual history (Box 11-5, page 548).
4. Review the peripheral blood smear (see Figs. 5-1 through 5-5).
5. Determine electrolytes, blood urea nitrogen (BUN), and creatinine for baseline purposes.

include an increased extraction of oxygen from the hemoglobin molecule, thereby shifting the oxyhemoglobin dissociation curve to the left, and an increased cardiac index co/m^2 as a result of an increase in heart rate and stroke volume. Patients who become symptomatic either have had a short-term loss of blood, have severe, chronic anemia, or have concurrent diseases that are exacerbated by the anemia and the decrease in oxygen delivery.

III. **Categories of anemia**

By using the data gleaned from the basic evaluation described in Box 5-1, the clinician assigns the anemia to one of three major categories, based on the size of the erythrocytes and the amount of hemoglobin in each erythrocyte. Although there is some overlap, each category has a different differential diagnosis, evaluation, and management outline. The three categories are hypochromic microcytic anemias, macrocytic anemias, and normochromic normocytic anemias. Underlying conditions and evaluative tools for each category are listed in Table 5-2.

IV. **Hypochromic microcytic anemia**

Hypochromic microcytic anemias are relatively common. The underlying conditions and specific tests for the further evaluation of these anemias are given in Table 5-2. The four specific forms of hypochromic microcytic anemia that are further discussed subsequently are iron-deficiency anemia, anemia of chronic disease, thalassemia, and hemoglobinopathies.

A. **Iron-deficiency anemia**

1. The **underlying pathogenesis** of iron-deficiency anemia is a chronic loss of blood, and therefore iron, from

T A B L E 5-1
Normal Values for Blood Parameters in the Evaluation of Anemia

Parameter	Normal Range
Mean corpuscular volume (MCV)	80–94 fL
Mean cell hemoglobin (MCH)	27–31 pg/cell
Red blood cell count	4.0–6.0 million
Reticulocyte count	1%–2%
Reticulocyte index [Reticulocyte count × (Hct./45%)]	1.0–1.5
White blood cell count	5,000–10,500 cells/mm^3
Platelet count	150,000–450,000/mm^3
Stool guaiac	Negative

any site in the body. Iron is requisite for the synthesis of hemoglobin; therefore, a deficiency in this cationic metal will result in the decreased production of erythrocytes and the onset of anemia. The most common origins of blood loss are from the gastrointestinal (GI) tract (most frequently from colon carcinoma and recurrent peptic ulcer disease) and, in a menstruating woman, menstrual blood loss.

2. The **specific manifestations** of iron-deficiency anemia include a guaiac-positive stool or excessive menstrual losses and koilonychia ("spoon nails") or cheilosis (skin cracking at the corners of the mouth).

3. The **evaluation** includes performing iron studies. Iron studies are quite important in the evaluation. As the serum iron is decreased, the total iron-binding capacity (TIBC) is normal to increased, transferrin saturation is <30%, and serum ferritin is decreased. Uterine and GI sources of blood loss must be evaluated with a pregnancy test, pelvic examination, and/or imaging of the GI tract. Three different approaches to imaging the GI tract are available:

   a. Flexible proctosigmoidoscopy, air-contrast barium enema examination, and an upper GI series, or
   b. Colonoscopy and an upper GI series, or
   c. Colonoscopy and esophagogastroduodenoscopy.

4. The **management** includes: iron replacement therapy (i.e., FeSO$_4$, 325 mg p.o., t.i.d.) for 2–3 months. A follow-up hematocrit determination and reticulocyte count in 2 weeks are indicated. Any GI lesion must be managed specific to its diagnosis and location. (See section on Gastrointestinal Bleeding in Chapter 2, page 110, for further discussion.)

T A B L E 5-2
Categories of Anemia

Type	Underlying Causes	Evaluation May Include
Hypochromic microcytic	Iron deficiency Anemia of chronic disease Thalassemia Plumbism (lead) Hypothyroidism	Serum iron TIBC Transferrin saturation Sickledex screen test RBC, elevated in thalassemia HB electrophoresis Serum lead, in children Bone marrow (Prussian blue stain for iron stores) TSH
Macrocytic	B_{12} deficiency Folate deficiency Hypothyroidism Ethanolism Reticulocytosis	LDH, total bilirubin B_{12} level Folate level Liver-function tests Ethanol use/abuse history TSH Bone marrow examination
Normochromic normocytic	Acute hemorrhage Chronic renal failure Acute hemolysis Aplastic anemia Monoclonal gammopathies	BUN, creatinine Coombs test Haptoglobin, LDH, and total bilirubin Serum free hemoglobin SPEP (serum protein electrophoresis) ESR (erythrocyte sedimentation rate) Glucose-6-phosphate dehydrogenase level; only in patients at risk and after the hemolysis has resolved Bone marrow examination

B. **Anemia of chronic disease**
   1. The **underlying pathogenesis** is a decreased production of erythrocytes due to a decreased ability of the bone marrow to produce erythrocytes. The materials necessary for erythrocyte production are present, but the inflammatory process, by a not completely understood mechanism, depresses erythropoiesis.
   2. The **specific manifestations** are attributable to the underlying chronic disease process.
   3. The **evaluation** of this type of anemia includes determining iron indices, which will reveal a decreased serum iron level, decreased TIBC, a normal to elevated serum ferritin level, and a normal transferrin saturation.
   4. The **specific management** is focused on determining the underlying cause and effectively managing that process. $FeSO_4$ replacement is not indicated.
C. **Thalassemia**
   1. The underlying pathogenesis is a deficiency in either the α or β components of the hemoglobin molecule. The normal hemoglobin molecule has two α and two β chains. If the patient is completely deficient in α or β chains, the condition is, respectively, α- or β-**thalassemia major.** α-Thalassemia major leads invariably to death in utero, whereas β-thalassemia major leads to severe anemia, extramedullary hematopoiesis with HbF and a decreased life span of the patient. An incomplete deficiency in α or β chains is termed α- or β-**thalassemia minor.** α-Thalassemia (i.e., a deficiency in α chains, is common in people of Asian descent, whereas β-thalassemia, or a deficiency in β chains, is common in people of African or Mediterranean descent. In α- or β-thalassemia minor, there are no pathologic consequences of the decreased hematocrit and hemoglobin.
   2. There are no specific outward **manifestations** of thalassemia minor, either α or β. Most patients with thalassemia major die early in life.
   3. The **evaluation and management** of **thalassemia minor** entail making the diagnosis and then reassuring the patient that the condition is "normal" for the patient. The iron studies are all normal, as are virtually all other tests, including a negative sickle cell screen (Sickledex). A hemoglobin electrophoresis in β-thalassemia minor will reveal an increased quantity of hemoglobin A_2. The only other clue to the diagnosis is that these patients invariably have an elevated RBC count. Although treatment is beyond the scope of this text, bone marrow transplantation is effective in the therapy for β-thalassemia major.

D. **Hemoglobinopathies**
   1. The **underlying pathogenesis** of these disorders is a change in the functional structure of the hemoglobin molecule.

   Hemoglobin is a complex protein. Any change in the primary structure of hemoglobin will result in significant changes in its function and usefulness. A change in one amino acid can decrease the life span of the molecule and thus of the erythrocyte. Moreover, such a change can significantly decrease the ability of the molecule, and thus the ability of the erythrocyte, to perform its life-sustaining functions of transporting oxygen to and carbon dioxide from the tissues.

   The sixth amino acid on the β chain is the site of common pathologic changes and as such is a defining feature in the three most common types of adult hemoglobin: A, S, and C.

   a. **Hemoglobin A:** The normal hemoglobin molecule. The amino acid at β position 6 is the uncharged valine (pKa = 7.2).

   b. **Hemoglobin S:** Hemoglobin that if homozygotic (SS), results in sickle cell disease, but if heterozygotic (SA or SC), results in either sickle cell trait (SA) or the disease of hemoglobin SC. The amino acid at β position 6 is the negatively charged molecule, glutamic acid (pKa = 7.0).

   c. **Hemoglobin C:** Hemoglobin that, if homozygotic (CC), results in death early in life, but if heterozygotic (SC or AC) results in either the disease of hemoglobin SC or the benign AC hemoglobin. The amino acid at the β position is the positively charged molecule, lysine (pKa = 7.4).

   2. The **specific manifestations and evaluation** are based on the specific hemoglobinopathy. In all cases, the overall evaluation, as listed in Box 5-1, and hemoglobin electrophoresis are clearly indicated. The Sickledex screen is positive, and serum iron studies are normal. Because the life span of these cells is decreased, there is a compensatory erythropoiesis, and therefore the reticulocyte count is invariably quite elevated, between 10% and 20%. The three most common hemoglobinopathies are SC disease; SA, sickle cell trait; and SS, sickle cell disease.

   a. **SC disease** is a fairly uncommon hemoglobinopathy in which 45% of the hemoglobin is S, 45% is C, and 10% is F. The peripheral smear reveals target cells and sickle cells. Refer to Fig. 5-1. The patient may have mild pain crises but is otherwise relatively asymptomatic. Also, unlike SS disease, autosplenectomy will rarely occur, and thus splenomegaly is often evident.

  b. **SA (i.e., sickle cell trait)** is a disease in which 40%–45% of the hemoglobin is S, 50% is the normal A, and 5% is F. This form is virtually always asymptomatic. The peripheral smear is relatively normal; if anemia is present, it is quite mild. The spleen is normal in size.

  c. **SS disease (i.e., sickle cell anemia)** is the classic and most severe form. Of the hemoglobin, 90% to 95% is S, with a small proportion of hemoglobin F. The peripheral smear reveals sickle cells (see Fig. 5-1). The patient has recurrent splenic infarctions early in life, or autosplenectomy, the spleen is never palpable in an adult. A classic manifestation of SS disease is the sickle cell pain crisis.

  Pain crises occur when, for some reason, there is sludging of blood flow to specific areas of the body, resulting in relative ischemia. Precipitants include an antecedent viral infection or anything that can result in intravascular volume depletion. The patient has excruciating axial skeleton bone pain, usually deep and boring in nature, and may have findings of intravascular volume depletion.

3. The **specific management** of sickle cell–related syndromes includes preventing crises and infections. Pain crises may be a significant manifestation of SS

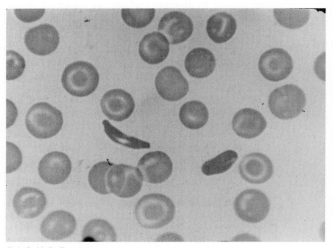

F I G U R E   **5-1**
Sickle cell and target cells on peripheral blood smear; consistent with the diagnosis of hemoglobin S-C.

B O X   5-2

Specific Management of Sickle Cell–Related Syndromes

Management

1. Administer Pneumovax and *Haemophilus influenzae* vaccine at time of presentation in adults.
2. Provide yearly influenza A vaccination.
3. Provide folate supplementation, 5 mg p.o., q. a.m.
4. Instruct the patient to stop smoking.
5. Watch for and rapidly intervene in any pain crises.
6. Obtain a hematology consult for SS disease.
7. Determine the hematocrit and reticulocyte count every 6 months and with any change in the clinical condition of the patient.
8. Manage any acute crises, as described in text.

and at times SC disease. In addition, as the result of the rapid turnover of cells, the patient can become deficient in cofactors, especially folate, which may further exacerbate the anemia. Furthermore, there can be splenic dysfunction, which can result in an increased risk of infections. Box 5-2 lists specific modalities integral to the management of sickle cell–related syndromes.

   a. The immediate **management** of a pain crisis involves keeping the patient hydrated with i.v. fluids, supplying supplemental oxygen by nasal cannula, and administering narcotic analgesia. This is a major morbid problem and can result in many admissions to the hospital for management. High-dose steroids (1 g methylprednisolone) i.v. at time of admission and at 24 hours has been reported markedly to decrease the manifestations of pain crises.

   b. Other interventions that can be performed include exchange transfusion and the use of hydroxyurea.

   i. In exchange transfusion, a unit of the patient's blood is removed and replaced with a unit from a patient with hemoglobin A (α_2, β_2). The goal is to give the patient normally functioning erythrocytes. This can be performed before a surgical procedure or during a particularly severe pain crisis. This has the risks of hepatitis and other blood-borne pathogens and should be reserved as a "last-ditch" effort.

ii. Another exciting potentially beneficial agent is hydroxyurea. This must be used under the direction of a hematologist. This agent has been demonstrated to increase the level of HbF (α_2, γ_2), fetal hemoglobin, thus decreasing the level of HbS and decreasing the intensity and frequency of pain crises. Obviously, this has a number of potentially significant side effects and should be monitored closely.

4. Crises, nonpain

In addition to pain crises, other crises can occur in sickle cell syndromes. These include the aplastic, hyperhemolytic, and sequestration crises. These are relatively rare, and thus only the **aplastic crisis** is discussed here. The normal reticulocyte count in sickle cell anemia is 10%–20%; therefore, anything <10% may be indicative of impending aplastic crisis. The most common reasons for aplastic crises include deficiencies in one or more cofactors, especially folate, or any systemic, including viral, infection. The clinician must watch for the development of this crisis type.

V. Macrocytic anemias

In a **macrocytic anemia,** the mean corpuscular volume (MCV) of the erythrocytes is >94. Macrocytic anemias are not uncommon. The differential diagnosis includes processes that are eminently treatable and quite curable. The underlying causes and specific tests for the further evaluation of these anemias include those listed in Table 5-2. Two specific forms of macrocytic anemia are discussed: vitamin B_{12} deficiency and folate deficiency.

A. Vitamin B_{12} deficiency

A deficiency in this essential cofactor and vitamin, cyanocobalamin, will result in a macrocytic anemia.

1. The **pathogenesis** relates to the physiologic function of vitamin B_{12} in the body and the GI absorption of this cofactor.

a. Physiology. Cyanocobalamin acts as a cofactor for several enzymatic reactions.

i. Thymidine synthesis: Coenzyme B_{12} is required to synthesize thymidine from uridine. The thymidine is required for DNA synthesis and therefore for mitosis and meiosis. Therefore, all tissues that have cells with rapid turnover (e.g., hematopoiesis, skin, mucous membranes, and the mucosa of the GI tract) are affected. Both B_{12} and folate are required for this process.

      ii. **ʟ-Methylmalonyl-CoA mutase:** B_{12} is preferred for this required reaction (i.e., the mutase to form succinyl CoA from ʟ-methylmalonyl CoA. If B_{12} deficient, the alternate reaction uses a hydrolase to produce methyl malonic acid.

      iii. **Methionine synthase:** Methionine is synthesized from homocysteine. Both B_{12} and folate are required for this reaction.

   b. **Gastrointestinal absorption.** GI absorption of vitamin B_{12} has been well elucidated. Vitamin B_{12} occurs in high concentrations in meat, especially red meat. Once ingested, it is bound in the stomach to intrinsic factor, a chemical produced by antral parietal cells and absorbed exclusively in the terminal ileum. Origins of B_{12} deficiency include nutritional deficiency (rare because the storage pool of B_{12} lasts ≤2 years); deficiency of intrinsic factor as the result of pernicious anemia or gastric/antral resection; or decreased absorption at the terminal ileum, either as the result of inflammatory bowel or surgical resection.

2. The **specific manifestations** of vitamin B_{12} deficiency relate to its physiologic functions and include not only chronic anemia but also a smooth tongue (atrophic glossitis) as a result of loss of tongue papillae (Fig. 5-3), and a decreased sensation to vibration and decreased position sense with an ataxic gait as a result of loss of highly myelinated axons in dorsal columns of the spinal cord. The peripheral smear will reveal hypersegmented polymorphonuclear cells, large platelets, and macroovalocytes (see Fig. 5-2). In addition, the increased homocysteine levels may be an independent factor in the development of accelerated atherosclerotic disease.

3. The **specific evaluation and management** include the steps listed in Box 5-1 and in Table 5-2. Serum levels of B_{12}, folate, lactate dehydrogenase (LDH), and total bilirubin should be determined. If the serum cyanocobalamin level is <221 pmol/L, it is diagnostic of B_{12} deficiency. Further tests include an elevated serum homocysteine and serum methylmalonic acid levels. If the patient is B_{12} deficient:

   a. Administer vitamin B_{12}, 1,000 μg i.m., now and once a day for 4 days, and then once weekly for 4 weeks, followed by 1,000 μg i.m. once monthly for life.

   b. Monitor the reticulocyte count and potassium level. The reticulocyte count should markedly increase with replacement of B_{12}, whereas the potassium levels may and often do precipitately decrease as the result of the reticulocytosis.

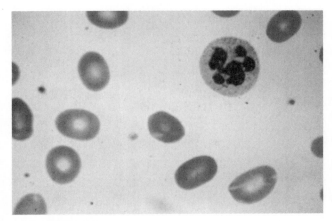

F I G U R E   5-2
Peripheral smear showing profound macrocytic anemia in a patient
with vitamin B_{12} deficiency as a result of pernicious anemia. Note the
large erythrocytes, paucity of platelets, and a hypersegmented
polymorphonuclear cell.

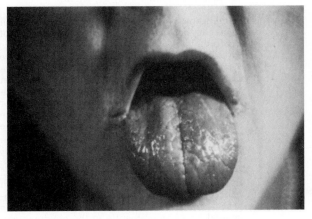

F I G U R E   5-3
Atrophic glossitis in a patient with vitamin B_{12} deficiency as a
result of pernicious anemia. Note loss of tongue papillae as
indicated by the shiny and smooth tongue surface.

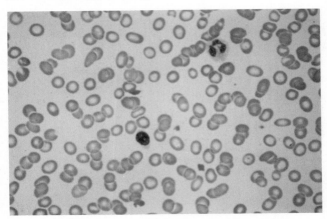

FIGURE 5-4
Peripheral smear showing rouleaux, i.e., abnormal stacking of erythrocytes. This individual had an IgG monoclonal gammopathy.

    c. Supplementation with iron and folate is indicated. Supplementation should be provided during the phase of reticulocytosis (i.e., approximately over the first 4–6 months of B_{12} repletion).

B. Folate deficiency
    1. The pathogenesis relates to the physiologic function of folate in the body and to the GI absorption of this cofactor.
        a. Physiology. Folate acts as a cofactor, in this case as a direct source of methyl groups. In several biochemical reactions, it serves this function, the most important one being the synthesis of deoxyribonucleic acid (DNA). Folate is required as a cofactor for synthesis of thymidine from uridine and the synthesis of methionine from homocysteine. See discussion of these activities in preceding B_{12} section.
        b. Gastrointestinal absorption. GI absorption of folate has been well elucidated. Folates are found in many foodstuffs but occur in particularly high concentrations in leafy green vegetables. Once ingested, folate is absorbed in the small intestine in general, and predominantly in the proximal jejunum. Deficiency of folate is a result of nutritional defect, especially in chronic ethanol abusers. In addition, malabsorption may occur at the level of the small intestine.

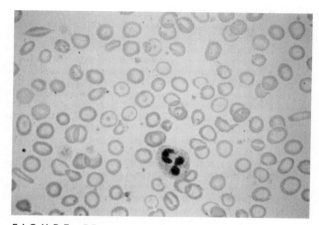

F I G U R E   5-5
Peripheral smear from a patient with profound hypochromic microcytic anemia as a result of iron deficiency. Note marked decrease in pigment (hemoglobin) within the erythrocytes.

2. The **specific manifestations** of folate deficiency reflect its physiology and include chronic anemia. Unlike in cyanocobalamin deficiency, there are no neurologic manifestations associated with folate deficiency. The peripheral smear will reveal hypersegmented polymorphonuclear cells, large platelets, and macroovalocytes (see Fig. 5-2).

3. The specific evaluation and management of folate deficiency include the steps listed in Box 5-1 and Table 5-2. Serum levels of B_{12}, folate, LDH, and total bilirubin should be determined. Homocysteine levels in the serum are also elevated.

    a. If the serum B_{12} is normal and the serum folate is low, replete the folate with folate, 3–5 mg p.o., once daily.

    b. As with B_{12} replacement, the reticulocyte count and potassium should be closely monitored.

VI. Normochromic normocytic anemia

Anemias in which the MCV and the mean corpuscular hemoglobin (MCH) of the erythrocytes are within normal range are quite common. The underlying causes and specific evaluative tests for these anemias include those items listed in Table 5-2. Although the differential diagnosis is broad, only the normochromic normocytic anemia associated with chronic renal failure and multiple myeloma is discussed here.

A. **Chronic renal failure**
1. The **underlying pathogenesis** of this anemia relates to the endocrine function of the kidneys. In the normal state, the hormone erythropoietin is released when the kidneys sense a decrease in the intravascular volume. This hormone directly stimulates the normoblasts, with resultant reticulocytosis. This endocrine function of the kidneys becomes embarrassed and is clinically significant when there is a modest to marked overall impairment of renal function (i.e., the creatinine clearance rate is <20 mL/min).
2. The **specific manifestations** are minimal until the anemia is quite marked. It is not uncommon for a patient to have a hematocrit in the low to middle 20% range without any significant manifestations of such a degree of anemia. The paucity of symptoms and signs results from the slow progression and chronicity of the anemia, which allows compensatory mechanisms to take effect, and from the development of an acidosis, which further shifts the oxyhemoglobin dissociation curve to the left, increasing and optimizing the extraction of oxygen from hemoglobin by the tissues. The peripheral smear will reveal anemia with some spur cells (echinocytes).
3. The **specific evaluation and management** include the steps listed in Box 5-1 and in Table 5-2. In addition, the cause of the renal failure must be determined and managed (see Chapter 3, page 179). Furthermore, the initiation of erythropoietin is an effective modality in management. This recombinantly synthesized molecule is homologous to the natural human hormone and is quite effective. The goal is to increase the hematocrit and maintain it in the 30%–33% range.

B. **Multiple myeloma**
1. The **underlying pathogenesis** is the development of a neoplastic clone of B lymphocytes and therefore of plasma cells. This clone of plasma cells causes mischief by growing and replacing the bone marrow, with resultant pancytopenia and functional hypogammaglobulinemia, bone resorption via an osteoclast-activating factor (OAF) produced by the plasma cells, and a specific gamma globulin produced by the cell clone. This protein is monoclonal and is categorized by subtype (i.e., IgA, IgG, IgE, or IgM) and by type of light chain present, λ or κ. IgG is the most common type of gammopathy; IgM is quite rare but is a specific syndrome (i.e., Waldenstrom's macroglobulinemia).
2. The **specific manifestations** include those attributable to the replacement of the bone marrow by the malignant neoplastic clone (i.e., the pallor of anemia, pete-

chiae of thrombocytopenia, and the increased risk of
infection as the result of leukopenia and functional
hypogammaglobulinemia). The accelerated bone loss
will manifest with compression fractures of the back
(i.e., vertebrae), fractures of the long bones, and symptomatic hypercalcemia. Finally, the hypergammaglo-
bulinemia will result in the potential for increased
viscosity and a functional decrease in the gamma globulin needed for infections. This results in an increased
risk of infection with encapsulated bacteria, especially *Streptococcus pneumoniae* and *Haemophilus
influenzae*. Renal failure is also a component resulting
from the protein in the tubule.

3. The **overall evaluation and management** includes the
tests listed in Box 5-1 and Table 5-2. The serum protein electrophoresis (SPEP) will reveal a monoclonal
gammopathy (spike); the peripheral smear will reveal
rouleaux (see Fig. 5-4); the urinary protein electrophoresis (UPEP) will reveal Ig or light chains in the urine;
the immunoglobulin analysis will determine the specific type; the patient should have creatinine, BUN,
calcium, PO_4, and albumin tests; and finally, a skeletal
survey looking for any lytic lesions should be performed. If there are any mental-status examination
changes, the serum calcium and viscosity should be
closely monitored. Any evidence of hyperviscosity is
best treated with plasmapheresis; any hypercalcemia
treatment discussed in Chapter 9, page 485; and any
fractures are best treated with local radiation therapy.
A bone marrow aspiration to determine the percentage
of plasmacytes should be performed to confirm the
diagnosis. If multiple myeloma is indeed present (i.e.,
anemia, monoclonal gammopathy, >10% plasmacytes on bone marrow, renal insufficiency, and/or
hypercalcemia), it mandates referral to oncology for
initiation of systemic chemotherapy: usually melpha-
lan and prednisone or VAD (see Table 5-10). The patient should also receive Pneumovax and *H. influenzae* vaccines.

VII. Consultation

Problem	Service	Time
Pancytopenia	Hematology	Urgent
Anemia of undetermined etiology	Hematology	Urgent
Hemoglobinopathies	Hematology	Elective
Chronic renal failure	Nephrology	Elective
Multiple myeloma	Hematology	Required

VIII. Indications for admission:
Any evidence of hemodynamic
instability, any sickle cell anemia crisis, or an acute loss of
blood, either by hemorrhage or hemolysis.

Excessive Bleeding States

Effective hemostasis is complex and integral to the survival of any human being. Hemostasis is the ability of the blood and its components to patch leaks in blood vessels. The leak is usually acquired as a result of trauma. By patching the acquired defect, hemostasis prevents the loss of fluid and blood from the intravascular tree. The patch so formed is a clot or thrombus.

Thrombus generation involves several sets of proteins and one formed element (platelets) in the blood. The proteins are grouped into the intrinsic and extrinsic coagulation cascades that, when either or both are activated, form the protein **thrombin.**

The intrinsic coagulation cascade consists of factors VIII, IX, and X and is activated by any breakdown of plasma membrane, such as endothelial breakdown. The extrinsic coagulation cascade consists of factors II, V, VII, IX, and X.

Platelets are the formed elements in the blood that are involved in thrombus formation. Concurrent with thrombin formation, platelets, through a mechanism involving the large protein, von Willebrand factor (VWF), will adhere to any area of endothelial breakdown. This results in the activation of and aggregation with other platelets. This platelet aggregate with the early thrombin fibrils is termed a primary thrombus. The primary thrombus matures by the development of covalent linkages between thrombin molecules to form the stable secondary thrombus.

I. **Overall manifestations**

The **overall manifestations** of excessive bleeding include the dermatologic findings of petechiae (red, nonblanching macules on the skin), purpura (nonblanching patches), and ecchymoses. Hematologic manifestations may include recurrent epistaxis (nosebleeds), hemarthroses, and upper or lower gastrointestinal (GI) bleeding. The patient may report episodes of frank hematuria (blood in urine), and women may describe menorrhagia (heavy menstrual flow) or menometrorrhagia (abnormal menstrual bleeding between normal periods). The time of onset and whether the condition has been present since youth or is of recent onset are important because one can thus differentiate congenital from acquired coagulation defects. The patient must be questioned about the use of anticoagulants, especially heparin or warfarin, and the use of the antiplatelet agent aspirin.

Once the clinical diagnosis of an excessive bleeding state has been made and the evaluations listed in Box 5-3 have been performed, the coagulopathy (excessive bleeding state) can be subcategorized into one of three overall groups. These groups are discussed subsequently.

II. **Elevated prothrombin time (PT)**

A. The **underlying pathogenesis** is a decrease in the production or effectiveness of the factors in the extrinsic coagulation pathway. These coagulation factors include factors II, V, VII, IX, and X. A deficiency of these coagulation factors may be acquired as a result of vitamin K deficiency or of severe hepatic dysfunction.

1. A **deficiency in vitamin K,** a vitamin required for the production of all of the extrinsic coagulation factors except factor V, will manifest with an elevated PT and an increased bleeding tendency. The differential diagnosis includes entities that decrease vitamin K absorption in the ileum or its effectiveness in coagulation-factor synthesis. Therefore, malnutrition (especially of leafy green vegetables), or any malabsorption syndrome, or the use of the oral anticoagulant warfarin will decrease vitamin K stores and increase PT.

2. **Severe hepatic dysfunction.** All of the coagulation factors of the extrinsic pathway are produced in the liver, including factor V. Therefore, severe liver disease results in an increased PT and an increased bleeding tendency.

B. The **specific manifestations** of excessive bleeding due to an increased PT are similar to those listed under I. In addition, there is a history of Coumadin (sodium warfarin) use, poor nutrition, or ileal disease, or manifestations of severe hepatic insufficiency (see section on End-Stage Hepatic Dysfunction in Chapter 2, page 97).

C. Further **evaluation** includes making the clinical diagnosis and performing the tests listed in Box 5-3. One can differentiate vitamin K deficiency from liver failure by the following measures.

1. Administer 10 mg of vitamin K subcutaneously or 1 mg vitamin K i.v. If the PT increase is the result of vitamin K deficiency of any cause, the PT will correct, whereas in liver failure, the PT increase will not correct.

2. The plasma level of factor V, which is not dependent on vitamin K, will be normal in vitamin K deficiency but low in liver disease.

3. Liver function test (LFT) results are usually normal in vitamin K deficiency but abnormal in hepatic failure.

4. If surreptitious warfarin use is suspected, the plasma warfarin level should be determined.

D. The **management** of excessive bleeding due to an isolated increased PT includes determining the underlying cause and treating that specific entity.

1. If the patient is bleeding acutely, administer FFP immediately to give coagulation factors and reverse the coagulopathy, unless an inhibitor is present.

2. If the condition is due to vitamin K deficiency, provide supplemental vitamin K and instruct the patient to eat leafy green vegetables. If the deficiency is due to malabsorption, administration of vitamin K, 10 mg p.o. or s.c., q.d., may be required.

3. In patients with liver failure, vitamin K supplementa-

B O X 5-3

Basic Evaluation and Management of an Increased Bleeding Tendency

Evaluation

1. Determine the platelet count, the prothrombin time, (PT) and activated partial thromboplastin time (aPTT). These values are central to further evaluation and management.
2. Determine the complete blood cell (CBC) count for baseline purposes.
3. Determine the bleeding time reproducibly to quantify the coagulopathy.
4. Elicit the family history. If there is any family history of excessive bleeding, a family tree specific to the problem of excessive bleeding should be made.
5. Determine the age at onset of the increased bleeding tendency, which will help differentiate an acquired defect from a congenital defect.
6. Determine the patient's nutritional status. Estimate the quantity of leafy green vegetables that the patient ingests. Leafy green vegetables are rich in vitamin K.
7. Elicit the medication history, including the use of prescribed and over-the-counter agents.
8. Easily and rapidly to differentiate an acquired inhibitor from a factor deficiency, mix the patient's plasma 1:1 with fresh frozen plasma (FFP). If a factor deficiency is present, the coagulopathy will correct; if an acquired inhibitor is present, no correction occurs.

Management

1. FFP can be used on an emergency basis to control most coagulopathies (except inhibitors). FFP is rich in all factors required for coagulation; therefore, it can be used in any condition causing an extrinsic or intrinsic coagulation deficit. Because it is a blood product and there is an inherent risk of transmitting blood-borne pathogens including hepatitis with transfusion, its use should be reserved for clear emergencies. Insofar as is possible, use specific factor concentrates if the deficiency type is known.
2. Instruct the patient not to use aspirin until the coagulopathy has been defined and corrected.

tion can be attempted but is usually of little utility. The liver disease must be treated to correct the coagulopathy.

4. If any invasive procedures are planned, the PT must be decreased to <15 seconds. If the PT is increased as the result of warfarin, the clinician can use one of three methods to decrease the PT:

   a. Instruct the patient not to take the warfarin for 2–3 days before the procedure **and/or**

   b. Administer 0.5–1.0 mg vitamin K i.v., 4 hours before the procedure **or**

   c. If the procedure is emergent, FFP may be administered.

   If the PT is increased as the result of hepatic dysfunction, FFP may be administered before the procedure.

III. **Increase of the activated partial thromboplastin time (aPTT)**

A. The **underlying pathogenesis** is a decrease in the production or effectiveness of factors in the intrinsic coagulation pathway. These factors include VIII, IX, and X. A deficiency in these coagulation factors may be either congenital or acquired.

   1. The **differential diagnosis** of congenital deficiencies in these intrinsic coagulation factors and thus an elevated aPTT includes the X-linked recessive hemophilia A (factor VIII deficiency), the X-linked recessive hemophilia B (factor IX deficiency), the dysfibrinogenemias, and von Willebrand's disease (a deficiency of VWF, a large protein that is necessary for factor VIII function and platelet adhesion).

   2. The **differential diagnosis** of acquired deficiencies in these intrinsic coagulation factors and thus an elevated aPTT includes the use of heparin or the development of the pathogenic entity disseminated intravascular coagulation (DIC).

B. The **specific manifestations** of this group are similar to those listed under I. In addition, there is a history of hemarthroses, which are quite classic for factor VIII or IX deficiency states; furthermore, a history of heparin use is helpful in defining the process.

C. The further **evaluation** of this subgroup includes making the clinical diagnosis and performing the tests listed in Box 5-3. One can differentiate congenital from acquired disorders by the clinical history in virtually all cases. The specific evaluation is dependent on this differentiation.

   1. **In a presumed congenital deficiency:**

      a. Determine plasma levels of factor VIII and factor IX.

      b. Perform a ristocetin aggregation test for VWF deficiency. Normal platelets aggregate in vitro in the presence of the chemical ristocetin, but platelets from patients with von Willebrand's disease do not aggregate in vitro in the presence of ristocetin. A caveat to this test is that it measures aggregation; however, in vivo, the platelet dysfunction in von Willebrand's disease is one of adhesion. Adhesion is not easily measured, but aggregation can be measured reproducibly.

2. **In the acquired deficiency** states (i.e., heparin use and DIC):

   a. "DIC" panel of aPTT, PT, platelets, fibrinogen, and FDP (fibrin degradation products). In DIC there is an increase in the PT, aPTT, FDP, and a decrease in platelets and fibrinogen.

   b. If there is any question in differentiating heparin use from hypofibrinogenemic states (e.g., DIC), one can measure the thrombin time (TT) and perform the reptilase test.

      i. The TT measures the time required to convert fibrinogen to fibrin and is increased in patients with low or dysfunctional fibrinogen states (e.g., DIC) and in heparin use.

      ii. The reptilase time is the TT measured by using reptilase, a coenzyme that is not affected by heparin; therefore, the reptilase time is increased in low or dysfunctional fibrinogenemia states but not increased in heparin use.

D. The **management** of this group includes determining the underlying cause and treating that specific entity.

   1. **Hemophilia A**

      a. To treat emergently, and if no factor VIII concentrate is available, use FFP.

      b. Factor VIII concentrate should be used therapeutically to treat any bleeding and prophylactically before any procedure. The goals of therapy include:

         Minor bleeding: To attain >25% of normal plasma levels.
         Major bleeding: To attain >50% of normal plasma levels.
         Preoperatively: To attain a 100% level initially, and then >50% for 10 days.

      c. The usual **dosage** is 60 units/kg i.v. initially, and then 20–30 units/kg i.v. for 10 days.

   2. **Hemophilia B**

      a. To treat emergently, and if no factor IX concentrate is available, use FFP.

   b. Factor IX concentrate should be used therapeuti-
      cally to treat any bleeding and prophylactically
      before any procedure. The goals of therapy are sim-
      ilar to hemophilia A, as previously described.
   c. The usual **dosage** is 80 units/kg i.v. initially, and
      then 30–40 units/kg i.v. for 10 days.
3. von Willebrand's disease
   a. 1-Deamino-8-d-arginine vasopressin (DDAVP)—A
      synthetic vasopressin analog that releases stored
      factor VIII:ag multimers from the endothelium. (in-
      creases VWF and VIII release).

   Dosing regimen:
      Initial: 0.3 μg/kg in 50 mL of normal saline in-
      fused intravenously over 30 minutes.
      Maintenance: 0.3 μg/kg in 50 mL of normal sa-
      line infused intravenously over 30 minutes,
      once per day as long as the patient is at risk
      for bleeding.

   b. Cryoprecipitate—a blood product that is rich in
      factor VIII:ag multimers.

   Dosing regimen:
      Initial: 1 bag/10 kg administered as i.v. bolus.
      Maintenance: 1 bag/10 kg administered as i.v.
      bolus once per day as long as the patient is at
      risk for bleeding.

   Either one of these—DDAVP or cryoprecipitate—can be used immediately for bleeding or as
   prophylaxis before a surgical procedure.
4. Heparin use. If the patient is bleeding, discontinue
   heparin. Heparin anticoagulation can be rapidly reversed with protamine sulfate if the bleeding is significant. The **dose** of protamine is 1 mg i.v./100 U of
   heparin given over 8 hours.
5. DIC. Determine the underlying cause. Often the patient has impending or clinical septicemia, usually
   with gram-negative organisms. The clinician must aggressively determine and treat the underlying cause.
IV. Increased bleeding time (BT)
   A. The underlying pathogenesis is a decrease in the produc-
      tion, life span, or effectiveness of the formed elements
      involved in thrombus formation, the platelets. Platelet
      dysfunction may result from a quantitative deficiency of
      platelets (i.e., thrombocytopenia as defined by a platelet
      count of <150,000/mm^3) or from a qualitative defect in
      platelets.
      1. The **differential diagnosis** of the quantitative disor-
         ders (i.e., thrombocytopenia) includes disorders that

decrease production of platelets and disorders that increase peripheral destruction.

  a. Disorders that decrease the production of platelets in the bone marrow include aplastic anemia, megaloblastic processes (vitamin B_{12} or folate deficiency), myelophthistic processes (i.e., the replacement of bone marrow with tumor or granulomatous infection), or amegakaryocytic thrombocytopenia (i.e., the primary loss of megakaryocytes within the bone marrow).

  b. Disorders that result in premature peripheral destruction—that is, a decrease in the normal 9-day life span of the platelet—include the immune-mediated process of autoimmune thrombocytopenia purpura (ITP), systemic lupus erythematosus (SLE), Evans' syndrome (autoimmune hemolysis and autoimmune thrombocytopenia), and drug-related thrombocytopenia.

  2. The **differential diagnosis** of qualitative disorders includes anything that decreases the platelet's ability to perform its two fundamental functions in thrombus formation—adhering to the endothelium and aggregating. These include the acquired entities of aspirin use and uremia and the congenital entities of von Willebrand's disease, Glanzmann's thrombasthenia, and Bernard–Soulier syndrome. The most common cause is aspirin use.

B. The **specific manifestations** of this group are similar to those listed under I. In addition, there is a marked number of petechiae, as these skin and mucous membrane manifestations are quite specific for quantitative and qualitative platelet disorders. A history of aspirin use can be helpful in defining the process.

C. The further **evaluation** of this subgroup includes making the clinical diagnosis and performing the tests listed in Box 5-3. Specific evaluations include measuring levels of platelet-associated antibodies, IgM, IgG, and drug-specific antibodies; reviewing the peripheral smear; and determining serum folate and vitamin B_{12} levels. A bone marrow examination may be considered but is not mandatory.

D. The **specific management** of thrombocytopenia is based on the degree of the deficit and the underlying cause.

  1. If there is any evidence of bleeding, or if surgery is contemplated, or if the platelet count is <10,000/mm^3, platelet transfusions are indicated. The dosage of random-donor platelets is 1 pack/10 kg of patient's body weight. Each random-donor platelet pack should raise the peripheral count by 10,000/mm^3. Transfusion of human leukocyte antigen (HLA)-typed platelets is effective but extremely expensive, requires an active and large blood bank, and is time consuming for the donor of the platelets. Thus HLA-matched platelets should be reserved for refractory cases.

2. If the process is thought to be immune mediated, discontinue the potentially offending medications and initiate a course of steroids. The steroid dose is either prednisone, 60–80 mg p.o., once per day, or methylprednisolone (Solumedrol), 40 mg q.8hr i.v., either with a slow taper. The steroid taper should be titrated to the platelet count.

   a. If the patient is not bleeding, transfusion with platelets in patients with immune-mediated processes is of little benefit because of the rapid peripheral destruction of normal host and donor platelets.

3. Until stabilized, platelet counts should be determined daily. After the steroid taper begins, less frequent measurement is acceptable.

4. Aspirin is contraindicated.

V. Consultation

Problem	Service	Time
Elevated PT unresponsive to vitamin K	Hematology	Urgent
Elevated aPTT, except for heparin use	Hematology	Urgent
Thrombocytopenia	Hematology	Urgent/emergent

VI. Indications for admission: Any active bleeding, any consumptive coagulopathy such as DIC, or any profound thrombocytopenia (i.e., platelet count $<20,000/mm^3$).

Breast Malignancy

The normal breast is composed of multiple glands that, under appropriate hormonal stimulation, lactate (produce milk). The milk produced flows to the nipples through ducts. The epithelium lining these ducts is the source of the vast majority of malignant neoplastic lesions in the breast.

I. The **underlying pathogenesis** of breast malignancy is not completely known; however, certain endocrine and genetic factors are involved.

Specific risk factors for the development of breast malignancy include the endocrine factors of an early onset of menarche (before age 12 years), a late menopause (after age 50 years), the long-term use of high-dose estrogens, and a late first completed pregnancy (after age 30 years). Genetic risk factors include, prominently, a family history of breast cancer or in a first-degree female relative (mother, daughter, or sibling). A final risk factor is a personal history of breast carcinoma in the contralateral breast.

The incidence of this malignant neoplastic lesion is very high. In 1987 ~130,000 new cases of breast carcinoma were diagnosed in the United States and western Europe. The incidence and death rate for this malignancy are, in women, second only to those of bronchogenic carcinoma. Based on various epidemiologic calculations, a woman has a 1 in 9 risk of developing this malignancy in her lifetime.

II. **Screening tests:** Refer to Table 16-3, page 710

III. The **specific evaluation and management** of a lump discovered on palpation or by mammography include the following schemes. These schemes are put into effect before the diagnosis of breast carcinoma has been made. See also, Chapter 11, page 525: Breast mass/lump.

A. **Clinically suggestive lumps**

If the lump is in any way suggestive of a neoplastic lesion, the patient should be referred expeditiously to a general surgeon with experience in breast disorders for an excisional biopsy. Characteristics of the lump that increase the suspicion for malignancy include painlessness, firmness (even to the point of being hard), concurrent ipsilateral axillary lymph node enlargement, and the mammographic demonstration of minute calcifications within its substance. Patient characteristics that increase the suspicion for malignancy include any of the risk factors for breast carcinoma development described.

B. **Clinically benign lumps**

If the lump is clinically benign, it can be followed up with a repeated physical examination in 1 month and a mammogram at that time. The defining physical features of a benign lump include the absence of any features listed under A that would define a suspicious lesion and, if it is in a young patient, the lump is intermittently tender, especially waxing and waning in discomfort and size during the menstrual cycle, and there are no microscopic calcifications in the lump detected mammographically. If on repeated examination the lump has not resolved or if there is any suspicion for malignancy, referral to a surgeon is indicated for excisional biopsy. *Caveat:* The threshold for biopsy should be low.

C. **Surgical options**

Once the decision to perform an excisional biopsy is made, the surgeon, primary care physician, and the patient should decide how to proceed if the frozen-section results of the excisional biopsy are positive for carcinoma. It is at this time, before the procedure and before the diagnosis is histopathologically confirmed, that the strategy for surgical management must be determined.

If the lump is histopathologically demonstrated to be carcinoma, the surgical options include:

1. A modified radical mastectomy with axillary dissection, in which the entire breast along with the underlying pectoralis muscle and the adjacent axillary lymph nodes are resected in one piece; or
2. A lumpectomy with axillary dissection and postoperative adjuvant irradiation, in which the breast lump is resected and, in a concurrent procedure, the axillary nodes are dissected and resected. Postoperative local adjuvant irradiation is mandatory, even if the lesion is a localized ductal carcinoma in situ.

IV. **Evaluation and staging** of histopathologically diagnosed carcinoma

The evaluation and staging of clinically and histopathologically diagnosed (via biopsy) breast carcinoma usually occur after a definitive surgical intervention. The evaluation and staging are based on the natural history of the disease. Early metastases of breast carcinoma are to the lymph nodes. If the primary lesion is in the outer quadrants of the breast, disease will spread to the ipsilateral axillary lymph nodes, whereas if the primary lesion is in the inner quadrants of the breast, disease will spread to the ipsilateral mediastinal nodes. In advanced disease, metastases occur to the supraclavicular lymph nodes, liver, lungs, brain, and/or bones. Components in the evaluation and staging of the carcinoma are listed in Box 5-4.

V. The **overall management** of breast carcinoma entails effectively screening for breast lesions, making the diagnosis early, using the described strategies, and effecting appropriate surgical intervention. After surgery and staging, the clinician assesses the risk for disease recurrence and thus the need for further nonsurgical therapy. Furthermore, there are tests for several markers that may be performed on the tumor; these indicate a more aggressive tumor.

A. **Minimal risk**

There is no evidence of metastatic disease, including no metastatic disease in the ipsilateral axillary lymph nodes. Specific histopathologic markers on the tumor may indicate a less aggressive tumor. After the surgical procedure, no adjuvant chemotherapy is needed.

B. **Moderate risk**

Either one to three lymph nodes are positive for metastatic carcinoma without any other evidence of metastatic disease or the specific histopathologic markers on the tumor demonstrate an aggressive tumor. Although the tumor has been surgically resected, there is the risk for micrometastatic disease, and therefore, adjuvant chemotherapy is indicated.

BOX 5-4

Overall Evaluation and Staging of Breast Carcinoma

Evaluation

1. Bilateral mammography should already have been performed in the evaluation of a breast mass.
2. Obtain chest radiographs in PA and lateral views to stage the disease, looking especially for any nodules in the pulmonary fields.
3. Perform LFTs, including alkaline phosphatase, LDH, aspartate aminotransferase (SGOT), alanine aminotransferase (SGPT), and total bilirubin. If any of these indices is elevated, disease may have metastasized to the liver. Further evaluation with computed tomography (CT) of the abdomen may be indicated.
4. Perform a radionuclide bone scan to look for any "hot spots," areas of increased uptake in bone indicative of metastatic disease.
5. If there is any hepatomegaly or if any LFT test results are abnormal, perform abdominal CT to look for space-occupying lesions consistent with metastatic disease.
6. All biopsy specimens must be tested for estrogen and progesterone receptors. The presence or absence of these receptors on the tumor is an integral factor in determining further management.
7. If there is any neurologic deficit, perform CT of the head to look for any space-occupying lesion consistent with metastatic disease.

Staging

The overall staging is important not only in prognosis but also in determining the best modalities to use in addition to surgery in the treatment of breast carcinoma. The TNM (tumor, node, metastases) staging system is listed in Table 5-3.

C. **High risk**

There is documented metastatic disease outside the axillary lymph nodes, or more than four lymph nodes are positive for disease. Not adjuvant but therapeutic chemotherapy and/or hormonal intervention is needed.

T A B L E 5-3
TNM Staging Classification of Breast Carcinoma

Stage	Description
T1	Lesion size: <2 cm in diameter
T2	Lesion size: 2 cm to 5 cm in diameter
T3	Lesion size: >5 cm in diameter
T4	Lesion fixed to the chest wall and/or skin
N0	No nodal metastases
N1	Mobile axillary nodes
N2	Axillary nodes fixed to the skin and/or fascia
N3	Supraclavicular nodes
M0	No distant metastases
M1	Any distant metastases

VI. Chemotherapy and hormonal therapy

A. Chemotherapy (See Tables 5-9 and 5-10)

Adjuvant or therapeutic chemotherapy includes regimens of CMF (cyclophosphamide, methotrexate, and 5-FU) or regimens based on anthracycline (e.g., Adriamycin). Adjuvant regimens are of shorter duration but not necessarily of lower intensity than therapeutic regimens.

B. Hormonal therapy

Endocrine manipulation includes the use of the antiestrogen agent tamoxifen, which is effective in controlling metastatic disease in estrogen receptor (ER)–positive patients. Tamoxifen is most useful in postmenopausal women with ER-positive, metastatic disease. The dosage of tamoxifen is 10 mg/day p.o. A potential side effect is hypercalcemia in patients with metastatic disease to the bones.

VII. Consultation

Problem	Service	Time
Any suspicious lesion	General surgery	Urgent
Adjuvant local irradiation	Radiation oncology	Urgent (if a lumpectomy with axillary node dissection is planned)
Adjuvant or therapeutic chemotherapy is indicated	Medical oncology	Urgent

VIII. Indications for admission: Scheduled admissions for the initiation of chemotherapy or for surgical intervention.

Bronchogenic Carcinoma

I. The **underlying pathogenesis** of bronchogenic carcinoma is unclear, but the cells of origin of the malignant neoplastic growth are in the lung tissue and have been postulated to be from a common stem cell or from malignant transformation of mature cells in the airways, the alveoli, or the neuroectoderm—Kulchitsky's cells. Thus there can be significant diversity in the histopathologic types of bronchogenic carcinomas.

   A. The **risk factors** for the development of all bronchogenic carcinomas except the specific non–small-cell carcinoma, adenocarcinoma, include smoking of any tobacco product, smoking marijuana, exposure to asbestos fibers, and exposure to heavy metals or irradiation. Smoking of tobacco and exposure to asbestos synergistically increase the risk of bronchogenic carcinoma development.

   The **risk factors** for adenocarcinomas include any process that results in scarring or fibrosis of the lung tissue, irradiation, and exposure to asbestos. Adenocarcinoma has been referred to as "scar carcinoma."

   B. The incidence of these malignant neoplastic disorders is high and increasing at an alarming rate. This entity is the most common cause of cancer and cancer-related deaths in the United States and probably in the western world. In 1988 >150,000 new cases of bronchogenic carcinoma were diagnosed in the United States alone.

II. The **overall manifestations** of bronchogenic carcinoma are usually quite minimal until late in the disease course. These manifestations can be as a direct result of the tumor in the lung or of metastatic disease; they may also occur as paraneoplastic syndromes.

   A. **Manifestations attributable to the tumor**

   Manifestations directly attributable to the tumor include a cough that is chronic or subacute, intermittent hemoptysis, unintentional weight loss, and a history of recurrent pneumonias in the same lobe. Further manifestations include wheezing localized to the affected areas and chest radiographic findings of a nodule (<4 cm in diameter), a mass (>4 cm in diameter), or a persistent radiographic infiltrate. Other manifestations that may occur as a direct result of locally advanced disease include those described subsequently.

      1. **Horner's syndrome,** which manifests with the triad of unilateral miosis, unilateral ptosis, and unilateral anhydrosis, all as a result of tumor in the ipsilateral upper lobe that directly invades the ipsilateral superior cervical ganglion. This ganglion supplies sympathetic innervation to the ipsilateral face and head.

2. The development of a brachial plexopathy, which manifests with weakness (paresis), pain, paresthesias, and dysesthesias, all as a result of tumor in the ipsilateral upper lung that has invaded the brachial plexus.

B. **Manifestations of metastatic disease**
These manifestations include bone pain, especially in the low back, and even pathologic fractures, all as a result of bony metastases. Furthermore, neurologic deficits and hepatomegaly can develop as a result of metastatic disease to the brain or liver.

C. **Manifestations of paraneoplastic syndromes**
Several of these syndromes are discussed in the specific discussion of small-cell and non–small-cell carcinoma.

III. **Screening**
Bronchogenic carcinoma would be a perfect disorder for a screening examination. Unfortunately, no effective screening technique, including scheduled chest radiography, is useful in the detection of this malignant disorder.

IV. The **overall evaluation** and staging of these lesions include assessing the probability that bronchogenic carcinoma is present, based on findings on chest radiographs and clinical observations, especially in patients with a moderate to high risk-factor profile. In many respects, the overall evaluation is quite similar to that described for a solitary pulmonary nodule (see Chapter 4). The overall evaluation is listed in Box 5-5.

V. **Specific evaluation and management** by tumor type
The specific evaluation, natural history, staging, and management of the various primary bronchogenic carcinomas are best outlined if the lesions are divided into two broad categories, small-cell carcinoma and non–small-cell carcinoma.

A. **Small-cell carcinoma** is a unique but common form of bronchogenic carcinoma, possibly derived from cells of neuroectoderm origin.

1. **Manifestations**
The **specific manifestations** of small-cell carcinoma include those listed in section II. This specific type of neoplasm will often manifest with a paraneoplastic syndrome. In fact, the paraneoplastic syndrome is the initial manifestation of this lesion. These paraneoplastic syndromes include but are not limited to the following:

a. The **syndrome of inappropriate antidiuretic hormone secretion (SIADH),** with resultant hyponatremia. The hyponatremia may be marked and may result in delirium, lethargy, and seizures.

b. The syndrome of **ectopic adrenocorticotropic hormone (ACTH),** with resultant increased skin pigmentation and findings of hypercortisolism. The

B O X 5-5

Overall Evaluation of Suspected Bronchogenic Carcinoma

Evaluation

1. If a solitary pulmonary nodule is discovered, see the section on Solitary Pulmonary Nodule in Chapter 4, page 238.
2. Take a thorough history and perform a physical examination, with emphasis on the findings listed under II.
3. Obtain chest radiographs in PA and lateral views, a central component of the evaluation. The radiographs are useful in demonstrating the size of the lesion and the presence or absence of concurrent manifestations such as pleural effusions or hilar enlargement.
4. Obtain sputum for cytology, AFB smear, and Gram stain q. a.m. for 3 days. The cytologic findings, if positive, will clinch the diagnosis, and further invasive evaluation is usually unnecessary. Negative cytologic findings, however, do not rule out a malignant neoplastic lesion.
5. If pleural fluid is accessible, perform thoracentesis for diagnostic purposes (see section on Pleural Effusions, Chapter 4, page 216). The cytologic findings on the pleural fluid, if positive for a malignant, neoplastic lesion, will clinch the diagnosis and in most cases obviate the need for other invasive evaluation.
6. Perform CT imaging of the lesion with and without contrast media. This imaging technique demonstrates the extent of local disease: the size of the mass, any mediastinal lymph node enlargement, and any concurrent pleural disease.
7. If the previous steps do not produce a histopathologic diagnosis, more-invasive evaluation is indicated.
   a. If the lesion is peripheral in location, percutaneous needle biopsy under CT guidance should be performed by a radiologist with expertise in this procedure.
   b. If lesion is central, bronchoscopy for biopsy of the lesion should be performed by a pulmonologist.

(continued)

B O X   5-5 *(continued)*

8. Perform pulmonary function tests (PFTs), including FEV_1, FVC, and arterial blood gases. PFTs are particularly important if any surgical intervention for resection of the lesion is being considered, as an FEV_1 of <1.5 L is a contraindication to pneumonectomy.
9. Determine levels of serum calcium, phosphorus, albumin, electrolytes, and a CBC with differential for baseline purposes. These indices are important, as several of the malignant neoplastic lesions can manifest with hypercalcemia and/or profound hyponatremia as a result of a paraneoplastic syndrome.
10. Differentiate the tumor type into one of two groups: small-cell carcinoma or non–small-cell carcinoma. The specific evaluation and management are based on this differentiation.

secondary hypercortisolism will manifest with truncal obesity, hypertension, hyperglycemia, hypokalemia, and hypernatremia.

c. **Eaton–Lambert syndrome,** a diffuse, myasthenia-like muscle weakness that, unlike myasthenia gravis, improves with repeated motor activity.

2. **Natural history**
   Small-cell carcinoma grows rapidly and metastasizes early and significantly: to adjacent lung tissue, the contralateral lung, the bones, bone marrow, brain, liver, or adrenal glands.

3. The **specific evaluation** of this entity includes the steps listed in Box 5-5 and making the histopathologic diagnosis. Evaluation is based on the natural history of the tumor and is tantamount to staging. Evaluation entails a CT imaging of the head, the thorax, and abdomen. Further evaluation includes performing a bone scan and bone-marrow aspiration.

4. The **staging** of small-cell carcinoma entails categorizing the disease as limited or extensive. In the limited stage, tumor is restricted to one hemithorax; in the extensive stage, disease is demonstrated outside the affected hemithorax. The stage is a marker for prognosis and also aids in therapeutic decision making.

5. The **management** of small-cell carcinoma is based on disease stage at the time of presentation and on the fact that it is a malignant neoplasm that responds to chemotherapy. In the limited stage, this tumor is

potentially curable. Therefore therapeutic intervention must be aggressive. Chemotherapy regimens include etoposide (VP-16) and cisplatin; or cyclophosphamide, doxorubicin, and vincristine; or cyclophosphamide, doxorubicin, and etoposide (VP-16). Chemotherapy results in complete remission in 85%–95% of cases of limited disease; 65%–85% of cases of extensive disease. Chemotherapy will also palliate any local manifestations. Long-term responses (i.e., 5-year survival) is bleak—2%–8% for limited disease; 0%–1% for extensive disease.

A caveat to management is that a solitary pulmonary nodule that has been resected and diagnosed to be small-cell carcinoma should be treated, at a minimum, as limited disease. Therefore, unlike in a solitary pulmonary nodule that is non–small-cell carcinoma, adjuvant chemotherapy is indicated in small-cell carcinoma.

B. Non–small-cell carcinoma

Non–small-cell carcinomas include adenocarcinomas, squamous cell carcinomas, and large-cell anaplastic carcinomas. Each of these malignant neoplasms is biologically distinct, but from a clinical point of view, all behave and respond to therapy in similar ways, and as such are discussed together.

1. The **specific manifestations** of these lesions include those listed under I. Non–small-cell carcinomas often manifest with a paraneoplastic syndrome, which may be the initial manifestation of a lesion. The paraneoplastic syndromes include but are not limited to the following:

   a. The syndrome of ectopic secretion of a **parathormone (PTH)-like** substance with resultant hypercalcemia. This will often manifest with polyuria, polydipsia, constipation, intravascular volume depletion, lethargy, and even coma.

   b. The development of **hypertrophic pulmonary osteoarthropathy,** which manifests with bilateral clubbing and a diffuse, symmetric, polyarticular, small-joint arthritis (see Figs. 4-1 and 4-2, page 206).

2. **Natural history**

   Non–small-cell carcinomas grow quite slowly and metastasize first to the local mediastinal lymph nodes, and then to bone and liver.

3. The **specific evaluation** of non–small-cell carcinoma includes the steps listed in Box 5-5 and making the histopathologic diagnosis. Evaluation is based on the natural history of the tumor and is tantamount to staging. Evaluation entails CT imaging of the thorax and

T A B L E 5-4
TNM Staging Classification of Non–Small Cell Carcinomas

Stage	Descriptors
T1	Mass <3 cm in diameter
T2	Mass ≥3 cm in diameter and/or there is extension to the hilum
T3	T2 and the presence of atelectasis and/or pleural effusion
N0	No nodal metastases
N1	Hilar nodes present
N2	Mediastinal nodes present
M0	No extrathoracic metastases
M1	Any extrathoracic metastasis

abdomen and, if clinically indicated, of the head. Further evaluation includes performing a bone scan to look for bony metastases.

4. **Staging**

The staging of non–small-cell carcinomas is best done by the TNM (tumor, node, metastases) method (Table 5-4).

5. **Management**

The management of non–small-cell carcinoma is based on disease stage at the time of presentation and on the fact that these lesions are refractory to irradiation and chemotherapy. After disease has spread from the primary site, the condition is essentially incurable. Therefore early-stage lesions, especially those that are a solitary pulmonary nodule, should be treated aggressively surgically, but for advanced disease, only palliative therapy is indicated (see Table 5-11). Thus irradiation should be saved until the patient has become symptomatic (i.e., the disease can be palliated).

VI. **Prevention**

Prevention is a major factor in the management of bronchogenic carcinoma. Instructing the patient to discontinue smoking tobacco and developing strategies to minimize exposure of people to second-hand smoke and to carcinogenic fibers (e.g., asbestos) are of paramount importance.

VII. **Consultation**

Problem	Service	Time
CT-directed biopsy of peripheral lesion	Radiology	Urgent
Bronchoscopy for central lesion	Pulmonology	Urgent

Bronchogenic carcinoma	Oncology	Required
Superior vena cava syndrome	Radiation oncology	Emergent
Any solitary pulmonary nodule in a high-risk surgery patient	Cardiothoracic	Urgent

VIII. **Indications for admission:** Any symptomatic paraneoplastic syndrome, active pneumonia, severe side effects of chemotherapy, Horner's syndrome, a superior vena cava syndrome.

Colon Carcinoma

I. The **underlying pathogenesis** of colon carcinoma is not completely clear, but it is known that colon adenocarcinoma usually develops from adenomatous polyps in the colon. These polyps are lesions in which there is the nonmalignant neoplastic growth of the colonic mucosa. Such polyps may be pedunculated or sessile. They grow slowly and can transform into malignant neoplastic disease (i.e., colon adenocarcinoma). The risk factors for polyp development are essentially the same as for the development of colon adenocarcinoma. Two chromosomal abnormalities have been associated with the development of colon carcinoma: the adenomatous polyposis coli (APC) gene and the deleted in colon cancer (DCC) gene. The APC gene on chromosome 5, when deleted or mutated, results in familial polyposis syndrome; the DCC gene on chromosome 18q, when deleted, is associated with the development of sporadic colon carcinoma.

A. **Risk factors** include the presence of adenomatous polyps in the colon, in general, and the polyposis syndromes, many of which are hereditary, in specific. Several polyposis syndromes are described in Table 5-5. Other risk factors include a low-fiber, high-fat diet and the inflammatory bowel disorder, ulcerative colitis. Ulcerative colitis is independent of polyps in the development of colon adenocarcinoma.

B. The **incidence** of colon cancer is high in North America and western Europe. Various sources reported an overall incidence of almost 50 cases per 100,000 population per year in the U.S. population older than age 30 years. Moreover, colon cancer is second only to bronchogenic carcinoma as a cause of cancer-related death in the United States today.

II. The **overall manifestations** of colon carcinoma depend on the stage of the disease and the antecedent risk factors.

A. **Early manifestations**

The disease process is minimally symptomatic until quite late in its course. Adenomatous polyps, even those with areas of carcinoma in situ, usually manifest with intermittently guaiac-positive stools and only rarely become symptomatic. The exception to the paucity of early manifestations is if the antecedent disease process is ulcerative colitis. In the case of ulcerative colitis, bloody diarrhea, fevers, and abdominal pain are usually quite evident; in fact, the patient usually already has that diagnosis.

B. Late manifestations

Manifestations of advanced colon adenocarcinoma include constipation, obstipation, melena, hematochezia, weight loss, a pale color to the skin and mucous membranes due to anemia, and occasionally findings referable to large-bowel obstruction (i.e., diffuse abdominal pain, tympanic abdominal distention, and a significant decrease in flatus).

III. Screening tests

Screening tests for colon carcinoma and colon polyps include stool guaiac examinations and flexible proctosigmoidoscopy. The screening test is based on the fact that adenomatous polyps and early colon adenocarcinomas bleed intermittently.

A. Recommended screening schedule—See Table 16-3, page 710.

B. Subsequent studies based on screening results

1. When a stool guaiac screen is positive, further evaluation is indicated. The evaluation entails either flexible proctosigmoidoscopy and an air-contrast barium enema examination, or colonoscopy.

2. If flexible proctosigmoidoscopy or the air-contrast barium enema examination discloses one or more polyps, full colonoscopy and biopsies of all polyps are indicated.

3. The histopathology of these lesions is of paramount import. If adenocarcinoma is demonstrated, further evaluation and management are indicated, whereas if a nonmalignant adenomatous polyp is demonstrated, follow-up colonoscopy in 1 year is indicated.

4. If ulcerative colitis is demonstrated, yearly surveillance colonoscopy is indicated starting 10 years after the initial diagnosis. Multiple biopsy specimens should be obtained, especially of any suspicious looking areas.

IV. Evaluation and staging

Evaluation and staging are based on the natural history of the disease. The malignant neoplastic disease starts as a focus of malignant transformation (i.e., carcinoma in situ) in the polyp and, with growth, invades the colonic wall. Early metastases of the carcinoma are to the local lymph nodes, to the liver via the portal venous system, and later to the lungs, bone, and brain.

T A B L E 5-5
Polyposis Syndromes

Syndrome	Genetics	Components
Familiar polyposis syndrome	Autosomal dominant Mutated APC gene (adenomatous polyposis coli) on chromosome 5	Multiple (>100) adenomatous and villous polyps in colon and the upper gastrointestinal tract (ascending and descending) Increased risk of colon adenocarcinoma
Gardner's syndrome	Autosomal dominant Mutated APC gene (adenomatous polyposis coli) on chromosome 5	Multiple (>100) adenomatous polyps Skeletal osteomata Sebaceous cysts Lipomas Neoplasia of the thyroid/adrenal Neoplasia of the biliary tree Desmoid tumor (i.e., fibromatosis of the mesentery) Increased risk of colon carcinoma Congenital hypertrophy of retinal pigment epithelium

Turcot's syndrome	Autosomal recessive	Multiple (>100) adenomatous polyps Supratentorial glioblastomas including glioblastoma multiforme Increased risk of colon adenocarcinoma
Peutz–Jegher's syndrome	Autosomal dominant	Mucucutaneous pigmentation in nose, lips, buccal mucosa, hands, and feet Harmartomatous polyps in the GI tract, most common in the small intestine Increased risk of duodenal carcinoma Mild increase in risk of colon carcinoma
Hereditary polyposis colorectal cancer syndrome	Autosomal dominant	<100 adenomatous polyps Mainly on right/ascending colon Increased risk of colon carcinoma

A. **Evaluation**

Once the histopathologic diagnosis has been made by biopsy of a polyp via flexible proctosigmoidoscopy or colonoscopy, the overall evaluation is tantamount to a staging evaluation. Components of evaluation and staging are listed in Box 5-6.

B. The staging of colon adenocarcinoma is described in Table 5-6. The prognosis is related to stage: the later the stage, the poorer the prognosis. Preoperative staging will demonstrate only extracolonic metastases and thus only dichotomizes the staging into Dukes' D and non–Dukes'

B O X   5-6

Overall Evaluation of Known Colon Adenocarcinoma

Evaluation

1. Colonoscopy, if not yet performed, is necessary to look for any metachronous lesions. The reasoning is that if one carcinoma or polyp is discovered, there is an increased risk of concurrent colonic lesions.

2. A serum carcinoembryonic antigen (CEA) level should be determined at baseline. An elevated CEA level is a marker for disease regression or recurrence. A normal CEA level, however, does not rule out metastatic or recurrent disease.

3. Obtain chest radiographs in PA and lateral views to look for any nodules that might be consistent with metastatic colon carcinoma. The classic pattern is one of multiple nodular lesions in both pulmonary fields.

4. Determine the CBC count for baseline purposes and to look for any evidence of an iron-deficiency anemia.

5. Perform LFTs to look for any abnormal elevations that might be consistent with metastatic disease to the liver. The classic pattern is one of a moderate increase in GGT and alkaline phosphatase levels and a mild increase in AST, ALT, and LDH levels.

6. Perform CT of the abdomen if there is any clinical evidence of hepatomegaly or any LFT abnormalities. CT is used to look for any metastatic disease to the liver. The classic pattern is one of multiple space-occupying lesions in the liver.

T A B L E 5-6
Astler–Coller Modification of the Dukes' Staging Classification

Stage	Definition	Prognosis (5-Year Survival)
A	Limited to mucosa	95%
B1	Extends to the muscularis propria, lymph nodes negative	80%
B2	Extends through the entire wall; lymph nodes negative	70%
C1	Extends to the muscularis propria; lymph nodes positive	50%
C2	Extends through the entire wall; lymph nodes positive	30%
D	Distant metastases	10%

D lesions. Further Dukes' staging requires analysis of the surgical specimen.

V. The **overall management** of colon carcinoma entails screening for the lesions, especially in patients at high risk, and making the diagnosis expediently via invasive endoscopy and biopsy. Once the diagnosis is made, the management schemes differ according to whether the stage of the cancer is non–Dukes' D or Dukes' D.

A. **Non–Dukes' D lesions**

All non–Dukes' D lesions demand surgical intervention. Surgical interventions include hemicolectomy on the side involved by the adenocarcinoma or a total proctocolectomy in polyposis syndromes or ulcerative colitis. Surgical intervention in the early stages is essentially curative. If the stage is B2 or C, adjuvant chemotherapy may be of benefit. Adjuvant therapy includes 5-FU and levamisole and is indicated for B2 and C disease. Recent reports demonstrate that in colon carcinoma, the expression of the DCC gene (allelic loss of chromosome 18q), predicts a poorer prognosis. This is particularly true in stage B2 disease.

B. **Dukes' D lesions**

All Dukes' D carcinomas are candidates for chemotherapy. Although the response rates are low (10%–15%), some significant partial and even complete remissions can occur with chemotherapy. The most commonly used regimens include 5-FU and leucovorin (leucovorin augments activity and toxicity of 5-FU). Surgical intervention in stage Dukes' D disease is indicated only for palliation.

V. Consultation

Problem	Service	Time
Dukes' B2 and C lesions	Oncology	Postoperatively: required
Dukes' D lesions	Oncology	At time of diagnosis: urgent
All non–Dukes' D lesions	General surgery	Urgent

VI. **Indications for admission:** Evidence of bowel obstruction, or for scheduled surgical interventions.

Hodgkin's Disease and Non-Hodgkin's Lymphoma

Lymphoid tissue consists of lymphocytes and cells of the reticulo-endothelial system and is normally present in various collections in every organ system of the body. Among the most common collections of such tissue are the lymph nodes. The functions of normal lymphoid tissue include acting as a line of host defense against invading pathogens and as a repository of the cells of humoral and cell-mediated immunity, B lymphocytes and T lymphocytes, respectively. Hodgkin's disease is a specific form of malignant lymphoproliferative transformation of this lymphoid tissue. See Table 5-7 for specifics on non-Hodgkin's lymphoma.

The **incidence of Hodgkin's disease** is bimodal, with a sharp peak in the population in the third decade of life and a lesser peak in the sixth decade.

I. **Underlying pathogenesis**
The **underlying pathogenesis** of this malignant lymphoproliferative disease is unknown, but one of the postulated mechanisms involves a viral infection. The virus that has been most highly correlated with the development of Hodgkin's disease is the DNA virus of Epstein–Barr. The cell type that becomes malignant is similarly unknown but is postulated to be a stromal or a reticuloendothelial cell within the lymph node that manifests histopathologically as a **Reed–Sternberg cell.**

II. **Overall manifestations**
The overall **clinical manifestations** of Hodgkin's disease are variable and depend on the site of lymph node–tissue disease and the stage of the disease at the time of presentation. Early in the course of the disease, the patient may be asymptomatic, presenting to the physician only with a "lump in the neck" or "enlarged glands." On examination there often is lymph node enlargement with a rubbery texture.

In advanced disease, B symptoms may appear. B symptoms have staging implications and, when present, are consistent with an advanced stage and portend a poorer progno-

T A B L E 5-7
Non-Hodgkin's Lymphoma

Classes	% of Diseases	Types	Survival	Treatment
I Low grade	40%	Small lymphocytic Follicular small cleaved cell Follicular mixed small cleaved cell	5–7 yr	Radiation
II Intermediate grade	40%	Follicular, large cell Diffuse, small cell, cleaved cell Diffuse, mixed, large, cleaved, and noncleaved cell	2–5 yr	CHOP or BACOP
III High grade	20%	Diffuse large cell immunoblastic Lymphoblastic Small noncleaved (Burkitt's)	6–18 mo	CHOP or BACOP

B-cell markers: 85% of all NHL
T-cell markers: 15% of all NHL

sis. B symptoms include an unintentional weight loss of >10 pounds, drenching night sweats, and/or fevers, especially fevers with a fever curve of the Pel–Ebstein pattern (i.e., clusters of multiple spikes separated by several days without fever).

III. **Screening**

There are no effective screening techniques for this disease.

IV. **Overall evaluation and staging**

   A. **Evaluation**

   The overall evaluation is based on the natural history of the disease. This malignant lymphoproliferative disease starts in one lymph node group and spreads contiguously to other lymph node groups. Once the histopathologic diagnosis has been made via biopsy, further evaluation, ostensibly for staging, includes the steps described in Box 5-7.

   B. **Staging**

   By using the results and data gleaned from the evaluation described in Box 5-8 and the information regarding B symptoms, it is quite easy to stage the disease. In Hodgkin's disease, as in many other malignant conditions, the stage is important in determining prognosis and directing therapy—radiation, chemotherapy, or both. The stages of Hodgkin's disease are listed in Table 5-8.

V. **Overall management**

   The overall management of Hodgkin's disease entails making the diagnosis and staging the disease by using the outline given in Box 5-8 and Table 5-10. Aggressive treatment with early and mandatory oncology consultation is indicated. Referral to general surgery for lymph node biopsy also is indicated.

T A B L E 5-8
Stages of Hodgkin's Disease

Stage I: Disease in one lymph node group on one side of the diaphragm

Stage II: Disease in more than one lymph node group on one side of the diaphragm

Stage III: Disease in more than one lymph node group on both sides of the diaphragm

Stage IV: Extralymphatic involvement (i.e., in the liver or bone marrow)

NOTE: Each stage may be further qualified by A, denoting absence of B symptoms, or B, denoting presence of B symptoms such as unintentional weight loss, drenching night sweats, and episodic fevers (see text).

B O X 5-7

Overall Evaluation and Staging of Presumed Hodgkin's Disease

1. Biopsy of an accessible lymph node should be performed by a general surgeon. The biopsy can be incisional or excisional, and the specimen must be sent for histopathologic analysis. The pathologist should be informed of the clinical suspicion that the patient may have Hodgkin's disease.
2. Determine the CBC count with differential for baseline purposes and to look for any concurrent anemia. It is quite uncommon to have a leukocytosis or left shift.
3. Perform LFTs for baseline purposes. Elevated transaminase levels may be indicative of hepatic involvement by the lymphoproliferative disease.
4. Obtain chest radiographs in PA and lateral views for staging purposes, as the mediastinum is a common site of Hodgkin's-related lymphadenopathy.
5. Determine serum LDH and uric acid levels at baseline. Any lymphoproliferative disorder may, as a result of increased cell turnover, be accompanied by elevated levels of this catabolite of purine bases.
6. Perform a direct Coombs' test, especially in patients with anemia, as Hodgkin's disease may result in Coombs'-positive hemolytic anemia.
7. Obtain CT scans of the thorax, abdomen, and pelvis as part of the staging evaluation. The CT scans demonstrate, and grossly define, any lymphadenopathy in the mediastinum, the periaortic areas, or the retroperitoneal areas. Furthermore, CT is excellent for demonstrating any concurrent hepatomegaly or splenomegaly.
8. Bilateral bone marrow aspirates and trephine biopsies are indicated for staging. If Hodgkin's disease is present, it is, by definition, stage IV disease. Bone marrow aspirates are obtained bilaterally to increase the sensitivity of the testing procedure.

A. **Management strategies** (see Tables 5-9 and 5-10)
   1. Mantle irradiation can be used for stage IA and IIA disease if the disease is above the diaphragm. The radiation field includes cervical and mediastinal lymph nodes and the spleen.

2. Total body irradiation is used in stage IIA disease if the disease is below the diaphragm.

3. Chemotherapy is indicated in most patients with B symptoms or if the disease is stage III or IV. Chemotherapy regimens include either MOPP (mechlorethamine, vincristine, procarbazine, and prednisone) or ABVD (doxorubicin, bleomycin, vinblastine, and dacarbazine). ABVD is superior to MOPP and is equal to ABVD/MOPP but with fewer side effects.

B. **Side effects** include radiation-related xerostomia and hypothyroidism, chemotherapy-related infertility, and late, an increase in risk of leukemia.

C. Concurrent therapy includes allopurinol, 300 mg p.o. q.d. to prevent the purine/uric acid–related problems of tumor lysis syndrome, renal insufficiency, and/or gout.

VI. **Consultation**

Problem	*Service*	*Time*
Any suggestive lymph nodes	General surgery	Urgent
Hodgkin's disease	Oncology	Urgent

VII. **Indications for admission:** Initiation of chemotherapy under the direction of a medical oncologist.

Prostate Carcinoma

I. **Underlying pathogenesis**
The **underlying pathogenesis** is development of a malignant neoplastic disorder of the prostate, usually one of adenocarcinoma. This is now the second most common cause of cancer-related death in men.

II. **Specific manifestations**
The **specific manifestations** are quite minimal until the disease is relatively advanced. The manifestations of moderate to advanced disease include urinary tenesmus, hesitancy, and even incontinence, as the result of overflow incontinence of urine (see page 156). If advanced with metastatic disease, there may be bone pain as a result of bony metastases and/or neurologic deficits as a result of cord compression, cauda equina syndrome, or peripheral neuropathy as a result of entrapment at the egress of the nerve from the vertebral column (Box 5-8).

III. Overall **evaluation and management**
The overall evaluation and management include making the diagnosis at an early, treatable phase by performing the screening examinations of prostate-specific antigen (PSA) or digital rectal examination (see Chapter 16, Screening and Prevention). If there are one or more urologic symptoms (i.e.,

B O X 5-8

Overall Evaluation and Management of Prostate Carcinoma

1. Screen for prostate disease as appropriate (see Table 16-3).
2. If there are any symptoms or signs of prostate carcinoma (e.g., urinary tenesmus, dribbling, frequent small voids, recurrent UTIs) and/or if the prostate is diffusely enlarged or has one or more firm nodules, and/or if the PSA is >10:
   a. Urinalysis with microscopic examination.
   b. Postvoid residual; if > 100 ml, keep Foley catheter in urinary bladder.
   c. Refer to a GU subspecialist for biopsy of prostate, with US guidance. If a nodule is present, perform a biopsy on this specifically.
3. If prostate carcinoma is diagnosed, stage with CT of pelvis, chest radiograph, PA and lateral, and bone scan to assess for pelvic lymph node enlargement, chest metastases, and bony metastases, respectively.
4. a. If local disease and patient has <10-year life expectancy overall, conservative treatment (see text).
   b. If local disease and patient has >10-year life expectancy overall, surgery with radical prostatectomy or pelvic irradiation.
   c. If there are lymph nodes positive for metastatic disease, treat as if advanced.
   d. If advanced disease is present, treat with hormonal manipulation and monitor for development of complications (see text).
5. Perform a Gleason stage/grade on tumor.
6. Monitor PSA, neurologic examination, and query patient for bone pain on a q.6 month basis.
7. Treat any concurrent UTI as necessary; see Chapter 3, page 171.

hesitancy, frequency, recurrent urinary tract infections, or urinary tenesmus), a thorough urologic examination is mandatory. In prostate carcinoma, the PSA is often >10. The digital rectal examination (DRE) may or may not reveal a firm nodule in and/or adjacent to the substance of the gland, or the gland may be diffusely enlarged.

IV. **Treatment**

The **treatment** of prostate carcinoma, especially that of local-ized, asymptomatic disease, is undergoing a significant de-gree of evolution, and developments will change quite rap-idly. The specifics in treatment include those listed in Box 5-8 and in the following discussion.

A. If life expectancy for the patient is <10 years and there is localized, asymptomatic disease, conservative treatment with watchful waiting or antiandrogen therapy is indi-cated, as the vast majority of cases will not lead to the death of the patient.

B. If life expectancy for the patient is >10 years and there is localized disease, the goal is to cure the disease (i.e., to remove all cancer). The treatment options here include radical prostatectomy or pelvic radiation therapy. The 10-year survival rates for these two procedures are quite similar. The radical prostatectomy is now performed by using a nerve-sparing, retropubic route that preserves erectile function. The side effects and incidence include blood loss, incontinence of urine in 5%–10%, and impo-tence in 30%–40% of cases. Mortality rates are 0.5% in many series for this procedure. Pelvic radiation therapy side effects include proctitis, cystitis, and scrotal edema (incidence of 30%–40%).

C. If at the time of radical prostatectomy, there are lymph nodes positive for disease (obtained through pelvic lymphadenectomy and assessed by frozen section before beginning the radical prostatectomy), the management should be that of advanced prostate disease, as there is little evidence to demonstrate benefit to the patient by pelvic radiation.

D. If there is advanced disease (i.e., bony metastases or lymphadenopathy), hormonal treatment is indicated. Objective outcomes include symptomatic relief and a decrease in PSA. Methods of hormone therapy include:

1. Orchiectomy: outpatient procedure performed under local anesthesia.

2. Diethylstilbestrol (DES): 3 mg p.o., q.d. (>3 mg results in a marked increase in cardiovascular side effects; <3 mg has a decreased efficacy).

3. Gonadotropin-releasing hormone antagonists (e.g., leuprolide acetate), which result in a decreased LH and therefore a marked decrease in testosterone. The dose of leuprolide is 7.5 mg (depot) i.m., q.d.

4. Flutamide: acts by blocking the binding of testoster-one to intracellular receptors. The dose of flutamide is 250 mg p.o., t.i.d.

(text continued on page 309)

TABLE 5-9
Chemotherapeutic Agents

Agent	Mechanism of Action	Excretion	Side Effects	Indications

Bleomycin	Intercalates with DNA
	Generates free radicals
		Renal	Pulmonary fibrosis
			Risks include:
			  a. Age >70
			  b. Antecedent lung disease
			  c. Concurrent irradiation
			  d. Cumulative dose >400 mg/M^2
			Minimal myelosuppression
			Nausea and vomiting
				Hodgkin's disease
				Testicular carcinoma
				Squamous cell carcinoma of head and neck
				Non-Hodgkin's lymphoma

Busulfan (Myleran)	Alkylating agent Decreases the replication of DNA	Renal	Myelosuppression Pulmonary suppression	Chronic myelogenous leukemia (CML), >90% response rate
Chlorambucil	Alkylating agent Decreases the replication of DNA	Renal	Myelosuppression	Chronic lymphocytic leukemia (CLL)
2-Chlorodeoxy-adenosine	Inhibits enzymes used in DNA repair; leads to programmed cell death (apoptosis)		Neutropenia Lymphopenia	Waldenstrom's macroglobulinemia
Cisplatin (CDDP)	Alkylating agent	Renal	Severe nausea and vomiting Renal tubular damage Acute tubular necrosis Type IV renal tubular acidosis	Testicular carcinoma Squamous cell carcinoma of the head and neck

(continued)

TABLE 5-9 (continued)

Agent	Mechanism of Action	Excretion	Side Effects	Indications
Cyclophosphamide (Cytoxan) and ifosphamide	Alkylating agent	Renal, catabolized by the liver before excretion	Myelosuppression Reversible alopecia Hemorrhaghic cystitis (prevented by adequate urine output and MESNA, a competitive inhibitor of the active catabolite of cyclophosphamide, thereby decreasing hemorrhaghic cystitis) Nadir 10–14 days	Non-Hodgkin's lymphoma Acute lymphocytic leukemia Multiple myeloma
Cytosine arabinoside (ARA-C)	Decreases DNA via the competitive inhibition of DNA polymerase by the active catabolite, cytidine triphosphate (CTP)	Renal	Myelosuppression, nadir 5–7 days Mild hepatitis Cerebellar dysfunction with profound ataxia	Acute nonlymphocytic leukemia
Dactinomycin	Intercalates DNA	Renal	Myelosuppression, nadir 21 days after Nausea and vomiting Reversible alopecia	Wilms' tumor Choriocarcinoma Testicular carcinoma
Daunorubicin and doxorubicin (Adriamycin)	Intercalates with DNA; generation of free radicals	Hepatic	Myelosuppression, nadir at 10–14 days Reversible alopecia	ANLL Breast carcinoma Sarcoma

Drug	Mechanism		Toxicity	Indications
			Nausea and vomiting Myocardial damage with resultant systolic heart failure; cumulative dose 550 mg/M^2	Hodgkin's disease
DTIC	Intercalates DNA	Renal	Nausea and vomiting; severe and at times dose limiting Myelosuppression, can be prolonged	Malignant melanoma Sarcoma Hodgkin's and non Hodgkin's lymphomas
Etopside (VP-16)	Generation of free radicals, which break the structure of DNA	Renal	Myelosuppression	ANLL Small cell carcinoma Hodgkin's disease Non-Hodgkin's disease
Fluorouracil (5-FU)	Interferes with DNA synthesis by serving as a pyrimidine analog to DNA synthesis Antimetabolite	Liver	Stomatitis: prevented by having patient suck on ice chips during and for 30 min after the infusion	Adjuvant chemotherapy for stage B2 and C colon CA, used with levamisole Therapeutic chemotherapy for Dukes' D colon CA, used in combination with leucovorin Squamous cell carcinoma of head and neck Breast carcinoma

(continued)

TABLE 5-9 (continued)

Agent	Mechanism of Action	Excretion	Side Effects	Indications
Hydroxyurea	Inhibition of ribonucleoside diphosphate reductase, which decreases synthesis of deoxyribose from ribose and therefore decreases synthesis of DNA	Renal	Severe leukopenia Megaloblastic anemia	CML Polycythemia rubra vera
Melphalan	Alkylating agent	Renal	Mild, dose-related myelosuppression	Multiple myeloma Ovarian carcinoma Malignant melanoma ALL
Mercaptopurine (6-MP)	Antimetabolite; purine analog that inhibits the conversion of inosinic acid to adenylic acid, thus decreasing synthesis of DNA	Xanthine oxidase	Leukopenia Jaundice Hyperuricemia	
Methotrexate	Antimetabolite; inhibits the enzyme dihydrofolate reductase. The product of the reaction catalyzed by this enzyme, tetrahydrofolate, is a necessary cofactor to convert uridylic acid to thymidylic acid, thus decreasing the synthesis of DNA	Renal	Leukopenia Stomatitis Mucosal sloughing Cirrhosis	Choriocarcinoma ALL Hodgkin's Non-Hodgkin's Mycosis fungoides Breast carcinoma Sarcoma

Drug	Classification	(Toxicity)	Side Effects	Indications
Mitomycin C	Alkylating agent	Hepatic	Myelosuppression with a delayed and severe anemia Mucositis Hemolytic uremic syndrome	GI carcinoma
Nitrosureas: carmustine (BCNU) and lomustine (CCNU)	Alkylating agents	Renal	Severe nausea and vomiting Delayed and prolonged myelosuppression, may have a 3–6 week nadir	Glioblastoma multiforme Hodgkin's Non-Hodgkin's Small-cell CA
Paclitaxel (Taxol)	Promotes the development of very stable microtubules and therefore, results in cell death by interfering with normal microtubular dynamics	Hepatic	Neutropenia Severe peripheral neuropathy (stocking/glove)	Ovarian CA Breast CA Lung CA
Procarbazine	Alkylating agent	Renal	Delayed and prolonged myelosuppression, may last up to 4–6 weeks Neurotoxic Some monoamine oxidase inhibition, therefore, patient must avoid tyramine-containing foodstuffs	Hodgkin's disease Small-cell CA Malignant melanoma

(continued)

Agent	Mechanism of Action	Excretion	Side Effects	Indications
All-trans retinoic acid	Binds to intranuclear receptor, which then allows the cell to differentiate from the malignant clone into a mature cell clone, specifically M3	Hepatic	Headache Hypertriglyceridemia Pseudotumor cerebri Retinoic acid syndrome: a. Weight gain b. Pulmonary infiltrates c. Pleural effusions	M3, ANLL
Streptozocin (Zanosar)	Alkylating agent	Renal	Renal tubular damage Rare myelosuppression	Pancreatic islet tumors Carcinoid Non-Hodgkin's lymphoma
Vincristine (Oncovin)	Blocks mitosis by binding to microtubules requisite for mitosis	Hepatic	Alopecia Neurotoxicity, peripheral neuropathy and constipation are common SIADH Minimal myelosuppression	ALL Small-cell CA Hodgkin's disease Non-Hodgkin's disease
Vinblastine (Velban)	Blocks mitosis by binding to microtubules requisite for mitosis	Hepatic	Myelosuppression, nadir 7–10 days	Testicular carcinoma Hodgkin's disease

Hormones

Dexamethasone (Decadron)	Decreases edema Lymphocytotoxic	Renal	Cushing's type syndrome	Intracranial METS Cord compression from METS Replacement for adrenal insufficiency (prednisone or hydrocortisone better) Part of virtually all regimens to treat leukemia/lymphoma
DES (Diethylstilbesterol)	Estrogen agent Decreases androgen activity	Hepatic	Decreased libido Impotence If >3 mg/day: a. DVT/PTE b. MIs Dose: 1–3 mg/day	Prostate carcinoma
Flutamide	Nonsteroidal antiandrogen agent–blocks binding of testosterone to its intracellular receptors (there is an increase in LH and testosterone, no receptors)	Hepatic	Impotence	Prostate CA
Leuprolide acetate	Gonadotropin-releasing hormone agents; decrease in LH, an initial mild increase in testosterone and then a marked decrease in testosterone	Hepatic	Impotence	Prostate carcinoma

T A B L E 5-10
Standard Chemotherapeutic Regimens and Indications

MOPP	Hodgkin's lymphoma
Mechlorethamine	
Oncovin (vincristine)	
Procarbazine	
Prednisone	
ABVD	Hodgkin's lymphoma
Adriamycin (doxorubicin)	
Bleomycin	
Vinblastine	
Dacarbazine	
COPP	Non-Hodgkin's lymphoma
Cyclophosphamide	
Oncovin (Vincristine)	
Procarbazine	
Prednisone	
BACOP	Non-Hodgkin's lymphoma
Bleomycin	
Adriamycin (doxorubicin)	
Cyclophosphamide	
Oncovin (vincristine)	
Prednisone	
CHOP	Non-Hodgkin's lymphoma
Cyclophosphamide	
Hydroxydaunomycin	
Oncovin (vincristine)	
Prednisone	
CVP	Non-Hodgkin's lymphoma
Cyclophosphamide	
Vincristine	
Prednisone	
VAD	Multiple myeloma
Vincristine	
Adriamycin	
Dexamethasone	
CAV	Small-cell carcinoma
Cyclophosphamide	
Adriamycin	
Vincristine	
CMF	Breast carcinoma
Cyclophosphamide	
Methotrexate	
5-Fluorouracil	

TABLE 5-11
Palliative/Analgesia/Antinausea Agents in Cancer Pain

Agent	Duration	Usual Dosage	Indications
Acetaminophen (Tylenol, others)	4–6 hr (short)	650 mg p.o./PR, q.4–6hr	Mild pain Fever
Ibuprofen (Motrin, Advil, others)	6–8 hr (intermediate)	400–800 mg p.o., q.6–8hr	Mild pain Concurrent inflammation
Acetaminophen, 325 mg, and codeine, 30 mg (Tylenol #3)	4–6 hr (short)	One tablet, p.o., q.4hr	Moderate pain
Acetaminophen, 325 mg, and codeine 60 mg (Tylenol #4)	4–6 hr (short)	One tablet p.o. q.4hr	Moderate pain
Acetaminophen, 325 mg, and oxycodone, 5 mg (Percocet)	4–6 hr (short)	One tablet p.o., q.4hr	Moderate pain
Morphine sulfate	4 hr (short)	15–30 mg p.o., q.4hr Titrate upward q.8–12hr in increases of 25%–50% until analgesia is achieved	Severe pain
Hydromophone (Dilaudid)	4 hr (short)	2–4 mg p.o., q.4 hr Titrate upward q.8–12hr in increases of 25%–50% until analgesia is achieved	Severe pain
MS-contin	12 hr (long)	Initial 30–60 mg p.o., q.12 hr Use with a short-acting agent, the dose of the short-acting 1/2 that of total 12-hr dose long-acting agent	Severe pain

(continued)

Agent	Duration	Usual Dosage	Indications
Roxanol SR	8 hr (intermediate)	Initial 30–60 mg p.o. q.8hr Use with a short-acting agent, the dose of the short-acting 1/2 that of total 12-hr dose long-acting agent	Severe pain
Fentanyl (Sublimaze Duragesic, others.)	30–60 min	Transdermal delivery, apply patch q.24hr Initial dose: 25 μg/hr; increase to maintenance of 75–525 μg/hr patch	Severe pain
Nausea			
Prochlorperazine (Compazine)	6 hr	10–25 mg p.o./PR, q.6hr	Mild to moderate nausea
Triethylperazine (Torecan)	6 hr	10 mg p.o./PR q.6hr	Mild to moderate nausea
Ondansetron (Zofran)	6–8 hr	4–8 mg p.o. q.8hr	Moderate/severe nausea
Combination of:			
Lorazepam (Ativan)	6–8 hr	1–2 mg p.o./i.m./i.v. q.6hr	Moderate/severe nausea
Metoclopramide (Reglan)	6–8 hr	5–10 mg p.o./i.m./i.v. q.6hr	Moderate/severe nausea
Diphenhydramine (Benadryl)	6–8 hr	25–50 mg p.o./i.m./i.v. q.6hr	Moderate/severe nausea
Marijuana	4–6 hr	Inhale	Moderate/severe nausea
Xerostomia			
Pilocarpine	6–8 hr	5 mg p.o. t.i.d. at mealtime; increases saliva	Xerostomia secondary to radiation treatment of squamous cell carcinoma of Hodgkin's disease

(text continued from page 298)

The patient must be monitored for the development of lower extremity weakness, for if this develops, one must evaluate for and rule out spinal cord compression. If suspected, one must perform, in addition to a thorough physical examination, an MRI of the area of spine suspected to be involved. If epidural disease is demonstrated, the patient should receive high-dose glucocorticoids (e.g., dexamethasone, 10 mg i.v., and then 4 mg i.v., q.6hr, with concurrent hormonal therapy or ketoconazole, 400 mg p.o., q.8hr. Referral to a neurosurgeon for decompression or to radiology for radiation therapy is indicated on an emergent basis. Palliative therapy for bony metastases with radiation therapy and/or effective pain management are indicated (see Table 5-11). No effective chemotherapeutic regimens are known.

IV. **Consultation**

Problem	*Service*	*Time*
Prostate nodule	GU	Required
Elevated PSA	GU	Required
Localized disease life span > 10 years	GU/RT	Required
Spinal cord compression	RT	Emergent
Advance of disease	H-O	Required

Bibliography

Anemia

Beutler E: The common anemias. JAMA 1988;259:2433–2437.

Brittenham GM, et al: Efficacy of deferoxamine in preventing complications of iron overload in patients with thalassemia major. N Engl J Med 1994;331:567–573.

Charache S, et al: Effect of hydroxyurea on the frequency of painful crises in sickle cell anemia. N Engl J Med 1995:332:1317–1322.

Clementz GL, Schade SG: The spectrum of vitamin B-12 deficiency. Am Fam Pract 1990;41:150–161.

Davenport J: Macrocytic anemia. Am Fam Pract 1996:53:155–162.

Fischer SL, Fischer SP: Mean corpuscular volume. Arch Intern Med 1983;143:282–283.

Hansen R, et al: Failure to suspect and diagnose thalassemic syndromes. Arch Intern Med 1985;145:93—94.

Konatey-Ahulu F: The sickle cell diseases: clinical manifestations including the sickle cell crisis. Arch Intern Med 1974;133:611.

Platt OS, et al: Pain in sickle cell disease. N Engl J Med 1991;325:11–15.

Steinberg MH, Dreiling BJ: Microcytosis: its significance and evaluation. JAMA 1983;249:85–87.

Sumner AE, et al: Elevated methylmalonic acid and total homocysteine levels show high prevalence of vitamin B_{12} deficiency after gastric surgery. Ann Intern Med 1996;124:469–476.

Witte DL, et al: Prediction of bone marrow iron findings from tests performed on peripheral blood. Am J Clin Pathol 1986;85:202–206.

Excessive Bleeding States

American Society of Hematology ITP practice guideline panel: diagnosis and treatment of idiopathic thrombocytopenic purpura. Am Fam Pract 1996;54:2437−2447.

Bone RC: Modulators in coagulation in sepsis. Arch Intern Med 1992;152:1381−1389.

Burns TR, Saleem A: Idiopathic thrombocytopenic purpura. Am J Med 1983;75:1001−1007.

George JN, Shattil SJ: The clinical importance of acquired abnormalities of platelet function. N Engl J Med 1991;324:27−38.

Holmberg L, Nilsson IM: Von Willebrand's disease. Clin Haematol 1985;14:461−488.

Hoyer LW: Hemophilia A. N Engl J Med 1994;330:38−47.

Kasper CK, et al: Hematologic management of hemophilia A for surgery. JAMA 1985;253:1279−1283.

Lind SE: Prolonged bleeding time. Am J Med 1984;77:305−311.

Breast Malignancy

AMA Council on Scientific Affairs: Mammographic screening in asymptomatic women aged 40 years and older. JAMA 1989;261:2535−2542.

Basset LW, Butler DL: Mammography and early breast cancer detection. Am Fam Pract 1991;43:547−557.

Chittoor SR, Swain SM: Adjuvant therapy in early breast cancer. Am Fam Pract 1991;44:453−462.

Eddy DM: Screening for breast cancer. Ann Intern Med 1989;111:389−399.

Fisher B, et al: Systemic therapy in patients with node-negative breast cancer. Ann Intern Med 1989;111:703−712.

Fisher B, et al: Lumpectomy compared with lumpectomy and radiation therapy for the treatment of intraductal breast cancer. N Engl J Med 1993:328:1581−1586.

Harris JR, et al: Breast Cancer. N Engl J Med 1992;327:473−480.

Harris JR, et al: Breast Cancer. N Engl J Med 1992;327:390−398.

McGuire WL, et al: Prognostic factors and treatment decisions in axillary-node negative breast cancer. N Engl J Med 1992:326:1756−1761.

Legha SS: Tamoxifen in the treatment of breast cancer. Ann Intern Med 1988;109:219−228.

Weiss RB, et al: Adjuvant chemotherapy after conservative surgery plus irradiation versus modified radical mastectomy. Am J Med 1987;83:455−462.

Bronchogenic Carcinoma

Brower M, et al: Treatment of extensive stage small cell bronchogenic carcinoma. Am J Med 1983;75:993−1000.

Bunn PA, et al: Chemotherapy alone or chemotherapy with chest radiation therapy in limited stage small cell lung cancer. Ann Intern Med 1987;106:655−662.

Cohen MH: Signs and symptoms of bronchogenic carcinoma. Semin Oncol 1974;1:183−187.

Eddy DM: Screening for lung cancer. Ann Intern Med 1989;111:232−237.

Johnson BE, et al: Non-small cell lung cancer. Am J Med 1986;80:1103−1110.

Johnson DH, et al: Thoracic radiotherapy does not prolong survival in patients with locally advanced, unresectable non-small cell lung cancer. Ann Intern Med 1990;113:33−38.

Ihde DC: Chemotherapy of lung cancer. N Engl J Med 1992:327:1434−1441.

Colon Carcinoma

Bulow S: Colorectal polyposis syndromes. Scand J Gastroenterol 1984;19:289–293.

Dodds WJ: Clinical and roentgen features of the intestinal polyposis syndromes. Gastrointest Radiol 1976;1:127–142.

Fletcher RH: Carcinoembryonic antigen. Ann Intern Med 1986;104:66–73.

Hansen RM: Systemic therapy in metastatic colorectal cancer. Arch Intern Med 1990;150:2265–2269.

Jen J, et al: Allelic loss of chromosome 18q and prognosis in colorectal cancer. N Engl J Med 1994;331:213–221.

Krook JE, et al: Effective surgical adjuvant therapy for high risk rectal carcinoma. N Engl J Med 1991;324:709–715.

Moertel CG: Chemotherapy for colorectal cancer. N Engl J Med 1994;330:1136–1142.

Provenzale D, et al: Risk for colon adenomas in patients with rectosigmoid hyperplastic polyps. Ann Intern Med 1990;113:760–763.

Ransohoff DF, Lang CA: Screening for colorectal cancer. N Engl J Med 1991;325:37–41.

Rustgi AK: Hereditary gastrointestinal polyposis and nonpolyposis syndromes. N Engl J Med 1994;331:1694–1702.

Shibata D, et al: The DCC protein and prognosis in colorectal cancer. N Engl J Med 1996;335:1727–1732.

Hodgkin's Disease

Buzaid AC, et al: Salvage therapy of advanced Hodgkin's disease. Am J Med 1987;83:523–531.

Fuller LM, Hagemeister FB: Hodgkin's disease in adults: stages I and II. In: Fuller LM, Hagemeister FB, Sullivan MP, Velasquez WS, eds. Hodgkin's disease and non-Hodgkin's lymphomas in adults and children. New York: Raven Press, 1988:230–246.

Gibbs GE, et al: Long-term survival of patients with Hodgkin's disease. Arch Intern Med 1981;141:897–900.

Kaplan HS: Hodgkin's disease: biology, treatment, prognosis. Blood 1981;57:813.

Prostate Cancer

Byrne TN: Spinal cord compression from epidural metastases. N Engl J Med 1992;327:614–620.

Catalona WJ: Management of cancer of the prostate. N Engl J Med 1994;331:996–1004.

Palliation

Cancer Pain Guideline Panel: Management of cancer pain: adults. Am Fam Pract 1994;49:1853–1868.

Levy MH: Pharmacologic treatment of cancer pain. N Engl J Med 1996;335:1124–1132.

Mosser KH: Transdermal fentanyl in cancer pain. Am Fam Pract 1992;45:2289–2295.

Weissman DE, et al: Handbook of cancer pain management. Madison: Wisconsin Cancer Pain Initiative, 1990.

Chapter 6

Infectious Diseases

Bacterial Skin Diseases

Descriptions of and treatments for common bacterial skin diseases are presented in Table 6-1.

Bite Wounds

I. **Human bite wounds**
Bite wounds inflicted by humans are a not uncommon problem.
A. **Mechanisms**
There are basically two mechanisms through which a human bite wound is incurred: indirect and direct.
1. In the **indirect** method, injuries are incurred by hitting or cutting the hand, fingers, or knuckles on another person's teeth. This method is commonly associated with a fist fight.
2. **Direct** bite wounds occur when another person directly bites the patient. Direct bite wounds commonly occur on the fingers, hands, genitals, and breasts.
B. The **underlying pathogenesis** of disease in human bite wounds involves damage resulting in skin breakdown, damage to adjacent soft-tissue structures, and exposure to infectious agents from the mouth and body secretions (e.g., saliva). Infectious agents include bacterial and viral agents.
1. The two requisite components in the development of bacterial skin infections are a disruption of the normal integrity of the skin and a source of bacteria.
a. The bacteria normally present on the skin of the patient result in infection when the integrity of the skin is disrupted. These include the aerobic gram-positive coccal organisms of the genera *Streptococcus* and *Staphylococcus*.
b. The bacteria present in the assailant's mouth may cause infection in the bite victim. Anaerobic bacte-

T A B L E 6-1
Bacterial Skin Infections

Disease	Clinical Findings	Organism	Treatment
Impetigo	Superficial skin infection Pruritic Significant oozing and crusting can occur Highly contagious; patient may autoinfect other parts of skin by touching originally infected area Types: a) Vesiculopustular type (yellow colored) b) Bullous type c) Ecthyma: An ulcerative type of impetigo that is quite deep	*Streptococcus* or *Staphylococcus* *Staphylococcus aureus* with phage	Contact isolation Mupirocin (Bactroban) 2% applied q.i.d. to affected skin Dicloxicillin, 250–500 mg p.o. q.6hr for 7–10 days, *or* cephalexin (Keflex), 500 mg p.o. q.i.d. for 7–10 days Hydroxyzine; 25 mg p.o. q.i.d. prn for pruritus
Erysipelas	Superficial infection that is sharply demarcated Usually has significant rubor, tumor, dolor, and calor Usually unilateral on the face No vesicles Nonpruritic Has associated systemic signs and symptoms: fever, chills, nausea	*Streptococcus*	Penicillin, 600,000–1,200,000 units i.v. q.4hr, *or* erythromycin, 500–1,000 mg i.v. q.6hr Usually should admit patient Watch for rapid dissemination Contact isolation Infectious disease consultation

(continued)

TABLE 6-1 (continued)

Disease	Clinical Findings	Organism	Treatment
	Can rapidly disseminate through the skin, subcutaneous tissues, and blood Even in immunocompetent hosts may be life threatening		
Folliculitis	Area of pus and erythema in and adjacent to hair follicle Single or multiple Patient may autoinfect during shaving	Staphylococcus aureus	Mupirocin (Bactroban) 2% q.i.d. for 5–7 days
Furuncle	Deep abscess due to folliculitis Very painful; also called "boil"	Staphylococcus aureus	Erythromycin, 500 mg p.o. q.i.d. for 7 days, or cephalexin, 500 mg p.o. q.i.d. for 7 days, or dicloxicillin, 250–500 mg p.o., q.i.d. for 7 days Avoid "squeezing" lesion Incise and drain when "mature"
Carbuncle	Multiple interconnecting abscesses Usually on neck and back Often recurrent Diabetes mellitus is a predisposing factor for this sequela of folliculitis	Staphylococcus aureus	As for furuncle, and screen for and aggressively manage diabetes mellitus
Hidradenitis suppurativa	Chronic infection of apocrine glands of axillae or inguinal areas	Staphylococcus spp.	As for furuncle; usually requires surgical drainage and debridement

| Cellulitis | Multiple abscesses and nodules develop in axillae and inguinal areas
Develops in postpubertal period
Deeper skin infection
Nonpitting edema with other signs of inflammation
Usually less well demarcated
Predisposition includes:
a) Lacerations or any skin break
b) Bites, human or animal (see Bite Wounds, page 312)
c) Lower extremity edema
d) Tinea infections (cracks in skin)
e) Diabetes mellitus
f) Intravenous drug use | *Streptococcus*
Staphylococcus aureus
Anaerobes
Specific pathogens in bites | If severe:
Admit
Blood cultures
Leading-edge aspirate and Gram stain of little value
Incise and drain any abscess
Minimize handling of area (keep elevated)
If bite, see Bite Wounds, page 312
Treat underlying tinea infection, if present
Antibiotics:
Ampicillin–sulbactam (Unasyn), 1.5–3.0 q.6hr/i.v. *or*
Clindamycin, 900 mg q.8hr i.v. and an aminoglycoside
If not severe:
Elevation
Cephalexin (Keflex), 500 mg p.o. q.i.d. for 10 days, and/or clindamycin, 600 mg p.o., t.i.d. for 10 days
For both:
Tetanus toxoid, if indicated (Table 6-2)
Debride any necrotic tissue
Control blood glucose |

ria are common if the assailant has gingival disease, as massive quantities of anaerobes would be present. Another bacterium, unique to the human mouth, that can cause bite-related wound infections is the gram-negative rod *Eikenella corrodens*. The gram-positive rod *Clostridium tetani*, the bacterial organism that results in tetanus, also can be transmitted.

2. The two requisite components for the transmission of viral agents from the assailant to the victim are a disruption of the normal integrity of the skin and a source of virus. The source of any virus is the bodily secretions of the assailant. These viruses include, but are not limited to, hepatitis B and the human immunodeficiency virus (HIV).

C. **Evaluation and management**
The **specific evaluation and management** of human bites include the steps listed in Box 6-1.

II. **Domestic animal bite wounds**
Bite wounds inflicted by domestic animals are more common than bite wounds inflicted by humans.

A. **Mechanism**
There is basically one mechanism of incurring a bite wound from an animal: by a direct bite. The most common domestic animals in the United States, and therefore the most common sources of animal bites, are dogs and cats. Common sites of animal bite wounds are the fingers, hands, face, and feet.

B O X   6-1

Overall Evaluation and Management of Bite Wounds, Human or Animal

Evaluation

1. Examine the patient's bite wound for adjacent soft tissue or structural damage (e.g., tendon damage if the bite is in the finger or wrist). Clean the wound vigorously and debride all necrotic tissue in and adjacent to the wound. Determine who or what bit the patient and when the bite wound occurred.

2. If the wound is clean and if the patient is seen within 24 hours of the bite, one can safely primarily close the wound with sutures.

(continued)

B O X 6-1 *(continued)*

3. If there is any evidence of infection or if the wound is >24 hours old, healing should be by secondary intent.
4. If cosmesis is a concern or if there is a large defect or any significant concurrent damage, referral to plastic surgery is indicated.
5. In all cases of human bite wounds, a serum HIV and hepatitis panel should be obtained from the assailant and the victim.
   a. If at risk, hepatitis gamma globulin or, if available, hepatitis B immune globulin and hepatitis B vaccine should be administered to the patient (see section on Hepatitis in Chapter 2, page 112).
   b. If the assailant is HIV positive, manage the bite as for a needle stick (see section on HIV Infection, page 325).

Management

1. Administer, as necessary, tetanus toxoid (see Table 6-2).
2. Antibiotics are indicated in all cases. Regimens can include one of the following:
   a. Ampicillin–clavulanic acid (Augmentin), 500 mg p.o., b.i.d., for 7 days, or
   b. A second-generation cephalosporin [e.g., cefuroxime (Ceftin), 500 mg p.o., b.i.d.] for 7 days, or
   c. Ciprofloxacin, 500 mg p.o, b.i.d., and clindamycin, 600 mg p.o., t.i.d., for 7 days. (Ciprofloxacin has minimal antibacterial activity against anaerobes.)
3. Follow-up should be quite close, and sutures, if placed, should be removed in 3–5 days. Any signs of infection should result in immediate opening of the wound and removal of the sutures.
4. In all cases of animal bites, the risk of rabies in the animal should be assessed. If at risk, the animal should be observed and, as necessary, destroyed for diagnostic purposes. The definitive method of diagnosing rabies in these animals is by demonstrating via microscopy the presence of Negri bodies in the hippocampus. If there is any suspicion that the animal is rabid, rabies vaccine should be administered to the patient. Table 6-3 provides specifics in the administration of and indications for the rabies vaccine.

T A B L E 6-2
Tetanus Immunizations

1. If patient was never immunized and has a dirty wound:
     a. Administer TIG (tetanus immune globulin), 250 IU
        i.m., and
     b. dT (diphtheria + tetanus toxoid) i.m.
2. If patient was immunized in the past and has a dirty
   wound:
     a. Administer a dT booster i.m., if the last booster was
        given >5 years before presentation
3. Every adult should have dT booster every 10 years

Modified from: CDC. Recommendations of the Immunization Practice Advisory Committee: Diphtheria, Tetanus, and Pertussis: Guidelines for vaccine prophylaxis and other preventive measures. MMWR 1985;34:405–414, 419–426.

 B. **Pathogenesis**
    The **underlying pathogenesis** of disease in animal bite wounds involves damage resulting in skin breakdown, damage to adjacent soft-tissue structures, and exposure to infectious agents from the mouth and body secretions (e.g., saliva) of the animal. Infectious agents include bacterial and viral agents.
    1. The two requisite components in the development of bacterial skin infections are a disruption of the normal integrity of the skin and a source of bacteria. **Dog bites** usually are avulsive wounds associated with significant areas of adjacent crush injury. **Cat bites,** invariably puncture-type wounds, may penetrate deep into the soft tissue.
       a. The bacteria normally present on the skin of the patient may result in infection when the integrity of the skin is disrupted. These include the aerobic gram-positive coccal organisms of the genera *Streptococcus* and *Staphylococcus*.
       b. The bacteria present in the animal's mouth may cause infection in the bite victim. Bacteria include the gram-negative rod *Pasteurella multocida*, the gram-negative rod DF-2 (*Capnocytophaga* spp.), and some anaerobes. Anaerobes are less a problem in animal bites relative to human bites. *Clostridium tetani*, the bacterial organism that results in tetanus, can be transmitted by animal bites.
    2. The viral agent that can be transmitted by animal bites is rabies virus.
 C. **Evaluation and management**
    The **specific evaluation** and management of animal bites include the steps listed in Box 6-1.

T A B L E 6-3
Rabies Vaccination

Domestic animal bites
1. If the animal is healthy and has received a rabies vaccine, observe the animal for 10 days. If the animal remains asymptomatic, no vaccination for the patient is needed
2. If the animal is rabid, or if it has escaped capture and cannot be observed, administer rabies vaccine to the patient. See dosing schedule below

Non–domestic animal bites
1. Bites from skunks, bats, fox, coyotes, and racoons require the initiation of rabies vaccine
2. Rabbits, rodents, squirrels, and livestock rarely have rabies; however, one must check with the lock Public Health Service for further information on these animals in the community. Rabies vaccine need not be administered

Schedule of administration for rabies vaccine
1. Rabies immune globulin (RIG), 20 mg/kg; half of the dose at the wound site, half of the dose i.m.
2. HDCV (human diploid cell vaccine) i.m., on the following days (after bite):
    Day 0
    Day 3
    Day 7
    Day 14
    Day 28
    Report the bite to the Public Health Service
Destroy the rabid animal

Modified from: CDC. Recommendations of the Immunization Practices Advisory Committee of the U.S. Public Health Services. Rabies Prevention, United States, 1984. MMWR 1984;33:393–402, 407–408.

III. Consultation

Problem	Service	Time
Infection refractory to antibiotics	Infectious diseases	Urgent
HIV risk high	Infectious diseases	Required
Bite to face	Plastic surgery	Urgent
Large wound	Plastic surgery	Urgent
Concurrent tendon or nerve damage	Plastic surgery	Urgent
Suspected rabies	Public Health Service	Urgent

IV. **Indications for admission:** Few. If plastic surgery is needed, admission is usually required.

Bacterial Endocarditis

Prophylactic measures for the prevention of bacterial endocarditis are presented in Table 6-4.

HIV Infection (HIV-1 and HIV-2)

I. **Epidemiology**

Over the past fifteen years both the incidence of infection with HIV and the incidence of the disease process resulting from this infection, acquired immunodeficiency syndrome (AIDS), have significantly increased around the world. The pandemic has a worldwide incidence of 13,000 cases/day. It is becoming more and more a disease of the poor and undereducated peoples of the world and the United States. There are >30 million people infected worldwide with the highest prevalences in sub-Saharan Africa and Southeast Asia, and the lowest in the industrialized nations of the world. Furthermore, almost 160,000 people in the United States have AIDS. In 1995, HIV became the leading cause of death among American men aged 25–44 years. Finally, a more diverse group of people are becoming infected with HIV. No longer is HIV/AIDS restricted to homosexual men or intravenous drug users in urban centers. In fact, in the

T A B L E   6-4
Endocarditis Prophylaxis

Cardiac lesions in which prophylaxis is indicated:

Prosthetic cardiac valves, metallic or bioprosthetic	High-risk lesion
Surgically constructed systemic–pulmonary shunts	High-risk lesion
Congenital heart malformations **except ASD**	High-risk lesion
Rheumatic heart disease	High- or low-risk lesion
Idiopathic hypertrophic subaortic stenosis (IHSS)	Low-risk lesion
History of bacterial endocarditis	High-risk lesion
Mitral valve prolapse with mitral regurgitation	Low-risk lesion

Procedures in which prophylaxis is indicated, if the patient has one or more of the above lesions:

Dental procedures inducing gingival bleeding
Professional cleaning

(continued)

T A B L E   6-4 (continued)

Dental extractions
Endodontic procedures
Tonsillectomy
Bronchoscopy, especially if rigid, and/or if biopsies are to be performed
Incision and drainage of any abscess in the oral cavity
Cystoscopy
Any prostatic surgery
Vaginal hysterectomy
Any colonic surgery
Any urinary tract surgery
Sclerotherapy for esophageal varices
Esophagogastroduodenoscopy (EGD) with biopsy
Flexible/rigid proctosigmoidoscopy with biopsies
Colonoscopy

Antibiotic regimens (1990):

A. Dental and respiratory procedures:
  Low-risk lesions
      Amoxicillin, 3 g p.o., 1 hr before and 1.5 g p.o., 6 hr after the procedure,
          or
      Erythromycin, 1 g p.o., 1 hr before and 500 mg p.o. 6 hr after the procedure,
          or
      Clindamycin, 600 mg p.o., 1 hr before and 300 mg p.o., 6 hr after the procedure
  High-risk lesions
      Ampicillin, 2 g i.v., and gentamicin, 1–1.5 mg/kg i.v., 1 hr before and 8 hr after the procedure,
          or
      Vancomycin, 1 g i.v., 1 hr before, over the hour before the procedure
B. Genitourinary and/or gastrointestinal procedures, all lesions:
      Ampicillin, 2 g i.v., and gentamicin, 1–1.5 mg/kg i.v. 1 hr before and 8 hr after the procedure,
          or
      Vancomycin, 1 g i.v. over 1 hr, and gentamicin, 1–1.5 mg/kg i.v., both 1 hr before the procedure and 12 hr after the procedure
      These regimens also are recommended in the prevention of periprocedure prosthetic joint infections.

Modified from: Prevention of bacterial endocarditis: Recommendations of the American Heart Association. JAMA 1990;264:2919–2922.

United States, the incidences of infection have increased in women and minorities but have declined in men and in homosexual populations. Twenty-five percent of the cases in the United States in 1995 were heterosexually transmitted. These data alone begin to reflect the gravity and magnitude of this problem in the fields of public health and professional health care.

II. Pathophysiology

The human immunodeficiency virus is an RNA virus of the lentivirus family. HIV uses the enzyme reverse transcriptase and the host cell's mechanisms to produce, by the process of reverse transcription, DNA specific to the virus. Once the DNA specific to the virus is produced, it can be stored in the nucleus of the host cell, or the host cell's mechanisms can be used to produce, by transcription, either new RNA viral particles or messenger RNA. This mRNA may then, again through host-cell mechanisms, be translated to produce specific proteins. One or more of these specific proteins result in the death of the host cell itself.

A. Disease mechanisms

HIV enters the body via blood or body secretions. Once in the body, the virus may enter any cell, but it has a propensity to infect cells of the immune system (i.e., monocytes and lymphocytes) in general and T-cell lymphocytes in specific.

1. HIV has a particular affinity for **lymphocytes bearing the CD4** receptor on their surface, as this receptor aids viral entry into the cell. The cells with CD4 receptors on their surface are known as T-helper lymphocytes and they become depleted by infection and eventual destruction. They are of central importance to **cell-mediated immunity (CMI).** T-helper cell depletion results in increased susceptibility of the patient to infections by opportunistic organisms. These include a diverse set of viral, fungal, bacterial, and parasitic organisms that would not cause infection in an immunocompetent patient.

2. HIV also has a propensity to infect monocytes and macrophages, thus forming an effective reservoir for the virus.

3. HIV can produce damage and manifestations through mechanisms independent of cell-mediated immunity. This is particularly evident in the central nervous system (CNS), where HIV causes direct neuronal infection and eventual cell death, with resultant dementia.

B. Transmission

Transmission of the virus, and therefore of the disease, occurs by direct contact of a patient's blood or body secretions with the blood or body secretions of a person infected with HIV. Any human can become infected with HIV and develop AIDS, but certain activities are associated with a higher risk of infection. These include, but are not limited to, the following:

1. Unprotected anal, oral, or vaginal sex with multiple partners, heterosexual or homosexual.
2. Unprotected sexual intercourse with an HIV-positive person.
3. Intravenous drug abuse.
4. Blood transfusions outside the United States or during the years 1977 to 1985 inside the United States. The risk of HIV transmission from a transfusion of blood in the United States today is extremely low (i.e., 1:45,000).
5. Unprotected sexual intercourse with a person who has a recent or past history of sexually transmitted disease, such as purulent urethritis, purulent cervicitis, or genital herpes.

III. **Natural history and overall manifestations of HIV infection**
   A. **Acute period**
      There is usually an acute viremia that, in a minority of cases, results in an infectious mononucleosis-like syndrome of exudative pharyngitis, myalgias, arthralgias, and fevers, but is self-limited and resolves in days to weeks. The HIV antibody test is nonreactive.
   B. **Quiescent period**
      In the quiescent period, the patient is asymptomatic. The virus has infected and remains in the cells designed to destroy it, the cells of the immune system. The largest reservoir of virus is the cells of the monocyte–macrophage lineage. During the quiescent period, the patient is HIV antibody reactive and infectious. The quiescent period is variable in duration, but theoretically may last for years to decades. In adults, the average time between infection and the development of AIDS is 11 years (range, 5 to >20 years).
   C. **Symptomatic period**
      In the symptomatic period, the virus has destroyed a significant quantity of T-helper lymphocytes. This decrease in T-helper cells results in cell-mediated immunosuppression, and the patient develops opportunistic infections. The HIV-antibody test is reactive, and the patient is infectious. Symptomatic HIV infection effectively defines AIDS (see subsequent discussion).
   D. **HIV-2:** Analogous to HIV-1 but has significant differences. It is rarely transmitted perinatally and has a prolonged quiescent period.

IV. **Evaluation of an asymptomatic patient**
   The evaluation of an asymptomatic patient at risk for HIV infection includes obtaining a history for the specific risk

factors. The history and physical examination should also look for any early infectious manifestations that are harbingers of early immunocompromise, such as recurrent herpes zoster in a young patient or the development of oral thrush. Another important evaluative tool is the serum HIV-antibody titer.

A. **Indications** for determining the serum HIV-antibody titer
   1. The patient has any of the known risk factors for the transmission of infection.
   2. The patient has sustained a needle-stick injury (Box 6-2).

B. **Rationale**
   The reasoning behind determining the serum HIV-antibody titer in such patients is not only to confirm the diagnosis but also to put into effect preventive and therapeutic interventions.
   1. **Preventive interventions,** which should be taught to all humans, not only to those who are HIV-antibody reactive, include the following:
      a. The institution of safe sexual practices, including the use of condoms. The clinician should reinforce that abstinence or monogamy with complete fidelity are the only true forms of safe sex.
      b. No sharing of needles by people who abuse drugs intravenously. The clinician should reinforce that the best way to prevent this form of transmission is to discontinue i.v. drug abuse.
   2. **Therapeutic interventions.** Some recent and compelling evidence from the National Institutes of Health indicates that early intervention with AZT in selected asymptomatic HIV-infected patients does slow the progression of HIV infection to AIDS.

C. **Protocol**
   The serum HIV-antibody test consists of two separate tests, both of which are highly sensitive and specific. The two tests should be performed in a specific sequence.
   1. The first test uses the **enzyme-linked immunosorbent assay (ELISA)** method to detect the presence of antibody in the patient's serum. This is a fairly inexpensive test and is quite useful as a first-line screening test. If this test is negative, it should be repeated twice at 6-month intervals, and patient measures to prevent viral transmission should be reinforced. Because the test specificity, although high, is not 100%, any positive result must be confirmed by a second test, the Western blot technique.
   2. The **Western blot examination,** when positive, has a specificity of virtually 100%, thereby minimizing the false-positive rate. If this test is positive, the patient should undergo the overall evaluation and management described in Box 6-3.

BOX 6-2

Management of Needle Sticks

Management

1. Minimize the risk of needle sticks. Place used needles in a "sharps" box, do not recap them, and never leave needles lying around. Wear latex gloves when examining any patient.
2. If a needle stick occurs:
     i. Immediately cleanse the wound with copious amounts of soap and water.
    ii. Assess the risk of the patient for HIV.
   iii. If the HIV status of the patient is unknown: Obtain HIV and hepatitis A, B, and C panels. See Table 2-14 (page 119).
    iv. If the HIV status of the patient is positive (known at outset), obtain hepatitis panel from patient.
     v. Obtain HIV, hepatitis panel, baseline CBC, electrolytes, and liver-function tests (LFTs) on caregiver.
    vi. Perform a pregnancy test on the caregiver, if appropriate.
   vii. Administer tetanus toxoid, if indicated, to the caregiver.
  viii. Administer hepatitis B gamma globulin i.m. to the caregiver if the patient is hepatitis B positive and the caregiver has no hepatitis B antibody.
    ix. If the patient is known to be HIV positive, initiate azidothymidine (AZT), 200 mg p.o. t.i.d. and 3TC 150 mg p.o. b.i.d. for 4 weeks, or if high risk, i.e., large amount of blood with a high HIV titer, AZT 200 mg t.i.d. p.o., 3TC 150 mg p.o. b.i.d. and Indinavir 800 mg t.i.d. for 4 weeks.
     x. Determine CBC, electrolytes, and renal function at 6 weeks, 12 weeks, 6 months, and 12 months.
    xi. Determine HIV antibody titer at 3, 6, and 12 months.
   xii. Use contraception for at least the first 3 months after exposure.
3. A young patient has had the onset of recurrent herpes zoster or oral thrush.
4. To confirm HIV infection in a patient with an opportunistic infection and thus, by definition, has AIDS.

B O X 6-3

*Overall Evaluation and Management of Newly
Diagnosed HIV Infection*

Evaluation

1. Take a thorough history and perform a physical examination, focusing on sexual practices and partners.
2. Determine the complete blood cell count with differential analysis for baseline purposes.
3. Determine the platelet count for baseline purposes.
4. Determine levels of alkaline phosphatase, LDH, total bilirubin, AST, ALT, and GGT to document the overall functioning of the liver at baseline.
5. Determine electrolyte, BUN, creatinine, and glucose levels for baseline purposes.
6. Determine albumin, calcium, PO_4, and magnesium levels for baseline purposes.
7. Perform the serum VDRL test to rule out concurrent infection with syphilis.
8. Obtain hepatitis A, B, and C panels to rule out concurrent infection with or past exposure to viral hepatitis.
9. Determine serum titers of cytomegalovirus (CMV) and *Toxoplasma* at baseline. If in the future an acute infection with one of these agents is suspected, a baseline titer will be of great clinical utility.
10. Obtain chest radiographs in PA and lateral views for baseline purposes and to rule out any concurrent infiltrates.
11. Perform urinalysis for baseline purposes.
12. Perform a PPD skin test with controls (Table 4-15, page 245) to determine if the patient has been exposed to mycobacterial disease and if the patient is anergic. If the patient does not react to any of the applied skin tests, he or she is, by definition, anergic. Anergy is a significant manifestation of cell-mediated immunocompromise.
13. Determine CD4 counts. This is a pivotal test in that there is a clear correlation between the number of CD4 T cells and rate of progression to AIDS: the lower the CD4 count, the faster the progression to AIDS. This is still one of the most reproducible methods of measuring cell-mediated immunity. Furthermore, the absolute number of T-helper cells—

(continued)

B O X 6-3 (continued)

the CD4 count—may yet be used as a marker for the initiation of therapy, as follows:

a. If the CD4 count is >500 cells and/or the viral load is <500/mL, follow up the counts every 4–6 months. No intervention is required.

b. If the CD4 count is <500 cells or if the viral load is 500–5000/mL, initiate one of the following regimens: AZT and dideoxyinosine (ddI) or AZT and dideoxycytidine (ddC) or AZT and 3TC or if the viral load >5000/mL AZT and 3TC and a protease inhibitor. Follow up the CBC and renal function on a biweekly basis and then on a bimonthly basis. Follow up the CD4 counts every 4–6 months. AZT, once initiated, should be continued indefinitely. See Table 6-6 for doses.

c. If the CD4 count is <200 cells, initiate *Pneumocystis carinii* prophylaxis with TMP-sulfamethoxazole (Bactrim DS, one tablet p.o., q.d.) or inhaled pentamidine every 2 weeks; initiate herpes simplex prophylaxis with acyclovir, 200 mg p.o., b.i.d., and initiate prophylaxis for mycobacterial diseases with rifabutin, or better, with clarithromycin, 500 mg p.o., b.i.d. These regimens, once initiated, should be continued, as tolerated, indefinitely.

14. Another, potentially more important discriminator in HIV-disease prognosis is the direct measurement of HIV-1 in the plasma (i.e., the viral load). A patient with HIV-1 RNA concentrations of >5,000 HIV molecules/mL have a much poorer prognosis than do those patients with HIV-1 RNA concentrations <5,000 HIV molecules/mL. This discriminating feature was independent of CD4 count; if the CD4 was >500 but the viral load was >5,000, the prognosis was poor. Viral load must be repeated at 4 weeks and then q 3–6 months to assess treatment efficacy.

Management

1. Immunizations
   a. Pneumovax, polyvalent.
   b. Influenza A.
   c. Hepatitis B (see section on Hepatitis in Chapter 2).

(continued)

B O X   6-3 *(continued)*

2. Education
   a. "Safe sex" techniques (e.g., condoms).
   b. No sharing of needles.
   c. No sharing of toothbrushes or razors.
3. Stage the disease by using the scheme in Table 6-5. Staging is useful in prognosis and in treating the patient.
4. Obtain an infectious diseases consult.

---

       a. If the Western blot is negative, it should be repeated, along with the ELISA assay, in 4 months.
       3. If there are any questions as to the interpretation of these tests, an infectious diseases consult to aid in interpretation should be sought.

V. Early management

In the early stages of HIV infection, the primary care physician will be managing these patients. A subspecialist should be consulted early in the course of the disease, but the overall management until late in the disease will be orchestrated by the primary care physician. See Box 6-3.

VI. Manifestations of HIV infection

The specific manifestations, along with their evaluation and the management of AIDS, are very diverse but can be classified into the following scheme.

A. Pulmonary manifestations

Pulmonary manifestations virtually all occur as a result of opportunistic infections caused by HIV-induced immunocompromise. The three most common opportunistic infections involving the lungs are *Pneumocystis carinii* infection, mycobacterial infections, and CMV infections. The immunocompromised patient is at risk for infection by a diverse set of pathologic agents, including the common community-acquired pathogens. Thus in addition to the following discussion, the reader is referred to the section on Community-Acquired Pneumonitis in Chapter 4 for further information and a discussion of pneumonia.

    1. *Pneumocystis carinii.* This protozoan organism may be present in the lungs of a normal patient but does not cause disease. In the cell-mediated immunosuppressed patient, especially a patient with HIV-induced immunocompromise, these organisms proliferate and result in life-threatening opportunistic infection. This infection is extremely common in AIDS patients.

T A B L E *6-5*
Classification System for HIV Infection

A. CD-4 T-lymphocyte categories

Category 1: >500 cells/μL
Category 2: 200–499 cells/μL
Category 3: <200 cells/μL

B. Clinical Categories of HIV

Category A
Asymptomatic HIV
Persistent generalized lymphadenopathy
Acute HIV infection
Category B: CMI deficits
Bacillary angiomatosis
Thrush
Recurrent vulvovaginal candidal infections
Cervical dysplasia (moderate to severe)
Carcinoma in situ of cervix
Hairy leukoplakia
Diarrhea >1 month
Herpes zoster
Immune-mediated thrombocytopenia (ITP)
Pelvic inflammatory disease
Peripheral neuropathy
Category C: AIDS-defining
Candida of bronchi
Candida of the esophagus
Invasive cervical carcinoma
Coccidiomycosis
Cryptococcosis
Cytomegalovirus (CMV) infection
CMV retinitis
HIV encephalopathy
Herpes simplex virus esophagitis
Histoplasmosis
Isosporiasis
Kaposi's sarcoma
Lymphoma—Burkitt's or immunoblastic types
CNS lymphoma
Mycobacterium avium complex
Mycobacterium tuberculosis
Pneumocystis cariini
Recurrent pneumonitis
Progressive multifocal encephalopathy
Recurrent Salmonella septicemia
Toxoplasmosis
Wasting syndrome

MMWR: 1993 Revised classification system for HIV Infection.

a. The **specific manifestations** of *P. carinii* infection include dyspnea, decreased exercise tolerance, and a nonproductive cough. Often the patient will have crackles in the lungs and fevers, but there may be surprisingly few signs on physical examination.

b. The **specific evaluation** of this disorder entails having an appropriate clinical suspicion in a patient with the specific manifestations of *P. carinii* infection and who is, or is suspected to be, HIV positive. Chest radiographs and arterial blood gas determinations are indicated in all cases. The chest radiograph usually shows a diffuse interstitial infiltrate, and the arterial blood gas values usually reveal hyperventilation with a respiratory alkalosis, and hypoxemia with an increased $A-aO_2$ gradient. An additional specific examination is bronchoscopy with bronchoalveolar lavage (BAL) for *P. carinii* organisms or other potential concurrent processes or causes of interstitial pneumonitis, including CMV viral titers and mycobacterial smears and cultures.

c. The **specific management** includes admitting the patient to the hospital, providing supplemental oxygen to keep P_aO_2 >65 mm Hg, and initiating empirical treatment. Effective therapeutic regimens include TMP/sulfa, or pentamidine, or dapsone (see Table 6-6 for dosages). The antibiotics should be initiated even before confirmatory bronchoscopy is performed.

Administration of steroids to patients with severe *P. carinii* pneumonitis offers a clear advantage in short-term survival and in quality of life, as measured by an increased exercise tolerance. The indications for steroid use early in the course of the disease include severe disease as manifested by an increased $A-aO_2$ gradient, decreased P_aO_2, and decreased O_2 saturation. Specific regimens include methylprednisolone, 40–60 mg i.v., q.8hr, for 5 days, or prednisone, 60 mg p.o., q.A.M. for 5 days, either followed by a tapering dose of prednisone.

d. **Prophylaxis.** Once treated, all of these patients require long-term prophylaxis with TMP-sulfa, inhaled pentamidine, or dapsone (see Table 6-6 for dosages and potential side effects).

2. **Mycobacteria.** Please refer to Chapter 4 section, and Tables 4-14 through 4-17.

3. **Cytomegalovirus.** This DNA virus is transmitted by blood and body secretions. CMV infection is quite common but underrecognized because it is often subclinical. This is a systemic infection to which the

patient was exposed in the past and now, as a result of HIV-induced immunocompromise, it has become reactivated.

a. The **specific manifestations** include shortness of breath, a quite nonproductive cough, and subjective fevers, chills, and night sweats. Examination usually discloses tachypnea, tachycardia, and a low-grade fever. Auscultation of the lungs reveals diffuse crackles. Otherwise there is a paucity of cardiac or pulmonary signs.

b. The **specific evaluation** of CMV infection entails having an appropriate clinical suspicion in a patient with specific manifestations and who is, or is suspected to be, HIV positive. Chest radiographs and arterial blood gas determinations are indicated in all cases. The chest radiograph usually shows a diffuse interstitial infiltrate. Arterial blood gas values reveal hyperventilation with a respiratory alkalosis, and hypoxemia with an increased $A-aO_2$ gradient. A further specific examination is bronchoscopy with BAL to determine CMV titers and to look for other concurrent processes or causes of interstitial pneumonitis, including *P. carinii* and mycobacterial smears and cultures.

c. The **specific management** includes admission to the hospital, providing supplemental oxygen to keep P_aO_2 >65 mm Hg, and initiating empiric treatment. Effective therapy includes, once CMV titers are positive, the immediate initiation of DHPG (ganciclovir), 5 mg/kg given i.v. over 1 hour q. 12h for 21 days, then q day long term.Once therapy is initiated, it is for the long term, and therefore a catheter must be placed for permanent i.v. access, such as a Hickman catheter. Because the concomitant use of AZT with DHPG is relatively contraindicated, the diagnosis of CMV must be confidently made before committing the patient to long-term DHPG.

   CMV retinitis is a significant problem that may be concurrent with or antedate the pneumonitis. Therefore, an ophthalmology consult should be obtained to look for and to diagnose early CMV retinitis. DHPG is also used to treat this entity and should be limited when CMV retinitis is diagnosed (see Table 6-6 for dosages). The therapy is, again, long term. An alternative agent for the treatment of CMV infections is foscarnet. This agent has been demonstrated to be effective in the therapy of CMV and has several advantages over DHPG: it can be used concurrent with AZT, and data suggest that it may have an inherent anti-HIV effect and prolong overall patient survival.

TABLE 6-6
Medications Commonly Used in the Treatment of HIV or AIDS

Agent	Indications	Dosing	Mechanism	Side Effects
Acyclovir	Prophylaxis for HSV Treatment of HSV pneumonitis/encephalitis	400 mg p.o. b.i.d. 5–10 mg/kg i.v. q 8 hour	Thymidine synthetase inhibitor	Tremors Mild renal dysfunction
Amphotericin B	Treatment of disseminated fungal infections	0.5–1.0 mg/kg/day i.v. to 2 grams, then 0.5 mg/kg/day i.v. 2 times/wk		Wheezing Chills Hypocationemia (K, Mg) Renal failure Type I renal tubular acidosis To prevent wheezing and chills, the patient should be pretreated with: a) Diphenhydramine (Benadryl), 25–50 mg p.o./i.v., and b) Acetaminophen, 1 g p.o., and c) Hydrocortisone, 25–50 mg i.v., all before infusion
Azidothymidine (AZT) (Zidovudine) (Retrovir)	HIV positive, asymptomatic CD4 < 500 HIV positive, symptomatic AIDS *Follow CD4 and HIV-RNA viral load, q 4–6 weeks	300 mg p.o. b.i.d. or 200 mg p.o. t.i.d.	Antireverse transcriptase; inhibits HIV replication	Nausea, vomiting Headache; pancytopenia Melanonychia Hyperpigmentation Significant myopathy

Drug	Indication	Dose	Mechanism	Side effects
Atovaquone	Treatment of *Pneumocystis carinii* pneumonitis	750 mg p.o. b.i.d. with meals	Stops the de novo synthesis of pyrimidines	Diarrhea
Clindamycin-primaquine	Treatment of *Pneumocystis carinii*	Clindamycin 600 mg i.v./p.o. q.8hr and Primaquine 15 mg p.o. of base q AM		Diarrhea Hemolysis in patients with G-6-PD deficiency
Clarithromycin	Disemminated MAC	500 mg p.o. b.i.d.		Well tolerated; dysguesia
Clotrimazole (Mycelex troches)	Prophylaxis and treatment of thrush	10 mg 5 times/day		Minimal
Dapsone	Prophylaxis of *Pneumocystis carinii*	100 mg p.o. q.d.		Anemia Rash Increased methemoglobinemia Severe peripheral neuropathies Elevated amylase
Didanosine (ddI) (Videx)	HIV, asymptomatic HIV, symptomatic *Follow-up with CD4 and RNA viral load	200 mg p.o. b.i.d. (empty stomach)	Antireverse transcriptase; inhibits HIV replication	Very few
Fluconazole	Treatment of cryptococcal meningitis	200 mg p.o. q.d.		
Foscarnet	CMV retinitis	Induction: 60 mg/kg i.v. q.8hr for 3 wk; then Maintenance: 90 mg/kg i.v. q.d., indefinitely	Viral DNA polymerase inhibitor	Seizures Hypomagnesemia Hypocalcemia Renal dysfunction
Flucytosine	Treatment of *Cryptococcus* (adjuvant)	37.5 mg/kg p.o. q. 6hr		Pancytopenia
Gancyclovir (DHPG)	Treatment of CMV retinitis and pneumonitis	5 mg/kg/day i.v. or 1 g p.o. t.i.d.	Guanine nucleoside analogue	Granulocytopenia Thrombocytopenia AZT relatively contraindicated

(continued)

333

T A B L E 6-6 *(continued)*

Agent	Indications	Dosing	Mechanism	Side Effects
Indinavir (Crixivan)	HIV; follow RNA viral load q. 4 weeks	800 mg p.o. t.i.d. with extra water but not food	Protease inhibitor	Pancytopenia
Itraconazole	Treatment of virtually any and all nonmeningeal fungi, including: Blastomycosis Coccidiomycosis Histoplasmosis Paracoccidio mycosis Sporotrichosis	200 mg p.o. b.i.d., needs an acid milieu to be absorbed; administer with a cola drink	Attacks the ergosterol; the main sterol in the fungal cell membrane	Minimal
Lamivudine (3TC) (EPIVIR)	HIV, asymptomatic See text	150 mg p.o. b.i.d.	Nucleoside analog reverse transcriptase inhibitor	Pancreatitis Headache
Megestrol acetate	AIDS-related Cachexia	200 mg p.o. q.i.d.	Unknown	Minimal Slight increase in risk of DVT
Nystatin	Treatment of thrush	400,000–600,000 units q.i.d. by swish and swallow		Minimal
Pentamidine	Prophylaxis for *P. carinii*	300 mg by hand-held nebulizer every 2–4 wk		Hypoglycemia
	Treatment of *P. carinii*	4 mg/kg i.v. q.d. for 21 days		

Drug	Indication	Dose	Mechanism	Side effects
Pyrimethamine sulfadiazine	Prophylaxis for *T. gondii*	Pyrimethamine, 50 mg, q.D p.o., and sulfadiazine 1 g p.o. q.i.d.	Antimetabolite	Rash Stevens–Johnson syndrome Cytopenias To minimize SE administer leucovorin (folinic acid), 10 mg/day p.o.
	Treatment dose *T. gondii*	Pyrimethamine, 100 mg p.o. q.d. for 2 days, then 50 mg p.o. q.d. and sulfadiazine, 1–2 g p.o. q.i.d. for 4–6 wk		
Saquinavir	HIV; follow RNA viral load q.4 weeks	600 mg p.o. t.i.d. 2 hr after meals	Protease inhibitor	Pancytopenia
Trimethoprim sulfamethoxazole	Prophylaxis for *P. carinii*	Bactrim DS, one tablet p.o. thrice weekly	Inhibits DNA synthesis	Rash Anaphylaxis Stevens–Johnson syndrome Pancytopenia
	Treatment of *P. carinii*	15–20 mg/kg/day i.v. in 6-hour dosing, using the trimethoprim component for dosing		

B. **Neurologic manifestations**

Neurologic manifestations of HIV infection can result from the direct effects of the virus on the nervous system or from immunocompromise, with a resultant increased risk for and incidence of opportunistic infections in the CNS. A brief discussion of both the direct and indirect manifestations of HIV involving the CNS is presented.

1. **Direct HIV infection**
   a. The **underlying pathogenesis** of direct damage to the nervous system by HIV is as follows. This usually occurs only when he CD4 count is <200. The virus crosses the blood–brain barrier, usually via cells of the monocyte–macrophage lineage. Once in the central or peripheral nervous system, the virus directly infects the neurons themselves. Infected cells die, resulting in the loss of irreplaceable neurons.
   b. The **natural history** involves a slowly and irreversibly progressive course. Because virtually all patients with AIDS have a direct neuronal infection with the virus, the prevalence of this process is very high among patients with AIDS.
   c. The **specific manifestations** of these entities thus include those related to the actual loss of neuronal tissue in the central or peripheral nervous systems. These manifestations can be quite variable and depend on the relative damage to various parts of the central and peripheral nervous systems. The manifestations vary from a dementing process with associated spasticity as the result of cortical neuronal loss to a peripheral neuropathy as the result of loss of peripheral neurons.
      i. A dementing process manifests with a slowly progressive loss of memory, both short term and long term; a decrease in cognitive ability; and disorientation. The patient can develop seizures, spasticity, tremor, or Parkinson-like manifestations if the neuronal destruction affects the basal ganglia.
   d. The **specific evaluation** entails making the clinical diagnosis and excluding all potentially treatable causes or exacerbating processes. This includes excluding any concurrent opportunistic infection (see the following), obtaining a serum VDRL, and, if reactive, performing a lumbar puncture and VDRL on the cerebrospinal fluid (CSF) to rule out neurosyphilis; in addition a β_2-microglobulin on the CSF should be performed and will be increased in HIV-related dementia; performing thyroid function tests; and obtaining a serum B_{12} level; CT/

magnetic resonance imaging (MRI) scans of the brain will demonstrate diffuse brain atrophy.

e. The **specific management** includes treating the HIV infection, diagnosing and treating any reversible opportunistic intracranial infections, and treating any reversible causes of a dementing process. If the process is the result of HIV, supportive care and structuring of the patient's environment are of therapeutic assistance.

2. **Toxoplasmosis.** This is a disease process due to a eukaryotic opportunistic parasite, *Toxoplasma gondii.*

   a. **Transmission and natural history.** Like other opportunistic organisms, *T. gondii* results in disease only in patients with antecedent immunosuppression. The CD4 count is invariably <200. The portal of entry or exposure is thought to be the respiratory mucosa. Once exposed, the immunosuppressed patient may develop an intracerebral or retinal infection, or both. Cats are vectors, and disease may be acquired as a result of exposure to infected cat feces.

   b. The **specific manifestations** of toxoplasmosis include recurrent generalized headaches that, over days to weeks, progressively worsen in intensity, frequency, or duration. Concurrent with the headaches are, quite invariably, fevers, chills, and occasional night sweats. The patient may have delirium or seizures. The seizures, if present, not uncommonly have a focal component and may be followed by postictal localized paresis or plegia— Todd's paralysis.

   c. The **specific evaluation** of toxoplasmosis includes having the appropriate clinical suspicion in a patient with known or suspected HIV infection. The evaluation includes:

      i. Perform serum *Toxoplasma* antibodies.

      ii. The patient should undergo head imaging.

         (a) The first imaging technique should be a computed tomography (CT) scan with and without contrast. CT of the head in a patient with toxoplasmosis lesions will demonstrate multiple, relatively small (1–2 cm in diameter) lesions with peripheral ring contrast enhancement.

         (b) If the CT scan is normal and the suspicion for a space-occupying lesion remains, MRI of the head should be obtained. MRI of the head is the most sensitive imaging technique for toxoplasmosis lesions, because

MRI is the most specific and sensitive technique for imaging of processes that affect the white matter.

iii. An ophthalmologic consultation for a retinal examination to look for concurrent toxoplasmosis retinitis should be obtained.

iv. A lumbar puncture can be considered, unless an intracranial mass makes the risk of herniation high. The CSF obtained should be submitted for routine tests (see section on Meningitis in Chapter 14) and a *T. gondii* antibody titer.

v. Admission to the hospital as well as consultation with infectious diseases and neurosurgery should be performed in an expedient fashion.

d. **Management**

i. Antibiotic regimens that are effective immediately against toxoplasmosis should be initiated empirically. These regimens include pyrimethamine, 100 mg p.o., q.d., for 2 days, and then pyrimethamine, 25–50 mg p.o., q.d., and sulfadiazine, 4–8 g p.o., q.6h., and, to minimize pancytopenia, leucovorin (folinic acid), 5–10 mg/day p.o. (not folic acid, as this inhibits pyrimethamine activity). This regimen should be continued for a duration of 6 weeks (see Table 6-6).

ii. **Prophylaxis.** Once the diagnosis is secured, either by a high clinical suspicion, increased toxoplasmosis titers, or direct biopsy of a lesion, lifelong prophylactic therapy is required. This regimen includes pyrimethamine, 25–50 mg p.o., q.d., and sulfadiazine, 1 g p.o., q.i.d., or clindamycin, 600 mg p.o., q.d., along with folinic acid, 5 mg/day p.o. Finally, dapsone and pyrimethamine are effective agents in such prophylaxis (see Table 6-6).

3. **Cryptococcosis** is a disease process that is due to the eukaryotic opportunistic fungal organism, *Cryptococcus neoformans.*

a. **Transmission and natural history.** Like all opportunistic organisms, *C. neoformans* results in disease only in patients with antecedent immunosuppression. The CD4 count is invariably <200. The portal of entry or exposure is thought to be the respiratory mucosa. Once exposed, the patient can develop a localized pneumonitis or a solitary intracranial mass infection. In either case, the result is spread to the leptomeninges, which invariably results in severe leptomeningitis.

b. The **specific manifestations** of cryptococcosis include the subacute onset of recurrent generalized headaches, fevers, and chills. The symptoms then progress to delirium and/or generalized tonic–clonic seizures. On examination, there are often the meningeal signs of nuchal rigidity, Brudzinski's sign, and/or Kernig's sign. In a small minority of cases, the process manifests with focal neurologic findings: cranial nerve palsies.

c. The **specific evaluation and management** of this entity include having the appropriate clinical suspicion in a documented or suspected HIV-positive patient. After a history and physical examination looking for any focal sensory or motor deficits, the patient should undergo head imaging.

   i. The first imaging study should be a CT scan, with and without contrast. CT of the head in a patient with cryptococcal lesions will demonstrate multiple, relatively small (1–2 cm in diameter) lesions with peripheral ring enhancement.

   ii. A lumbar puncture should be considered, unless an intracranial mass makes the risk of herniation high. The CSF obtained should be submitted for routine tests, a *T. gondii* antibody titer, an India ink stain for cryptococcal organisms (the organism, but not the peripheral capsule, will stain), and by latex agglutination, a cryptococcal antigen titer.

   iii. Admission to the hospital should be performed as well as consultation with infectious diseases and neurosurgery in an expedient fashion.

   iv. A chest radiograph to look for a nodule or infiltrate consistent with a cryptococcal infection should be obtained.

   v. Serum cryptococcal antigen and blood cultures should be obtained.

   vi. Antibiotic regimens that are effective against this opportunistic infection include amphotericin B, 0.5–1.0 mg/kg/day i.v., on a daily basis to a total dose of 2 g, and, concurrently, flucytosine, 37.5 mg/kg p.o. q. 6hr, or fluconazole, 200–400 mg p.o., q.d., until the dose of amphotericin has reached 2 g. While the patient is taking amphotericin B, the clinician must closely monitor renal function and cations, as hypokalemia and a decreased serum magnesium level often develop, and must monitor CBC frequently (i.e., one to two times per week).

d. **Prophylaxis.** Once the diagnosis is secured, lifelong prophylactic therapy is required. This prophylactic regimen includes amphotericin B, 40 mg

> i.v., two to three times per week, or fluconazole,
> 100–200 mg p.o., q.d. to q.o.d., lifelong. The am-
> photericin B regimen requires the placement of
> a Hickman catheter and close monitoring of the
> cation, renal, and fluid status of the patient.
>
> 4. **Mycobacterial**–See Chapter 14 (Neurology section:
>   meningitis, page 658) and Chapter 4 (Pulmonary sec-
>   tion: mycobacterial, page 242)

C. Gastrointestinal manifestations
The **gastrointestinal (GI) manifestations** of HIV and
AIDS are very diverse. The virus itself can directly damage the GI tract, and much more commonly, can indirectly increase the risk of opportunistic infections involving any area of the GI tract. The two manifestations of
HIV-related GI disease are diarrhea and dysphagia/ody-
nophagia. The reader is referred to these specific sections
in Chapter 2 (pages 86 and 82, respectively).

VII. Consultation

Problem	Service	Time
HIV positive	Infectious diseases	Required
Any opportunistic infection	Infectious diseases	Urgent/emergent
Any intracranial lesion not diagnosed by "routine" tests	Neurosurgery	Emergent/urgent
Interstitial pneumonitis	Pulmonology	Urgent/emergent bronchoscopy
Intractable diarrhea	Gastroenterology	Required, for flexible proctosigmoidoscopy
Odynophagia not responsive to antifungal agents	Gastroenterology	Urgent for EGD

VIII. Indications for admission: New interstitial pneumonitis in
an HIV-positive patient, severe vomiting with intravascular
volume contraction, any neurologic manifestations of HIV,
or any evidence of profound diarrhea.

Sexually Transmitted Diseases

Sexually transmitted diseases (STDs) are extremely common in
the United States today. As a group, these diseases have several
disconcerting and malignant features. First, the incidence of disease, in the United States and the world, is quite high and in some
cases increasing. Second, there is a significant morbidity and even
mortality in patients who are undiagnosed and thus untreated.

Third, STDs are disease processes that can be overlooked by physicians who are not attuned to the manifestations of STDs. Finally, HIV is spread through the same mechanisms as are other STDs, and HIV has a disconcertingly high prevalence in patients with other STDs.

I. **Sexual history**

The sexual history is an integral component of the overall history but may be quite challenging to obtain, even when the patient's complaint may be due to an STD.

A. **Historic information**

The history consists of the physician querying the patient regarding very personal, intimate, and potentially embarrassing activities. These include:

1. The patient's selection of partners, including sexual orientation [i.e., if the partners are of the same sex (homosexual), the opposite sex (heterosexual), or of either sex (bisexual)].

2. The number of sexual partners over a given period.

3. Specific sexual practices, including vaginal intercourse, anal intercourse, receptive anal intercourse, oral sex (including fellatio and/or cunnilingus), and the use of erotic devices.

4. The patient's knowledge of and use of barrier methods and/or "safer sex" techniques, in general, and condoms, in specific.

5. If the patient has had sexual contact with anyone who is HIV positive or at high risk for being HIV positive. High-risk groups include people who abuse i.v. drugs or who are promiscuous, whether homosexual, bisexual, or heterosexual.

B. **Tips for history taking**

Helpful tips in obtaining a sexual history include the following:

1. Explain to the patient the importance of an accurate history.

2. Reassure the patient that the questions are not meant to embarrass.

3. The queries should be asked in a matter-of-fact manner.

4. The physician must be comfortable asking the patient these questions.

5. The questions, as in all history taking, should begin with general queries and move on to specifics.

6. The physician should become cognizant of and use, when appropriate, the slang terms for various anatomic structures or activities. A penis may be referred to as "my nature," masturbation as "mashing" or "beating off," fellatio as "a blow job" or "giving head." The use of these terms may make the patient under-

B O X   6-4

Overall Evaluation and Management of a Suspected STD

Evaluation

1. Obtain a sexual history, central to the evaluation and management (see text).
2. Assess the patient's risk for HIV (see section on HIV Infection, page 320).
3. Perform a physical examination, looking for any rashes or any evidence of purulent pharyngitis in the oropharynx, and/or purulent discharge of the genitourinary system. In all males, a GU and rectal examination is mandatory; in all females, a pelvic and rectal examination is mandatory.
4. Perform chlamydial cultures of the cervix in females and of the urethral orifice in males.
5. Perform a gonococcal (GC) smear and culture of the cervix in females and of the urethral orifice in males. If pharyngitis or proctitis is clinically suspected, perform GC cultures from those sources. The culture should be swabbed onto the Thayer–Martin or New York City agar at the time of specimen procurement.
6. Obtain a serum VDRL in all patients. If reactive, confirm with FTA-abs and treat as described in the text (page 348).
7. Determine the serum HIV antibody titer in all patients at risk.
8. Obtain a hepatitis B panel in all patients at risk.
9. Obtain a Tzanck smear of any painful vesicular lesions to look for multinucleated giant cells, a finding indicative of herpes simplex infection.
10. Perform a dark-field examination on scrapings from any painless, raised lesions present. Such a lesion is consistent with a chancre. The dark-field analysis is a microscopic assessment used to diagnose primary syphilis.
11. Perform a urine pregnancy test in all women who have not previously undergone a hysterectomy or bilateral oophorectomy. This test is mandatory.

B O X 6-4 *(continued)*

Management

1. Antibiotic regimens
   a. Treatment for *Neisseria gonorrhoeae*
      Ceftriaxone, 250 mg i.m., in one dose, or
      *Amoxicillin, 3 g, and probenicid, 1 g p.o., in one dose, or
      Spectinomycin, 2 g i.m., in one dose (the agent of choice for GC proctitis).
      *NOTE: Ceftriaxone is the drug of choice in communities in which the resistance of *N. gonorrhoeae* to penicillin and penicillin analogs is >1%.
      AND
   b. Treat *Chlamydia* infections. Because GC and non-GC urethritides co-occur in 50%–60% of cases, both must be treated concurrently. Therefore, in addition to the GC treatment, a regimen for *Chlamydia* should be instituted. These regimens include:
      Tetracycline, 500 mg p.o., q.i.d., for 10 days, or
      Doxycycline, 100 mg p.o., b.i.d., for 10 days, or
      Erythromycin, 500 mg p.o., q.i.d., for 10 days.
      Azithromycin, 1,000 mg p.o., for one dose (take on an empty stomach).
2. Treat genital herpes simplex with acyclovir, 200 mg p.o., five times per day for 10 days.
3. Foster prevention. Educate patient in safe sexual practices (monogamy, barrier methods) or abstinence.
4. Report all cases to the Public Health Service.

stand your queries and even make her or him more comfortable.

7. Have the patient describe in his or her own words the activities and symptoms (Box 6-4).

II. Bacterial diseases

Bacteria that can cause STDs include *Neisseria gonorrhoeae*, *Chlamydia trachomatis*, and *Treponema pallidum*. These organisms are the causative agents in the vast majority of symptomatic STDs. Each is discussed subsequently.

A. *Neisseria gonorrhoeae*

This gram-negative intracellular diplococcus results in a significant percentage of symptomatic STDs in the United States and the world. It is transmitted by the exchange of infected body fluids and can be transmitted during any sexual activity. It infects and affects the mucosal surfaces of any part of the body. The vast majority of symptomatic cases involve the male urethra or female cervix, but the pharynx and rectum can also be affected. The manifestations, complications, evaluation, and management of specific syndromes caused by this pathogenic bacterium include the following:

1. **Urethritis in males**
   a. The **specific manifestations** of this entity include a fairly acute onset of moderate to severe dysuria with associated hesitancy, urgency, and pyuria. There are usually no associated fevers or hematuria. Patients often complain that a yellow discharge is present in the underpants or on bedlinen in the morning. A history of unprotected intercourse in the proximate past can usually be obtained from the patient. **Complications** of this infection include transmission to others and the development of systemic disease, which may manifest with a monoarticular arthritis.
   b. The **specific evaluation and management** of this entity entail making the clinical diagnosis by performing the examinations and management steps outlined in Box 6-4. Cultures should be plated onto agar medium at the time of specimen procurement. *Chlamydia* infections should, in most cases, be concurrently treated.

2. **Cervicitis or urethritis in females**
   a. The **specific manifestations** of this entity include a fairly acute onset of a moderate amount of yellow vaginal discharge with concurrent pruritus, a burning sensation, or pain in the vaginal area. There often are associated dyspareunia (pain during coitus) and a mild to moderate dysuria with associated hesitancy, urgency, and pyuria. There usually are no associated fevers or hematuria. A history of unprotected intercourse in the proximate past can usually be obtained from the patient.
   b. The **complications** of this infection include:
      i. Transmission to others.
      ii. The development of systemic disease, which manifests with a monoarticular arthritis.
      iii. The development of pelvic inflammatory disease (PID). PID is the infection and resultant purulent inflammation of the fallopian tubes by the underlying bacterial pathogen. The pathogen may be either *N. gonorrhoeae* or *C. trachomatis*. The natural history of this specific complication is the development of an acute tubal abscess, septicemia, and spread of

infection to the upper peritoneum with resultant peritonitis. This peritonitis, also known as perihepatitis or the Fitz-Hugh–Curtis syndrome, can lead to intraabdominal abscess formation and death.

    iv. A long-term complication of PID is scarring of the fallopian tubes with a resultant increased risk of infertility or tubal pregnancy.

c. The **specific evaluation and management** of this entity entail making the clinical diagnosis by performing the examinations and management steps outlined in Box 6-4. Cultures should be plated onto agar medium at the time of specimen procurement. *Chlamydia* infections should, in most cases, be concurrently treated.

    i. If the patient has any evidence of adnexal fullness on pelvic examination or any evidence of systemic dissemination (e.g., fevers), further specific evaluation and management include:

        (a) A CBC count to look for anemia or leukocytosis.

        (b) Ultrasound of the pelvis to look for an abscess in the fallopian tubes.

        (c) Consultation with and probably admission to the gynecologic service is indicated. See also Chapter 11, Pelvic mass (page 541).

    ii. Once PID is suspected or diagnosed, the initiation of parenteral antibiotics (e.g., Cefoxitin 2.0 g q.6hr i.v. and doxycycline 100 mg i.v./p.o. q. 12hr until afebrile for 48 hours, then doxycycline 100 mg p.o. b.i.d. for 14 days).

3. Pharyngitis

a. The **specific manifestations** of this entity include the fairly acute onset of a moderate to severe sore throat. Often the patient has concurrent urethral or cervical manifestations, as described previously. A history of unprotected intercourse and fellatio in the proximate past is generally present. Examination discloses purulent pharyngitis with marked cervical lymphadenopathy. Complications of this infection include transmission to others and the development of systemic disease, which may manifest with a monoarticular arthritis.

b. The **specific evaluation and management** of this entity entail making the clinical diagnosis by performing the examinations and management steps outlined in Box 6-4. Cultures should be plated onto agar medium at the time of specimen procurement. *Chlamydia* infections should, in most cases, be concurrently treated. Once GC pharyngitis is suspected or diagnosed, the initiation of parenteral antibiotics (e.g., ceftriaxone, a third-generation cephalosporin), is indicated. If indeed it is GC pharyngitis, it usually responds rapidly to the ceftriaxone.

4. **Proctitis**

a. The **specific manifestations** of this entity include the fairly acute onset of moderate to severe perianal and/or rectal discomfort that is exacerbated by defecation. It is not uncommon in heterosexual or homosexual patients who practice anal intercourse, especially receptive anal intercourse. It is not uncommon for the patient to have concurrent urethritis or cervicitis, depending on sexual practices. A history of unprotected intercourse in the proximate past is generally present. Examination discloses marked tenderness in the rectal vault. Complications of this infection include transmission to others and the development of systemic disease, which manifests with a monoarticular arthritis.

b. The **specific evaluation and management** of this entity entail making the clinical diagnosis by performing the examinations and management scheme outlined in Box 6-4. Cultures should be plated onto agar medium at the time of specimen procurement. Chlamydia should, in most cases, be concurrently treated. Once GC proctitis is diagnosed or suspected, treatment is with regimen described in Box 6-4. The strain of *N. gonorrhoeae* that is associated with this entity is markedly resistant to β-lactams, and thus the drug of choice is spectinomycin, 2 g i.m. for one dose.

B. *Chlamydia trachomatis*

This is an atypical bacterium that results in a significant percentage of symptomatic STDs in the United States and the world; in fact, it is one of the most common causes of STDs in the world today. The organism is transmitted by the exchange of infected body fluids and can be transmitted during any sexual activity. It can infect and affect the mucosal surfaces of any part of the body. The vast majority of asymptomatic and symptomatic cases involve the male urethra or female cervix. The manifestations, complications, evaluation, and management of specific syndromes caused by this pathogenic bacterium are described subsequently.

1. **Urethritis in males**

a. The **specific manifestations** of this entity cover a wide spectrum, ranging from the fairly acute onset of moderate to severe dysuria with associated hesitancy, urgency, and pyuria, quite similar to gono-coccal urethritis, to virtually no symptoms even when the disease is acute. There usually are no associated fevers or hematuria. Unlike in GC ure-thritis, patients rarely report that a yellow dis-charge is present on underpants or on bedlinen in the morning. A history of unprotected intercourse in the proximate past can usually be obtained from the patient. Complications of this infection include transmission to others and the development of epididymitis with abscess formation in the future.

   b. The **specific evaluation and management** of this entity entail making the clinical diagnosis by per-forming the examinations and management steps outlined in Box 6-4. Urethral culture for *Chla-mydia trachomatis* and urethral smear and culture for *N. gonorrhoeae* are indicated. Cultures should be plated at the time of specimen procurement. If there is any suspicion of concurrent GC, it should be concurrently treated. Once the condition is diag-nosed or suspected, treatment should be with the regimen given in Box 6-4.

2. **Cervicitis or urethritis in females**
   a. The **specific manifestations** of this entity range from the fairly acute onset of a moderate amount of yellow vaginal discharge with pruritus in the vaginal area with a modest amount of associated dyspareunia and a mild to moderate dysuria with associated hesitancy, urgency, and pyuria, all quite similar to gonococcal urethritis, to virtually no symptoms even when the disease is acute. Women most often have minimal to no symptoms. There usually are no associated fevers or hematuria. A history of unprotected intercourse in the proxi-mate past can usually be obtained from the patient.

   b. The **complications** of this infection include:
      i. Transmission to others.
      ii. The **development of PID.** PID is the infection and resultant purulent inflammation of the fal-lopian tubes with the underlying bacterial pathogen. The pathogen can be either *N. gonor-rhoeae* or *C. trachomatis*. The natural history of this specific complication is the develop-ment of an acute tubal abscess, septicemia, and spread of the infection to the upper peritoneum with resultant peritonitis. This peritonitis, also known as perihepatitis or Fitz-Hugh–Curtis syndrome, can lead to intraabdominal abscess formation and death.
      iii. A chronic complication of PID is scarring of

the fallopian tubes with a resultant increased risk of infertility or tubal pregnancy.

iv. The complication of neonatal chlamydial pneumonitis or conjunctivitis can occur in neonates born of mothers who deliver vaginally when the disease is active.

c. The **specific evaluation and management** of this entity entail making the clinical diagnosis by performing the examinations and management steps outlined in Box 6-4. Urethral culture for *C. trachomatis* and urethral smear and culture for *N. gonorrhoeae* are indicated. Cultures should be plated at the time of specimen procurement. If there is any suspicion of concurrent GC, it should be concurrently treated. Once the condition is diagnosed or suspected, treatment should be with the regimen listed in Box 6-4.

i. If the patient has any evidence of adnexal fullness on pelvic examination or any evidence of systemic dissemination (e.g., fevers), further specific evaluation and management include the following steps.

(a) A CBC count to look for anemia or leukocytosis.

(b) US of the pelvis to look for an abscess in the fallopian tubes.

(c) Consultation with and probably admission to the gynecology service are indicated. See Chapter 11, Pelvic Masses (page 541).

ii. Once PID is suspected or diagnosed, the initiation of doxycycline 100 mg p.o. b.i.d. for 14 days and, to empirically cover for GC, parenteral antibiotics (e.g., ceftriaxone, a third-generation cephalosporin) is indicated.

iii. All pregnant woman who have evidence of or are at risk for *Chlamydia* infection should undergo the examinations listed in Box 6-4. Specific therapy for *Chlamydia* infection is more difficult, and management should be undertaken with consultation by the patient's obstetrician.

C. *Treponema pallidum*

This non–Gram-staining spirochetal organism causes the local and systemic disease called syphilis or lues venereum. This STD, although still uncommon, has been increasing in incidence in the United States. The organism is transmitted by the exchange of infected body fluids and can be transmitted during any sexual activity. It can infect and affect the mucosal surfaces of any part of the body. The vast majority of asymptomatic and symptomatic cases initially involve the male urethra or female vulva. The manifestations, complications, evaluation, and management are best described by categorizing the disease in one of the well-described discrete stages, based on the natural history of this infectious disease process.

1. **Primary lues**
    a. The **specific manifestations** of this temporal stage of treponemal infection are the result of the initial exposure and infection. These manifestations occur 1–2 weeks after exposure. They are limited to the development of a **chancre,** an indurated, painless lesion with raised borders and a central depression (Fig. 6-1). The chancre develops in an area of sexual contact, usually the vulva, penis, scrotum, or oral mucosa. The lesion is self-limited, resolving spontaneously, without sequelae, in 7–10 days. It is, however, a lesion in which transmission of the spirochete is highly likely if intimate contact is made with another person (i.e., it is highly infectious).
    b. The **specific evaluation and management** of this entity entail making the clinical diagnosis by performing the examinations and management steps outlined in Box 6-4. A **serum VDRL** and a **scraping** of the **lesion's base** for dark-field assessment should be performed for diagnostic purposes. Once the diagnosis is made, therapy should be initiated.

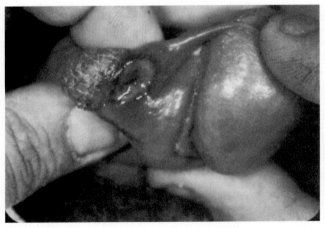

F I G U R E 6-1
The chancre of primary lues venereum. (Patient's fingers; examiner must wear gloves)

The therapy for primary lues is penicillin G benzathine, 2.4 million units i.m. once, or doxycycline* 100 mg p.o. b.i.d. for 14 days (see Table 6-7).

2. **Secondary lues**
   a. The **specific manifestations** of this temporal stage of treponemal infection result from systemic dissemination of the spirochetes after the initial infection in a host who has not been effectively treated. These manifestations occur 6–8 weeks after exposure, and thus ~4–6 weeks after chancre resolution. They include low-grade fever, fatigue, night sweats, and one or more of the following dermatologic manifestations:
      i. A generalized, painless, erythematous macular rash that involves the soles and palms.
      ii. A self-limited, painless, generalized papular rash, called **condyloma lata.** This phase of lues venereum is self-limited and lasts up to several weeks. Many times this phase is only modestly symptomatic. The specific lesions of condylomata lata also have treponemes present and are infectious in nature.
   b. The **specific evaluation and management** of this entity entails making the clinical diagnosis by performing the examinations and management steps outlined in Box 6-4. A serum **VDRL** as well as a scraping of the lesional base of a papule in condyloma lata for dark-field assessment should be performed for diagnostic purposes. Once the diagnosis is made, therapy should be initiated. The therapy for secondary lues is penicillin G benzathine, 2.4 million units i.m., q week for 3 weeks, or doxycycline* 100 mg p.o. b.i.d. for 14 days (see Table 6-7).

3. **Latent lues**
   a. The **specific manifestations** of this temporal stage of treponemal infection are as the result of the host controlling and in some cases effectively eradicating the body of the spirochetes, in a host who has not been effectively treated. This stage, by definition, begins at the termination of the manifestations of the secondary lues phase and may continue for life. As this is defined to be a "latent" period, there are no clinical manifestations of disease. The patient may, in the sexual history, relate a history of a chancre that was not treated. The latent stage can be further divided into two subgroups, early and late.

* contraindicated in pregnancy.

T A B L E 6-7
Regimens for the Treatment of Syphilis (Lues Venereum)

Syndrome	Drug of Choice	Alternate Regimens
Primary lues Secondary lues Early latent lues	Penicillin G benzathine, 2.4 million units i.m.	Doxycycline 100 mg p.o. b.i.d. for 14 days
Late latent lues	Penicillin G benzathine, 2.4 million units i.m. once a week for 3 wk	Doxycycline 100 mg p.o. b.i.d. for 28 days
Neurosyphilis Cardiovascular lues	Penicillin G, 2–4 million units i.v. q.4hr for 10 days	Doxycycline 100 mg p.o. b.i.d. for 28 days

(Based on: CDC treatment guidelines for sexually transmitted disease. MMWR 1989;38[Suppl]:5.)

      i. Early latent—The first year after the exposure to the disease.

      ii. Late latent—>1 year after exposure to the disease.

    b. The **specific evaluation and management** of this entity entail making the clinical diagnosis by performing the examinations and management steps outlined in Box 6-4. A serum VDRL and a serum FTA-abs are indicated. It is not uncommon for the VDRL to become nonreactive in the latent stage; however, the FTA-abs remains reactive permanently. If the patient has latent lues, a lumbar puncture to obtain CSF for a VDRL test must be performed to rule out asymptomatic neurosyphilis (see subsequent discussion). Once the diagnosis is made, therapy should be initiated.

      i. The therapy for early latent lues is penicillin G benzathine, 2.4 million units i.m., once, or doxycycline 100 mg p.o. b.i.d. for 14 days (see Table 6-7).

      ii. The therapy for **late latent lues** requires a more intensive course of antibiotics (i.e., penicillin G benzathine, 2.4 million units i.m., once weekly for 3 consecutive weeks, or doxycycline 100 mg p.o. b.i.d. for 28 days (see Table 6-7).

  4. Tertiary lues. This temporal stage of treponemal infection is as the result of the infection becoming clinical again after a variable period of subclinical latency. The manifestations of tertiary lues can begin years to decades after the primary infection. The manifestations of this stage of the disease are effectively and clinically divided into several subtypes relating to the location of manifestations. The patient with tertiary lues venereum may have one or more of the following manifestations, including more than one type of neurosyphilis. These include gummatous, cardiovascular, and neurosyphilis. **Gummatous** is the presence of one or more chronic nodules; VDRL is often negative but the FTA-abs is reactive; **cardiovascular** lues: there is a thoracic aortic aneurysm and the development of aortic insufficiency, confirmed by echocardiogram and clinical examination; **neurosyphilis** is as described in Table 6-8. Treatment modalities for each of these is in Table 6-8.

III. **Viral diseases**

Viral organisms that cause STDs include herpes simplex II, hepatitis A virus, hepatitis B virus, the HIV, and human papillomavirus (HPV).

A. **Herpes simplex II**

This DNA virus causes a significant percentage of symptomatic STDs in the United States and the world. It is transmitted by the exchange of infected blood and body fluids and can be transmitted during any sexual activity. It can infect and affect the mucosal surfaces of any part of the body. The vast majority of symptomatic cases involve the male glans and shaft of the penis or female vulva, but the pharynx and rectum can also be infected or affected.

1. The **specific manifestations** include the acute onset of clusters of vesicular lesions that are very painful (Fig. 6-2). The vesicular lesions remain for 7–10 days and then spontaneously resolve. The virus is present in very high concentrations within these vesicles; therefore, the vesicular lesions are very infectious.

2. **Natural history.** The virus remains in the ganglia of the cutaneous nerves supplying the infected area. At various times after the initial infection, there can be a recurrence, which manifests very similarly to the initial infection with clusters of vesicular lesions. Whenever the disease is active—that is, whenever vesicular lesions are present—the disease is transmissible.

3. The **specific evaluation and management** entail making the clinical diagnosis by examination and performing the tests described in Box 6-4. It is usually not necessary to perform a Tzanck smear on all cases,

T A B L E 6-8
Syndromes of Neurosyphilis

Syndrome	Manifestations	Cerebrospinal Fluid Findings	Management
Asymptomatic	No specific manifestations History of untreated STD or chancre	VDRL reactive Mild increase in protein Cell count normal	See Table 6-7
Tabes dorsalis	Sensory neuropathy to fine touch, position, and vibration in a "stocking–glove" distribution Diffusely decreased deep tendon reflexes Argyl–Robertson pupil: constricts normally to accommodation, but not to direct or consensual light	VDRL reactive Mild increase in protein Cell count normal	See Table 6-7 Refer to occupational therapy
Meningovascular	Generalized headaches Low-grade fevers Cranial nerve defects, unilateral or bilateral, including peripheral cranial nerve VII and XII deficits Mild to modest neck stiffness; rarely any acute meningeal signs	VDRL reactive Mild increase in protein Marked increase in number of cells with a predominance of lymphocytes	See Table 6-7
General paresis	Insidious, progressive onset of dementia	VDRL reactive Mild increase in protein Mild increase in number of cells, mainly lymphocytes	See Table 6-7

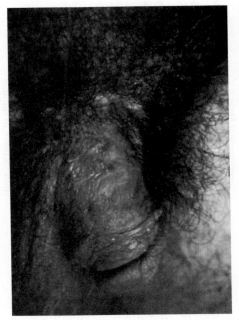

F I G U R E   6-2
Clusters of vesicles and erosions in this painful rash of herpes simplex
genitalis.

as the clinical diagnosis is often quite straightforward.
The specific management includes that described in
Box 6-4. Acyclovir, 200 mg p.o., five times a day,
for 10 days, decreases the duration and intensity of
symptoms, decreases the duration of the vesicles, and
thus decreases the duration of infectivity. It is not a
curative regimen and is most effective in the first episode of herpes simplex infection. There is no advantage to acyclovir ointment. In addition, if the patient
has a significant number of recurrences, long-term
acyclovir in the suppressive dose of 400 mg p.o., b.i.d.,
is indicated.

B. Other viruses

The reader is referred to the section on Hepatitis in Chapter 2 (page 112) for a discussion of viral hepatitis, to the
section on HIV Infection, page 320, for details on that
disease process, and to the section on Viral Skin Infections in Chapter 8 for a discussion of HPV infection.

IV. Consultation

Problem	Service	Time
Latent or tertiary lues	Infectious diseases	Urgent
HIV positive	Infectious diseases	Required
Condyloma latum	Dermatology	Elective
Cardiovascular lues	Cardiology	Urgent
Adnexal mass	Gynecology	Urgent
Evidence of systemic spread of GC	Gynecology	Emergent
Pregnancy concurrent with STD	Ob/Gyn	Urgent
Painful scrotal mass	Urology	Emergent
Any STD	Public Health	Required

V. Indications for admission: Neurosyphilis, evidence of cardiovascular lues venereum, adnexal mass on pelvic examination, evidence of ectopic pregnancy, and evidence of systemic spread of *N. gonorrhoeae.*

Bibliography

Bacterial Skin Infections
Hook E, et al: Microbiologic evaluation of cutaneous cellulitis in adults. Arch Intern Med 1986;146:295–298.
Reagan D, et al: Elimination of coincident *Staphylococcus aureus* nasal and hand carriage with intranasal application of mupirocin calcium ointment. Ann Intern Med 1991;114:101–106.
Suss SJ, Middleton DB: Cellulitis and related skin infections. Am Fam Pract 1987;36:126–136.
Wheat LJ, et al: Diabetic foot infections. Arch Intern Med 1986;146:1935–1940.

Bite Wounds
Fishbein DB, et al: Rabies. N Engl J Med 1993;329:1631–1638.
Goldstein E, Richwald G: Human and animal bite wounds. Am Fam Pract 1987;36:101–109.
Klein M: Nondomestic mammalian bites. Am Fam Pract 1985;32:137–141.
Marcy SM: Infections due to dog and cat bites. Pediatr Infect Dis 1982;1:351–356.
Suwanagool S, et al: Pathogenicity of *Eikenella corrodens* in humans. Arch Intern Med 1983;143:2265–2268.

Bacterial Endocarditis
American Heart Association: Prevention of bacterial endocarditis. JAMA 1990;264:2919–2922.
Baltch AL, et al: Bacteremia in patients undergoing oral procedures. Arch Intern Med 1988;148:1084–1088.
Dewitt DE, et al: Endocarditis in injection drug users. Am Fam Pract 1996;53:2045–2049.

HIV Infection

Barnes PF, et al: Tuberculosis in patients with human immunodeficiency virus infection. N Engl J Med 1991;324:1644–1650.

Bartlett JG: Protease inhibitors for HIV infection. Ann Intern Med 1996;124:1086–1088.

Bloom J, Palestine A: The diagnosis of cytomegalovirus retinitis. Ann Intern Med 1988;109:963–969.

Broder S, et al: Antiretroviral therapy in AIDS. Ann Intern Med 1990;113:604–608.

Carpenter CCJ, et al. for the International AIDS study—U.S.A.: Antiretroviral therapy for HIV infection in 1996. JAMA 1996;276:146–154.

Cesarman E, et al: Kaposi's sarcoma-associated herpesvirus-like DNA sequences in AIDS-related lymphomas. N Engl J Med 1995;332:1186–1191.

Collier AC, et al: Treatment of HIV infection with saquinavir, zidovudine and zalcitabine. N Engl J Med 1996;334:1011–1017.

Como JA, et al: Oral azole drugs as systemic antifungal therapy. N Engl J Med 1994;330:263–273.

Coombs RW, et al: Association of plasma HIV type-1 RNA level with risk of clinical progression in patients with advanced infection. J Infect Dis 1997;176:940.

Delta Coordinating Committee: Delta: a randomised double-blind controlled trial comparing combinations of zidovudine plus didanosine or zalcitabine with zidovudine alone in HIV-infected individuals. Lancet 1996;348:283–291.

Drew WL, et al; Oral ganciclovir as maintenance treatment for CMV retinitis in patients with AIDS. N Engl J Med 1995;333:615–620.

Gabuzda D, Hirsch M: Neurologic manifestations of infection with human immunodeficiency virus. Ann Intern Med 1987;107:383–391.

Gemson DH, et al: Acquired immunodeficiency syndrome prevention. Arch Intern Med 1991;151:1102–1108.

Hirsch MS, et al: Therapy for HIV infection. N Engl J Med 1993;328:1686–1695.

Laskin OL, et al: Ganciclovir for the treatment and suppression of serious infections caused by cytomegalovirus. Am J Med 1987;83:201–207.

Makadon HJ: Assessing HIV infection in primary care practice. J Gen Intern Med 1991;6(suppl):S2–S7.

Martin MA, et al: A comparison of the effectiveness of three regimens in the prevention of *Pneumocystis carinii* pneumonia in HIV-infected patients. Arch Intern Med 1992;152:523–528.

Mellors JW, et al: Prognosis in HIV-1 infection predicted by the quantity of virus in plasma. Science 1996;272:1167–1170.

Mellors JW, et al: Prognosis in HIV-1 Infection predicted by the quantity of virus in plasma. Science 1996;272:1167–1170.

Miles SA: Diagnosing and staging of HIV infection. Am Fam Pract 1988;38:248–256.

MMWR: 1993 Revised classification system for HIV infection. MMWR 1993; 1992; 41(RR-17):1.

Montaner J, et al: Corticosteroids prevent early deterioration in patients with moderately severe *Pneumocystis carinii* pneumonia and the acquired immunodeficiency syndrome (AIDS). Ann Intern Med 1990;113:14–20.

Palestine AG, et al: A randomized, controlled trial of foscarnet in the treatment of cytomegalovirus retinitis in patients with AIDS. Ann Intern Med 1991;115:665–673.

Pierce M, et al: A randomized trial of clarithromycin as prophylaxis against disseminated *Mycobacterium avium* complex infection in patients with advanced acquired immunodeficiency syndrome. N Engl J Med 1996;335:384–391.

Powderly WG, et al: A controlled trial of fluconazole or amphotericin B to prevent relapse of cryptococcal meningitis in patients with the acquired immunodeficiency syndrome. N Engl J Med 1992;326:793–798.

Small PM, et al: Treatment of tuberculosis in patients with advanced human immunodeficiency virus infection. N Engl J Med 1991;324:289–294.

Tarantola DJM et al: Global expansion of HIV infection and AIDS. Hosp Pract 1996;31:63–79.

Vinson RP, Epperly TD: Counseling patients on proper use of condoms. Am Fam Pract 1991;43:2081–2085.

Sexually Transmitted Diseases

Boslego JW, et al: Effect of spectinomycin use on the prevalence of spectino-mycin-resistance and of penicillinase-producing *Neisseria gonorrhoeae*. N Engl J Med 1987;317:272–278.

Guinan M: Oral acyclovir for treatment and suppression of genital herpes simplex virus infection. JAMA 1986;255:1747–1757.

Hart G: Syphilis tests in diagnostic and therapeutic decision making. Ann Intern Med 1986;104:368–376.

Hutchinson C, et al: Characteristics of patients with syphilis attending Balti-more STD clinics. Arch Intern Med 1991;151:511–516.

Kirchner J: Syphilis—an STD on the increase. Am Fam Pract 1991;44:843–854.

Morgan R: Clinical aspects of pelvic inflammatory disease. Am Fam Pract 1991;43:1725–1732.

Pruessner HT, et al: Diagnosis and treatment of chlamydial infections. Am Fam Pract 1986;34:81–92.

Romanowski B, et al: Serologic response to treatment of infectious syphilis. Ann Intern Med 1991;114:1005–1009.

Schwarcz SK, et al: National surveillance of antimicrobial resistance in *Neisseria gonorrhoeae*. JAMA 1990;264:1413–1421.

Stone K, et al: Primary prevention of sexually transmitted diseases. JAMA 1986;255:1763–1767.

Stott GA: New macrolide antibiotics: clarithromycin and azithromycin. Am Fam Pract 1992;46:863–869.

—D.D.B.

Chapter 7

Musculoskeletal Disorders

Monoarticular Arthritis

All mobile joints in the body are lined with the simple squamous epithelium, synovium. The synovium in the normal healthy state produces a small amount of fluid that functions as a lubricant for the joint. An inflammation of this lining or its adjacent structures within the joint is entitled synovitis, or, more colloquially, arthritis. If the arthritis involves only one joint, it is called monoarticular arthritis.

By definition, acute arthritis is the onset of specific findings within 2 weeks of presentation, whereas chronic arthritis consists of findings present for >2 weeks at the time of presentation (Box 7-2).

I. **Crystal-induced arthropathies**

These are not uncommon processes in which crystals of various chemical composition are deposited in the synovium of one or more joints with resultant acute arthritis.

A. **Gout**

1. The **underlying pathogenesis** is an increased total body uric acid level that sometimes manifests with an increased serum uric acid level. Uric acid is a catabolite of the purine nucleosides. The rapid shift in serum uric acid levels, either an increase or a decrease, can precipitate deposition of sodium monourate crystals in a synovial space. The crystals induce inflammation by several mechanisms, including prostaglandins and leukotrienes. The most clearly understood mechanism is the release of crystal chemotactic factor (CCF) from PMNs. The increased total body uric acid levels may result from one or more of the following processes:

a. Excessive consumption of foods rich in purines and uric acid.

(text continues on page 363)

BOX 7-1

Overall Evaluation and Management of Discomfort, Pain, or Dysfunction of a Joint

1. Query the patient as to any antecedent trauma.
2. If any trauma or risk of fracture, radiograph(s) of the affected joint(s) is (are) mandatory.
3. **Finger/hand/wrist, specific:**
   a. Perform range of motion (ROM), passive and active (°):

DIP	Flexion	80
	Extension	0
PIP	Flexion	120
	Extension	0
MCP	Flexion	90
	Extension	0
	Abduction	25
	Adduction	0
Wrist	Flexion	80
	Extension	70
	Ulnar deviation	30
	Radial deviation	30
	Circumduction	45
Thumb IP	Extension	0
	Flexion	80
Thumb MCP	Extension	0
	Flexion	30
Thumb MC/	Circumduction	30
scaphoid	Flexion	60
	Extension	0
	Adduction	0
	Abduction	90

   b. Inspect and palpate the joints for deformity and/or contractures of the DIP, PIP, or MCP.
   c. Palpate the MCP palmar aspect for clicking of a trigger finger.
   d. Inspect fingers, wrist, tendons, and hand for ganglion and/or Dupuytren's contracture.
   e. Palpate the snuffbox and perform Finkelstein's (passive ulnar deviation of the hand) for de Quervain's tenosynovitis.
   f. Neurologic examination:
   Radial nerve
   i. Sensory: Radial/dorsal side
   ii. Motor: Extension of the wrist and digits

   (continued)

B O X   7-1 (continued)

Ulnar nerve
   i. Sensory: Ulnar side
   ii. Motor: Flexion of digits 4 and 5
       Abduction and adduction of digits (i.e., interosseus muscles)
       Thumb adduction
Median nerve
   i. Sensory: Radial palmar side
   ii. Motor: Thumb flexion
       Flexion of digits 2 and 3
       Thenar eminence
   g. **Tinel's sign** (i.e., tapping over an area). If over the palmaris longus area, and tingling develops, it is consistent with **carpal tunnel syndrome;** if over the loge de Guyon, and tingling develops over the lateral hand, it is consistent with **Guyon's tunnel** syndrome.
   h. Management: see Table 7-1 (page 364).
4. **Elbow specific**
   a. Perform ROM, passive and active (°)

Extension	0
Flexion	160
Pronation	90
Supination	90

   b. Palpate the olecranon, cubital tunnel, ulnar epicondyle, radial epicondyle, and the joint space itself for swelling/effusion.
   c. Perform Tinel's sign over the cubital tunnel: if tingling is over the ulnar side, **cubital tunnel syndrome**
   d. Management: see Table 7-2 (page 368).
5. **Shoulder specific**
   a. Perform ROM, passive and active (°)

External rotation	90
Internal rotation	90
Extension	50
Flexion	180
Abduction	180
Adduction	50

   b. Palpate the shoulder structures: sternoclavicular joint, acromioclavicular joint, glenohumeral joint and the rotator cuff, and more superficial muscles.

(continued)

B O X 7-1 (continued)

    c. Perform Yergason's (i.e., flexion and supination of the elbow and forearm) and palpate over the bicipital groove.

    d. Passive versus active abduction of the shoulder at the glenohumeral joint:

        If passive and active are limited, supraspinatus tendinitis.

        If active limited only, supraspinatus tear.

    e. Apley's from above and below:

        If internal rotation is limited, subscapularis damage.

        If external rotation is limited, intraspinatus and/or teres minor damage.

    f. Management: see Table 7-3 (page 370).

6. **Hip specific:**

    a. Perform ROM, passive and active (°)

Knee straight	Flexion	90
	Extension	15
	Abduction	45–60
	Adduction	30
Knee flexed	Flexion	120
	Extension	0
	Abduction	40
	Adduction	40

    b. FABERE test: the patient passively flexes, abducts, and externally rotates at the hip so that lateral malleolus touches the knee. This localizes the site of discomfort for further evaluation.

    c. Palpate the thigh and greater trocanteric and ischiogluteal bursae.

    d. Tinel's over the lateral inguinal area: if tingling over the anterior thigh, meralgia paresthetica.

    e. Management: see Table 7-4 (page 374).

7. **Back specific**

    a. Perform ROM, active and passive (°)

Extension	30
Flexion	75–90
Lateral binding	30, left and right
Rotation	30, left and right

    b. Perform a urinalysis

    c. Palpate over the paraspinous muscles and the spinous processes

(continued)

B O X   7-1 *(continued)*

    d. Neurologic examination

S1	Sensory	Plantar foot	
	Motor	Plantar flexion at ankle	
L5	Sensory	Dorsal foot	
	Motor	Dorsiflexion at ankle	
L4	Sensory	Anterior thigh	
	Motor	Extension at the knee/quadriceps muscle	

    e. FABERE test, as above in hip

    f. Perform Schober test, i.e., mark a site 5 cm above the posterior superior iliac spine with the patient standing erect, and then remeasure with active flexion: should increase in length.

    g. Management: see Table 7-5 (page 375).

8. **Knee specific**

    a. Perform ROM, passive and active (°)

Extension	5
Flexion	130
Abduction/Adduction	Minimal
Internal/External rotation	Minimal

    b. Varus/Valgus: articulation between the tibia and femur

    c. Q-angle: angle between two lines, one from the anterior superior iliac spine to the center of the patella, and the other line from the center of the patella to the anterior tibial tuberosity. If the angle is increased, indicative of patellar-tracking dysfunction, i.e., the milieu for the patellofemoral syndrome.

    d. Check for an effusion by ballottement of the patella, bulge sign, and fluid displacement.

    e. Anterior drawer: with the knee at 90°, attempt to draw the tibia anteriorly.

    f. Lachman's: with the knee at 30°, attempt to pull the proximal tibia anteriorly.

    g. McMurray test: passive flexion and extension of knee with the foot internally and externally rotated; if a click or pain, consistent with meniscal tears.

    h. Valgus and varus stress at 30° of flexion: laxity is indicative of MCL or LCL damage.

    i. Management: see Table 7-6 (page 378).

(continued)

B O X 7-1 (continued)

9. **Foot/Ankle specific**
   a. Perform ROM, passive and active (°)

      Tibiotalar joint
      Dorsiflexion at ankle   20
      Plantarflexion at ankle   45
      Subtalar joints
      Inversion of foot (great toe up)   30
      Eversion of foot (great toe down)   20
      Supination (foot lateral side down)   20
      Pronation (foot medial side down)   30

   b. Palpate and inspect structures: lateral ankle, medial ankle, fibular head, MTP joints, plantar aspect of calcaneus, Achilles' tendon, retrocalcaneal bursal area, and the toes.
   c. Perform Tinel's over the tarsal tunnel, inferior to the medial malleolus
   d. Squeeze test: Pain upon squeezing the proximal fibia and fibula together may indicate syndesmotic tear involving interosseus membrane.
   e. Observe gait: determine whether there is a proprioceptive and/or steppage gait present.
   f. Management: see Table 7-7 (page 382).

(text continued from page 358)

   b. A partial or total congenital deficiency of the enzyme hypoxanthine-guanine phosphoribosyl transferase, an enzyme necessary for the catabolism of purines.
   c. Saturnine gout, in which the ingestion of substances high in lead [e.g., moonshine with lead (plumbism)] will lead to renal failure and gout.
   d. Lymphoproliferative disorder with increased nuclear catabolism and thus purine release and uric acid increase.

2. The **specific manifestations**, in addition to those described in Box 7-2 (page 389), include the predilection of gout for certain joints. These joints include the first metatarsophalangeal (MTP) joint (podagra), the knee joint (gonogra), and the wrist (chiragra). The patient rarely has any associated systemic manifestations and is virtually always afebrile.

3. The **specific evaluation** of this entity includes making the diagnosis by performing crystal analysis on the

(text continues on page 386)

T A B L E 7-1
Hand/Wrist: Specific Clinical Syndromes

Swan neck/bou- tonnière de- formity	Damage to the tendons at and around the PIP joint Volar plate rupture as the result of trauma (stepping on) or syno- vitis from RA: *swan neck* Dorsal tendon damage as result of trauma (laceration), or teno- synovitis from RA: *boutonnière*	*Swan neck:* PIP hyperextension contracture, DIP flexion con- tracture *Boutonnière:* PIP flexion con- tracture, DIP hyperextension contracture	Acutely, splint the finger(s) NSAIDs Treat any underlying arthritis (see section on polyarticu- lar arthritis) (page 397)
Mallet finger	Traumatic avulsion of finger extensor tendon Trauma related hyper- flexion of DIP	Attitude of flexion at the DIP No active full extension at DIP Passive full extension of DIP	Acutely, buddy splint in full extension Treat early to prevent chronic sequelae
Boxer's fracture	Simple fracture of the 5th metacarpal, in the diaphysis The result of hitting ob- ject with a closed fist	Acute onset of pain and tender- ness on the ulnar aspect of the hand after appropriate trauma Examine for any defects in the ul- nar artery or nerve	Clinical diagnosis Radiographs confirm the di- agnosis (Fig. 7-1) Splint hand and wrist OT/PT consult Referral to orthopedics

Trigger finger	Inflammation at the site where the profunda flexor tendon passes through the superficial tendon, at the MCP joint Incidence increases with increasing age	*Triggering:* snapping sensation of the digit on flexion/extension *Locking:* reversible inability to extend the affected digit, usually at the PIP joint	Clinical diagnosis Radiographs are unnecessary Splint the finger(s) NSAIDs If severe, consider triamcinolone, 10 mg, in the area of the MCP pulley OT consult
Ganglion	Collections of fluid within the synovium in and adjacent to tendon sheaths	Soft, at times fluctuant, nontender lesions in and about the tendons and tendon sheaths of the hand and wrist Wax and wane Well defined	Monitor, no specific treatment necessary May consider aspiration of the cyst If cyst is symptomatic or if there is a resultant neuropathy, refer to surgery
Dupuytren's contracture	Progressive idiopathic contracture of the palmar fascia with resultant contractures Related to ethanol or recurrent trauma (e.g., hypothenar hammer)	Flexion contracture of the digits with fibronodular areas in the contractured palmar fascia Unable passively or actively extend the affected digits	If severe, refer to plastic surgery for release of the contracture
de Quervain's disease	Nonspecific inflammation of tendons in the anatomic snuffbox Precipitating factors: Trauma Pregnancy Occupational	Tenderness over the snuffbox including the tendons of the Extensor pollicus longus Extensor pollicus brevis Abductor pollicus longus Manifestations exacerbated by knitting or peeling vegetables Positive *Finkelstein's sign*	NSAIDs (Table 7-8, page 393) Splint wrist in mild dorsiflexion with radial deviation of the thumb Refer to orthopedics

Wrist-drop hand	Radial nerve palsy Radial nerve damaged by humeral fracture or by a Colles' fracture *Radial nerve:* • Wrist and finger extensors • Thumb extension and abduction • Sensation to dorsum of hand: 1, 2, and 3	Numbness over the dorsum of the hand Weakness of the wrist and digit extensors Atrophy of the dorsal forearm muscles	Clinical diagnosis Confirm via nerve conduction/EMG Refer to orthopedic surgeon OT/PT consult
Carpal tunnel	Median nerve dysfunction Median nerve damaged by entrapment at the carpal tunnel usually as the result of occupational or systemic disorders, e.g., Diabetes mellitus Hypothyroidism RA *Median nerve:* • Thumb flexion • Finger flexion, digits 2 and 3 • Thenar atrophy	Numbness over plantar hand Weakness of thumb flexion Weakness of digits 2, 3 flexors Atrophy of the thenar muscles *Tinel's sign* over carpal tunnel *Phalen's sign* positive *Flick test* positive	Clinical diagnosis Confirm by nerve conduction/EMG Refer to orthopedic surgeon OT/PT consult

| Ulnar tunnel/ loge de Guyon | Ulnar nerve dysfunction Ulnar nerve damaged by entrapment at the ulnar tunnel: ulnar aspect of the wrist in area of the hamate and pisiform Entrapment may occur here *Ulnar nerve:* • Adduction of thumb • Abduction/adduction of the digits • Sensation on ulnar aspect of hand | Numbness over the ulnar aspect of hand and wrist Weakness of adduction/abduction of the digits Weakness of the finger flexors of digits 4 and 5 *Tinel's over the loge de Guyon* Atrophy of the interosseous muscles | Clinical diagnosis Confirm by nerve conduction/EMG Refer to orthopedic surgeon OT/PT consult |

T A B L E 7-2
Elbow: Specific Clinical Syndromes

Syndrome	Pathogenesis	Manifestations	Evaluation and Management
Medial epicondylitis (golfer's elbow)	Inflammation of the common origin of forearm flexor muscles	Acute, recurrent tenderness over medial epicondyle Limited forearm flexion May be recurrent, especially after repetitive activities like vacuuming or foreswing of golf	History and physical examination No need for radiographs NSAIDs (Table 7-8, page 393) Avoidance of the activity (i.e., rest) PT/OT consults If severe and recurrent, consider injection of the area with 10 mg triamcinolone
Cubital tunnel syndrome	Entrapment of ulnar nerve in cubital groove/tunnel (i.e., the anatomic site between the medial epicondyle and the olecranon) Entrapment is as the result of trauma, infiltration, or edema Diabetes mellitus Hypothyroidism	Tingling in the ulnar aspect of the forearm and hand, dorsal and palmar aspects *Tinel's sign* positive over the cubital tunnel Atrophy and weakness of flexor carpi ulnaris, interosseous, thumb adductors, and the flexors of fingers 4 and 5	As in medial epicondylitis, and Referral to orthopedic surgery for release of the entrapment may be necessary Fasting blood glucose TSH Calcium/albumin, plasma

Condition	Description	Clinical features	Management
Olecranon bursitis	Inflammation of the olecranon bursa: Trauma Tophi Rarely, infection	Painful or painless swelling olecranon may be fluctuant If hot and red, think infection If with yellow papules, think tophi	As in medial epicondylitis, and If *high suspicion* for infectious bursitis: Perform a needle aspirate and send fluid for Gram's stain culture and crystals If PMNs and Gram's positive organisms: Drain all the material and initiate cephalexin, 500 mg p.o., q.i.d. for 7–10 days If negative birefringent crystals: colchicine for 4 weeks, 2 weeks into the colchicine, start allopurinol 300 mg p.o., q.d., long term If *low suspicion* of infection: Adhesive wrap and initiation of an NSAID
Lateral epicondylitis	Noninfectious inflammation of the common origin of the extensor muscles adjacent to the lateral epicondyle	Tender lateral epicondyle Painful, limited to extension of the wrist Recurrent after knitting, repeated handshaking, backhand swing of tennis	As described for medial epicondylitis

TABLE 7-3
Shoulder: Specific Clinical Syndromes

Anterior glenohumeral dislocation (Fig. 7-2)	The anterior displacement of the head of the humerus from the glenohumeral joint Usually as the result of forced hyperextension (e.g., pitching or serving at tennis)	Acute onset of severe shoulder pain and decreased ROM *Position of arm: "dead arm"* • If the head is lateral/inferior to coracoid: *subluxed* • If the head is medial to coracoid: *dislocated* Must assess the arterial and nerve function of the involved upper extremity	Assess and document the nerves of the upper extremities Radiograph to document the entities and rule out any fracture Reduction of the dislocation (two steps) or subluxation (one step); may be performed by a primary care MD if so trained; otherwise, orthopedic surgeon Effective analgesia is mandatory Immobilize the joint in a sling PT consult/orthopedics consult
Acromioclavicular separation (Fig. 7-3)	Trauma in which there is an inferoposterior thrust put on the shoulder (e.g., running into a door or being tackled by a football linebacker)	Acute, trauma-related severe pain on the lateral clavicle The lateral clavicle is separated from the acromion • 1st degree: pain/tenderness • 2nd degree: tenderness, springing • 3rd degree: completely separated	Clinical diagnosis Radiographs of shoulder/clavicle Immobilize in a sling Refer to orthopedics on an urgent basis NSAIDs Acutely, ice

Sternoclavicular separation	Significant trauma to the chest and chest wall (e.g., rapid-deceleration MVA in which patient hits steering wheel)	Severe pain and swelling at the sternoclavicular joint Clicking sound at the joint with movement of the upper extremity Medial clavicle displaced anteriorly from the sternum	Clinical diagnosis Radiographs of clavicle, chest, and shoulder are indicated to confirm the diagnosis and document any concurrent fracture(s) or pneumothorax Emergent referral to orthopedics Immobilization and effective analgesia are required
Clavicular fracture	Direct trauma to the shoulder or anterior chest wall, usually as the result of a fall	Pain and decreased ROM of upper extremity Palpable fracture of the clavicle Patient unable to abduct or elevate the entire upper extremity	Clinical diagnosis Radiographs to confirm and look for concurrent fractures Physical therapy consult Orthopedics consult
Bicipital tendinitis	Inflammation of the long head of the biceps in the bicipital groove Usually as the result of new or overuse of the shoulder in a throwing activity (e.g., overhand pitching)	Pain over the bicipital groove Positive *Yergason's sign*, i.e., pain on flexion of the elbow and supination of forearm	Clinical diagnosis Proscription of overhead activity Place the arm in a sling with elbow flexed and shoulder movement minimized NSAIDs (Table 7-8, page 398) PT/OT for Codman exercises, i.e., arm dangled in front and passively moved side to side and in increasing sized circles If no improvement, consider referral to orthopedics

(continued)

Supraspinatus tendinitis	Inflammation of this, the major muscle of the rotator cuff	Lateral pain and tenderness	Clinical diagnosis
	If this is chronic it becomes calcified; hence calcific tendinitis bespeaks chronicity	Tenderness may extend anteriorly	Radiographs are of benefit as there may be concurrent lesions
	May be as the result of a tear or as the result of an osteophyte on the acromion	Painful *abduction,* limited at a level <90 degrees, both active and passive	NSAIDs (Table 7-8, page 393)
			Proscription of overhead activity
	Supraspinatus: Abduction first 30 degrees		Rest
	Infraspinatus/teres minor: external rotation	Decreased/painful external rotation	PT consult for Codman exercises (see above, page 371)
	Subscapularis: internal rotation	Decreased/painful internal rotation	Referral to orthopedic surgeon
			Injection of the shoulder with 15 mg triamcinolone may be indicated

| Rotator cuff tears | This is a tear in one or more of the tendons/muscles of the rotator cuff
The quantity of force required is dependent on the health of the patient: young, healthy, significant force; older, debilitated, minimal force
Supraspinatus: abduction first 30 degrees
Infraspinatus/teres minor: external rotation
Subscapularis: internal rotation | Acute pain and tenderness in lateral shoulder
Severe pain in younger; minimal pain in older individuals
Active abduction is decreased but passive abduction normal
Decreased abduction in first 30 degrees
Decreased/painful external rotation
Decreased/painful internal rotation | Clinical diagnosis
Radiographs are of benefit as there may be concurrent lesions
NSAIDs (Table 7-8, page 393)
Proscription of overhead activity
PT consult for Codman exercises (see above; page 371)
MRI and referral to orthopedics, especially in young individuals |

TABLE 7-4
Hip: Specific Clinical Syndromes

Femoral neck fracture	Traumatic fracture	Pain and tenderness in the hip Ecchymosis and Grey Turners of the ipsilateral hip/flank No range of motion of hip Lower extremity is shortened and externally rotated Quite common	Radiographs confirm the fracture Must monitor the CBC as bleeding is not uncommon Traction of the lower extremity Analgesia with Toradol or narcotics (Table 7-8, page 393) Emergent referral to orthopedics for open reduction and internal fixation (ORIF)
Ischiogluteal bursitis	Inflammation of the bursa, usually as the result of trauma Bursa is between the gluteal muscles and the ischium May cause sciatica	Acute onset of pain in the buttock Exacerbated by sitting/Valsalva Pain worse at night One etiology of sciatica FABERE demonstrates pain in buttock	Clinical diagnosis Heating pads/pillow locally NSAIDs (Table 7-8, page 393) Short- and long-term PT
Greater trochanteric bursitis	Inflammation of the bursa, usually as the result of trauma Bursa is on the lateral hip at the greater trochanter	Tenderness over the posterior aspect of the greater trochanter FABERE with tenderness at that location	Clinical diagnosis Radiographs are normal NSAIDs (Table 7-8, page 393) Inject with triamcinolone, 10–20 mg, if refractory to therapy
Osteoarthritis	Recurrent trauma, to the joint Trauma Obesity Hip dislocations	Pain in the inguinal area Decreased ROM and crepitus Patient keeps leg in adduction flexion and external rotation Trendelenburg's sign positive on the affected side (atrophy) FABERE with tenderness	Clinical diagnosis Radiographs demonstrate osteophytes and a decrease in joint space Use a cane NSAIDs (Table 7-8, page 393) PT Referral to orthopedics

T A B L E 7-5
Back: Specific Clinical Syndromes

Musculoskeletal/ligamentous sprain	Actual stretching and tearing of the muscles and ligaments in the back	Acute onset of low back pain Unilateral > bilateral Rarely with sciatica Tearing sensation at time of trauma Lifting a heavy object, then stiffness and pain in back Examination with spasm and pain No radicular findings/no neurologic deficits	Rest NSAIDs (Table 7-8, page 393) Warmth PT for ROM and Williams exercises Lift objects by using the muscles of the thighs and legs
Herniated disk	Acquired herniation of an intervertebral disk; results in impingement or entrapment of nerve roots Most common sites of herniation: L3/L4:L4 root L4/L5:L5 root L5/S1:S1 root *Sciatic nerve* is L5 and S1 *Femoral nerve* is L4	Acute onset of low back pain with radiation into the foot Pain is especially present in the posteriolateral thigh *Examination:* Weakness of dorsiflexion: L5 Weakness of plantarflexion: S1 Decreased ankle reflex: S1 Weakness of knee extension: L4 Decreased quadriceps reflex: L4	Clinical diagnosis Radiographs of lumbar spine MRI of back to look for site of herniation if no improvement after 6 weeks of conservative therapy Surgery may be necessary if motor defects develop but not for sensory defects alone Patient should sleep on side with knees flexed, pillow between knees PT consult

(continued)

T A B L E 7-5 *(continued)*

| Vertebral compression fracture | Loss of height of an individual vertebral body (i.e., compression of the body)
Trauma-related, or
Osteoporosis, or
Osteomyelitis, or
A *neoplastic* process (i.e., multiple myeloma or metastatic adenocarcinoma)
Thoracic: osteoporosis
Lumbar: neoplasia, osteomyelitis
May have concurrent epidural disease | If acute fracture, there is an acute onset of bilateral pain at the site of the fracture, pain may be quite severe with discrete tenderness to percussion
Loss of height of patient with an accentuated thoracic kyphosis are common: "dowager's hump" in osteoporosis
Fever and pain worse at night is consistent with osteomyelitis
There may be *cauda equina* manifestations with decreased anal sphincter tone and motor weakness in neoplastic or osteomyelitis | Clinical diagnosis
Localize lesion
Look for and define any neurologic defects
Radiographs of affected area
MRI of affected area
Blood cultures
ESR
If *osteomyelitis,* biopsy and antibiotics (vancomycin and AMG i.v.)
If *neoplasia,* biopsy and oncology referral/radiation therapy consult
If *trauma,* orthopedics referral
Prevention of osteoporosis, see chapter 11 (page 535) for specifics
Bone scan/gallium scan (Bone scan "hot" in both infectious and neoplastic disease; gallium "hot" only in infectious disease) |

Facet disease	Degenerative disease of the facet joints; results in an acquired anterior subluxation of a vertebral body on an adjacent body (i.e., spondylolisthesis)	Chronic and/or recurrent low back pain, may have manifestations of sciatica or even of cauda equina if the subluxation is significant	Clinical diagnosis Lumbar radiograph MRI Conservative treatment If severe, consider injection of triamcinolone to the facet joint guided by CT imaging Referral to orthopedics
Ankylosing spondylitis	Seronegative polyarticular arthritis Affects the central (axial) skeleton more than peripheral (appendicular) skeleton	Bilateral pain on ambulation (i.e., "neuroclaudication") Significant morning stiffness Straightening of the back: *Schober's sign* present Tender over the SI joints Decreased chest expansion with breathing *FABERE* with SI pain	Clinical diagnosis NSAIDs (Table 7-8, page 393) Radiographs of pelvis and lumbar spine (sacroiliitis) Referral to rheumatology See section, polyarticular arthritis (page 397)

T A B L E 7-6
Knee: Specific Clinical Syndromes

Suprapatellar bursitis/ plicatis	Trauma-related effusion in the suprapatellar plica "Houseperson's knee"	Large effusion in the plica Quite non- to minimally tender Effusion is doughy The effusion is in the area above the patella and deep to the distal quadriceps	Clinical diagnosis Radiographs of little benefit Needle aspiration of the bursa is of benefit
Infrapatellar bursitis	Inflammation of the bursa deep to the patellar ligament Mild, recurrent trauma to the infrapatellar area; recurrent kneeling: "clergyman's knee"	Tender area deep to the patellar ligament with mild fullness	Clinical diagnosis Radiographs are of little benefit NSAIDs (Table 7-8, page 393) Limit the kneeling by patient
Pes anserine bursitis	Inflammation of the pes anserine bursa; this bursa is adjacent to the insertions of the sartorius, gracilis, and semimembranous muscles (goose foot) Usually trauma-related, usually in runners	Tender area 4 cm inferior to the medial condyles at the pes anserine	Clinical diagnosis Radiographs of little use Change running pattern NSAIDs (Table 7-8, page 393)

Anterior cruciate tear	Partial or complete tear of the anterior cruciate ligament (ACL) ACL attaches to the tibia anteriorly Results from trauma pushing the tibia anteriorly and valgusly Often as a part of *unhappy triad:* a. Medial meniscus b. Medial collateral ligament c. ACL	Pain and swelling with effusion in the knee Laxity of knee *Anterior drawer positive* *Lachman's test positive*	Clinical diagnosis If large effusion, arthrocentesis, usually a hemarthrosis Radiographs are important as fractures may be present Analgesia Knee immobilization Crutches Referral to orthopedics MRI of knee
Posterior cruciate tear	Partial or complete tear of the posterior cruciate ligament (PCL) PCL attaches to the tibia posteriorly Results from trauma pushing the tibia posteriorly	Pain and laxity of the knee Effusion not uncommon Positive *posterior drawer*	Clinical diagnosis Radiographs are important as fractures may be present Analgesia Knee immobilization Crutches Referral to orthopedics MRI of the knee

(continued)

TABLE 7-6 *(continued)*

Medial meniscal tear	Partial or complete tear of the meniscus (i.e., the cartilage in the knee joint) Knee locking and clicking Trauma via skiing	Pain and swelling over the joint line Mild swelling *Medial McMurray test*	Clinical diagnosis Radiographs are important Analgesia Knee immobilization MRI of knee NSAIDs (Table 7-8, page 393) PT/OT
Lateral meniscal tear	Partial or complete tear of the meniscus (i.e., the cartilage in the knee joint) Knee locking and clicking	Pain and swelling over the joint line Mild swelling *Lateral McMurray test*	Clinical diagnosis Radiographs are important Analgesia Knee immobilization MRI of knee NSAIDs (Table 7-8, page 393) PT/OT
Medial collateral ligament tear	Partial or complete tear of the ligament Significant valgus trauma	Pain and swelling over the condyles Mild swelling *Valgus stress test* positive	Clinical diagnosis NSAIDs (Table 7-8, page 393) Knee immobilization PT/OT If mild, conservative treatment, but if present for >6 weeks, MRI and orthopedics consult

| Lateral collateral ligament tear | Partial or complete tear of the ligament Significant varus trauma | Pain and swelling over the lateral condyles Mild swelling *Varus stress* test positive | Clinical diagnosis NSAIDs (Table 7-8, page 393) Knee immobilization PT/OT If mild, conservative treatment, but if present for >6 weeks, MRI and orthopedics consult |
| Patellofemoral syndrome | Dysfunctional tracking of the patella relative to the knee *Risks:* • Increased Q angle • Women • Posterior cruciate tear • Weak quadriceps muscle, especially after trauma and immobilization | Anterior pain Significant crepitus of the knee Swelling *Increased Q angle* Weakness of the vastus obliquus medialis (VOM) Apprehension test present If severe, lateral subluxation of the patella | Clinical diagnosis NSAIDs (Table 7-8, page 393) Prevention and treatment with isometric exercises to strengthen the quadriceps muscle, especially the VOM |

TABLE 7-7
Foot/Ankle: Specific Clinical Syndromes

Lateral sprain	Injury of forced inversion and supination (e.g., twisting the ankle to the side)
	Three ligaments may be damaged:
	  a. Calcaneofibular
	  b. Anterior talofibular
	  c. Posterior talofibular
	May have a *syndesmotic injury* (i.e., a dislocation of the fibula/tibia), with an increase in risk of compartment syndrome
		Lateral pain, swelling, tenderness at and inferior to the lateral malleolus
		Anterior drawer sign: the calcaneus may be drawn anteriorly on the tibia
		Concurrent tenderness over fibular head may indicate a proximal fibular fracture
		A *positive squeeze test:* squeeze the fibula/tibia together may result in pain and is consistent with a syndesmotic tear, i.e., one involving the interosseous membrane
			Radiographs are indicated to look for fibula/tibia dislocation, and/or avulsion fractures
			12 hours of ice/cool
			Wrap with adhesive tape (ACE wrap)
			NSAIDs, including Toradol (Table 7-8, page 393)
			Application of a posterior splint to the joint
			Crutches for 10–14 days
			Refer to OT/PT
			If there is a fracture, a syndesmotic injury or dislocation of the tibia/fibula: refer to orthopedics

Medial sprain	Injury of forced eversion and pronation Ligament damaged is the deltoid Much less common than lateral sprain	Medial pain, swelling and tender at and below the medial malleolus Syndesmotic injury more common, therefore, squeeze test very important	As for lateral sprain, see above

Jones' fracture	Acute trauma to the foot with forced inversion Simple fracture of base of the 5th metatarsal	Acute onset of lateral foot pain, swelling, tenderness Decreased ROM of tibiotalar joint and ecchymosis Often there are concurrent manifestations of a lateral sprain	Radiographs are indicated Wrap with adhesive tape (ACE wrap) NSAIDs, including Toradol (Table 7-8, page 393) Application of a posterior splint to the joint Crutches for 21–28 days Refer to orthopedics
Tarsal tunnel syndrome	Damage to or inflammation of the tarsal tunnel, a structure inferoposterior to the medial malleolus This results in an entrapment of the posterior tibialis nerve The posterior tibialis nerve is a branch of S1, sensory to plantar foot; motor to intrinsic muscles of the foot	Paresthesiae and numbness to the plantar foot Weakness of toe flexion, adduction, and abduction Tinel's is positive when applied to the inferior aspect of medial malleolus	History and physical examination EMG and nerve conduction confirms Rest with splinting NSAIDs (Table 7-8, page 393) Referral to surgery for release if severe and/or recurrent Must be diagnosed early to prevent neuropathic sequelae
Foot-drop syndrome	Dysfunction of the common peroneal nerve, usually in the proximal fibular region	Steppage or foot-drop gait Weakness to ankle dorsiflexion Atrophy of the anterior leg and dorsal foot muscles	History and physical examination EMG and nerve conduction confirms NSAIDs (Table 7-8, page 393)

(continued)

TABLE 7-7 (continued)

Foot-drop syndrome *(cont.)*	Common peroneal nerve provides sensory to the dorsum of foot; motor to toe and foot dorsiflexors Etiologies: Trauma Diabetes mellitus Infiltrative processes	Decreased sensation to the dorsum of the foot	Must be diagnosed early to prevent neuropathic sequelae PT to provide exercises for anterior compartment Podiatry for special shoes
Hammertoes	Ill-fitting shoes	Acquired deformity in which there is an MTP contracture in hyperextension, PIP contracture of flexion, and a normal DIP Invariably a corn on the affected toe	Clinical diagnosis No radiographs are needed Prevention Referral to a podiatrist for shoes and potential surgery
Bunion	Inflammation of the bursa over and medial to the great toe Concurrent with a hallux valgus Result of ill-fitting shoes	Tenderness over the MTP joint especially of the great toe, especially the dorsomedial aspect The great toe is laterally displaced Corn or callus is often present at base of hallux valgus	Radiographs demonstrate an increased angle between first and second metatarsals (angle is <10 degrees normally) NSAIDs (Table 7-8, page 393) Referral to a podiatrist Special shoes and/or podiatric surgery may be necessary

Plantar fasciitis	Inflammation of the plantar fascia as the result of small tears in the fascia related to overuse	Plantar/medial pain in the affected foot/feet Often in active runners First-step phenomenon, the first step after a prolonged rest (e.g., on awakening or after sitting for a time) is most painful then decreases with subsequent steps Usually bilateral Most specific tenderness at the plantar calcaneus	Clinical diagnosis Radiographs demonstrate an osteophyte on plantar calcaneus, 50% Proscribe running for 5–7 days NSAIDs (Table 7-8, page 393) Refer to podiatry if severe
Achilles tendinitis	Inflammation of the Achilles tendon, i.e., the gastrocnemius tendon Repetitive microtrauma via jumping on hard soles Common in runners	Tenderness in and about the Achilles tendon Manifestations are increased with exercise relieved with rest Tenderness throughout the tendon May have concurrent retrocalcaneal bursitis, i.e., swelling and tenderness 3–4 cm superior to the calcaneus	Clinical diagnosis Limitation of running (i.e., rest) Application of a 3/8" posterior heel pad prevents recurrence Prevention via gastrocnemius-stretching exercises NSAIDs (Table 7-8, page 393)

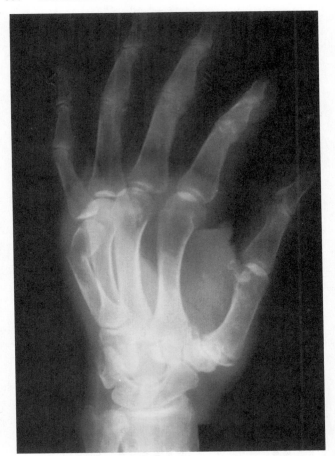

FIGURE   7-1
Boxer's fracture, i.e., a simple, slightly displaced fracture of the
diaphysis of the fifth metacarpal.

(text continued from page 363)

synovial fluid. The crystal chemical type is sodium
monourate. These crystals have the physical property of negative birefringence, as demonstrated on
polarizing microscopy. The crystals are very rare in
prosthetic joints. Their polarizing properties are that
the crystals oriented parallel to the light are yellow,

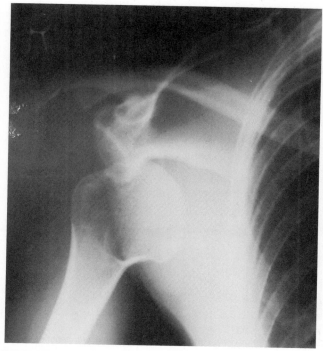

F I G U R E 7-2
Radiograph of shoulder, AP. Anterior dislocation of the humerus from the glenohumeral joint. Note the position of the humeral head inferior and even slightly medial to the coracoid process.

whereas those oriented perpendicular to the light are blue. Their polarizing properties are as follows:
  a. Crystals parallel to the light: yellow crystals.
  b. Crystals perpendicular to the light: blue crystals.
4. The **specific management** of gout includes making the clinical diagnosis and initiating intervention immediately (see Box 7-3 (page 392)) and then preventing recurrence of the disease process. Long-term therapy for gout is based on several modalities to prevent future attacks; once a patient has an episode of acute gout, he or she will desire never to experience another. Preventive modalities include the abortion of an acute attack with colchicine or a nonsteroidal antiinflammatory drug (NSAID), an overall adjustment in risk-factor profile, and initiation of allopurinol.

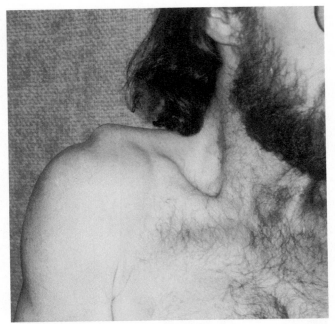

F I G U R E 7-3
Shoulder, anterior view: Third degree acromioclavicular separation.

a. **Abortion of acute attacks.** This preventive method is effective, easy, and obviates long-term, potentially life-long, daily medication. The abortion of an acute attack can be done with an NSAID, but the best agent to use is colchicine. The patient is instructed to take a dose of colchicine by mouth as soon as the attack starts and to use the regimen described in Box 7-3 (page 392).
b. Decrease weight if obese and decrease ethanol use, both of which will decrease the risk of gout attacks.
c. **Allopurinol**
   i. **Mechanism of action:** Agent is a xanthine oxidase inhibitor (i.e., it decreases the production of uric acid in the catabolism of purines).
   ii. **Dose:** 300 mg p.o., q.d. In patients with renal insufficiency, the dosage must be adjusted downward to 100 mg p.o., q.d.
   iii. **Indications:** Limited, because aborting attacks is the prophylactic **treatment** of choice. In a minority of cases, however, allopurinol must

B O X 7-2

Overall Evaluation of Monoarticular Arthritis

Evaluation

1. Take a history and perform a physical examination. The classic findings of inflammation involving the affected joint are quite easily demonstrated. These findings include *tumor* (swelling), *dolor* (pain), *rubor* (redness), *calor* (warmth), and decreased ROM of the involved joint. The patient may have a history of antecedent trauma or of similar manifestations in the same or different joint in the past. An effusion may be present in the affected joint.
2. Obtain radiographs in two views of the affected joint to look for fractures, chondrocalcinosis, and soft-tissue swelling (see Fig. 7-4).
3. Arthrocentesis of the affected joint is mandatory. The following laboratory tests should be performed on the fluid in all cases (Fig. 7-5):
   a. Gross assessment: bloody versus clear versus purulent.
   b. Crystal analysis by using a polarizing microscope (see page 386).
   c. Gram stain of fluid, looking for polymorphonuclear (PMN) cells and bacteria.
   d. Culture and sensitivity testing of fluid.
4. Immobilize the joint acutely if there is any evidence of trauma.
5. Categorize the process as crystal-induced, traumatic, or infectious.

be initiated and continued. These include patients with recurrent gouty attacks, patients with hypoxanthine guanine phosphoribosyl transferase (HGPRT) deficiency, patients who have concurrent uric acid nephrolithiasis, patients with tophaceous gout, and patients who have or are being treated for lymphoproliferative disorders.

    iv. **Side-effect profile:** Limited. Side effects include the rare cases of hepatic dysfunction, usually mild in nature.

    v. **Goals of use:** Not only the prevention of gouty attacks and uric acid nephrolithiasis, but also the maintenance of the serum uric acid level in the 6- to 8-mg/dL range.

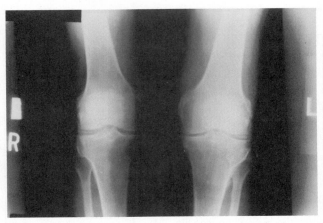

FIGURE 7-4
Radiograph of the knees, AP. The presence of calcium within the lateral compartments of the knees is consistent with the chondrocalcinosis of pseudogout.

   vi. **Caveat:** During the first 2–3 weeks of therapy, the serum and body uric acid levels may paradoxically increase, with resultant increased risk of gouty attacks; thus colchicine or an NSAID must be administered for the first 2 weeks of therapy with allopurinol.
 d. **NSAIDs** (see Table 7-8)
   i. The **mechanism of action, dosages,** and **side effects** are described in Table 7-8 (page 393).
   ii. The **duration** of therapy is 4–6 weeks and/or 2 weeks after the initiation of long-term therapy [i.e., allopurinol (if long-term therapy is indicated)].
   iii. A **caveat to therapy** with one of these agents is that these agents are nonspecific in their antiinflammatory effects. Therefore one must have evidence, based on arthrocentesis, to rule out any infectious origin before initiating this treatment, which could easily mask but not treat an infection.
 e. **Intraarticular steroids**
   This **modality** is clearly effective. It should be reserved for patients with arthrocentesis-proven monoarticular gout who cannot take anything by mouth or who have relative or absolute contraindications to colchicine and an NSAID. Dose depends on the size of the joint. In small joints (e.g., the metatarsophalangeal joint): 5–10 mg triamcinolone; in large joints

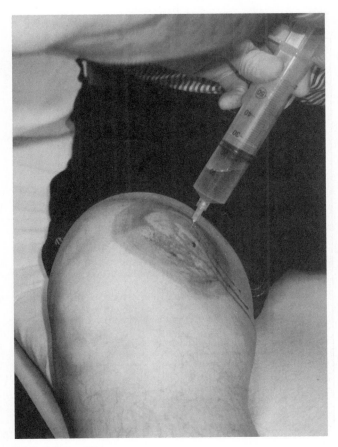

F I G U R E   7-5
Arthrocentesis procedure of knee. Using sterile technique, the needle is
inserted into the joint space immediately deep to the patella. This is a
knee with massive effusion as the result of a Charcot joint.

        (e.g., the knee): 35–50 mg triamcinolone should be
        intraarticularly administered.
  B. Pseudogout
      1. The **underlying pathogenesis** is the acute precipita-
         tion of calcium pyrophosphate crystals in the synovial
         space. The crystals induce inflammation by several
         mechanisms, including the release of prostaglandins

B O X 7-3

Management of Acute Gout

Management

1. **Colchicine**
   a. The **mechanism of action** of this highly effective **modality** in the **treatment** of acute gout is that it inhibits the release of CCF from PMNs, thus specifically inhibiting inflammation in gout. This agent is only mildly effective in the treatment of pseudogout.
   b. **Dosage**
      i. **Oral:** The vast majority of patients can receive colchicine in the oral form. The dosage is 0.6 mg p.o., now, repeated hourly until one of three things occurs: relief of symptoms, a total of six doses has been given, or diarrhea occurs. If relief occurs, continue dose of 0.6 mg p.o., b.i.d. If there is no response, rethink the diagnosis and attempt an NSAID (see Table 7-8, page 393).
   c. **Side effects** include diarrhea, which can be severe and dose limiting.
   d. The **duration** of therapy is 4–6 weeks and/or 2 weeks after the initiation of long-term therapy [i.e., allopurinol (if chronic therapy is indicated)].
   e. A **caveat to therapy** is that colchicine is specific for gout; therefore, if relief occurs, it is tantamount to a diagnosis of gout.
   f. A further caveat is the observation that the longer it takes to start the **treatment** after onset of symptoms, the longer it takes to effect relief.

and leukotrienes from PMNs. The underlying reason for the precipitation of such crystals is not completely known, but certain disease processes have been associated with it. These include primary hyperparathyroidism, secondary hyperparathyroidism, and chronic mild hypercalcemia of any cause.

2. The **specific manifestations** are similar to those listed in Box 7-2 (page 389). The patient rarely has significant systemic manifestations and rarely, if ever, has a fever.
3. The **specific evaluation** of this entity includes making the diagnosis by performing crystal analysis on the

TABLE 7-8
Nonsteroidal Anti-Inflammatory Agents

Agent	Mechanism of Action	Dose	Side Effects
Acetylsalicylic acid (aspirin)	Cyclooxygenase inhibition Decreases prostaglandin levels systemically	600 mg p.o., t.i.d. (therapeutic range 150–300 μg/ml) in serum	Tinnitus Metabolic acidosis
Ibuprofen (Motrin)	Same	400–800 mg p.o., t.i.d.	Gastropathy Nephropathy
Piroxicam (Feldene)	Same	20 mg p.o., q.d.	Gastropathy Nephropathy
Naproxen (Naprosyn)	Same	500 mg p.o., q.12 hr	Gastropathy Nephropathy
Magnesium choline salicylate (Disalcid)	Same	Two 750-mg tablets b.i.d.	Gastropathy Decreased risk of gastropathy relative to other agents
Toradol (Ketorolac)	Same	30–60 mg i.m., repeat q. 30–60 minutes times 2	Gastropathy Nephropathy

synovial fluid. The crystal chemical type is calcium pyrophosphate. These crystals have the physical property of positive birefringence on polarizing microscopy. Their polarizing properties are that the crystals oriented parallel to the light are blue, whereas the crystals oriented perpendicular to the light are yellow. Furthermore, the evaluation should include determining the serum calcium, phosphorus, and albumin levels. If the calcium level is increased, especially with a mild to modestly decreased serum phosphorus, an intact PTH (parathormone) level should be determined to rule out hyperparathyroidism (see page 485).

4. The **specific management of pseudogout** includes making the clinical diagnosis and initiating intervention immediately (see Box 7-2) and then preventing recurrence of the disease process. In the acute disease, the drug of choice is an NSAID (see Table 7-8, page 393), as the efficacy of colchicine in pseudogout is significantly less than in gout. The **long-term therapy** of pseudogout is based on several modalities that are helpful in preventing future attacks; once a patient has had an episode of acute pseudogout, he or she will desire never to experience another. Preventive modalities include aborting an acute attack with an NSAID and effective diagnosis and treatment of any of the associated or secondary causes (see Chapter 9).

II. **Inflammatory, nonseptic arthritis**
Polyarticular inflammatory arthritides of a chronic or acute nature (e.g., rheumatoid arthritis) can and do present with one joint affected before progressing (see section on Polyarticular Arthritis, page 397).

III. **Septic arthritis**
A. The **underlying pathogenesis** is bacterial infection of the synovial lining of the affected joint. The route of infection can entail hematogenous spread, contiguous spread from an adjacent cellulitis, bursitis, or osteomyelitis, or traumatic or iatrogenic invasion of the joint space by a compound fracture involving the joint, or by arthrocentesis. The most common organisms that cause septic arthritis are *Neisseria gonorrhoeae, Haemophilus influenzae, Streptococcus* spp., and *Staphylococcus* spp.

1. *Neisseria gonorrhoeae*
This gram-negative diplococcus is the most common organism to cause infectious arthritis in adults. The **natural history** is one in which there is, via sexual contact and transmission, an antecedent untreated gonococcal urethritis, proctitis, cervicitis, or pharyngitis with a concomitant bacteremia. The organism

spreads hematogenously to the joint space, where inflammation/infection occurs.

   2. *Haemophilus influenzae*
      This gram-negative coccobacillus is uncommon in adults but one of the most common causes of infectious arthritis in children. The **natural history** is one of contiguous spread of *H. influenzae* to the joint from an adjacent area of epiphyseal osteomyelitis or by hematogenous spread from another source. This is becoming more and more uncommon now that effective prophylaxis with the *Haemophilus influenza* vaccine is being used.

   3. *Streptococcus and Staphylococcus*
      These gram-positive cocci in chains and clusters, respectively, are not uncommon causes of septic arthritis. The **natural history** is development by contiguous spread, either from an adjacent cellulitis or infectious bursitis or by introduction of organisms via arthrocentesis (rare) or, more commonly, by trauma (e.g., a compound fracture).

   4. Other quite uncommon pathogens include mycobacterial arthritis and blastomycosis-related arthritis.

B. The **specific manifestations** of this entity, which is also known as infectious arthritis, include, in addition to those described in Box 7-2, the systemic features of fevers, chills, night sweats, and, quite often, an antecedent history of dysuria and pyuria. This origin can result in severe sequelae, including loss of joint function and even death. Therefore, the diagnosis must be effectively ruled out in all patients with monoarticular arthritis. The sternoclavicular joint is more commonly involved in i.v. drug abusers.

C. The **specific evaluation** includes the steps described in Box 7-2 and making the diagnosis by Gram stain and culture of the synovial fluid. In virtually all cases, the diagnosis can be made from the Gram stain. If the organism is thought or diagnosed to be *N. gonorrhoeae,* examination and gonococcal cultures by using Thayer–Martin plate media of the urethra, cervix, pharynx, and rectum are indicated.

D. The **specific management** of infectious arthritis includes making the diagnosis by using the evaluative tools listed previously and intensive therapy, including the following measures:

   1. **Complete drainage** of the fluid from the joint. If the fluid reaccumulates, as it often will, repeated needle drainage is necessary. Placement of a surgical drain may be needed to completely and effectively drain the joint.

2. **Immobilize** the affected joint with appropriate splintage.
3. **Consultation** with orthopedics and infectious diseases experts is mandatory.
4. Initiation of **parenteral antibiotics,** including
   a. If *Neisseria gonorrhoeae* is suspected or diagnosed: ceftriaxone, 1–2 g i.v., q.12hr, for 10 days (see section on Sexually Transmitted Diseases in Chapter 6, page 340, for other mandatory concurrent antibiotic treatment).
   b. **If gram-positive cocci:**
      Vancomycin, 1 g i.v., q.12hr, should be initiated and used until culture and sensitivity of the pathogen demonstrate that it is sensitive to methicillin, at which time the regimen may be changed to nafcillin, 2 g i.v., q.8hr, or cefazolin, 2 g i.v., q.8hr, and an aminoglycoside for 10 days.
      In patients who are penicillin allergic, vancomycin should be continued.
   c. If *H. influenzae:* ampicillin, 2 g i.v., q.8hr, or cefuroxime, 1.5 g i.v., q.8hr, for 10 days.

IV. **Hemarthrosis**
   A. The **underlying pathogenesis** is, in the vast majority of cases, traumatic damage to the intrinsic structures of the joint. The classic example is hemarthrosis associated with an acute tear of the anterior cruciate ligament of the knee. Spontaneous (non–trauma-related) hemarthrosis can occur as a result of hemophilia A or hemophilia B, in which bleeding into the joint can occur at any time and without any antecedent trauma.
   B. The **specific manifestations** of this entity include, in addition to those described in Box 7-2, an antecedent history of recent trauma to the joint. There are rarely any systemic manifestations, and the patient is invariably afebrile.
   C. The **evaluation** includes that described in Box 7-2. It is necessary to obtain radiographs of bones around the joint. Usually there is little doubt as to the diagnosis, as the synovial fluid is grossly bloody; however, the fluid should be sent for all of the routine studies listed in Box 7-2, especially joint-fluid culture to rule out concurrent or early infectious arthritis. Further assessment includes a detailed orthopedics examination of the affected joint and determining the platelet count, prothrombin time (PT), and activated partial thromboplastin time (aPTT) to rule out concurrent coagulopathy.
   D. The **specific management** of a hemarthrosis includes making the diagnosis and initiating intensive therapy, including the following steps:

1. Complete drainage of the joint of all fluid. Repeat arthrocentesis as necessary to keep the joint free of excess fluid.
2. **Immobilize** the affected joint with appropriate splintage.
3. **Consult orthopedics** on an urgent/emergent basis.
4. Initiate effective analgesia, including narcotics as necessary.
5. If the underlying cause is hemophilia, see section on Excessive Bleeding States in Chapter 5 (page 268) for further evaluation and management.

V. **Consultation**

Problem	*Service*	*Time*
Infectious arthritis	Orthopedics	Urgent
Crystal-induced arthritis	Rheumatology	Elective
Fracture	Orthopedics	Required
All	Physical therapy	Elective

VI. **Indications for admission:** Septic arthritis, uncontrolled coagulopathy, or concurrent fracture of the bone involved in the articulation.

Polyarticular Arthritis, Acute or Chronic

The synovium, the simple squamous epithelial lining of the joint, may become inflamed as a result of a systemic inflammatory process or damaged by chronic trauma. As with monoarticular arthritis, the difference between acute and chronic polyarticular arthritis is based on the duration of symptoms—< or >2 weeks—at the time of presentation.

I. **Overall manifestations**
   The **overall manifestations** of polyarticular arthritis include those resulting from joint inflammation and those resulting from systemic inflammatory or from noninflammatory disease itself.
   A. **Joint manifestations**
      The **manifestations** of joint inflammation include the classic findings of *tumor* (swelling), *dolor* (pain), *rubor* (redness), *calor* (warmth), and loss of function. The pattern of joint involvement can be stratified by using certain qualifying features. These features, which can be used to aid in the diagnosis of the underlying systemic disease, include:
      1. **The number of joints involved.** Involvement of two to four joints is pauciarticular arthritis, whereas involvement of more than four joints is termed polyarticular arthritis.
      2. The degree of symmetry of joint involvement. Various

disease processes have varying degrees of symmetry (i.e., the concurrent involvement of the same joints on contralateral sides).
3. The size of the joints involved. Some disease processes predominantly involve small joints (e.g., hands) or large joints (e.g., axial skeleton).

B. **Systemic manifestations**

The **systemic manifestations** can include those specific to the underlying disease itself, which are discussed subsequently, and the presence of the constitutional findings of fevers, easy fatigability, malaise, and stiffness of the joints, especially morning stiffness. As a rule of thumb, inflammatory arthritides (e.g., rheumatoid arthritis, Lyme disease) often have the systemic findings of malaise, fevers, and significant morning stiffness, whereas noninflammatory processes (e.g., osteoarthritis) manifest with pain but without any systemic findings.

C. **Emergencies** in inflammatory polyarticular arthritis
   1. **Atlantoaxial subluxation** (i.e., C1/C2)
   2. **Stridor** as the result of synovitis at the cricoarytenoid joint [i.e., true vocal cord (fixed in adduction)]
   3. Septic arthritis
   4. **Scleritis** (i.e., pericorneal inflammation/injection with eye tenderness and anterior chamber uveitis) may result in scleromalacia perforans and rupture of the globe
   5. **Tendon rupture,** most commonly on extensor aspect of hand or volar plate of fingers
   6. Acute **entrapment neuropathies** (e.g., carpal tunnel syndrome, loge de Guyon syndrome)
   7. Rupture of a Baker's cyst: knee or shoulder

II. **Rheumatoid arthritis**

A. The **underlying pathogenesis** is an immunologically mediated systemic disease that produces chronic inflammatory and destructive arthritis. The immune-mediated process can be demonstrated with a reactive rheumatoid factor (RF) test. Furthermore, several human leukocyte antigen (HLA) types have been associated with severe rheumatoid arthritis: HLA-DR1 and HLA-DR4. Some **variant syndromes** will have different immune-mediated mechanisms and will be RF negative [see Table 7-9 (page 402): Rheumatoid variant syndromes]. There are four overall types of **seropositive (RF-positive) rheumatoid arthritis** in terms of **natural history:**
   1. *Self-limited with and acute onset*: Rare, resolves in 6–12 months
   2. *Palindromic rheumatism* with acute exacerbations and long remissions: May resolve or may proceed to evolve into symmetric, chronic polyarthritis

3. *Chronic symmetric polyarthritis* with fatigue and with recurrent flares: This is the most common type of rheumatoid arthritis. The manifestations and sequelae range from mild to severe; 20% will develop joint nodules

4. *Malignant rheumatoid arthritis:* Severe erosive, destructive rheumatoid arthritis with a leukocytoclastic vasculitis; Sjögren's and Felty's syndrome along with mononeuritis multiplex and visceral ischemia are all common in this form.

B. The **specific manifestations** of this disorder can be divided into those occurring early in the course of the disease and those occurring later.

1. **Early manifestations** include an insidious onset of fatigue, morning stiffness, and arthralgias with an associated symmetric arthritis, initially involving the small joints. The first joints involved are in the digits of the hands and feet (i.e., the PIP and DIP joints). Furthermore, there can often be the acute development of nontender rheumatoid nodules over the extensor surfaces in 20%–40% of patients.

2. The **late manifestations** are sequelae of the inflammatory processes and include, but are far from limited to, ulnar deviation of the digits, joint contractures, and the development of "swan neck" deformities in the digits of the hands and feet (the PIP joint is hyperextended, the DIP has a flexion contracture) or boutonnière deformities (the PIP has a flexion contracture, and the DIP is hyperextended).

3. **Systemic manifestations** include the development of *entrapment neuropathies,* e.g., carpal tunnel syndrome; ulnar tunnel syndrome; tarsal tunnel syndrome; *fevers; Sjögren's,* which manifests with dry eyes, dry mouth, and enlargement of the salivary and lacrimal glands and an increased risk of lymphoproliferative disorders; *pulmonary manifestations,* which range from multiple nodules to bronchiolitis obliterans; *episcleritis,* i.e., a red dot in the cornea, minimal risk of side effects; *scleritis* with manifestations of red eye, pericorneal injection, anterior uveitis and treated with topical glucocorticoids; *atlantoaxial subluxation/dislocation* with manifestations of bilateral upper-extremity paresthesiae; *inflammation of the true vocal cord* (cricoarytenoid articulation) so that it is in adduction with resultant stridor; and finally, *rheumatoid arthritis–related vasculitis.* The *vasculitis* is a rare, life-threatening acute complication, long-standing RF-positive nodular type rheumatoid arthritis, which will result in *mononeuritis multi-*

plex, i.e., a peripheral neuropathy, infarction of the mesentery, and leukocytoclastic vasculitis. This is treated with systemic glucocorticoids (60–80 mg prednisone) and cyclophosphamide, 2–4 mg/kg/day, p.o.

  C. The **evaluation** of this disorder includes making the clinical diagnosis with the tools described in Box 7-4.

  D. The **specific management** includes rest, both overall and of the affected joints. One modality is to splint those joints that have active disease. In all cases, the patient should be referred to physical therapy for initiation of ROM exercises. NSAIDs (see Table 7-8, page 393) should be initiated. In all cases, especially when there is evidence of active, erosive disease, refer the patient to a rheumatologist for the initiation of **treatment** with disease-modifying antirheumatoid agents. These include those listed in Table 7-11 (page 404).

III. Osteoarthritis

  A. The **underlying pathogenesis** of this disorder is an idiopathic degenerative noninflammatory arthritis that is nonsystemic. Predisposing factors include trauma to the joints, Legg–Calvé–Perthes disease of the hips, and obesity.

  B. The **specific manifestations** of this very common disorder, which has a prevalence of 20%–30% in the geriatric population, include chronic and/or recurrent dull pain in any or all joints. The most commonly involved joints

---

B O X 7-4

Overall Evaluation of Polyarticular Arthritis

Evaluation

1. Take a thorough history and perform a physical examination, with particular emphasis on the history of any recent skin rashes, sore throat, exposure to ticks, exposure to hepatitis B, or past manifestations of inflammatory bowel disease. On physical examination, look for the presence of any rashes or erythema, nodules in the skin, conjunctivitis, pharyngitis, nodules over tendons, or tender hepatomegaly. Furthermore, a thorough examination of all joints is mandatory, looking for decreased ROM, inflammatory findings, and contractures.

(continued)

B O X 7-4 (continued)

2. Based on these findings, stratify the arthritis into inflammatory and noninflammatory types. The inflammatory arthritides produce systemic manifestations and all of the signs of inflammation, whereas the noninflammatory arthritides cause only pain and loss of function. The schemas for evaluation are based on this and include:
   a. **Noninflammatory and inflammatory**
      i. **Arthrocentesis** of any joint with an effusion to rule out any crystal-induced or septic arthritis.
      ii. Serum uric acid, calcium, phosphorus, albumin levels.
      iii. **Radiographs** of affected joints, especially if there is any loss of function, looking for any concurrent fractures and narrowing of the joint-space size.
      iv. **Chest radiographs** in posteroanterior (PA) and lateral views, looking for any mass that may represent a non–small-cell carcinoma causing the paraneoplastic syndrome, hypertrophic pulmonary osteoarthropathy.
      v. **Lyme titer,** serum; an enzyme-linked immunosorbent assay (ELISA) for antibodies to *Borrelia burgdorferi.* If immunoglobulin M (IgM) levels increased, indicative of recent infection.
      vi. **Hepatitis serology** (i.e., HbsAg, IgM Hbc and anti-HCV) and liver-function tests (LFTs) to rule out any recent hepatitis B or C infection that can, in its prodrome, manifest with such an arthritis.
   b. **Inflammatory only**
      i. **Erythrocyte sedimentation rate (ESR).** This nonspecific test for inflammation should be elevated if inflammatory.
      ii. Rheumatoid factor to aid in evaluation for rheumatoid arthritis. If negative, can still be a "rheumatoid variant" (Table 7-9, page 402).
      iii. Complete blood cell count with differential to look for concurrent autoimmune cytopenia.
      iv. Antinuclear antibody (ANA; see Table 7-10, page 403, for types and interpretation).
      v. Blood urea nitrogen (BUN) and serum creatinine to look for concurrent renal dysfunction.
      vi. Urinalysis with microscopic examination to look for concurrent renal dysfunction.

Syndrome	HLA-B27	Rheumatoid Factor	Appendicular Joints	Axial Skeleton	Associated Manifestations
Reiter's syndrome	Positive	Negative	Lower-extremity more involved than upper-extremity joints	Mild disease Asymmetric	Uveitis Conjunctivitis Urethritis Aortic insufficiency
Ankylosing spondylitis	Positive	Negative	Lower-extremity more involved than upper-extremity joints	Marked disease Symmetric Sacroiliitis	Aortic insufficiency
Psoriatic arthropathy	Negative	Negative	Upper-extremity more involved than lower-extremity joints	Mild disease Asymmetric	Psoriasis
Inflammatory bowel disease	Negative	Negative	Lower-extremity more involved than upper-extremity joints	Mild disease Symmetric	Crohn's disease Ulcerative colitis Sclerosing cholangitis Uveitis Aortic insufficiency

T A B L E 7-10
Types of Antinuclear Antibodies

Specific Antigen	Antigen Description	Associated Disease States and Sensitivity
ds DNA	Native, double-stranded DNA	Systemic lupus erythematosus Sensitivity: 70%
Histone	Protein associated with native, double-stranded DNA	Drug-induced DNA Sensitivity: 95% SLE Sensitivity: 70%
SS-A	Also known as Ro Nonhistone protein associated with RNA	Sjögren's syndrome Sensitivity: 80%–85% SLE Sensitivity: 15%–20%
SS-B	Also known as La Nonhistone protein associated with RNA	Sjögren's syndrome Sensitivity: 80%–85% SLE Sensitivity: 20%–25%
Sm	Smith antigen Nonhistone protein associated with RNA	SLE Sensitivity: 35%–40% Specificity: 95%—100%
Nucleolar	Intranuclear processor of ribosomal RNA	Progressive systemic sclerosis (scleroderma) Sensitivity: 45%–50%
Centromere	Protein to which the chromatids attach during meiosis and mitosis	Progressive systemic sclerosis (scleroderma) Sensitivity: 50%–60% CREST syndrome Sensitivity: 80%–90%
C-ANCA	Antineutrophilic cytoplasmic antibodies; "C" gives a pattern of granular staining in cytoplasm of neutrophils	Wegener's granulomatosis Specificity of C-ANCA: 95%–99% for Wegener's

are large joints and include the knees, hips, and hands.
The distribution can be symmetric or asymmetric. The
manifestations usually improve with activity or after a
hot bath. There is no associated stiffness or swelling of
the affected joints, nor are there any systemic manifesta-

TABLE 7-11
Agents to Modify Rheumatoid Arthritis*

Agent	Mechanism	Dose	Side Effects†	Specific Comments
Azathioprine (Imuran)	Immunosuppression	100 mg p.o., q. day	Pancytopenia Contraindicated in pregnancy	
Cyclophosphamide (Cytoxan)	Immunosuppression	Use only under direction of a rheumatologist	Hemorrhagic cystitis Pancytopenia	Excellent for: a. Wegener's granulomatosis b. Lupus cerebritis c. Lupus nephritis, severe
Cyclosporine	Cell-mediated immunosuppression	200 mg p.o., q. day	TTP-like syndrome Renal failure Hypertension	
Hydroxychloroquine (Plaquenil)	Antimalarial	400 mg p.o., q. day	Macular dysfunction with red/green color blindness occurring first Pancytopenia Rashes	Mild rheumatoid disease
Methotrexate	Immunosuppression	7.5 mg p.o., q. week	Pernicious cirrhosis Hypersensitivity pneumonitis Pancytopenia	Use agent early in course May be the best agent overall

Penicillamine	unknown	250 mg p.o., q. day, may increase slowly to 1000 mg/day p.o.	Membranous GNP Pancytopenia Myasthenia gravis
Gold	unknown	Auranofin, 6 mg p.o., q. day -or- Aurothioglucose, 10 mg i.m. 1st week, then 25 mg i.m. 2nd and 3rd weeks; then 50 mg i.m. q week to a total of 1 gr; then 25–50 mg i.m. q.2–3 weeks	Pancytopenia Rashes Membranous GNP Stomatitis
Steroids	Immunosuppression	*If severe:* Pulse dose of methylprednisolone (Solu-Medrol), 100–500 mg i.v., q. day for 3 days *If chronic:* Taper to 10 mg prednisone q. day	Last ditch effort Attempt to keep chronic steroid dose <10 mg/day Steroids are indicated for a. SLE b. Malignant RA (i.e., severe vasculitis with the rheumatoid arthritis)

1998 combination of choice: azathioprine, methotrexate, hydroxychloroquine.
*Should be used under direction of a rheumatologist.
†All are relatively or absolutely contraindicated in pregnancy.

tions. On examination, there often is the nonspecific finding of crepitus in the affected joints, especially at the base of the thumb. There usually are Bouchard's nodes (nontender nodules at the PIP joints) and/or Heberden's nodes (nontender nodules at the DIP joints of the digits of the hands and/or feet).

C. The **evaluation** of this entity includes making the clinical diagnosis with the tools described in Box 7-4. Laboratory findings in this type of arthritis are invariably normal, and thus routine laboratory evaluative tests for the clinical diagnosis of osteoarthritis are not indicated.

D. The **specific management** of this disorder includes rest of the affected joint(s), including the use of a cane if the joint affected is the hip or knee. Obese patients should lose weight. Referral to physical therapy for ROM exercises and muscle-strengthening exercises is indicated. For pain relief, especially to encourage activity, **acetaminophen** can be prescribed.

1. If the patient is refractory to this therapy, especially if one joint is significantly more symptomatic than the rest, injection of the affected joint with triamcinolone, 15–20 mg for a small joint, 35–50 mg for a large joint, is an effective **modality** that usually affords 3–6 months of relief. Before intraarticular glucocorticoids are administered, however, the patient must be informed that this **treatment modality** may accelerate the osteoarthritic process.

2. If **refractory manifestations** develop, referral to orthopedics for surgical intervention is indicated, involving replacement of the affected joint, especially if the joint is a hip or knee.

IV. **Systemic lupus erythematosus (SLE)**

A. The **underlying pathogenesis** is an autoimmune systemic disease that manifests with inflammation of many of the organ systems of the body, including the central nervous system (CNS), kidneys, hematologic system, and joints. The specific pathogenesis remains unclear, although there is a component of an abnormal immune surveillance system and a probable decrease in the overall number of T-suppressor cells relative to helper cells. The vasculopathy is as the result of immune complex deposition.

B. The **specific manifestations** of this not uncommon disorder include an insidious onset of fatigue; diffuse, symmetric arthralgias; fevers; and frothy urine as a result of proteinuria. Further manifestations can include recurrent Raynaud's phenomenon and recurrent aphthous ulcers in the mouth. The patient also often has pleuritic and pericardial chest pain as a result of inflammation of these mesothelial linings. On examination there may be a malar erythematous rash of the face, mild inflammation of some joints, especially the small joints of the hands and feet, and pitting edema, which can approach anasarca if the patient has developed nephrotic syndrome. The two most common manifestations are the **polyarthritis** and the **dermatitis**.

C. The **evaluation** of this entity includes making the clinical diagnosis with the tools described in Box 7-4 (page 400). The "screening test" for SLE is the ANA, which has a 95% sensitivity. The American Rheumatologic Association (ARA) criteria for the diagnosis of SLE are given in Table 7-12. Furthermore, refer to Chapter 3, Renal Disease for SLE-Related Acute Renal Failure (page 179) and (Table 3-7, page 169) on the WHO Classification of lupus nephritis.

D. The **specific management** is directed toward symptomatic relief and the **treatment** of the systemic disorder, which will help resolve the symptoms. As with other inflammatory processes, cornerstones of therapy include rest, initiation of NSAIDs, and referral to rheumatology and physical therapy in an expedient fashion. NSAIDs are best for serositis and arthritis manifestations. If there is evidence of an active glomerulonephritis (i.e., renal failure and red cell casts on urinalysis), consultation with

T A B L E 7-12
Criteria for Systemic Lupus Erythematosus

Cytopenias
   Anemia, may be Coombs positive
   Granulocytopenia
   Immune-mediated thrombocytopenia
Malar rash, erythematous
Serositis
   Peritonitis
   Pericarditis
   Pleuritis
Alopecia
Proteinuria, may be nephrotic range
Photosensitivity
RBC casts on urinalysis
Cerebritis, may manifest as psychosis or seizure disorder
Raynaud's phenomenon
Discoid lupus
False-positive VDRL
Recurrent aphthous-type ulcers
Positive serology, including ANA (see Table 7-10)

From Tan EM, et al. The 1982 revised criteria for the classification of systemic lupus erythematosus (SLE). *Arthritis Rheum* 1982;25:1271.

nephrology is indicated for assistance and for the potential of performing a diagnostic renal biopsy. Furthermore, in active disease, the initiation of high-dose glucocorticoids (e.g., prednisone, 60–80 mg p.o., q.d.) is clearly indicated.

1. Specific indications for **initiation of glucocorticoids** include:
   a. Severe serositis.
   b. Hemolysis (Coombs positive).
   c. Immune-mediated thrombocytopenia.
   d. Glomerulonephritis, especially membranous type.
2. Other immunosuppressive agents that can be initiated under the direction of a rheumatologist in patients with severe symptomatic SLE include high-dose pulse steroids (1 g methylprednisolone, i.v.), cyclophosphamide (Cytoxan), or hydroxychloroquine.
   a. **High-dose pulse steroids** and **cyclophosphamide** in:
      i. Lupus cerebritis
      ii. Severe, rapidly progressive, crescentic glomerulonephritis
   b. **Hydroxychloroquine** in a dose of 400 mg p.o., is especially effective if there is a significant component of discoid lupus (i.e., significant skin and mucosal involvement).

V. **Rheumatic fever**
   A. The **underlying pathogenesis** is a systemic immune-mediated illness occurring as a result of recent infection with group A β-hemolytic streptococci.
   B. The **specific manifestations** of this rare yet important entity include an antecedent exudative pharyngitis that was not treated with antibiotics but was recently clinically resolved. The patient now has a several-day history of fevers, constitutional signs and symptoms, the development of heart valve dysfunction as manifested by murmurs, and polyarticular arthritis. Other manifestations include those described as Jones' criteria (see Table 12-2, page 578).
   C. **Evaluation**
      The **specific evaluation** includes that described in Box 7-4 and obtaining a pharyngeal culture on the chance that β-hemolytic streptococci are present. Also, to document a recent streptococcal infection, a serum antistreptolysin antibody (ASO) titer should be obtained. Echocardiography to document valvular, myocardial, and pericardial function is indicated.
   D. **Management**
      The **specific management** includes initiation of NSAIDs and an antistreptococcal antibiotic, either penicillin or erythromycin, for 10 days. Once the diagnosis is made

or highly suspected, the patient will need long-term prophylaxis with penicillin. An effective regimen is benzathine penicillin (Bicillin) i.m., every 2 weeks, or erythromycin, 250 mg p.o., b.i.d. Finally, the patient will need
one of the "high-risk" prophylactic antibiotic regimens
for any invasive or dental procedures (see section on
Bacterial Endocarditis in Chapter 6, page 320).

VI. **Other causes of polyarticular arthritis**

    A. **Virus-related:** Polyarticular arthritis may be a compo-
nent of the prodromal phase of hepatitis B or C, Cox-
sackie-virus, or rubella. These are self-limited and result
in no long-standing rheumatologic events.

    B. **Lyme disease:** This infectious disease can, in its late,
untreated stages, manifest with chronic polyarticular arthritis (refer to Box 7-4, page 400). The patient often
vacationed at or lives in a geographic area where this
infection, caused by the spirochete *Borrelia burgdorferi,*
is endemic. These geographic areas include the north-
eastern and the upper midwestern areas of the United
States. A history of a tick bite, the rash of **erythema
chronicum migrans (ECM),** is the most common manifestation. ECM occurs days to weeks after a tick bite, is >5
cm in size, begins as a red macule that increases in size
with central clearing; this is different from the annular
lesion that occurs within hours of the tick bite: it is a
hypersensitivity reaction. In addition to the rash and
arthritis, the patient may have a peripheral cranial nerve
VII palsy (See Chapter 14, page 623), chronic meningitis,
and/or the development of atrioventricular (AV)-nodal
blocks. The **specific management,** after making the diagnosis or suspecting it, includes the initiation of antibiotics, either doxycycline, 100 mg p.o., b.i.d., and/or a sec-
ond- or third-generation cephalosporin [e.g., cefuroxime
(Ceftin), 500 mg p.o., b.i.d., or ceftriaxone 2.0 g i.v., q.d.]
for a duration of 10–21 days if early; longer duration
(4–6 weeks) of antibiotics if later in course. Consultations
with infectious diseases and rheumatology are clearly
indicated. In particularly perplexing cases, confirmation,
via a synovial biopsy sent for polymerase chain reaction
(PCR) DNA analysis of *B. burgdorferi,* is indicated.

    C. **Remitting seronegative symmetric synovitis with pitting
edema (RS3PE)** is a relatively uncommon idiopathic
form of arthritis. The **specific manifestations** include the
presence of pitting edema of the dorsum of the hands
and feet and small-joint symmetric synovitis; the process
is of acute onset. There are never any erosions in the
joints associated with the arthritis. The evaluation includes performing an RF measurement, which is negative, and the initiation of agents including aspirin or

an NSAID and hydroxychloroquine. Overall the affected patient has an excellent prognosis.

D. **Wegener's disease:** The **underlying pathogenesis** is one of the development of a necrotizing vasculitis involving small to medium-sized vessels. The organs most commonly involving include the respiratory tree and the kidneys. The **specific manifestations** include recurrent epistaxis, hemoptysis, and the development of recurrent sinusitis, nodules that cavitate in the pulmonary parenchyma, and crescentic glomerulonephritis. Evaluation includes that described in Box 7-4 (page 400) having an appropriate clinical suspicion and obtaining a c-ANCA (i.e., antineutrophil cytoplasmic antibody and biopsy of the sinus, lung tissue, or kidney). The c-ANCA is quite specific for active Wegener's granulomatosis. **Treatment** is quite effective with cyclophosphamide. Referral to rheumatology is clearly indicated.

E. **Still's disease:** The **underlying pathogenesis** is idiopathic. The **specific manifestations** include the development of acute arthritis with spiking intermittent fevers, a macular nonpruritic rash on the proximal limbs and trunk, which increases in intensity after a hot bath/shower; splenomegaly; and lymphadenopathy. Both small and large joints are involved and may have erosion development. The **evaluation** includes that in Box 7-4 (page 400) making the clinical diagnosis, obtaining an RF, which will be increased, and initiating a course of high-dose aspirin and/or NSAIDs. Referral to rheumatology is indicated.

VII. **Consultation**

Problem	Service	Time
Polyarticular arthritis	Rheumatology	Urgent
Rheumatoid arthritis—emergency	Rheumatology	Emergent

VIII. **Indications for admission:** Recurrent fevers of undetermined origin, acute renal failure, intensely active acute inflammatory disease, the acute onset of lupus cerebritis, or evidence of valvular failure in acute rheumatic fever.

Bibliography

Hand

American Society for Surgery of the Hand: The hand: examination and diagnosis. 2nd ed. New York: Churchill Livingstone, 1985.

Berg D, Worzala K, Pachner R: Advanced clinical skills with emphasis on physical diagnosis. Boston: Blackwell-Science, 1998.

Hoffman DF, Schaffer TC: Management of common finger injuries. Am Fam Pract 1991;43:1594–1607.

Jones JG: Ulnar tunnel syndrome. Am Fam Pract 1991;44:497–502.

Loder RT, Mayhew HE: Common fractures from a fall on an outstretched hand. Am Fam Pract 1988;37:327–338.

Elbow

Berg D, Worzala K, Pachner R: Advanced clinical skills with emphasis on physical diagnosis. Boston: Blackwell-Science, 1998.

Bernhang AM: The many causes of tennis elbow. N Y State J Med 1979;79:1363.

Shaffer B, et al: Common elbow problems, part 2: management specifics. J Musculoskel Med 1997;14:29–44.

Shoulder

Berg D, Worzala K, Pachner R: Advanced clinical skills with emphasis on physical diagnosis. Boston: Blackwell-Science, 1998.

Smith DL, Campbell SM: Painful shoulder syndromes: diagnosis and management. J Gen Intern Med 1992;7:328–339.

Zuckerman JD, et al: The painful shoulder: part I. Extrinsic disorder. Am Fam Pract 1991;43:119–128.

Zuckerman JD, et al: The painful shoulder: part II. Intrinsic disorders and impingement syndrome. Am Fam Pract 1991;43:497–512.

Back

Berg D, Worzala K, Pachner R: Advanced clinical skills with emphasis on physical diagnosis. Boston: Blackwell-Science, 1998.

Byrne TN: Spinal cord compression from epidural metastases. N Engl J Med 1992;327:614–619.

Deyo RA: Early diagnostic evaluation of low back pain. J Gen Intern Med 1986;1:328–338.

Deyo RA, et al: Herniated lumbar intervertebral disk. Ann Intern Med 1990;112:598–603.

Frymoyer JW: Back pain and sciatica. N Engl J Med 1988;318:291–300.

Jensen MC, et al: Magnetic resonance imaging of the lumbar spine in people without back pain. N Engl J Med 1994;331:693.

Hip, Thigh, and Bony Pelvis

Berg D, Worzala K, Pachner R: Advanced clinical skills with emphasis on physical diagnosis. Boston: Blackwell-Science, 1998.

Solomon L: Patterns of osteoarthritis of the hip. J Bone Joint Surg [Br] 1976;58:75–82.

Knee

Baugher WH, White GM: Primary evaluation and management of knee injuries. Orthop Clin North Am 1985;16(2):315–327.

Berg D, Worzala K, Pachner R: Advanced clinical skills with emphasis on physical diagnosis. Boston: Blackwell-Science, 1998.

Berg E, et al: Office diagnosis of knee pain. Patient Care 1990;24:48–78.

Butcher JD, et al: Lower extremity bursitis. Am Fam Pract 1996;53:2317–2324.

Hawkins RJ, et al: Acute patellar dislocations: the natural history. Am J Sports Med 1986;14:117–120.

Larsson LG, Baum J: The syndromes of bursitis. Bull Rheum Dis 1986;36:1–8.

Laskin RS, ed: Symposium on disorders of the knee joint. Orthop Clin North Am 1979;10(1):1.

Press JM, et al: Knee ligament injuries: making the diagnosis, restoring use. J Musculoskel Med 1996;13:14–25.

Rothenberg MH, Graf BK: Evaluation of acute knee injuries. Postgrad Med 1993;93:75–86.

Foot and Ankle

Berg D, Worzala K, Pachner R: Advanced clinical skills with emphasis on physical diagnosis. Boston: Blackwell-Science, 1998.

Cailliet R: Foot and ankle pain. Philadelphia: FA Davis, 1974.

Kavanaugh JH, et al: The Jone's fracture revisited. J Bone Joint Surg [Am] 1978;60:776–782.

Keene JS, Lange RH: Diagnostic dilemmas in foot and ankle injuries. JAMA 1986;256:247–251.

Mahowald ML: Examination of the foot in rheumatic disease. Postgrad Med 1986;79:258–261.

Rifat SF, et al: Practical methods of preventing ankle injuries. Am Fam Pract 1996;53:2491–2498.

Rubin A, et al: Evaluation and diagnosis of ankle injuries. Am Fam Pract 1996;54:1609–1618.

Swain RA, Holt WS: Ankle injuries. Postgrad Med 1993;93:91–100.

Monoarticular Arthritis

Baker DG, et al: Acute monoarticular arthritis. N Engl J Med 1993;329:1013–1019.

Freed JF, et al: Acute monoarticular arthritis: a diagnostic approach. JAMA 1980;243:2314.

Goldenberg DL, Reed JI: Bacterial arthritis. N Engl J Med 1985;312:764.

Popp JD, et al: New insights into gouty arthritis: Cont Intern Med 1995; 7:55–63.

Roberts WN, et al: Colchicine in acute gout. JAMA 1987;257:1920–1922.

Wolfe F: Gout and hyperuricemia. Am Fam Pract 1991;43:2141–2150.

Polyarticular Arthritis

Calin A: Degenerative joint disease. Am Fam Pract 1986;33:167–172.

Cash JM, et al: Second-line drug therapy for rheumatoid arthritis. N Engl J Med 1994;330:1368–1375.

Kelley WN, et al, eds: Textbook of rheumatology. Philadelphia: WB Saunders, 1978.

Mills JA: Systemic lupus erythematosus. N Engl J Med 1994;330:1871–1878.

Nadelman RB, et al: Comparison of cefuroxime, axetil, and doxycycline in the treatment of early Lyme disease. Ann Intern Med 1992;117:273–280.

Paget SA, et al: Current management and recommendations for rheumatoid arthritis. Cont Intern Med 1994;6:35–43.

Pinals RS: Rheumatoid arthritis: a pharmacologic overview. Am Fam Pract 1988;37:145–152.

Rahn DW, Malawista SE: Lyme disease: recommendations for diagnosis and treatment. Ann Intern Med 1991;114:472–481.

Smith CA, Arnett FC: Diagnosing rheumatoid arthritis: current criteria. Am Fam Pract 1991;44:863–870.

Tan EM: Antinuclear antibodies in diagnosis and management. Hosp Pract 1983;Jan:79–84.

Weiner SR: Emergencies in rheumatoid arthritis. Am Fam Pract 1984;29:127–131.

—D.D.B

Chapter 8

Dermatology

Acne Vulgaris

Acne vulgaris is a disorder of skin structures normally present in the skin, the pilosebaceous glands. These glands, located mainly in the skin of the face, upper back, and trunk, produce sebum, a lipoproteinaceous material that aids in skin moisturization. In acne, the pilosebaceous glands abnormally increase the production and content of fatty acids in sebum. The abnormal increase in sebum production is multifactorial. Underlying factors that influence its development include heredity and an increase in serum androgens during male puberty. Furthermore, androgen use for illicit or therapeutic purposes will increase sebum production.

In certain patients, the increase in sebum sets off a cascade of events. These events include (a) obstruction of the ducts of the pilosebaceous glands by keratin and the excess sebum, with resultant dilation of the gland, and (b) infection and inflammation of the obstructed gland and adjacent tissue by anaerobic bacteria, especially the species *Propionibacterium acnes*. Acne lesions will drain spontaneously but, if the inflammatory component was great, will heal with scarring.

I. **Overall manifestations**
   The **overall manifestations** include multiple lesions over the areas where pilosebaceous glands are located (i.e., the face, neck, upper back, and upper trunk). There are three discrete types of lesions—closed comedones, open comedones, and cystic lesions. Patients may have some of each, but one type usually predominates.
   A. **Closed comedo**
      This is a mildly tender papule with a whitish yellow center and mild erythema peripherally. It is commonly referred to as a **whitehead.** It occurs as a result of obstruction of the gland's duct with the accumulation of keratin and sebum.

B O X 8-1

Overall Evaluation and Management of Acne Vulgaris

Evaluation

1. The diagnosis is made clinically after a thorough history and physical examination. No special tests are required for diagnosis, nor is biopsy required.
2. No specific dietary changes are necessary, as there has been no documented association of acne with any foodstuff, including chocolate.
3. Limit face washing to twice per day. Excessive washing and picking at the face can exacerbate the acne.
4. Direct the patient not to squeeze the comedones.
5. If cosmetics are necessary, water-based ones should be used and should be washed off each evening before the patient retires.

Management of comedo-predominant acne

1. Benzoyl peroxide, 10% lotion or cream, may be applied to the affected skin b.i.d. This agent can be used as monotherapy and will control comedo-predominant acne in the majority of cases.
   a. This agent acts as a comedolytic agent, decreasing the fatty acid content of the sebum and decreasing the quantity of anaerobic bacteria in the affected gland.
   b. **Side effects** include drying of the skin, which can be dose limiting.
   c. Benzoyl peroxide is available as an over-the-counter agent.
2. **Tretinoin (topical retinoic acid),** 0.01%–0.025% gel, 0.05% liquid, or 0.05%–0.1% cream, may be applied to affected skin every other evening on retiring. Because the cream is the least irritating form, it is the form most commonly used for the **treatment** of comedo-predominant acne. It should be used for ≥6–12 weeks before any improvement can be expected. The patient should be instructed that there may well be an exacerbation of the acne early in the course of therapy. There is synergy in efficacy when **tretinoin** is used with **benzoyl peroxide**.
   a. This agent acts as a comedolytic.
   b. **Side effects** include significant skin drying, which can be dose and agent limiting.

(continued)

B O X 8-1 (continued)

Management of cystic/nodular-predominant acne

1. **Benzoyl peroxide,** 10% lotion or cream, may be applied to the affected skin b.i.d. This agent can be used as monotherapy and will control cystic/nodular-predominant acne in a minority of cases.
   a. This agent acts as a comedolytic agent, decreasing the fatty acid content of the sebum and decreasing the quantity of anaerobic bacteria in the affected gland.
   b. **Side effects** include drying of the skin, which can be dose limiting.
   c. Benzoyl peroxide is available as an over-the-counter agent.
2. **Topical antibiotics** are effective in the **treatment** of inflammatory nodular acne. Specific antibiotic agents include erythromycin, 3% cream; clindamycin, 1% cream; and tetracycline, 0.22% cream. Any of these agents is effective when applied to the affected areas b.i.d., as long as there is an inflammatory component to the acne.
   a. These agents are very effective when used with benzoyl peroxide. A product that combines a topical antibiotic with benzoyl peroxide is **Benzamycin 3%,** which combines erythromycin 3% and benzoyl peroxide 5%. This agent is applied to the skin b.i.d.
   b. Topical antibiotics treat the anaerobic infection and therefore decrease the inflammation.
   c. **Side effects** include irritation and drying of the skin.
3. **Systemic antibiotics** are effective and therefore indicated if the inflammatory component is marked or refractory to topical antibiotic therapy. Specific regimens include, in the acute setting, tetracycline, 500 mg p.o., q.i.d., for 14 days, or erythromycin, 250 mg p.o., t.i.d. to q.i.d., for 14 days, followed by long-term tetracycline, 250 mg p.o., once daily, or erythromycin, 250 mg p.o., once daily.
   a. Systemic antibiotics treat the bacterial infection and therefore decrease the inflammation.
   b. **Side effects** include the fact that tetracycline is contraindicated in pregnant women.

(continued)

B O X 8-1 (continued)

4. **Isotretinoin (Accutane),** a vitamin A derivative, can be used in the **treatment** of severe cystic/nodular acne refractory to other therapeutic modalities.
   a. The dosage is 0.5–1.0 mg/kg/day p.o., in a b.i.d. dosing for 16–18 weeks. The response rate is dramatic, as ≤90% of patients will respond after 4 months of therapy.
   b. The mechanism of action of this agent includes decreasing sebum production and local antiinflammatory effects.
   c. **Side effects** are significant and include severe drying of the skin, which can limit dose and even agent. The agent can cause an increase in serum triglycerides and has been associated with the development of hepatic dysfunction. Finally, isotretinoin is teratogenic, and therefore its use is **contraindicated** in **pregnant women.** In fact, it should not be used by any woman of childbearing age. Because of its side-effect profile, it should be reserved for the most severe cases of acne vulgaris.

B. **Open comedo**
This is a nontender papule with a central black area, commonly called a **blackhead.** It occurs as a result of the duct or "pore" opening and allowing some of the contents of the gland to drain externally.

C. **Cystic/nodular**
These lesions are nodular and are frequently accompanied by inflammation in and adjacent to them. The nodules may be quite tender and large, reaching 1–2 cm. They may exude purulent material, especially early in their time course. These lesions usually represent a progression from comedones and are the lesions that cause the most scarring (Box 8-1).

II. The **overall evaluation and management** include that described in Box 8-1.

III. **Consultation**

Problem	Service	Time
Refractory acne	Dermatology	Elective

IV. **Indications for admission:** None.

(Text continues on page 424)

Blistering Diseases (Table 8-1 and Fig. 8-1)

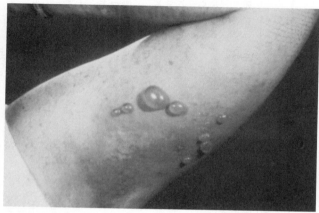

F I G U R E 8-1
Bullous pemphigoid on the right upper extremity.

Disease	Affected Areas/ Manifestations	Site of Cleavage	Histopathology	Associated Laboratory	Treatment
Pemphigus vulgaris Pemphigus foliaceus Pemphigus paraneo-plastica	Skin Mucous membranes Flaccid bullae Erosions	Intraepi-dermal	Acantholysis IgG and C3 to desmosomes	Antidesmo-somal anti-body assay positive HLA-A10	High-dose prednisone (60–80) *or* High-dose pulse steroids, e.g., 1 g methylpredniso-lone i.v. q.d. × 5 then, as the disease comes under control, add aza-thioprine 100 mg p.o. q.d., then wean from both Dermatology consultation Erythromycin, 250 mg p.o. q.i.d. (during active blis-tering)
Bullous pemphigoid (see Fig. 8-1)	Skin Mucous membranes Tense bulla Urticarial plaques	Subepi-dermal	IgG and C3 to basement membrane	Anti-basement membrane an-tibody pres-ent in serum	Similar to pemphigus vul-garis (See above)
Cicatricial pemphigoid	Face and scalp Tense blisters with scarring	Subepi-dermal	IgG and C3 to basement membrane	None	Similar to bullous pem-phigoid Chlorhexidine mouthwash q.12hr

	Clinical features	Level	Immunofluorescence	Additional	Treatment
	Severe gingival erosions and scarring External ocular vesicles and scarring				
Dermatitis herpetiformis	Skin, especially scalp, elbows, buttocks and knees Grouped vesicles/erosions	Subepidermal	IgA, linear deposits along the basement membrane and upper papillary dermis	HLA-B8/Dw3 Gluten-sensitive enteropathy 70% have IgA antiendomysial antibodies in the serum	Gluten-free diet Dapsone, 50 mg p.o. q.d. Dermatology consultation
Herpes gestationalis	Second trimester of pregnancy Tense blisters Target-like macules Truncal location Increased fetal mortality	Subepidermal	IgG and C3 to basement membrane		Prednisone, 60–80 mg p.o. q.d. or high-dose pulse steroids, i.e., 1 g methylprednisolone i.v. q.d. × 5 Dermatology consultation
Epidermolysis bullosa acquista	Generalized tense blisters Oral erosions Esophageal strictures	Subepidermal	IgG against Type VII collagen		Prednisone, 60–80 mg p.o. q.d. or high-dose pulse steroids, i.e., 1 g methylprednisolone i.v. q.d. × 5 Dermatology consultation

* In any and all cases, it is imperative to replete any intravascular volume fluid deficit, support the patient and, if significant bullous disease is present, to manage **as a burn patient.** Lactated Ringer's solution is the most appropriate for i.v. fluid repletion.

† **Indications for admission** include active disease, intravascular volume depletion, and any sign of bacterial superinfection.

Dermatitis (Table 8-2)

TABLE 8-2
Dermatitis

Disease	History and Physical Examination Findings	Treatment
Contact	Erythema with vesicles and blisters Weeping and crusting of affected areas Severe pruritus Can develop secondary bacterial infections Located on areas exposed to inciting agent (e.g., chemical, allergen, detergent) Asymmetric pattern of distribution (e.g., poison ivy) Poison ivy (*Toxicodendron radicans*)—"Leaves of three, leave them be.": Takes 3 weeks for resin to evaporate from any material.	a) Remove inciting agent b) Triamcinolone 0.1% b.i.d. to affected areas (Appendix, page 461) c) Calamine lotion b.i.d. to affected areas d) If lichenified, use ointment (greasy) e) If severe: prednisone, 40–60 mg p.o. q.d. for 10–14 days (tapering dose) f) Hydroxyzine (Atarax), 25 mg p.o. q.6hr prn for itching g) Prevention
Atopic (eczema)	Pruritic Symmetric distribution Distribution on face, neck, trunk; also on flexor surfaces of elbows and knees Can have lichenification of lesions Strong correlation with other atopic diseases Eosinophilia is common Special type: *eczema herpeticum*—herpes simplex viral infection superimposed on atopic dermatitis	a) Hydroxyzine (Atarax) 25–50 mg p.o. q.6hr prn for itching b) Triamcinolone 0.1% b.i.d. to affected areas c) Calamine lotion b.i.d. to affected areas d) Rarely severe enough to require oral steroids e) If eczema herpeticum, add parenteral acyclovir to above regimen (dose: 10 mg/kg/24 hr i.v. dosing by i.v. for 7–10 days) f) Dermatology consult

Drug-induced	Bright, erythematous rash Pruritic Begins on trunk and spreads to periphery Time course is different for each use of the agent (amnestic response): a) First use: onset 8–10 days after start b) Subsequent use: onset 1–3 days after start	a) Hydroxyzine (Atarax) 25–50 mg p.o. q.6hr prn b) Discontinue offending agent c) Triamcinolone 0.1% topical q.6hr (Appendix, page 461) d) Observe patient for other anaphylactic sign (bronchospasm, hypotension); if present, epinephrine SC is indicated (see Table 4-1, page 197) e) Systemic steroids rarely necessary in treatment f) Label patient "allergic" to that specific agent
Photo-dermatitis (sunburn)	Development of diffuse, confluent, nonraised, warm, erythematous rash on areas exposed to sunlight or other UV light sources Nausea and diarrhea Risk factors: a) Fair-skinned b) SLE	Prevention: a) Limit exposure to UV light b) Use sunscreens with SPF (sunprotective factor) >15 if in sun Treatment of acute burn: a) Topical steroids (e.g., triamcinolone 0.1% cream) b) Aspirin, 325 mg p.o. q.4–6hr c) If severe, prednisone, 40–60 mg p.o. q.d. for 5 days d) If **porphyria cutanea** tarda is a factor, chloroquine 125 mg p.o. 2× per week, and/or phlebotomy once monthly are effective in treatment
Seborrheic	Chronic and recurrent Papulosquamous lesions with a distribution adjacent to the hairline Pruritic, greasy appearing Many exacerbating and/or precipitating factors: a) Hormone changes b) Emotional stress c) Infections	Low-dose topical steroids, e.g., hydrocortisone 0.1% q.i.d. (Appendix, page 461) Selenium sulfide–containing shampoos (e.g., Selsun Blue, and others)

Erythemas (Table 8-3 and Fig. 8-2)

TABLE 8-3
Erythemas

Disease	Symptoms and Signs	Precipitating Factors	Biopsy and Laboratory Findings	Treatment
Erythema nodosum	Tender, erythematous, nodular lesions 1–10 mm in size. Extensor surfaces of the distal lower extremities	Streptococcal infections Coccidioidomycosis Mycobacterial infections Hepatitis B Lues venereum Sarcoidosis Ulcerative colitis Leukemia	Septal panniculitis (i.e., Ig and complement in the vessel wall betwixt the lobules of fat in the subcutaneous tissues)	a) Diagnose and treat underlying cause b) KI (potassium iodide), in saturated solution, 5–15 drops to nodules t.i.d.
Erythema multiforme (see Fig. 8-2)	Multiple wheals and papules. Symmetric in distribution. Can progress to toxic epidermolytic syndrome and involve mucous membranes (Stevens–Johnson syndrome). Occurs on palms and soles. Classically, "target" shaped lesions. "minor": one set of lesions. "major": multiple sets of lesions; may involve mucous membranes	*Mycoplasma* infections Herpes simplex (HSV) infections (as a late sequelae) Drug-related: Phenytoin TMP/sulfa Cell-mediated hypersensitivity to a diverse set of immunologic insults	Nonspecific Increased cold agglutinins in serum	a) Diagnose and treat the underlying cause b) If severe (Stevens–Johnson), treat as a burn: Admit to burn unit. Aggressively monitor for and replete fluid and electrolyte losses c) Acyclovir, 200 mg p.o., 5× per day, if HSV suspected × 10d d) Erythromycin, 500 mg p.o./i.v., q.6h., if *Mycoplasma* suspected × 10d

Erythema marginatum	Erythematous Rapidly spreading Flat, pale centers Raised red margins	Rheumatic fever (streptococcal infections)	Increased ASO titer in serum	e) Consider steroids p.o. or i.v. acutely, especially if major f) Dermatology consult Treat underlying infection (streptococcal) with appropriate antibiotics (usually penicillin based)
Erythema infectiosum	Erythematous, papular rash Trunk, back, face Central clearing present Fevers to 103°F Can have rhinorrhea, sore throat, other URI symptoms concurrently Slapped face appearance common Pediatric age group Also known as "fifth disease"	Parvovirus B-19	Nonspecific	Symptomatic and supportive Pregnancy precautions: pregnant women should be isolated from patients with this infection
Erythema chronicum migrans	Flat with central clearing Asymmetric Nonpruritic Trunk, back, thighs Occurs several days to weeks after a tick bite Can resolve, then recur in another area Concurrent arthalgias, neuropathy, and/or cardiac manifestations not uncommon	Lyme disease (Borrelia burgdorferi)	Elevated Lyme titer	See subsection "Other causes of polyarticular arthritis" in Chapter 7 (page 409)

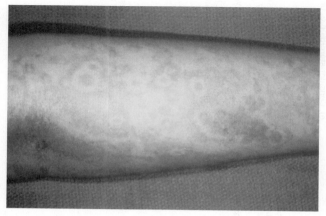

FIGURE 8-2
Erythema multiforme on the flexor surface of an upper extremity.

(text continued from page 416)

Nails

I. **Problems**
   Specific problems that can affect the fingernails or toenails
   are described subsequently.
   A. **Paronychia/eponychia**
      1. The **specific manifestations** of this entity include the
         acute onset of pain and swelling about the lateral nail
         fold unilaterally. If the proximal fold is involved, it
         is an eponychium. The patient usually has a history
         of trauma to the involved nail or of onychocryptosis
         ("ingrown nail") in the affected digit. Examination
         discloses redness, warmth, tenderness, swelling, and
         often an area of purulent material in and adjacent to
         the involved lateral nail fold.
      2. The **underlying pathogenesis** is growth of the nail
         plate into the lateral nail fold or otherwise irritating
         the lateral nail fold. Irritation can occur as a result of
         trauma, poor nail care, or a fungal infection involving
         the nail plate (onychomycosis). Causative organisms
         include the gram-positive cocci (e.g., *Streptococcus*
         spp. and *Staphylococcus* spp.).
      3. The **specific evaluation** of this problem includes mak-
         ing the clinical diagnosis and examining the patient
         for any concurrent processes, such as septic arthritis
         or cellulitis. Radiographs of the affected hand, foot,
         or digits are indicated only if there are any atypical

features, a history of antecedent trauma, evidence of a concurrent septic arthritis as manifested by a decreased range of motion of the DIP or PIP joints of the affected digit, or if the patient has diabetes mellitus.

4. The **specific management** includes warm soaks of the involved digit, antibiotics, and simple local surgery.

   a. Specific antibiotic regimens include either a 7-day course of cephalexin (Keflex), 500 mg p.o., q.i.d., or erythromycin, 250–500 mg p.o., q.i.d.

   b. If there is any evidence of fluctuance or if the lesion is severe, the area must be incised and drained by incising the lateral fold longitudinally.

B. **Subungual hematoma**

1. The **specific manifestations** of this entity include the acute onset of pain in the distal digit beginning immediately after crushing or pinching trauma to that digit. Examination discloses a reddish blue collection of blood beneath the nail plate in the nail bed itself and exquisite tenderness on minimal palpation of the affected nail plate.

2. The **underlying pathogenesis** is trauma resulting in the collection of blood beneath the nail plate, with resultant increased pressure in the distal digit.

3. The **specific evaluation** of this problem includes making the clinical diagnosis. Radiographs of the hand, foot, or digit are indicated only if there is evidence of trauma-related concurrent damage.

4. **Management**

   The central goal is to relieve the pressure and pain by incising the hematoma. Various methods may be used to achieve this goal. One of the easiest and most effective methods is to use a paper clip. The tip of the paper clip is bent perpendicularly, and then heated in a flame until the tip is red hot. This sterilizes the tip and allows easy passage of the tip through the nail plate. The clinician firmly and rapidly presses the red-hot tip through the nail plate into the hematoma. Once it is drained, the symptoms rapidly resolve.

   After the procedure, the nail plate will have a defect that will resolve in several weeks as the nail plate grows distally. The patient need only keep the wound clean. Antibiotics are not indicated unless a concurrent process is present.

C. **Onychomycosis**

1. The **specific manifestations** of this not uncommon problem include onychauxis (i.e., thickened nail plates), brittle nail plates, and easy fracturing of the affected plate (see Fig. 8-3). The process may be limited to one nail or may involve multiple nails. Examination frequently discloses erythema of the adjacent skin, cracking of the adjacent skin with concurrent

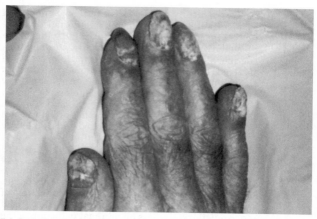

F I G U R E   8-3
Onychomycosis of the nail plates on all digits. Note loss of translucency, thickening, and distal breaking of the nail plates themselves.

flaking, or even vesicle formation, all as a result of a concurrent tineal infection. The risk of development of onychocryptosis and of a paronychium is increased in this process.

2. The **underlying pathogenesis** is a chronic infection with the fungal elements of a dermatophyte or *Candida* infection. There invariably is a long history of antecedent tineal skin infections and/or uncontrolled diabetes mellitus.

3. The **specific evaluation** of this problem includes making the clinical diagnosis by inspection of the affected nails. For diagnostic confirmation, one can perform a fungal culture by using Sabouraud's medium on a piece or fragment of the infected/affected nail.

4. The **specific management** includes the following measures.

   a. Application of **clotrimazole** (Lotrimin, Mycelex) 1% cream, b.i.d., to affected areas. This topical antifungal agent will not cure the onychomycosis but will treat the underlying tineal skin infections and thus prevent spread to other nails. The feet should be kept dry.

   b. **Systemic antifungals** are clearly indicated and may obviate the need for surgical intervention. These include:

      i. Itraconazole, 200 mg p.o., q.d. for 2–6 months (monitor liver function tests q. month)

-or-
    ii. Terbinafine, 250 mg p.o., q.d. Few side effects; duration of **treatment**: 1–2 months for fingernails/3–6 months for toenails.

D. Onychocryptosis
1. The **specific manifestations** of this relatively common process include pain and tenderness in the tissue in and adjacent to the lateral nail fold, with the lateral aspect of the nail plate embedded in the lateral nail fold.
2. The **underlying pathogenesis** is inappropriate growth of the nail plate into the lateral nail fold. **Risk factors** for the development of this process include trauma, onychomycosis, onychorrhexis, and onychauxis. It can in itself be a risk factor for the development of a paronychium.
3. The **specific evaluation** and management of this entity entail making the clinical diagnosis and, if the condition is significant, surgically removing the involved half of the nail plate.

E. Onychogryphosis
1. The **specific manifestations** of this entity include a grossly elongated nail that may develop a hooked configuration (Fig. 8-4). This is invariably due to lack of manicure or pedicure, quite often in a patient with poor hygiene.
2. The **specific evaluation and management** of this problem include making the clinical diagnosis and performing a manicure or pedicure of the affected nails.

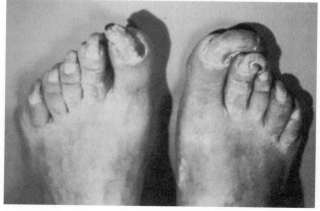

F I G U R E 8-4
Onychogryphosis of the nails of the feet.

> Pedicure of large toenails may be done by a podiatrist with a special technique.

II. Consultation

Service	Time
Podiatry	Elective

III. Indications for admission: No specific indications.

Neoplasia, Benign and Malignant

I. Basal-cell carcinoma (BCCA)

A. Incidence

BCCA is one of the most common forms of cancer in the United States today. More than 500,000 new cases are diagnosed per year. Furthermore, it is a malignant neoplasm that is increasing in incidence. **Risk factors** for its development include fair skin, increasing age, exposure to UV (A and B) light, and a history of irradiation exposure.

B. The **specific manifestations** include lesions appearing on skin areas that are frequently exposed to the sun (i.e., the face, head, and back of the neck). These lesions are papular, with a translucent quality. Invariably they have surface telangiectasias, and occasionally they ulcerate. They have been described as having a "pearly" margin (see Fig. 8-5).

C. Natural history

This malignant neoplasm, although it is very invasive and quite destructive by contiguous growth, rarely metastasizes. Therefore, whereas it is locally malignant and causes significant morbidity, it rarely causes death.

D. The **specific evaluation and management** include making the clinical and histopathologic diagnosis by performing the evaluative tests described in Box 8-2 (page 430). Any lesion potentially a basal-cell carcinoma, especially one that is pigmented and thus slightly suggestive of melanoma, must have an excisional biopsy.

    1. A specific type of surgical biopsy has been developed for BCCA. In **Mohs' surgical technique,** the surgeon shaves off layers of the tumor and sends each layer for frozen-section analysis to determine whether the margins of the excision are free of the tumor. This allows the surgeon to resect all of the tumor, while minimizing adjacent normal tissue removal.

    2. If there is a contraindication to surgical intervention or if the size of the tumor precludes surgical intervention, a **punch biopsy** for confirmation of the diagnosis followed by local irradiation should be performed. Local irradiation is an effective modality in the **treatment** and cosmetic effect, even with large BCCAs.

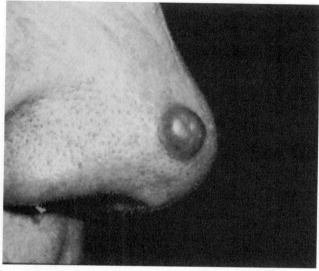

F I G U R E   8-5
Basal-cell carcinoma of the nose. Classic features include a smooth, pearly, translucent nodule with some telangiectasias within the lesion.

II. Squamous-cell carcinoma (SCCA)

A. Incidence

This not uncommon malignant skin neoplasm is increasing in incidence in the United States. **Risk factors** for its development include exposure to UV light, exposure to ionizing radiation, recurrent trauma to the skin, and the virus-related lesions of condyloma acuminatum and periungual warts. The specific virus is the DNA human papillomavirus (HPV). Two historic risks include the occupation of being a chimney sweep and/or the chronic exposure to or ingestion of arsenic.

B. The **specific manifestations** include lesions developing on the face, ears, or dorsum of the hands. The patient is seen with a nontender, solitary nodular lesion in the skin. The nodule invariably has a central necrotic-appearing ulcer and some peripheral erythema (Fig. 8-6). The lesion increases rapidly over weeks to months. The ulcer is often punched out with smooth edges. Multiple lesions usually occur in patients with more than one risk factor.

C. Natural history

These lesions may invade adjacent tissues and structures and also metastasize. Thus, unlike BCCA, this type of

---

B O X 8-2

*Overall Evaluation and Management of
Neoplastic Skin Disorders*

Evaluation

1. Examine the lesion, including inspection and palpation. In the vast majority of cases, a presumptive diagnosis can be made from the examination results.
2. If there is any suspicion that a lesion is malignant or premalignant, refer the patient to dermatology or general surgery for an excisional biopsy. Excisional biopsy usually allows complete resection of the lesion and therefore is diagnostic and therapeutic.
3. After the histopathologic characteristics of the lesion are known, stage the lesion. See discussion in the text for the natural and staging of each type of malignant neoplastic lesion.

Treatment

1. Starting at age 40 years, each person should have a thorough skin inspection and examination to screen for early lesions.
2. The major focus is on prevention. Many of the malignant and premalignant skin neoplasms can be prevented by limiting exposure to UV light. Tanning salons and sun exposure should be minimized. If sun exposure cannot be directly limited, the use of lotions with a sun protection factor (SPF) of >15 is strongly advised.

skin cancer can, if not treated early in its course, cause the death of the patient. These tumors metastasize to local lymph nodes early in the course of disease. Sites of later metastases include the bone, brain, liver, and lungs.

D. The **specific evaluation and management** include making the clinical and histopathologic diagnosis by performing the evaluative tests described in Box 8-2. Any lesion that is potentially SCCA must have a biopsy. Excisional biopsy is the procedure of choice. If performed early, it can be diagnostic and curative.

1. Once the diagnosis has been histopathologically confirmed, one must **stage** the disease. This consists of palpating any adjacent lymph nodes, performing liver function studies (LFTs), and obtaining a chest radio-

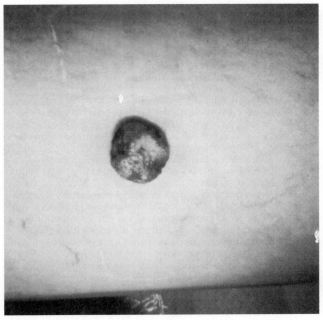

F I G U R E   8-6
Squamous-cell carcinoma on the upper extremity. Note the features of an ulcerated, nontender nodule.

graph. If there are any suggestive (i.e., indurated) lymph nodes, they should have biopsies. If there are any suspected areas on the chest radiograph or LFT abnormalities, further imaging with computed tomography (CT) of the suggestive areas should be performed.

2. If there is any evidence of metastatic disease, expedient referral to an oncologist is indicated. The management of metastatic SCCA is beyond the scope of this text.

III. Dysplastic nevus syndrome

A. Epidemiology

This syndrome, first described ~15 years ago by Clark et al., has an estimated prevalence of 2%–5% in the United States today. **Risk factors** for development are familial. The familial form is transmitted as an autosomal dominant trait. A sporadic form has been described that appears spontaneously.

B. The **specific manifestations** of dysplastic nevi are best described by comparing and contrasting them with benign nevi.

1. **Benign nevi,** present on every human being, usually are small (<5 mm in diameter); have sharp, well-defined boundaries with adjacent skin; are uniformly pigmented; are usually macular; and rarely have any pink hue to the pigment.

2. **Dysplastic** nevi are usually large (>5 mm in diameter); have irregular, ill-defined boundaries with adjacent skin; have a disorganized pigment; are usually papular; and quite often have pink hues in the pigment. On histopathologic analysis, there are irregular, atypical-appearing melanocytes within the dermis. Dysplastic nevi in general have a significant malignant potential.

C. **Natural history**

This syndrome results in multiple recurrent dysplastic nevi with a great potential for malignant transformation. There is a significant risk of the development of malignant melanoma, especially in patients with familial dysplastic nevus syndrome, in which the relative risk can be 50 times that of the general population.

D. The **specific evaluation and management** include making the clinical and histopathologic diagnosis by performing the evaluative tests described in Box 8-2. After the clinical diagnosis has been made, a thorough family history and even examination of family members for such lesions is required. Photographs of the patient's skin should be obtained using a digital camera at baseline and again every 4–6 months for comparison. Any suggestive lesion mandates an excisional biopsy, never a punch biopsy, as the lesion may be a malignant melanoma. The patient should be instructed to perform a monthly skin self-examination and to report any changes in the nevi.

IV. **Malignant melanoma**

A. **Incidence**

This malignant neoplasm of the skin is increasing in incidence. Specific **risk factors** for its development include fair skin; intense sunburns, especially as a child; a family history of melanoma; the presence of dysplastic nevus syndrome; and exposure to UV light.

B. The **specific manifestations** of this entity include a nevus with irregular borders, an irregular distribution of pigment within the nevus, or one that has increased in diameter. Although any of these changes in a nevus suggests a malignant melanoma (Fig. 8-7), suspicion is even higher if the patient has a history of dysplastic nevus syndrome. There are several clinical variations of malignant melanoma, which are described in Table 8-4 (page 434).

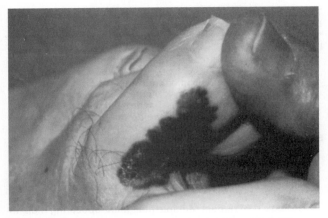

F I G U R E   8-7
Superficial spreading malignant melanoma of the left foot. Any
pigmented lesion on the palms of the hands or soles of the feet should
raise the suspicion that the lesion is malignant.

C. **Natural history**

Early in its course, the malignant lesion remains quite
superficial, with little to no invasion or metastatic potential. As the tumor grows, it invades deeper into the skin
and increases the incidence of metastatic spread. There
is a direct relation between depth of invasion and distant
metastases and an inverse relation between depth of invasion and survival. Thus the lesion is staged by depth
of penetration.

1. The two systems used in **staging malignant melanoma**
are the Clark and Breslow staging schemas. The **Clark
system** describes the depth relative to skin layer; the
Breslow system uses depth measured in millimeters.
A brief overview of these important staging systems
is given in Table 8-5 (page 435).

2. Distant metastases are to the regional lymph nodes,
liver, lungs, and the brain. It can and frequently does
metastasize to unique organs, including the myocardium and/or the wall of the small or large intestine.

D. The **specific evaluation and management** include making the clinical and histopathologic diagnosis by performing the evaluative tests described in Box 8-2 (page
430). After a thorough history and physical examination,
excisional biopsy of any suspected lesion is mandated.

1. The gold standard for staging malignant melanoma is
the Clark/Breslow levels; therefore, extensive imaging

T A B L E 8-4
Clinical Variants of Malignant Melanoma

Lentigo-maligna
  Location: Any skin areas that are recurrently exposed to UV light
  Gross manifestations: Flat, with irregular borders, various shades of brown and black pigment within the nevus
  Histologic description: Normal and malignant melanocytes within the basal area of the epidermis
  Mean age of patient at presentation: 70 years
Superficial spreading (see Fig. 8-7)
  Location: Any and all body surfaces
  Gross manifestations: Palpable lesion with irregular borders; asymmetric configuration of the lesion with multiple colors within the nevus itself: black, brown, and pink pigments
  Histologic description: Multiple malignant-appearing melanocytes within the epidermis
  Mean age of patient at presentation: 50 years
Nodular
  Location: Any and all body surfaces
  Gross manifestations: Palpable lesion; smooth borders; uniform black pigmentation with a surrounding area of decreased pigmentation
  Histologic description: Large numbers of malignant melanocytes with multiple areas of dermal invasion
  Mean age of patient at presentation: 45 years

of other organ systems is not indicated unless symptoms are referable to that area.

2. The **specific management** of metastatic malignant melanoma is beyond the scope of this text; however, some points can be made.

   a. No data indicate that radical dissection of regional lymph nodes is of any benefit to the patient in the short or long term. Therefore, this procedure is usually not indicated.

   b. There is a want of effective modalities, including radiation and chemotherapy, in the **treatment** of advanced malignant melanoma. As such, the major thrust in management is on **prevention** (primary prevention) and early detection (secondary prevention).

V. **Actinic keratoses**

   A. **Incidence**

   As with that of many other neoplastic dermatologic lesions, the incidence of this premalignant, albeit benign,

T A B L E 8-5
Clark Staging Systems for Malignant Melanoma

Clark level I
  Confined to the epidermis
  Breslow level, <0.75 mm
  0 metastases
  100% cure rate
Clark level II
  Penetrates the epidermal basement membrane into the papillary dermis
  Breslow level, <0.75 mm
  5% metastases
  95% cure rate
Clark level III
  Penetrates the epidermal basement membrane to a level at the junction of the papillary and reticular dermis
  Breslow level, 0.75–1.5 mm
  15%–25% metastases
  70% cure rate
Clark level IV
  Penetrates into the deep reticular dermis
  Breslow level, 1.5–3.0 mm
  40% metastases
  40%–50% cure rate
Clark level V
  Penetrates the entire thickness of both the epidermis and the dermis into the subdermal fat
  Breslow level, >3.0 mm
  70% metastases
  20% cure rate

neoplastic disorder is increasing. **Risk factors** for their development include UV light exposure, especially in individuals with fair skin, increasing age, and (of historic importance) the chronic ingestion of or exposure to arsenic.

B. The **specific manifestations** of these lesions include occurrence on the face, neck, dorsal aspects of hands, and forearms. There are four discrete variants, each with different clinical features.

   1. **Atrophic variant.** The lesion is dry, scaly, and rough. Lesions may be single or multiple and are usually <5 mm in diameter.

   2. **Hypertrophic variant.** These pink papules are well demarcated from the adjacent skin tissue. They often form cutaneous "horns" of keratin, a finding that, when present, is quite dramatic.

   3. **Bowenoid variant** (not Bowen's disease). The scaly,

red plaques can be quite large, >1 cm. They are well demarcated from the adjacent skin.

4. **Spreading variant.** These papules and plaques spread centrifugally from a central origin.

C. **Natural history**

Although the lesion is itself benign, it is premalignant for SCCAs.

D. The **specific evaluation and management** include making the clinical and histopathologic diagnosis by performing the evaluative tests described in Box 8-2 (page 430). If there is any suspicion for a BCCA or SCCA, excisional biopsy of the suggestive lesion is mandated. If there is no clinical suspicion for malignancy within the lesion, one of the following therapeutic modalities may be used.

1. **Cryosurgery.** Liquid nitrogen is applied to the lesion by using a cotton swab. This procedure effects excellent results, especially for smaller lesions.

2. **Shave biopsy.** After local anesthesia, the lesion is shaved off. This modality is excellent for diagnosis and **treatment**, especially of smaller lesions.

3. **5-Fluorouracil cream** (Efudex) applied b.i.d. for 4–6 weeks is quite satisfactory for the **treatment** of a large spreading actinic keratosis.

VI. **Seborrheic keratoses**

A. **Incidence**

These benign dermatologic lesions are extremely common. The prevalence approaches 100% in the elderly. **Risk factors** for development include familial factors. If familial, it is transmitted as an autosomal dominant trait. Other **risk factors** are the Leser–Trelat syndrome, which is a marked increase in seborrheic keratoses in association with an internal adenocarcinoma and, finally, increasing age.

B. The **specific manifestations** of these lesions include occurrence with a symmetric distribution on the trunk and proximal extremities. The lesions are often 1–1.5 cm in size, slowly increase in size over time, and are light brown to dark brown in color. They have a "stuck-on" appearance. They are nonpainful and nonpruritic.

C. **Natural history**

The lesions may remain constant or may slightly deepen in color or increase in size with time. These lesions are of the epidermis only and have no malignant potential.

D. The **specific evaluation and management** include making the clinical diagnosis by performing the evaluative tests described in Box 8-2 (page 430). Usually biopsy is not required, but if there is any question as to the diagnosis clinically, excisional biopsy should be performed. The specific modalities used to remove these lesions for cosmetic purposes include cryosurgery.

VII. Hemangiomas

This is a diverse group of benign lesions. Almost every human will, over the course of life, develop one or more of these lesions. A selected group of the most common types of hemangiomas is discussed here.

A. Spider hemangiomas

1. **Manifestations**

   These uncommon lesions are asymptomatic. The lesion consists of a pinhead-sized central vessel, usually an arteriole, with small vessels radiating centripetally from the center. It can be compared with a spider in appearance. Each lesion will blanch with the application of mild pressure. The lesions, which can be single or multiple, invariably occur on the skin of the shoulders and upper chest and back.

2. **Underlying causes** include severe hepatic dysfunction, pregnancy, and the use of relatively high-dose oral contraceptives.

3. The **specific evaluation** includes a urine pregnancy test in the appropriate patient. Abdominal examination and LFTs to look for signs of hepatic dysfunction are indicated in clinically appropriate patients. However, in most cases, no acute evaluation is indicated.

4. **Management**

   No **specific treatment** is necessary unless removal for cosmetic reasons is required. This is easily performed by electrosurgery. The electrosurgical probe on low current is placed into the central vessel.

B. Capillary hemangiomas

1. **Manifestations**

   These not uncommon lesions are asymptomatic. The lesion is a 3- to 5-mm red papule that may occur singly or in multiples on any skin surface, increasing in frequency with increasing age.

2. **Evaluation and management**

   No **specific evaluation** or intervention is required unless indicated for cosmetic purposes, in which case surgical excision or electrosurgical removal is effective.

C. Port-wine spots

1. **Manifestations**

   These relatively uncommon lesions are large, asymptomatic flat patches that may occur anywhere on the body. When they occur on the face, they are associated with the Sturge–Weber syndrome (i.e., a port-wine nevus with concurrent cerebellar and retinal hemangiomas). They are congenital and do not enlarge with increasing age.

2. **Evaluation**

   No **specific evaluation** is indicated unless Sturge–Weber syndrome is suspected, in which case a retinal examination looking for retinal hemangiomas and CT of the head looking for cerebellar hemangioma are indicated.

3. The **specific management** of the local lesion is cosmetic; however, few modalities have proved effective in providing cosmesis for large lesions. Referral to a plastic surgeon should be considered if the patient so desires.

VIII. **Consultation**

Problem	Service	Time
Any suspicious nevus	Dermatology	Required
Clinical suspicion for basal-cell carcinoma	Dermatology	Required
Clinical suspicion for squamous-cell carcinoma	Dermatology	Required
Clinical suspicion for malignant melanoma	Dermatology	Required
All skin lesions with a low clinical suspicion for malignancy	Dermatology	Elective

IX. **Indications for admission:** Few. Virtually all patients with malignant or nonmalignant neoplastic dermatologic disorders can be managed as outpatients.

Parasitic Infestations

I. **Scabies**
   A. The **specific manifestations** include severe pruritus affecting the trunk, back, and arms. The pruritus is especially severe at night. Epidemics may and often do occur because the organism that causes this entity is easily transmitted between individuals. Lesions from the infestation may occur on the skin anywhere on the body except for the head. On examination, the lesions are 1–3 mm in size and occur in straight lines, or "runs." An excellent place to look for these lesions is on sides of the digits. These lesions usually have areas of excoriation adjacent to them and may become pustular as a result of secondary bacterial infection.
   B. **Pathogenesis**
      The organism that causes this infestation is *Sarcoptes scabiei*. The organism burrows in the skin and causes the described lesions.
   C. The **specific evaluation** of this entity involves making the clinical diagnosis. If there is any question as to the diagnosis, a shave biopsy of one of the runs can be performed. On microscopic evaluation, the organism is often so demonstrated. A urine pregnancy test should be performed on all women of childbearing age.

D. Management

The **specific management** includes the following:

1. In all patients, one must treat any secondary bacterial infection with topical antibiotics (e.g., polymyxin B and bacitracin: Polysporin) and, if severe, with systemic antibiotics such as cephalexin (Keflex), 500 mg p.o., q.i.d., or dicloxacillin, 250 mg p.o., q.i.d., for 5 days.

2. All clothes and linen must be washed in hot water, >140°F, for 1–2 hours and then dried in a hot dryer for >20 min.

3. All family members must be treated concurrently.

4. **In nonpregnant adults:**

   a. Lindane (Kwell), 1% cream, is applied once to the entire body below the head and left on overnight. Lindane comes in 1% cream, lotion, or shampoo. It is contraindicated in pediatric or pregnant patients. Usually it is 100% effective.

   b. Alternatively, permethrin (Elimite), 5% cream, is applied once to the entire body except for the face and left on overnight. It is contraindicated in pregnant patients or those younger than 2 months. The advantages over lindane include the facts that it can be used in the hair and in younger patients. It is usually 95%–100% effective.

5. In children and pregnant women, crotamiton (Eurax), 10% cream or lotion, is used. The patient first bathes, and then applies the agent to all areas from the neck down. The process is repeated in 24 hr. It is >90% effective in eradicating the infestation.

II. Pediculosis (lice infestation)

A. The **manifestations** are specific to the site affected and include the acute onset of pruritus in the affected hair-containing areas. Examination discloses some erythema and excoriations about the hair infested with the organism. Furthermore, nits, or egg capsules, appear as whitish structures on the hair filaments. This organism is relatively easy to transmit and often will result in epidemics.

B. Pathogenesis

The organisms that cause this infestation include *Pediculus humanus capitis,* the head louse; *Pediculus humanus corporis,* the body louse; and *Phthirus pubis,* the genital hair louse, commonly called "crabs." The **underlying pathogenesis** is that the organism infests an area of hair-containing skin. The organism is transmitted by close body contact (i.e., it can be a sexually transmitted disease, or it can be transmitted by sharing combs or bed linen).

C. The **specific evaluation** of this entity involves making the clinical diagnosis by physical examination; presence of nits confirms the diagnosis.

D. The **specific management** includes the following:
1. In all patients, treat any secondary bacterial infection with topical antibiotics (e.g., polymyxin B and bacitracin: Polysporin) or, if severe, with systemic antibiotics such as cephalexin (Keflex), 500 mg p.o., q.i.d., or dicloxacillin, 250 mg p.o., q.i.d., for 5 days.
2. All clothes and linen must be washed in hot water (>140°F) for 1–2 hr, and then dried in a hot dryer for >20 min.
3. All family members must be treated concurrently.
4. In nonpregnant adults, **lindane (Kwell)** 1% cream, lotion, or shampoo, is applied to the affected hair and left on for 15–30 min. The nits should be combed out at 12 hr. This agent is contraindicated in pregnant women and children. The patient should be instructed to avoid mucous membranes with this substance.
5. In pregnant women and children, **pyrethrin, 0.3%,** or **piperonyl butoxide, 3%** (Nix, Rid, others), as a gel, shampoo, or solution, is applied to affected hair and adjacent skin, and then after 10–15 minutes washed out, with any nits concurrently combed out.

III. **Fleas**
A. The **specific manifestations** include the onset of generalized pruritus in a patient with a dog and/or cat at home. On examination, there may be multiple, tiny (1–2 mm) punctate lesions on the skin. The lesions are asymmetric in distribution and may occur anywhere on the skin surface. There may be, but not necessarily are, excoriations adjacent to the lesions. Often the patient relates that the pet has been excessively or incessantly scratching itself.
B. **Pathogenesis**
The organisms that cause this infestation include *Ctenocephalides felis,* in which the cat is the preferred host, and *Ctenocephalides canis,* in which the dog is the preferred host. The organism infests an area of hair-containing skin. The organism can be transmitted by sharing combs with an infested pet or by close contact with an infested pet. Humans are not the preferred host for these blood-sucking organisms.
C. The **specific evaluation and management** of this entity involve making the clinical diagnosis and treating the pet with an appropriate topical agent. This agent may be obtained over the counter or from a veterinarian.
1. The patient should steam clean all carpets and wash all linen in hot water and dry in a hot dryer for >20 minutes to kill any adult fleas and eggs.
2. Once the preferred host—the cat or dog—is treated, the infestation resolves. No other specific topical **treatment** is required for the patient.

(text continues on page 448)

Scaling Diseases (Table 8-6 and Figs. 8-8 and 8-9)

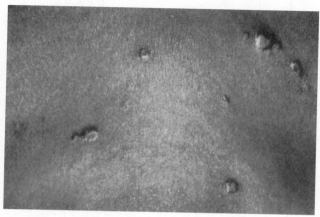

F I G U R E 8-8
Pruritic papules of lichen planus on the upper trunk.

Disease	History and Physical Examination Findings	Precipitating Factors or Events	Histopathology	Treatment
Lichen planus (Fig. 8-8, page 441)	Pruritic papules Symmetric distribution Mucous membranes and skin involved Violaceous appearing Wickham's striae present, i.e., white streaks on papular surface Koebner's sign present, i.e., lesions occur along linear scratch sites	Ulcerative colitis Vitiligo Graft-versus-host disease Medications Gold Quinine Tetracycline Streptomycin	IgG and C3 at basement membrane, and infiltration of T-cells into the dermis	Topical glucocorticoids (See Appendix, page 461) Discontinue or treat the underlying factor Dapsone 50 mg p.o. q.d. Psoralens with PUVA (long wave UV light) Referral to dermatology
Psoriasis (Fig. 8-9, page 444)	May secondarily blister Reddish plaques with scales Mild pruritus Nail pitting Asymmetric arthritis Koebner's sign present Scalp, elbows, and knees commonly affected, usually symmetric distribution Recurrent, chronic	Genetic predisposition: chromosome 17q HIV may cause a psoriasis-like rash	Hyperproliferation of epidermis and dermis Inflammation of the dermis and epidermis	Mild: a. Emollients, petrolatum-based, applied b.i.d. to plaques: 35% response rate b. Keratolytics, e.g., salicylic acid 2%–10%: softens the scaley layer of the plaque c. Coal tar used in shampoo to treat scalp psoriasis d. Topical steroids for short periods of time—1–2 weeks of high-dose steroid ointments, e.g., betamethasone (See Appendix, page 461)

	Clinical features	Associated	Diagnosis	Treatment
	Scales silvery Auspitz's sign—minute bleeding sites when a scale is removed	None	Nonspecific inflammation; biopsy is rarely needed	e. Calcipotriene ointment (50 µg/gram): A derivative of vitamin D *Severe:* a. Coal tar with concurrent UVB (300–320 nm) daily for 2–3 weeks is highly effective b. Methoxsalen 0.6 mg/kg p.o. 2hr before PUVA (320–340 nm) q.d. for 20 treatments—85% response rate c. Methotrexate 2.5–5.0 mg q.12hr for 3 doses q week d. Systemic steroids: Rarely used as risk of Cushing's and infection markedly increases; for acutely ill erythrodermic psoriasis
Pityriasis rosea	Spring and fall are periods of highest incidence Oval, scaly lesions Herald patch on trunk, followed by development of multiple patches on trunk, back, and chest			Diphenhydramine, 25–50 mg p.o. q.6hr Reassurance

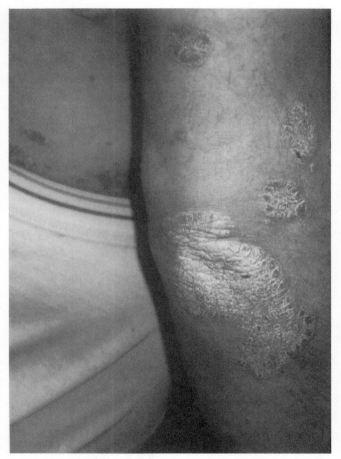

FIGURE 8-9
Scaly, mildly pruritic plaquelike lesions of psoriasis.

Fungal Skin Infections (Table 8-7 and Figs. 8-10 and 8-11)

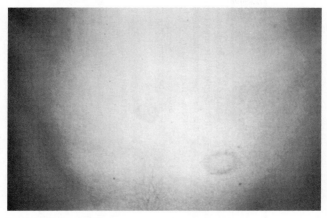

F I G U R E *8-10*
Tinea corporis on lower abdomen. Note the peripheral erythema with central clearing. Lesions are mildly pruritic.

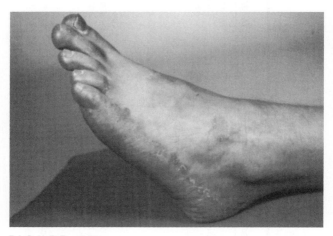

F I G U R E *8-11*
Tinea pedis on the left foot. Note the erythematous, scaly rash on plantar aspect of the foot.

TABLE 8-7
Fungal Skin Infections

Disease	History and Physical Examination	Diagnosis	Treatment
Tinea capitis	Scalp Multiple scaly areas with alopecia Mildly pruritic Kerion development: nodular pustule in the scalp	Microscopic analysis of hair pretreated with KOH, and/or fungal culture of hair	Itraconazole 200 mg p.o. q.d. for 6–8 wks Clotrimazole 1% to area b.i.d. If kerion present, use above and: KI, 5–10 drops p.o. q.d. for 10 days *and* Prednisone, 40 mg p.o. q.d. for 10 days *and* Dermatology consult
Tinea corporis (Fig. 8-10, page 445)	Pruritic Scaly, centrally clearing lesions with reddish margins Usually on trunk, back, thighs Asymmetric distribution Also known as ringworm	Scrape margins of lesion with a scalpel; add KOH to scrapings and look for hyphae	Clotrimazole 1% b.i.d. to affected areas If severe, fluconazole, 100 mg p.o. q.d. for 1 wk
Tinea cruris	Pruritic Intertriginous zones Sharply demarcated areas	KOH preparation of scrapings Clinical diagnosis	Loose-fitting underwear Absorbing powder (talc, Zeasorb, others) to affected areas

	Clinical Features	Diagnosis	Treatment
	Moist; some superficial skin breakdown can occur Usually occur in hot, humid weather		Clotrimazole 1% b.i.d. If severe, fluconazole, 200 mg p.o. q.d. for 14 days and wet compresses applied once daily, saturated with 1:10,000 $KMnO_2$
Tinea pedis or manuum (Fig. 8-11, page 445)	Erythema, pruritus Acutely can have small vesicles and weeping fissures develop in toe and finger webs Can develop onychomycosis	KOH preparation, look for hyphae	Absorbing powder (talc, Zeasorb, others) to affected areas Change socks daily Dry between toes Clotrimazole 1% b.i.d. Aluminum subacetate solution; soak feet for 20 min 3 times daily Clotrimazole 1% b.i.d.
Tinea unguium, i.e., onychomycosis	Toenails and/or fingernails friable, discolored, and brittle	Scrapings of nail with KOH, hyphae seen	Itraconazole 200 mg p.o. q.d. for 2–6 mo or more Terbinafine 250 mg p.o. q. A.M. for 4–10 mo; see page 425 Difficult to eradicate
Tinea versicolor	Macules, hypopigmented Trunk Mildly pruritic	Organism: *Pityrosporon orbiculare* (also known as *Malassezia furfur*) Clinical diagnosis Scrapings of affected areas with KOH, hyphae demonstrated	Lotion containing selenium sulfides* (e.g., Selsun Blue, others) q.d. for 1–2 wk Clotrimazole 1% b.i.d. to the affected area

* The appropriate use of selenium sulfide-containing lotion (1%–2.5%) is as follows. The patient should bathe and dry completely, then apply the lotion to all skin areas from the neck to the pubis and allow the lotion to dry. The lotion is washed off 2–4 hours later. This process is repeated on a weekly basis for 1–2 weeks. If fluconazole used, follow liver function test.

(text continued from page 440)

Urticaria (including insect stings; look also to Table 8-2: Dermatitis)

I. **Overall manifestations**

The **overall manifestations** of urticaria include the development of intensely pruritic wheals, commonly called hives, on any area of the skin. The lesions may be local or generalized. Often dermatographism is present. **Dermatographism** is demonstrated by gently scratching the skin surface with a pen cap or gloved fingernail. The scratching results in local erythema; therefore, one can actually "write" symbols or letters on the skin. The patient may have a history of angioedema. **Angioedema** is a phenomenon in which there is swelling of the deep tissues, often manifested as a swelling of the lips and other oropharyngeal mucous membranes. In severe cases, the angioedema can result in upper airway obstruction (Box 8-3).

II. **Classification of urticaria**

Urticaria may be classified into two categories, acute and chronic.

A. **Acute urticaria**

1. The **specific manifestations** of acute urticaria include the sudden onset of urticaria, which is invariably and intimately related temporally to a precipitating event. The patient may have a history of urticaria or of allergies to certain entities. Associated manifestations include hypotension, angioedema, and wheezing and shortness of breath as a result of bronchospasm.

2. The **underlying pathogenesis** is usually an immuno-globulin E (IgE)-mediated event in which the allergen stimulates production of IgE from B lymphocytes. The IgE, which is specific to that allergen, is incorporated into the plasma membrane of mast cells. If and when the allergen is presented again to the patient, it binds to the IgE on the mast-cell surface, which induces the release of histamine from the mast cell. Histamine acts on the smooth muscle of the airways and vasculature to cause the **specific manifestations** of **anaphylaxis,** i.e., urticaria, angioedema, bronchospasm, hypotension, and airway compromise.

3. **Precipitants**

The list of precipitants of acute urticaria is legion. A brief overview includes the following:

a. **Medications.** Virtually any medication can cause acute urticaria. Medications most commonly associated with urticaria include the β-lactam class of antibiotics (e.g., penicillin), the sulfa class of antibiotics, and the angiotensin-converting en-

B O X 8-3

Overall Evaluation and Management of Urticaria/Angioedema

Evaluation

1. ABCs (i.e., maintain the patient's airway, breathing, and cardiac function) via CPR and ACLS protocol.
2. Take a thorough history and perform a physical examination looking for the **specific manifestations** described in text.

Management

1. If there is any evidence of **anaphylaxis** (i.e., any bronchospasm, airway compromise, or hypotension), institute the following measures.
   a. Administer 0.3 mL epinephrine, 1:1000 s.c. or i.v. This can be repeated 2–4 times at intervals of 10 minutes.
   b. Administer the H_1-receptor antagonist diphenhydramine (Benadryl), 25–50 mg p.o., i.m., or i.v. Repeat in 30 minutes and every 4–6 hours thereafter as needed.
   c. Provide i.v. fluids with normal saline.
   d. Administer steroids in the form of a bolus of methylprednisolone (Solu-Medrol), 80 mg i.v.
   e. If there is any evidence of wheezing, administer a β_2-receptor agonist topically [e.g., metoproterenol (Alupent) or albuterol (Proventil)] or by hand-held nebulizer.
   f. Administer an H_2-receptor antagonist (e.g., cimetidine, 400 mg i.v., or ranitidine, 50 mg i.v., at the outset.
   g. Clean site of any site.

zyme inhibitor class of antihypertensive agents. The urticaria is usually generalized.
   b. Insect bites. Virtually all insect bites will result in local urticaria; however, certain patients experience generalized urticaria and even anaphylaxis. A bee or wasp bite will result in a localized urticarial reaction at the bite site in virtually all patients, and in a small but significant minority of patients, a generalized urticarial reaction occurs. Mosquito

bites result in a localized solitary urticarial lesion but virtually never a generalized urticarial reaction.

c. Foods and food additives, including dyes and preservatives, can result in localized angioedema and generalized urticaria.

4. The **specific evaluation** includes that described in Box 8-3 and making the clinical diagnosis.

5. **Management** includes determining the precipitating factor and identifying the patient as allergic to that factor. A Med-Alert bracelet stating this allergy should be prepared for the patient. If allergic to insect bites, the patient or a family member should obtain an Epi-Pen and be educated as to its use. Finally, all of these patients should have allergy consults for long-term follow-up.

B. **Chronic urticaria**

1. The **specific manifestations** of chronic urticaria include the fact that it is present for >2 weeks. The patient is unable to cite, even after extensive questioning, any overt precipitating event. The urticaria is usually generalized and can have associated angioedema. The patient may experience components of an acute anaphylactic reaction at any time during this process.

2. The **underlying pathogenesis** is a mediator-related effect on the smooth muscle of the bronchial airways or vasculature. The mechanism of mediator release is multifactorial and depends on the specific mediator. The most common mediators are histamine, usually via the IgE mechanism described previously; leukotrienes, prostaglandins; serotonin; and/or autoimmune-mediated dysfunction of the smooth muscle.

3. The **underlying causes** include vasculitis, C1-esterase deficiency, the prodromal phase of hepatitis B, medications, cold-induced, and idiopathic.

4. The **specific evaluation** includes making the clinical diagnosis and performing the evaluations described in Box 8-3. Further evaluation should be directed toward ascertaining and defining the underlying cause of the urticaria. These include obtaining serum electrolytes, blood urea nitrogen (BUN), and creatinine levels and urinalysis to look for any concurrent renal dysfunction or glomerulonephritis. Further **specific evaluation** includes obtaining an erythrocyte sedimentation rate (ESR), antinuclear antibody (ANA), rheumatoid factor (RF), CH50, C3, and C4 levels. The ESR, ANA, or RF titer may be evaluated in a vasculitis, whereas the complement levels may be concurrently decreased. Further **specific evaluation** can include ob-

taining a hepatitis B panel (IgM Hbs and HbsAg), plasma cryoglobulins, a plasma C1-esterase level, and a biopsy of one of the skin lesions.

5. The **specific management**, in addition to that described in Box 8-3, is directed toward the underlying cause. Specific interventions on a long-term basis include the following measures.

   a. H_1-receptor antagonists on an as-needed or scheduled basis. These can include diphenhydramine (Benadryl), 25–50 mg p.o., q.i.d., or hydroxyzine (Atarax), 25 mg p.o., q.i.d., or astemizole (Hismanal), 10 mg/day.

   b. H_2-receptor antagonists on a scheduled basis. These can include cimetidine (Tagamet), 400 mg p.o., b.i.d., or ranitidine (Zantac), 150 mg p.o., b.i.d.

   c. If predominantly cold-induced and not as the result of a cryoglobulinemia, cyproheptadine, 4 mg p.o., q.i.d., is effective. Recommend to the patient that the patient move to a warm climate and minimize exposure to cold.

   d. If severe and not related to hepatitis B, steroids (e.g., prednisone, 40–60 mg p.o., q.d.) may be of efficacy.

   e. If C1-esterase deficiency with acute angioedema, may administer methyltestosterone, 10 mg p.o., q.d.

6. **Prevention** should include:

   a. Watch for wasps.

   b. Prescribe and instruct patient to carry an Epi-PEN.

   c. Desensitization with venom immunotherapy.

III. **Consultation**

Service	Time
Allergy	Urgent

IV. **Indications for admission:** Any evidence of anaphylaxis, angioedema, or airway compromise.

Viral Dermatologic Lesions

I. **Herpes labialis**

   A. The **specific manifestations** of this entity include the acute onset of a unilateral, single group of vesicles on the perioral areas, including the lips. The vesicles last for ~2–3 days, crust over, and resolve in 7–10 days. The lesions are commonly referred to as fever blisters or cold sores. They may recur, with asymptomatic periods between episodes lasting up to several years. Events that precipitate these lesions include fever, any upper respiratory tract infection, trauma to the area, or generalized stress.

B. The **underlying pathogenesis** of herpes labialis is an infection of the perioral mucous membranes with the DNA virus, herpes simplex virus (80% are HSV-1; 20% are HSV-2). Most of the population becomes infected with the virus as children as the result of kissing of the child by a parent or sibling who has active infection. After the onset of vesicles, there is viral shedding for 5 days. After the acute vesicular stage, the virus becomes dormant in the sensory ganglion of the dermatome involved (i.e., the trigeminal ganglion), only to become recurrently symptomatic at a later date.

C. The **specific evaluation** includes making the clinical diagnosis from the history and physical examination findings. In the vast majority of cases, no further examinations are required, but if there is any question as to the diagnosis, a Tzanck smear of vesicular contents can be performed. The Tzanck smear will show large, bizarre, multinucleated cells, a finding consistent with HSV infection.

D. The **specific management** is usually minimal, as the infection is usually self-limited. A course of systemic acyclovir administered in a dose of 200 mg p.o., 5 times per day for 7 days, is effective in the therapy of HSV. Acyclovir decreases viral shedding and, therefore, the risk of transmission.

   1. As with other processes, prevention is important. Thus someone with active herpes labialis should never kiss anyone else until the lesions have resolved. Parents and grandparents should be educated to this fact, so as not to transmit this viral infection to infants, toddlers, and children.

   2. The clinician must monitor for and aggressively treat any complications. Two complications that can occur in patients with herpes labialis are keratitis and mucocutaneous herpes simplex.

      a. **Keratitis.** The acute onset of corneal inflammation concurrent with or after an episode of herpes labialis. This infection is severe and on fluorescein examination reveals a dendritic pattern of ulcerations on the cornea. If not aggressively treated, it leads to visual loss. See section on Red Eye in Chapter 13, page 605.

      b. **Mucocutaneous herpes simplex.** This occurs in patients who are immunocompromised, especially with any compromise of cell-mediated immunity, such as patients with acquired immunodeficiency syndrome (AIDS) or those undergoing chemotherapy for malignant neoplastic lesions. The infection may be unilateral or bilateral and consists of rapidly spreading vesicles of the skin and mucous membranes with concurrent painful sloughing of the superficial skin and mucosa. This can be caused by HSV-1 or -2 and requires aggressive **treatment.** If the patient has no other underlying reason for immunocompromise, the patient has, by definition, AIDS.

   i. The **specific management** includes placing the patient under blood and body fluid precautions, obtaining a serum human immunodeficiency virus (HIV) antibody level, and administering acyclovir, 200 mg p.o., 5 times per day for 14 days, or 10 mg/kg/24 hours i.v., in q.8hr dosing for 7–10 days, followed by long-term therapy with acyclovir, 200 mg p.o., q.A.M. indefinitely.

   ii. Refer to section on HIV Infection in Chapter 6, page 320.

II. Herpes genitalis

HSV-2 infection. Refer to section on Sexually Transmitted Diseases in Chapter 6, page 340.

III. Herpes zoster

   A. The **specific manifestations** of this entity include the acute onset of erythema and vesicles unilaterally in the region of a single dermatome (see Fig. 8-12). There usu-

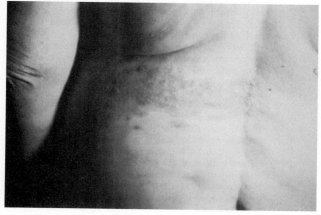

F I G U R E   8-12
Herpes zoster. Unilateral, painful, vesicular rash over one dermatome.

ally are associated hyperesthesia and significant pain. The vesicles last for 2–3 days and then crust over and slowly resolve over a 3–4 week period. Pain may last for a time after the lesions resolve and may lead to the chronic pain syndrome, postherpetic neuralgia. This entity is commonly called shingles.

B. The **underlying pathogenesis** of herpes zoster is infection with the same DNA virus that causes varicella (i.e., chicken pox). After the acute varicella infection, the varicella-zoster virus remains in the sensory ganglia of the spinal cord and cranial nerves. After a prolonged quiescent period, the virus is reactivated and the manifestations of zoster occur. Events that precipitate or are **risk factors** for the development of herpes zoster include increasing age, immunosuppression (e.g., with steroids, chemotherapy, or AIDS), and/or any generalized stress.

C. The **specific evaluation** includes making the clinical diagnosis from the history and physical examination findings. In the vast majority of cases, no further examinations are required.

D. The **specific management** includes the following measures.

   1. Administer acyclovir, 800 mg p.o., five times per day for 7–10 days. If initiated within 48 hours of the onset of vesicles, this will decrease the duration of viral shedding and symptoms of disease. In the rare case of acyclovir resistance (i.e., the virus does not have thymidine kinase), use **foscarnet** as an alternate agent. Concurrent early administration of prednisone also may afford palliation (e.g., prednisone, 60 mg p.o., q.d., for 1 week, 40 mg p.o., q.d., for the second week, and 20 mg p.o., for the third week.

   2. Place the patient on respiratory and contact isolation/pregnancy precautions. During the vesicular stage, it is transmissible, and anyone (including a fetus) who has not had varicella (chicken pox) is susceptible to infection.

   3. The **treatment** of postherpetic neuralgia includes the administration of narcotic agents as needed and the administration of topical capsaicin (Zostrix) cream, 0.025%–0.075% (start with low dose and slowly increase the concentration). This agent, applied to the dermatome after the acute lesions have healed, on a b.i.d. dosing for 10 days, increases substance P, thus increasing intrinsic analgesia at the level of the nerves. Finally, if pain is intractable, referral to a pain clinic is necessary.

IV. Varicella

   A. The **specific manifestations** of this entity include the acute onset of fever, malaise, mild rhinorrhea, and multi-

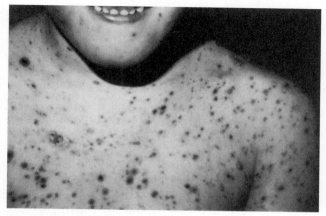

F I G U R E **8-13**
Varicella (chicken pox). Note the various crops of papules, which
evolve into vesicles. The vesicles in turn evolve into pustules, which
then crust over and heal.

ple vesicles. The vesicles become, in 3–4 days, pustules,
which subsequently rupture and crust over. These then
slowly resolve and heal without scarring for the next 5
days. A new group of vesicles, sometimes referred to as
individual crops, occurs every 2–3 days until several
crops of vesicles in various stages of evolution are present. The disease is usually self-limited and lasts for a
total of 14–18 days (i.e., four to five crops of lesions. The
lesions are usually painless but moderately pruritic in
the crust stage. The first crop usually occurs on the trunk,
with subsequent crops being progressively peripheral
(see Fig. 8-13).

B. The **underlying pathogenesis** of this acute viral infection
is a DNA herpesvirus. The virus is transmitted from another person with acute zoster or varicella by aerosol
to be inhaled by the patient. The incubation period is
~10–14 days after exposure.

C. The **specific evaluation** includes making the clinical diagnosis by history and physical examination. In the vast
majority of cases, no further examinations are required.

D. The **specific management** is, in the vast majority of cases,
symptomatic only. The patient can be afforded antipyretic and analgesic relief with acetaminophen and topical
use of calamine lotion applied b.i.d. The calamine lotion will decrease any pruritus. Salicylates should be

avoided, given the potential association of aspirin and viral syndrome with Reye's syndrome.

1. The clinician must watch for the development of complications, especially in older (>15 years) patients and those who are immunosuppressed. In such patients, the risk for complications, including mortality, is increased 25-fold. The most dramatic complication is pneumonitis.

   a. **Varicella pneumonitis** manifests with severe, diffuse interstitial infiltrates, an increased A-ao$_2$ gradient, hypoxemia, and dry cough, and can lead to respiratory failure and death.

   b. The **specific management** of varicella pneumonitis includes admission to the hospital, supportive care with oxygen, and the administration of parenteral acyclovir, 10 mg/kg hours in q.8hr divided doses. In the rare case of acyclovir resistance (i.e., the virus does not have thymidine kinase), use foscarnet as an alternate agent.

E. **Prevention** in adults is therefore extremely important. Any individual who is older than 15 years and has not had a case of chicken pox should have a varicella titer performed. If the antibody titer is minimal (i.e., no antibodies present), the individual should receive the varicella vaccination.

V. **Molluscum contagiosum**
   A. The **specific manifestations** of this entity include the insidious onset of and slow increase in the number of firm, painless papules on the trunk, face, arms, and genitals. Each of these lesions occurs on a narrow base [i.e., each one is umbilicated (see Fig. 8-14)]. There are no associated systemic symptoms or signs. The lesions last for weeks to months without significantly changing and then may spontaneously resolve, especially if there is minor trauma to specific papules.

   B. The **underlying pathogenesis** is a DNA virus in the poxvirus family infecting the skin. These lesions are transmitted by direct contact, either self to self (i.e., "autospread") or from one person to another.

   C. The **specific evaluation** includes making the clinical diagnosis by history and physical examination. In the vast majority of cases, no further examinations are required. If there is any question as to the diagnosis or if any lesion is different and/or suggestive of a malignant lesion, excisional biopsy must be performed.

   D. The **specific management** is minimal: these lesions either spontaneously resolve or disappear after minor trauma. Thus superficial trauma to each lesion with an electrosur-

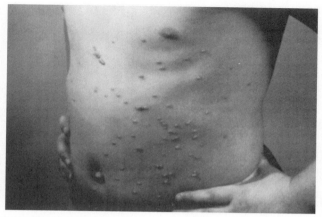

F I G U R E 8-14
Molluscum contagiosum on the trunk abdomen.

gical probe or with liquid nitrogen will safely and easily cure the lesions of this viral infection. Each lesion must be individually traumatized to effect resolution.

VI. **Condylomata acuminata**

  A. The **specific manifestations** of this entity include the insidious onset of single or multiple rough papules on or adjacent to the perianal, vulvar, perineal, scrotal, or penile skin. The lesions are usually asymptomatic and painless, even when large (see Fig. 8-15). The lesions increase in number and slowly enlarge in size from papular lesions to large, exuberant cauliflower-like lesions. Spontaneous regression of the lesions is uncommon. These lesions have been correlated with the development of the malignant neoplastic lesions including squamous-cell carcinoma and cervical carcinoma.

  B. The **underlying pathogenesis** is infection of the genital skin and mucous membranes by HPV, especially viral types 16 and 18. This is one of the most common sexually transmitted diseases in the United States today, and its incidence is increasing. Of concern is that a significant minority of these infections are in patients who have subclinical disease; however, this infection, even if not clinically demonstrable, can be transmitted by virtually any sexual activity.

  C. The **specific evaluation** includes making the clinical diagnosis by history and physical examination. If any le-

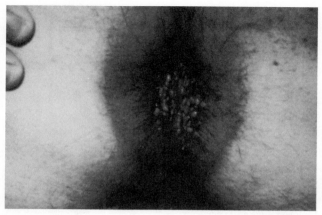

F I G U R E   **8-15**
Condylomata acuminata on the anal and perineal areas.

sion is atypical-appearing or suggestive of a malignant
lesion, excisional biopsy is mandated.

1. Often the examination should include stereoscopic
   microscope examinations of the affected areas. This
   technique can demonstrate smaller, earlier, and therefore easier-to-treat lesions. The stereoscope used is a
   colposcope if used to examine female subjects or an
   androscope and anoscope when used to examine
   male genitalia.

2. The use of **acetic acid** is another technique to demonstrate the extent of the condylomata and to demonstrate small, early lesions. Gauze saturated with 5%
   acetic acid (vinegar) is placed on the skin. The acetic
   acid will turn the condylomatous tissue white. When
   this is used in conjunction with stereoscopy, early,
   small lesions can be visualized and treated, by using
   the schemas described subsequently, with great precision.

D. The **specific management** includes basic education on
   methods of safe sex. Specific modalities used in the **treatment** of these lesions include the following:

   1. **Podophyllin,** 25% in benzoin. Apply this directly to
      the lesion, dry, and wash off 6–8 hours later. Anesthe-
      sia is not required. The mechanism of action is that
      it causes direct destruction/necrosis of the infected
      and normal tissue; therefore, one must be precise in

treatment. Treatment can be repeated every 1–2 weeks for three to four cycles. This treatment is 50%–80% effective, especially in small lesions.

2. **Trichloroacetic acid (TCA),** 50% and 80% solutions. This is one of the best modalities in the treatment of condylomata acuminata because, with proper instruction, the patient can self-apply it to the lesions. Anesthesia is not required. This agent causes direct destruction/necrosis of the infected and normal tissues; therefore, one must be precise in treatment.

   a. The 50% solution is applied to the lesion b.i.d. and allowed to dry. The duration of this regimen is for 3 consecutive days per week for 3 consecutive weeks.

   b. If no improvement occurs, the same procedure and schedule is used for the 80% solution. Because the solution causes significant necrosis of both infected and normal tissue, care must be taken to optimize precision in treatment.

3. **Surgery.** Direct surgical resection is indicated if the lesions have not responded to 6–8 weeks of aggressive topical treatment or if there is any suspicion of a concurrent neoplasm.

   a. **Direct surgical** resection is effective, with a cure rate of ≥90%.

   b. **Cryosurgery** with liquid nitrogen is also effective and can be applied by the primary care physician, but is not indicated if there is any suspicion of malignancy.

   c. Electrosurgery and laser ablation are effective but should not be performed, given the well-documented risk of aerosolization of the lesions with live virus with the potential to cause respiratory HPV infections, especially laryngeal nodules, in the physician or the patient.

VII. **Verruca vulgaris**

A. The **specific manifestations** include the insidious onset of papules on the skin of the distal upper or lower extremities. The papules have a rough texture, and their centers can develop minute black spots deep in the papule itself. These lesions are ubiquitous; the lifetime prevalence is virtually 100% for humans. These lesions, which are painless and virtually asymptomatic, are commonly known as warts. There are two major types of warts, the **common wart,** which occurs on the fingers, and the **plantar wart,** which is quite deep and occurs on the plantar aspects of the feet. These lesions can slowly increase in size and number but can, quite spontaneously, resolve. An increased incidence of SCCA has been reported in warts located adjacent to the nail folds (i.e., periungual warts).

B. The **underlying pathogenesis** is an infection of keratinized skin on the hands or feet with the DNA virus, HPV.

C. The **specific evaluation** includes making the clinical diagnosis by history and physical examination. If any lesion is atypical appearing or suggestive of a malignant lesion, excisional biopsy is mandated.

D. The **specific management** of these lesions is to destroy the wart with minimal damage to the adjacent tissue. It requires the destruction of the tissue deep into the dermis itself. One or more of several modalities can be used.

   1. **Cryosurgery** with liquid nitrogen to the wart itself. This procedure, by using a cotton swab to apply the liquid nitrogen to the lesion, must be repeated on a weekly basis until the wart is completely destroyed.

   2. **TCA in saturated solution.** Apply to base of wart by using a cotton swab, and allow to dry. Excise any destroyed tissue with scissors in 24 hours. Repeat the process on a daily basis until the wart is completely destroyed.

   3. **Salicylic acid,** 10% solution (Compound W). Apply to wart by using a cotton swab every evening for 7 days. Trim off the destroyed tissue each morning. This modality is clearly inferior in effectiveness relative to the previously described modalities.

VIII. **Consultation**

Problem	Service	Time
Any suspicious lesion	Dermatology	Urgent
Periungual wart	Dermatology	Required
Any evidence of HSV keratitis	Ophthalmology	Emergent
Condylomata acuminata refractory to treatment	General surgery	Required
Varicella pneumonitis	Infectious diseases	Urgent
Mucocutaneous HSV	Infectious diseases	Urgent

IX. **Indications for admission:** Parenteral acyclovir, or evidence of varicella pneumonitis.

Appendix

Selected Topical Glucocorticoids

Agent	*Fluorinated*	*Potency*
Hydrocortisone Cream: 0.25%, 0.5%, and 1% Ointment: 0.5% and 1% Lotion: 0.25%, 0.5%, and 1%	No	Low (I)
Triamcinolone (Kenalog) Cream: 0.1% Lotion: 0.1%	Yes	Low to moderate (II)
Triamcinolone (Aristocort) Cream: 0.5%	Yes	Moderate (II)
Fluocinonide (Lidex) Cream: 0.05% Ointment: 0.05%	Yes	High (III)
Amcinonide (Cyclocort) Ointment: 0.1%	Yes	High (III)
Betamethasone dipropionate (Diprolene) Ointment: 0.05%	Yes	High (III)

NOTE: Topical glucocorticoids that are fluorinated should not be used on the face, as they are associated with the development of telangiectases and other cosmetic sequelae. Ointment should be used if cracking of skin is present, as creams increase the itching.

Class I, lowest potency; class II, moderate potency; class III, high potency.

Bibliography

Acne Vulgaris
Bondi EE: Topical retinoid therapy. Am Fam Pract 1989;39:269–272.
Quan M, Strick RA: Management of acne vulgaris. Am Fam Pract 1988; 38:207–217.
Shalita AR, et al: Acne vulgaris. J Am Acad Dermatol 1987;16:410–412.

Blistering Diseases
Fine JD: Management of acquired bullous skin diseases. N Engl J Med 1995;333:1475–1483.
Heimbach DM, et al: Toxic epidermal necrolysis. JAMA 1987;257:2171–2175.
Imber MJ, et al: The immunopathology of bullous pemphigoid. Clin Dermatol 1987;5:81–89.
Stanley JR: Pemphigus. JAMA 1990;264:1714–1717.

Dermatitis
Buckley RH, Mathews KP: Common allergic skin diseases. JAMA 1982; 248:2611.

Hanifin JM: Atopic dermatitis. J Am Acad Dermatol 1982;6:1.
Shuster S: The aetiology of dandruff and the mode of action of therapeutic agents. Br J Dermatol 1984;3:236.

Erythemas

Horio T, et al: Potassium iodide in the treatment of erythema nodosum and nodular vasculitis. Arch Dermatol 1981;117:29.
Schosser RH: The erythema multiforme spectrum: diagnosis and treatment. Curr Concepts Skin Dis 1985;6:6.

Neoplasia

Beacham BE: Solar-induced epidermal tumors in the elderly. Am Fam Pract 1990;42:153–160.
Greene MH, et al: Acquired precursors of cutaneous malignant melanoma. N Engl J Med 1985;312:91–97.
Koh HK: Cutaneous melanoma. N Engl J Med 1991;325:171–182.
Rhodes AR, et al: Risk factors for cutaneous melanoma. JAMA 1987;258: 3146–3154.
Tobinick EL: Basal-cell carcinoma. Am Fam Pract 1987;36:219–224.

Parasitic Infestations

Brodell RT, Helms SE: Office dermatologic testing: the scabies preparation. Am Fam Pract 1991;44:505–508.
Burkhart CG: Scabies: an epidemiologic reassessment. Ann Intern Med 1983;98:498.
Witkowski JA, Parish LC: Scabies. JAMA 1984;252:1318–1327.

Scaling Diseases

Gardner SS, McKay M: Seborrhea, psoriasis, and the papulosquamous dermatoses. Primary Care 1989;16:739–763.
Greaves MW, et al: Treatment of psoriasis. N Engl J Med 1995;332:581–588.
Truhan AP: Pityriasis rosea. Am Fam Pract 1984;29:193–196.

Fungal Skin Infections

Brodell RT, et al: Office dermatologic testing: the KOH preparation. Am Fam Pract 1991;43:2061–2065.
Pariser DM: Superficial fungal infections. Postgrad Med 1990;87:205–212.

Urticaria

Matthews KP: Urticaria and angioedema. J Allergy Clin Immunol 1983;72:1.
Zamm AV: Chronic urticaria: a practical approach. Cutis 1972;9:27.

Viral Dermatologic Lesions

Arbesfeld DM, Thomas I: Cutaneous herpes simplex virus infections. Am Fam Pract 1991;43:1655–1664.
Bolton RA: Nongenital warts: classification and treatment options. Am Fam Pract 1991;43:2049–2056.
Carmichael JK: Treatment of herpes zoster and postherpetic neuralgia. Am Fam Pract 1991;44:203–210.

Ferenczy A: Diagnosis and treatment of anogenital warts in the male patient. Primary Care Cancer 1990;Sept:11–20.

Zazove P, et al: Genital human papillomavirus infection. Am Fam Pract 1991;43:1279–1290.

Wald A, et al: Suppression of subclinical shedding of herpes simplex virus type 2 with acyclovir. Ann Intern Med 1996;124:8–15.

Miller DM, et al: HPV: treatment options for warts. Am Fam Pract 1996;53:135–143.

Whitley RJ, et al: Acyclovir: a decade later. N Engl J Med 1992;327:782–788.

—D.D.B.

Chapter 9

Endocrine Disorders

Diabetes Mellitus

Diabetes mellitus is quite prevalent in the United States. If uncontrolled and unchecked, it can result in significant, even life-threatening acute and chronic sequelae, all of which are preventable with early diagnosis and intervention. The overall prevalence of disease in the U.S. population is ~5%.

The **pathophysiology** of diabetes mellitus is quite complex and is continuing to be elucidated. Pertinent is the physiology of energy generation and glucose catabolism. All cells in the body require energy and therefore substrates for energy generation. Although several substrates, including proteins, amino acids, and fatty acids, can serve this function of energy generation, the most efficient and effective substrate is glucose. In fact, glucose is required for normal cell function, especially neuronal function.

Glucose is a monosaccharide that is absorbed from foodstuffs through the gastrointestinal (GI) tract. For glucose to be used as a source of energy (as a substrate for energy production), it must cross into the cell. Cell entry is controlled by the hormone insulin. Insulin is a relatively small polypeptide that is secreted by the beta islet cells in the pancreas.

Once within the cells, glucose is catabolized by the glycolytic pathway and Krebs cycle and coupled with aerobic respiration to produce the basic energy molecule of the cell, adenosine triphosphate (ATP).

All hormones have target cells on which they effect change. Within the surfaces of these cells are specific receptors, which are requisite for hormone activity. The target cells for insulin are virtually all the cells of the body, and specific insulin receptors in the plasma membranes of these target cells are required for insulin activity and therefore the generation of energy from glucose.

The **pathophysiology** of diabetes mellitus is related to the interworking of insulin and its specific cell receptors. A deficiency in either or both can result in the basic features of diabetes mellitus and forms the basis of the classification paradigm used for diabetes mellitus.

I. Pathogenesis

Two basic, interdependent features of diabetes mellitus are an increase in glucose in the plasma and an overall marked decrease in intracellular glucose, the cell's major substrate for energy production. The result is the pathophysiologic paradox of effective cellular starvation in the setting of ample amounts of glucose in the fluids bathing the cells.

The starving cells turn to other, less optimal substrates for energy production—proteins, amino acids, and fatty acids. These substrates not only are less efficient in energy production but also are primarily for anabolism (i.e., the synthesis of structures) and not for catabolism.

A specific outcome of the utilization of fatty acids and to a lesser extent amino acids for energy generation is the development of ketone bodies. These small anionic molecules, which include β-hydroxybutyrate, acetoacetate, and acetone, produce a systemic metabolic acidosis with an elevated anion gap.

II. Classification

The **classification** of diabetes mellitus is based on the physiology. There are two different pathophysiologic categories of diabetes mellitus, insulin-dependent diabetes mellitus and non–insulin-dependent diabetes mellitus.

A. Insulin-dependent diabetes mellitus (IDDM)

IDDM is a deficiency, either actual or relative, in the hormone insulin. The central feature is insulinopenia. The receptors are usually normal or even upregulated (increased in quantity or effectiveness), but without insulin, glucose cannot enter the cell. The deficiency in insulin occurs as a result of destruction of beta islet cells within the pancreas itself. Causes of IDDM include the following conditions.

1. **Autoimmune destruction.** Certain human leukocyte antigen (HLA) types and the coincidence of IDDM with other autoimmune disorders support this pathophysiologic mechanism.

2. **Virus mediated.** This is probably an indirect but significant mechanism in which the beta cells are damaged or destroyed by the immune system's fight against a viral infection, usually paramyxovirus.

3. **Recurrent pancreatitis.** Recurrent pancreatitis will result in destruction of the exocrine and endocrine pancreas (see section on Pancreatitis in Chapter 2, page 69).

B. Non–insulin-dependent diabetes mellitus (NIDDM)

Non–insulin-dependent diabetes mellitus (NIDDM), unlike IDDM, is a problem not with insulin, but with the receptor on which it works. It is postulated that receptors are decreased in number or in effectiveness at or immediately adjacent to the receptor (i.e., postreceptor level). Data demonstrate that the defect is in the insulin-related synthesis of glycogen (glucose transport phosphorylation) in each cell, thereby decreasing the glucose use by the cell and increasing plasma glucose. Insulin resistance in these patients involves all cells; however, the most significant site of resistance is in the cells of skeletal muscle. This results in the ultimate paradox of effective cellular starvation in the setting of excessive glucose and excessive insulin in an obese patient. In NIDDM, the glucose will, to certain degrees, enter the cells, and therefore the degree of intracellular starvation is less. This decreases the use of fatty acids and proteins, and therefore ketone bodies are not formed. Therefore NIDDM is noninsulinopenic and usually is not ketotic; however, there is a subset of NIDDM patients, especially older patients who develop ketosis during acute decompensation but do not require long-term insulin. **Risk factors** for the development of NIDDM include truncal obesity. Obese patients have a decrease in the quantity or effectiveness of insulin receptors. Furthermore, NIDDM has a strong genetic basis. First-degree relatives of patients with NIDDM have a 40% lifetime risk of developing diabetes mellitus.

III. **Overall manifestations (Box 9-1)**

The **overall manifestations** of IDDM or NIDDM are based on the **pathophysiology.**

A. **Polyuria and polydipsia**

Polyuria is an increased frequency and volume of urination, and polydipsia is an increase in the quantity of fluid ingested as a result of an increased thirst. Nocturia, or frequent urination at night, is a nonspecific manifestation that can be a marker for polyuria. In a patient who cannot maintain thirst, intravascular volume depletion with its **specific manifestations** of orthostatic hypotension and tachycardia may develop. The **underlying pathogenesis** is significant hyperglycemia with resultant glycosuria (i.e., loss of glucose, and with it water, in the urine).

B. **Blurred vision.** The **underlying pathogenesis** is an increase in glucose and therefore of water within the lens itself, causing a change in the refractory profile of the lens and visual blurring.

C. **Recurrent dermatologic fungal infections**

1. Tinea cruris, severe.
2. Tinea pedis with onychomycosis.
3. Candidal balanitis, i.e., infection and inflammation of the foreskin in a male.
4. Candidal vaginitis.

(text continues on page 470)

BOX 9-1

Overall Evaluation and Management of Hyperglycemia

Evaluation

1. Take a history and perform a physical examination with emphasis on the following features.
   a. **Risk factors** for the development of diabetes mellitus, including a strong family history, obesity, a history of diabetes during pregnancy, current pregnancy, or Native American ancestry.
   b. Current medications, as certain medications can result in hyperglycemia, the most common being glucocorticoids.
   c. Any overt sequelae of diabetes mellitus (i.e., neuropathy or retinopathy). Query the patient and examine for any peripheral or autonomic neuropathies, such as carpal tunnel syndrome, ulnar tunnel syndrome, impotence, lack of sweating, or an inappropriate lack of tachycardia on arising. Funduscopy is mandatory at baseline to look for any proliferative or nonproliferative retinal changes.
   d. Assess for concurrent **risk factors** for the development of atherosclerotic disease or nephropathy. These include hypertension, a family history of early (i.e., onset before age 60 years) atherosclerosis, a history of hyperlipidemia, and clinical manifestations of hyperlipidemia (i.e., xanthelasma or xanthomas).
2. If the patient has no overt manifestations but is at risk for the development of diabetes mellitus, determine a screening fasting glucose level.
   a. The screening test result is abnormal and diagnostic of diabetes mellitus if the fasting glucose level is, on two separate occasions, >126 mg/dL.
   b. The screening test result is abnormal but not diagnostic of diabetes mellitus if the fasting glucose level is >115 mg/dL.
3. Other diagnostic markers for diabetes mellitus include:
   a. Diabetic ketoacidosis.
   b. Any random plasma glucose level >200 mg/dL.
   c. An abnormal response to a 50-g glucose oral glucose tolerance test in a pregnant female.

(continued)

B O X   9-1 (continued)

4. Determine electrolyte, blood urea nitrogen (BUN), and creatinine levels for baseline purposes. Look for a decrease in tco_2, potentially indicative of an acidosis.
5. Perform urinalysis, looking for proteinuria, ketonuria, or glycosuria. The dipstick is positive only when there is >360 mg albumin in the urine.
   If no protein on routine dipstick analysis, determine a urine albumin level via dipstick each year to look for microalbuminuria (i.e., >40 mg of albumin in the urine).
6. Obtain a 12-lead electrocardiogram (ECG) for baseline purposes.
7. Determine the blood pressure to look for concurrent hypertension. Hypertension is an independent risk factor for the development of nephropathy and atherosclerotic disease.
8. Obtain an ophthalmology consultation at baseline.
9. Obtain a baseline lipid panel, including triglycerides, total cholesterol, and high-density lipoprotein (HDL) cholesterol, looking for concurrent hyperlipidemia.

Management

1. Educate the patient in foot care, pedicures, and so forth.
2. Institute dietary modifications.
   a. Obese patients should lose weight. This will reduce any concurrent hypertension and, in NIDDM, will increase the number or activity of insulin receptors and increase the sensitivity of skeletal muscle to insulin.
   b. Obese patients should decrease their overall caloric intake.
   c. The fat content should be decreased to <30% of total calories.
   d. The carbohydrates should be increased to ~60% of total calories.
   e. The saturated fat content should be decreased to <10% of total calories.
3. Instruct the patient to exercise. Exercise is an integral component of management in that it aids in weight reduction, increases the number and sensitiv-

(continued)

B O X 9-1 *(continued)*

ity of insulin receptors, and increases HDL cholesterol.
  a. Isotonic or aerobic exercise is recommended as it
will increase cardiovascular performance, increase
HDL cholesterol, and decrease hypertension. The
exercise should be performed 3 times per week.
Swimming, walking, and cycling are the best.
  b. Isometric exercise is relatively contraindicated as
it can precipitate a retinal tear or intraocular hemorrhage in a patient with retinopathy.
4. A Med-Alert bracelet should be worn by all patients
with diabetes mellitus. The information should include the diagnosis and the agents used in glycemic
control.
5. Educate the patient in the manifestations and acute
treatment of **hypoglycemia**. Both the patient and the
spouse should receive this information. The manifestations of hypoglycemia include those secondary to
catecholamine release (i.e., diaphoresis, tachycardia,
and tremor) and those resulting from the hypoglycemia itself (i.e., confusion).
  a. The acute intervention in hypoglycemia is intake
of glucose. The best source of rapidly available
sugar is honey. The patient should always carry
some source of sugar, such as a candy bar or
sugar cube.
6. Educate the patient in finger-stick glucose determinations. Determining finger-stick glucose values at
home is useful to fine-tune the control of diabetes
mellitus and to confirm any episodes of hypoglycemia. Thus all patients should learn the skill of glucose monitoring by finger stick and have the equip-
ment, supplies, and glucometer readily available.
Monitoring need not be done daily in all cases; in
fact, in patients with type II diabetes mellitus, once
per week is adequate, unless the patient becomes
symptomatically ill.
7. **IDDM:** Initiate insulin. See text and Box 9-2 (page
472) for details.
  NIDDM: Initiate aggressive dietary and exercise interventions. May need to initiate oral hypoglycemic
agents and/or metformin or, in extremely difficult
cases, insulin. See text and Box 9-2 for specifics.

(continued)

B O X   9-1 (continued)

8. Outcomes/Goals of therapy:
   a. **General:** Prevent acute and chronic sequelae of uncontrolled diabetes mellitus.
   b. **IDDM:** Follow up with finger-stick glucose levels on q.A.M., q HS and 1 hour postprandial to keep the postprandial plasma glucose 140–200 mg/dL and to keep overall glucose >60 mg/dL.
   c. **NIDDM:** Follow up with a HbA1c level on a q 3- to 4-month period. Goal is to decrease the HbA1c to 7.0–7.5.

(text continued from page 466)
   D. **Manifestations specific to IDDM**
      These manifestations include the development of ketones with resultant high-anion-gap acidosis (Table 9-1: Causes of High AG Metabolic Acidosis), acetone on the breath, and deep, rapid (Kussmaul) respiration. The patient with IDDM often loses weight.
IV. **Overall management**
      The **overall management** of diabetes mellitus is directed toward several goals: optimally controlling serum glucose values without precipitating hypoglycemia, monitoring and attempting to prevent sequelae of diabetes mellitus, and min-

T A B L E 9-1
Causes of High Anion Gap Metabolic Acidosis

$$Anion\ gap = Na - (Cl + HCO_3)$$

$$Normal = 12-14$$

Methanol ingestion   This toxin will form formic acid via the enzyme ethanol dehydrogenase.
Ketone bodies   The bodies, β-hydroxybutyrate, acetoacetate, and acetone, can be formed in diabetic ketoacidosis, ethanol-related ketoacidosis, and starvation.
Lactate   This anion is produced in hypoperfusion states and sepsis.
Salicylates   Overdosage or overdose.
Uremia   Fixed acids (i.e., anions) are not effectively excreted.
Ethylene glycol   Ingestion of this constituent of antifreeze will result in the formation of glyoxylic acid and oxylic acid.
Paraldehyde usage

imizing other concurrent **risk factors** for the development of atherosclerotic vascular disease.

A. Glycemic control

Glycemic control is central to the management of diabetes mellitus. Keeping serum glucose levels <200 mg/dL minimizes polyuria, polydipsia, and other acute manifestations of hyperglycemia; in addition, the evidence is mounting that parsimonious glycemic control prevents the chronic sequelae of diabetes mellitus. However, there is always the potential of hypoglycemia, which can lead to morbid, even mortal events. The risk of hypoglycemia increases with the intensity of the control regimen and in patients who have problems with compliance. Therefore the degree of glycemic control must be tailored to the patient. In a patient who has no sequelae and is compliant, the goal should be euglycemia (i.e., fasting glucose levels of 80–100 mg/dL and postprandial glucose levels ≤140 mg/dL. In a patient with multiple existing sequelae or other medical problems that will limit life span, such as metastatic carcinoma, the goal should be glucose values in the range of 150–250 mg/dL. Regimens for glycemic control include the following.

1. If the patient has acutely decompensated diabetes mellitus, emergent intervention in glycemic control is indicated. See Box 9-2 for specifics in management of both DKA (IDDM) and HHC (NIDDM).

2. If the patient has IDDM, insulin is required to provide effective glycemic control on a long-term basis.

    a. Only human recombinant insulin should be administered. There are various trade names of human insulin, including Humulin and Novolin.

    b. The pharmacokinetics of subcutaneously administered human recombinant insulin are as follows:

    Regular
Peak effect:	2–4 hr
Duration:	6 hr

    NPH
Peak effect:	8–14 hr
Duration:	18–20 hr

    Ultralente
Peak effect:	12–16 hr
Duration:	24–28 hr

    c. The overall total dosage of insulin usually is ~0.5–1.0 unit/kg/day of human insulin.

    d. **Insulin-dosing regimens** are modeled to approximate the normal physiologic secretion of insulin from the pancreas. A regimen of a long-acting agent plus boluses of short-acting insulin is optimal. Several such regimens (i–v) can be used.

(text continues on page 477)

B O X 9-2

Overall Evaluation and Management of Acutely Decompensated Diabetes Mellitus

I. The **acute decompensation of diabetes mellitus** is a medical urgency/emergency that the primary care physician will see on a regular basis in practice. Often the decompensation will be in a patient who has a defined type of diabetes mellitus—either insulin-dependent (IDDM) or non–insulin-dependent (NIDDM), but it may be the sentinel manifestation of the disease. The **overall goals** in the evaluation and management of this problem, irrespective of the type of diabetes mellitus, include:

  A. Assessment of the volume status and the repletion of that volume deficit with 0.9 normal saline.

  B. Assessment for the presence and degree of acidosis and, if ketoacidotic, the administration of insulin, to stop ketone body production, thereby allowing the liver to catabolize them.

  C. Assess for and correct any and all electrolyte abnormalities.

  D. Determine, if possible, the underlying, *precipitating, or exacerbating event.* The history and physical examination will afford the clinician ample information to determine this event or process in the vast majority of cases. Factors may include:

    1. Sentinel event (i.e., this is the first manifestation of IDDM or NIDDM).

    2. Poor compliance with the regimen, either insulin or an oral agent.

    3. Intravascular volume depletion for whatever reason (e.g., gastroenteritis).

    4. New severe stressor:
      · Infection
      · Urinary tract infection
      · Pneumonitis
      · Skin/skin structure infection
      · Acute coronary syndrome
      · Trauma
      · Acute cerebrovascular accident
      · Surgery
      · New medication (e.g., glucocorticoids)

    5. Define the type of diabetes if new onset: IDDM has, invariably, ketones and acidosis;

(continued)

B O X 9-2 *(continued)*

therefore, acute decompensation is called diabetic ketoacidosis (DKA); NIDDM manifests with profound hyperglycemia and volume depletion but minimal acidosis and ketones is termed hyperosmolar hyperglycemic coma (HHC).

6. Arrange for appropriate long-term follow-up.

II. **Overall evaluation of acutely decompensated diabetes mellitus:**

A. Perform a physical examination with emphasis on:

1. Volume status: Assessed by determining the weight of patient, orthostatic parameters, concentration and volume of urine, and skin turgor and volume.
2. Smell breath for ketone bodies of DKA.
3. Examine the breathing pattern of Kussmaul's as manifestation of severe acidosis-DKA.
4. Determine the mental status of the patient.

B. Laboratory assessment:

1. Serum electrolyte, BUN, creatinine, and glucose
2. Calculate the anion gap. See Table 9-1 (page 470).
3. Serum ketone levels. Recall that only acetoacetate and acetone are measured by using the standard test for ketone bodies.
4. If suspicion is high for an acidosis, perform an arterial blood gas determination.
5. Measure thyroid-stimulating hormone (TSH) to screen for thyroid disease.
6. Serum PO_4, Mg, Ca, and albumin. PO_4 is particularly important, because a result of therapy is hypophosphatemia.
7. Complete blood count with differential count.
8. Urinalysis with microscopic analysis.
9. 12-lead ECG.
10. CK and LDH with isozymes may be indicated.
11. Blood cultures may be indicated if there is any evidence of infection.
12. Chest radiograph—PA and lateral.

C. Based on the history, physical examination, laboratory, and suspicion of an exacerbating or precipitating event: Determine the **type (DKA versus HHC)** and its **severity (severe versus mild)**.

(continued)

B O X   9-2 (continued)

Management is based on these two features and is discussed subsequently.

If severe diabetic ketoacidosis:

A. **Features:** Often the patient is volume depleted, severely ill, hypotensive, has Kussmaul-type respirations; often the patient's serum glucose is >500 mg/dL, serum and urine ketones present, and most salient to the diagnosis, has an increased anion gap metabolic acidosis, the serum pH may actually be <7.0!

B. **Specific management:**
   1. Outcomes to follow include hourly checks of blood pressure, urine output, K, PO_4, pH, and glucose.
   2. Establish two peripheral i.v. catheters:
      a. One i.v. catheter is for fluids and electrolytes.
         · Administer 1 L 0.9N saline at 300–500 mL/hr, then decrease to 200 mL/hr.
         · Attempt to replete 50%–60% of the volume deficit in the first 24 hours.
         · If there is any question regarding volume status and/or if the patient is hypotensive, one may consider the placement of a Swan–Ganz catheter.
         · Replete potassium (sliding scale)
           K: 3.2–3.6: 20 mEq i.v.
           K: 2.8–3.1: 40 mEq i.v.
           K: 2.6–2.7: 60 mEq i.v.
           K: <2.6: 60 mEq i.v. and call MD
         · Replete magnesium (sliding scale)
           Mg: 1.4–1.8: 1 g $MgSO_4$ i.v.
           Mg: 1.0–1.3: 2 g $MgSO_4$ i.v.
           Mg: <1.0: 2 g $MgSO_4$ i.v. and call MD
         · Replete phosphorus. If serum PO_4 is <1.5, consider giving some K as i.v. KPO_3.
         · HCO3 is not indicated unless the pH is <7.0 or the patient is hyperkalemic (see section on hyperkalemia, page 491)
         · Use this i.v. line for any other medications (e.g., antibiotics).
      b. The second i.v. catheter is for the exclusive use of human insulin:

(continued)

B O X 9-2 *(continued)*

- Administer 5–10 U of regular human insulin i.v. as a stat bolus;
- Initiate a drip of 2–10 U of regular human insulin/hour i.v.
- Goal is to decrease the serum glucose by a rate of 75–100 mg/dL/hr to a level of 300 mg/dL.

  When the serum glucose reaches 300 mg/dL:

  i. Check a concurrent HCO_3 and pH.
  ii. *If the HCO_3 is >18 and pH is >7.3:*
  - Change the i.v. fluids from 0.9NS to D5.45NS.
  - Administer 10 U regular human insulin s.c. and discontinue the insulin drip in 30–60 minutes
  - Either give the patient the original dose of insulin or initiate human regular insulin on a **sliding scale** based on finger-stick glucose determinations made q.4–6hr:

    <60 mg/dL: i.v. $D_{50}W$
    61–120 mg/dL: Status quo
    121–180 mg/dL: 2–4 U
    181–240 mg/dL: 4–6 U
    241–300 mg/dL: 6–9 U
    301–360 mg/dL: 10–13 U
    >360 mg/dL: Call MD and check HCO_3 and ABGs: If acidosis and ketosis have returned, restart the insulin drip; if no acidosis, administer 12 U of s.c. regular insulin and check again in 4 hours.

  iii. If the HCO_3 is <18 and the pH is <7.3:
  - Change fluids from 0.9NS to D5.45NS.
  - Continue i.v. human insulin to clear the ketone bodies; it is extremely important to continue aggressive use of human insulin during the 24 hours after achieving a glucose level of 250–300 mg/dL because the patient will remain ketotic even though the glucose has decreased. Without adequate insulin replacement during this critical time, the

(continued)

B O X   9-2 (continued)

liver is not able to clear the ketone bodies present.
- Monitor glucose and HCO_3 and pH; when >18 and >7.3: Perform that described in ii.
- Start routine insulin b.i.d./t.i.d. as described on page 471. If patient is ketotic, life-long human insulin is necessary.

If mild DKA:

A. **Features:** Patient may be mildly volume depleted, sick with gastroenteritis or other infection but not severely ill; no Kussmaul respiration; glucose may be >500 mg/dL, but the pH is >7.2 and HCO_3 is >15.

B. **Specific management:**
  1. Patient may well be able to be managed as an outpatient with close follow-up.
  2. I.v. fluids of 0.9NS for volume repletion.
  3. Initiate s.c. insulin: administer 10 U regular human insulin s.c.
  4. Goal is to treat and limit ketone body synthesis; keep glucoses in 200–300 mg/dL range.
  5. Finger sticks q.i.d. and urine ketones q.i.d. are indicated.

If hyperosmolar hyperglycemic coma (HHC):

A. **Features:** Profound intravascular volume depletion with a decrease in urine output, increase in urine concentration, hypotension, orthostatic hypotension, decreased level of consciousness; glucose in serum may reach 1,000–1,200 mg/dL level; there is little if any acidosis, but the anion gap may be and often is elevated even without any significant acidosis.

B. **Specific management:**
  1. Outcomes to follow include hourly checks of blood pressure, urine output, K, PO_4, pH, and glucose in serum.
  2. Establish i.v. access:
    - IVF to rehydrate the patient. The fluid of choice is 0.9NS at 500 mL/hr; replace the fluid so that 50%–60% of the volume is replaced in the first 24 hours. The glucose level will often decrease significantly with this intervention alone. The cornerstone of **treatment** of HHC is i.v. fluids.
    - The volume deficit may be 8–10 L in some of these patients.

(continued)

B O X 9-2 *(continued)*

3. Assess the serum for ketone bodies as they may be present in the acute, severe decompensation of NIDDM.
4. Insulin s.c. regular, human may be indicated but is not mandatory in all cases. Indications for s.c. insulin include:
   • Ongoing severe stressor:
     i. Infection
     ii. Acute coronary syndrome
     iii. Bowel obstruction
   • Ongoing vomiting, thereby precluding the effective initiation of oral hypoglycemic agents
   • The development of ketoacidosis (not just ketones, but ketoacidosis).
5. If the patient is rehydrated and able to take by mouth, may initiate the long-term therapy as an outpatient.

(text continued from page 471)

i. 10–20 units ultralente insulin s.c. q.A.M., and then a dose of regular insulin before each meal. The ultralente acts as the basal secretion of insulin from the pancreas. Glucose values must be closely monitored by a finger-stick method to keep the postprandial glucose values in the range of 140–180 mg/dL with no overall glucose values <80 mg/dL or >180 mg/dL.

Glycemic monitoring should include finger sticks q.i.d.: one at bedtime and others 30 minutes to 1 hour after each meal.

-or-

ii. **Twice-daily dosing regimen** with a mixture of NPH and regular insulin. The doses should be administered 30 minutes before breakfast and 30 minutes before supper. Two thirds of the total dosage is NPH and one third is regular insulin. Two thirds of the total dosage is taken before breakfast and one third before supper.

Monitoring for glycemia should include finger sticks q.i.d.: immediately before insulin dosing, at noon, and at bedtime. Goals for intensive therapy include fasting: 70–120 mg/dL; premeal, <180 mg/dL; and midsleep (3 A.M.) >65 mg/dL.

-or-

    iii. Twice-daily dosing regimen with premixed human NPH and regular insulin. Several pharmaceutical corporations make premixed NPH–regular human insulin (e.g., Novolin 70/30, which is 70% NPH and 30% regular human insulin). It is administered in a b.i.d. dosing regimen. As with other b.i.d. regimens, two thirds of the dose is taken in the morning, and one third is taken in the evening.

    -or-

    iv. Continuous insulin infusion via pump: Regular human insulin infused at a rate of 0.4–1.0 U/hr subcutaneously; may decrease it during the afternoon or before exercise to prevent hypoglycemia. Glucose values must be closely monitored by a finger-stick method to keep the postprandial glucose values in the range of 140–180 mg/dL with no overall glucose values <80 mg/dL or >180 mg/dL. This should be performed under the direction of an endocrinologist.

      Glycemic monitoring should include finger sticks q.i.d., including noon and bedtime.

    -or-

    v. For NIDDM: Exercise, diet, and oral hypoglycemic agents and/or metformin. See further discussion on the management subsequently. If fasting blood sugar (FBS) is recurrently >200 mg%, consider initiation of NPH insulin in a dose of 10 units q.HS s.c.

  e. Insulin adjustments when the patient is ill (for example, the patient has gastroenteritis manifesting with nausea, vomiting, anorexia, and diarrhea) include instructing the patient to institute the following measures:

    i. Follow plasma glucose and urine ketone values closely, if possible on a q.i.d. basis.

    ii. Hold regular insulin dose, continue NPM at half to three fourths of the baseline dose. The regular dose is resumed when the patient can resume regular oral intake of fluids and food.

    iii. Go to the hospital if orthostatic manifestations or ketonuria develop.

3. If the **patient has NIDDM,** glycemic control is based on increasing the number and activity of the insulin receptors and of decreasing diabetes-related sequelae. This is accomplished by the following methods.

  a. Weight reduction, if obese, and exercise. Exercise improves insulin use by increasing the activity of insulin-stimulated glycogen synthesis in skeletal muscle. These **modalities** are most effective for glycemic control in this type of diabetes mellitus.

b. **Oral hypoglycemic agents.** These agents can be initiated in patients who are unable or unwilling to lose weight. The oral hypoglycemic agents of choice are glipizide (Glucotrol) or glyburide (Diabeta, Micronase). Both of these agents increase the number and effectiveness of insulin receptors and are catabolized in the liver. Recent reports have demonstrated that the risk of hypoglycemia is lower with glipizide than with glyburide, so it is the preferred oral hypoglycemic agent. The range for total dosage is:

Glipizide, 5–40 mg/day. The doses can be q.A.M. or b.i.d. p.o.

Glyburide, 2.5–20 mg/day. The doses can be q.A.M. or b.i.d. p.o.

c. **Metformin:** In patients with NIDDM refractory to oral agents alone, this adjustment may stave off the need for insulin. This is a unique agent that acts in concert with an oral agent. It has several significant side effects, including the risk for development of lactic acidosis and is contraindicated in patients with significant renal dysfunction or hepatic dysfunction. The dose is 500 mg p.o., b.i.d., may increase the dose q 4–6 weeks to a maximum dose of 2.5 g/day.

d. Insulin in NIDDM is of use in some patients who are particularly vexing. Usually after 15–20 years of untreated NIDDM, insulin may be required to assist in glycemic control. The regimen is 0.3–0.4 U/kg NPH insulin administered q.HS. The dosing of q.HS is best to decrease the insulin-related increased appetite and weight gain.

e. Glycemic monitoring should include finger-stick glucose determinations every morning and hemoglobin A1c determinations every 6 months. The goal is to decrease the hemoglobin A1c level to 7.0%–7.5%. The hemoglobin A1c is the percentage of hemoglobin to which glucose is covalently bound. This is a long-term measurement of the overall glycemic control of the patient, as the life span of an erythrocyte is ~120 days. The hemoglobin A1c depends on the level of glucose in the plasma and the level of hemoglobin. Hemoglobin A1c values can be falsely decreased in:

   i. Anemia, owing to a decreased level of hemoglobulin.

   ii. Reticulocytosis, because these are young cells.

   iii. Hemoglobinopathies (e.g., SS/SC disease, as a result of the decreased life span of the cells).

B. **Controlling sequelae of diabetes mellitus**

The specific sequelae of diabetes mellitus are diverse, and include the following.

1. **Retinopathy**

a. The **underlying pathogenesis** is one of the abnormal thickening of the basement membrane of the capillaries and microvasculature. This abnormal thickening of the endothelial cells paradoxically makes the membranes more fragile and, more important, more permeable to fluids and proteins. This results in an abnormal leakiness and therefore a loss of proteins, including albumin, into the interstitium. This basement membrane change is a central feature of the microvascular changes that involve all capillaries of the body.

This serves as fertile ground for the first set of clinical manifestations of diabetic retinopathy: the *nonproliferative changes*. These changes consist of microaneurysms and hard exudates. The microaneurysms are small, adjacent to capillaries, particularly at branch points, the hard exudates are collections of protein in the retina that result from the loss of protein into the neural layers of the retina. This starts after ≥5 years of uncontrolled diabetes mellitus. The next stage of retinopathy is termed *proliferative retinopathy*. Uncontrolled diabetes mellitus results in further microvascular changes and damage, eventually resulting in soft-edged areas termed "cotton-wool" spots. In the process of healing, new vessels form at the periphery and within the soft exudates. These vessels are quite fragile and bleed, and there is resultant vitreous hemorrhage and the strong potential for visual deficit. The result is marked decrease in vision caused by:

• Soft exudates, especially if they involve the macula
• Vitreous hemorrhages
• Retinal detachment as the result of the clot formed by the vitreous bleed retracting and pulling upon the retina.

b. The **specific manifestations** of diabetic retinopathy are described in the pathogenesis section, above

The visual acuity is embarrassed in end-stage retinopathy if the nonproliferative or proliferative changes affect the macula or if it progresses to involve a significant percentage of the retina.

c. The **specific evaluation and management** include the steps outlined in Box 9-1 and prevention. There is conclusive evidence via the Diabetes Control and Complication Trial (DCCT) that tight glycemic control prevents the development of nonproliferative and proliferative retinopathy. The DCCT demonstrated that tight control of glucose in IDDM results in primary prevention of retinopathy and, although a modest worsening of retinopathy early, an overall significant improvement in tertiary prevention. Although not conclusive, significant data indicate that the same holds true in NIDDM. All diabetic patients must undergo a baseline and annual retinal examination by an ophthalmologist. Any proliferative changes can be successfully treated with laser photocoagulation. In this procedure, new, fragile vessels are destroyed before they can bleed and cause mischief. Any significant vision changes in a diabetic patient mandates a funduscopic examination and often a referral to ophthalmology.

2. **Neuropathy**
   a. The **underlying pathogenesis** is multifactorial and includes ischemia to the nerves as a result of the microangiopathic (i.e., capillary basement membrane thickening) and macroangiopathic (i.e., vascular) changes. The decreased perfusion results in damage and even infarction of parts of the peripheral nerves. A concurrent process is an abnormal accumulation of the sugar sorbitol in the peripheral neurons. The aldose reductase pathway will produce sorbitol in significant amounts in the presence of significant hyperglycemia. The sorbitol is incorporated into the peripheral nerves, autonomic nerves, and probably into the nerves of the GI tract, and results in significant and progressive neuronal dysfunction via progressive dysfunction of the Na/K ATPase.
   b. The **specific manifestations** of diabetic neuropathy are diverse, manifold, and dependent on what nerves are primarily involved: peripheral, autonomic, or GI tract.
      i. **Peripheral neuropathies** manifest with paresthesias, pain, hypesthesia, or dysesthesia, usually in a stocking or glove distribution. The distribution can be variable, but usually is greater distally than proximally. There can be discrete syndromes, including carpal tunnel syndrome, ulnar tunnel syndrome, and even tarsal tunnel syndrome. The pain may be debilitating.
      ii. **Autonomic neuropathies** manifest with impotence, decreased sweating, and a lack of tachycardia on arising. This can preclude the development of the classic secondary manifestations of

hypoglycemia (i.e., tremor, tachycardia, and diaphoresis).

iii. **Enteropathy,** or dysfunction of the GI tract, will
result in gastroparesis with resultant postprandial vomiting that can be quite debilitating to
the patient. Diabetes-related diarrhea may also
result.

c. The **specific evaluation and management** include
the steps listed in Box 9-1 and the following measures.

i. For **peripheral neuropathies, specific management** includes defining the lesions. If carpal tunnel, ulnar tunnel, or tarsal tunnel syndrome is
present, one can splint the joint and administer
an NSAID prn. If the neuropathy is recurrent,
surgical intervention may be indicated.

If no specific lesions can be localized and the
manifestations are severe, administer amitriptyline (Elavil), 25–50 mg p.o., q.HS, or capsaicin
(Zostrix), 0.025% topically b.i.d. Capsaicin is a
peripheral inhibitor of pain that interacts with
the pain transmitter, substance P. Aldolase reductase inhibitors (e.g., Tolrestat, 200 mg p.o.,
q.d.) are being studied and have provided some
good effect in preventing and treating peripheral
and autonomic neuropathies.

Referral to a pain clinic is indicated in severe
cases. A pain-control specialist is often an an-
esthesiologist with training in **modalities** for
pain control.

ii. For **autonomic neuropathies,** define the manifestations. If they are predominantly orthostatic
hypotension without tachycardia, instruct the
patient to rise slowly from a supine position.
Further **modalities** include above-knee hose applied to both lower extremities and minimizing
the use of medications that can exacerbate the
nontachycardic hypotension. Impotence is managed by looking for any reversible causes, such
as hypogonadism, and referral to a genitourinary
(GU) specialist.

iii. **For enteropathies,** the **specific evaluation and
management** include defining the lesion. Two
modalities for direct imaging of the pylorus are
the barium swallow, which demonstrates specific anatomic lesions about the distal stomach
or pylorus or problems with transit time across
the pylorus, and a radionucleotide-labeled meal,
to measure transit time across the pylorus. The

specific management includes frequent small meals and the initiation of the agent metoclopramide (Reglan), 5–10 mg p.o., q.6hr on a scheduled basis. Also, a trial of other agents (e.g., erythromycin, 250 mg p.o., t.i.d., or of cisapride, 5–10 mg p.o., q.i.d.) may be of benefit. Finally, teracycline in a dose of 500–1,000 mg at the start of each attack or loperamide (Imodium) may be effective in treatment.

3. **Nephropathy**

   a. The **underlying pathophysiology** of this sequel, the most common origin of end-stage renal disease (ESRD), is probably analogous to the pathophysiology of retinopathy: thickening of the basement membrane in the capillaries and microvasculature of the kidneys. This thickening is postulated to be a result of deposition of glycosylated proteins and other substances within the basement membranes. Histopathologic examination shows definite thickening of the mesangium and glomerular basement membrane. The quintessential example of this process is the Kimmelstiel–Wilson lesion (i.e., focal nodular sclerosis).

   The abnormal thickening results in an abnormal leakiness of the capillaries within the kidneys (i.e., the glomeruli of albumin). Therefore an early marker for the development of nephropathy is albumin loss in the urine. In IDDM, microalbuminuria (i.e., >40 mg/24 hr indicates that there is an 80% chance of the patient developing renal insufficiency; if <40 mg/24 hr, the chance is 4%. The **natural history** entails progressive increases in protein loss to the point of classic hypoalbuminemic nephrotic syndrome. The presence of microalbuminuria also is a risk factor for accelerated atherosclerotic disease. Of interest is that in addition to the glomerular damage, there is tubular dysfunction (e.g., type IV, hyperkalemic, renal tubular acidosis).

   A concurrent factor in the development of nephropathy is uncontrolled hypertension.

   b. The **specific manifestations** of nephropathy are diverse and dependent on the time of presentation. Early in the course, there are no **specific manifestations.** The earliest manifestation is microalbuminuria (i.e., >40 mg of albumin in the urine per 24 hours). This is a powerful marker for the development of nephrotic syndrome; there is an 80% risk of development of nephrotic syndrome in 5 years. Later in the **natural history** of the disease, frank proteinuria will develop. Further progression to frank nephrotic syndrome occurs with the classic manifestations of hypoalbuminemia, albuminuria and proteinuria, and edema.

c. The **specific evaluation and management** of nephrotic syndrome include prevention. Prevention is the cornerstone of management. It includes aggressive control of glucose levels and tight control of hypertension. The DCCT demonstrated that there is a significant decrease in the development of and progression to microalbuminuria and albuminuria in patients with tight glycemic control. Hypertension must be optimally controlled to prevent nephropathy. The drug of choice for hypertension control is that of one of the angiotensin-converting enzyme (ACE) inhibitors, if tolerated. Furthermore, there is some evidence that prescription of a low-protein (i.e., 0.8 g/kg) diet will retard the progression of nephrotic renal failure. Furthermore, exposure to nephrotoxic agents (e.g., iodide contrast agents) must be minimized. Once nephrotic-range proteinuria (>3 g protein/24 hr) is present, renal failure will eventually occur, usually within 5 years. All patients with nephrotic-range proteinuria should be referred to a nephrologist.

4. **Atherosclerotic disease** (also referred to as macrovascular disease).

a. The **underlying pathogenesis** is not completely understood. Both IDDM and NIDDM are associated with an increased risk for and acceleration of atherosclerotic disease. Diabetes mellitus results in a change in the lipid profile characterized by a decrease in HDL cholesterol, an increase in low-density lipoprotein (LDL) cholesterol, and an increase in triglycerides, all of which increase the risk of development of atherosclerotic disease. This results in the development of atheromatous plaques in the medium and large arteries of the body.

b. The **specific manifestations** are few until late in the course of the disease. The manifestations are diverse and depend on where specifically the plaques occur. The most common sites for symptomatic arterial plaques (i.e., narrowing) are the coronary arteries, where plaques manifest with angina pectoris and acute myocardial infarction; the cerebrovascular vessels, where plaques manifest with transient ischemic attacks (TIAs) and strokes; and the peripheral arteries, where plaques manifest with intermittent, exercise-related claudication and diabetic foot infections (see cellulitis, Table 6-1 Chapter 6, page 315). A recent article by Reiber et al. demonstrated that the following are **risk factors** for amputation in patients with diabetes mellitus:

- An arterial–brachial index (ABI) <0.45
- The absence of lower-extremity vibratory sensation
- Low-level HDL cholesterol
- No education in diabetic training

  c. The **specific evaluation and management** include making the clinical diagnosis, the **overall management** of diabetes mellitus (see Box 9-1, page 467), and controlling any concurrent increases of plasma lipids. Furthermore, it is important to define and then control any concurrent **risk factors** for atherosclerotic disease development: control hypertension and the hyperglycemia and instruct the patient to stop smoking.

V. **Consultation**

Problem	Service	Time
All diabetics	Ophthalmology	Required
Sudden decrease in vision	Ophthalmology	Emergent
All diabetics	Endocrinology	Elective

VI. **Indications for admission:** Acute decompensation of diabetes mellitus (e.g., diabetic ketoacidosis) and nonketotic hyperglycemic coma.

Hypercalcemia

The physiology of calcium homeostasis is relatively complex. The levels of this divalent cation are parsimoniously maintained by several interrelated and interdependent mechanisms. These involve vitamin D, a vitamin required for effective calcium absorption from the small intestine; the small intestine itself as an absorptive site; and the renal tubules, which are under the direct regulation of the hormone parathormone (PTH); and controls the excretory loss of calcium into the urine. Finally, bone plays a major role in that it is the largest store of inorganic calcium in the body and will, under the direction of PTH, release calcium by osteolysis. Thus the perturbations of increased levels of vitamin D, increased levels of PTH or a PTH-like substance, or any process that results in increased osteoclastic activity (i.e., osteolysis) can result in hypercalcemia.

I. **Overall manifestations**

Hypercalcemia is asymptomatic in the vast majority of cases. Manifestations, when present, include the onset of moderate to marked polyuria, polydipsia, constipation, and a change in the level of consciousness (lethargy, somnolence, or even coma) that is more conspicuous than an acute confusional state (i.e., delirium). There is often evidence of intravascular volume depletion (i.e., orthostatic hypotension and tachycardia), which develops after the patient is unable to ingest adequate amounts of fluids to maintain hydration and indicates impending coma. There is often an antecedent history of a malignant neoplastic process, either a carcinoma or multiple myeloma (Box 9-3).

II. **Underlying causes**

A. **Squamous-cell carcinoma of the primary site**

The most common sites of squamous-cell carcinoma are the lung and the head and neck.

1. The **underlying pathogenesis** is production by the tumor of a PTH-like substance that results in increased osteoclast activity (osteoclasts being derived from macrophage-type cells) and hence an increased bone resorption and hypercalcemia with an increased urinary calcium.

2. The **specific manifestations** are referable to the increased calcium level and to the tumor itself.

3. The **specific evaluation and management** include steps outlined in Box 9-3 defining, and if possible, controlling or curing the malignant squamous-cell carcinoma. Unfortunately, the tumor is invariably metastatic when associated with hypercalcemia, and therefore **treatment modalities** are of palliative benefit at best. **These modalities include:**

B O X   9-3

Overall Evaluation and Management of Hypercalcemia

Evaluation

1. Determine serum calcium and albumin levels. Following are normal calcium values (equivalent measures):
   8.0–10.2 mg/dL, or
   4.0–5.1 mEq/dL, or
   2.0–2.6 mmol/dL.
      The corrected (true) calcium level = 0.8 (4.0 − measured albumin) + measured calcium. (Units for calcium used are mg/dL.)

2. Determine the serum phosphorus level. If increased with hypercalcemia, it is suggestive of vitamin D intoxication, whereas if decreased with hypercalcemia, it is suggestive of primary hyperparathyroidism.

(continued)

B O X 9-3 *(continued)*

3. Obtain chest radiographs in PA and lateral views, looking for pulmonary masses.
4. Perform urinalysis to look for hematuria, an early marker for renal cell carcinoma.
5. Determine the erythrocyte sedimentation rate (ESR), which may be increased in a monoclonal gammopathy.
6. Obtain a complete blood cell count, looking for a normochromic normocytic anemia and rouleaux (Box 5-4), either of which is consistent with a monoclonal gammopathy.
7. If a gammopathy is suspected, perform serum protein electrophoresis (SPEP) and urine protein electrophoresis (UPEP).
8. Determine the intact, N-terminus PTH level. This is the biologically active form of PTH and is of most utility in measurement. Older assays for the C-terminal, nonintact PTH include the inactive catabolites of PTH and can, in the setting of renal failure, suggest false increased levels of the PTH.
9. Perform thyroid function tests, especially if the patient has clinical evidence of hyperthyroidism or hypothyroidism.
10. Obtain a 24-hour urine collection for calcium determination. The normal level is 200–300 mg/24-hour urine collection. In hypercalcemia, an increased urine calcium level is suggestive of a malignant neoplastic or paraneoplastic process, whereas a decreased urine calcium level is suggestive of primary hyperparathyroidism.
11. Determine serum vitamin D25-OH and D1,25-OH levels. Increased levels are consistent with vitamin D intoxication.

Management

1. Make the patient volume replete with 0.9 normal saline intravenously. Usually the patient has a 4–5 L volume deficit.
2. Use a loop diuretic [e.g., furosemide (Lasix)] if and when the patient becomes hypervolemic from the volume repletion.
3. Further management is specific to the underlying cause of the hypercalcemia.

   a. **Plicamycin (mithramycin),** administered parenterally. The dose is 25 μg/kg i.v., the usual dose being 1.25 mg i.v. for one dose. This agent has been demonstrated to inhibit osteoclastic activity.
   b. **Calcitonin,** the hormone produced in the physiologic state by the parafollicular (C) cells of the thyroid gland. Calcitonin decreases levels of serum calcium and can be administered to effect a decrease in serum calcium. The dose of human calcitonin is 0.5 mg q.d., s.c.; whereas, for salmon calcitonin the dose is 4 IU/kg s.c. q.12hr; follow serum calcium levels.
   c. **Gallium nitrate.** This rare earth metal is an exciting novel **modality** to decrease serum calcium. It decreases calcium levels through an undetermined mechanism. It should be used only under the direction of an oncologist.
   d. **Oral phosphates** (e.g., Neutraphos). If the phosphorus is low at baseline (i.e., <4 mg/dL), oral phosphates can be administered to decrease the serum calcium. The serum phosphorus level must be closely monitored and the agent discontinued when the serum phosphorus level is >5 mg/dL. This is because, if the calcium and phosphorus reach a certain level [i.e., the double product (calcium × phosphorus) is >55], there is a high risk of metastatic calcifications in the brain and soft tissues. This is only an adjunctive therapeutic modality.
   e. **Pamidronate disodium.** This biphosphonate agent is an effective inhibitor of osteoclast-mediated bone resorption. The dose is 15–90 mg i.v. infused over 4–24 hr in the acute setting.
B. **Lymphoproliferative disorders**
   The most common lymphoproliferative disorders are multiple myeloma and the lymphomas, either of which can manifest with hypercalcemia.
   1. The **underlying pathogenesis** is production by the tumor of a substance that increases bone resorption and increases hypercalcemia, with an increased urinary calcium level. The substance, osteoclastic-activating factor (OAF), is a lymphokine that stimulates osteoclasts to resorb bone. Recent reports indicate that calcitriol (1,25-OH vitamin D_3) made by the tumor clone also may contribute to the hypercalcemia.
   2. The **specific manifestations** are referable to the increased calcium level and to the tumor itself. Recurrent pathologic fractures, bone pain, rouleaux on a peripheral blood smear (see Fig. 5-4), anemia, and "B" symptoms—fevers, unintentional weight loss, and drenching

night sweats—are the classic manifestations. The urinary calcium level is usually increased.

3. The **specific evaluation and management** include the steps outlined in Box 9-3, defining, and if possible controlling or curing the malignant lymphoproliferative disorder. Further evaluative **modalities** include bone marrow biopsy and referral to hematology/oncology for more definitive intervention. The hypercalcemia is quite sensitive to therapy with steroids [e.g., methylprednisolone (Solu-Medrol), 60–80 mg i.v. q.8hr] and, in patients with no contraindications to their use, a trial of nonsteroidal antiinflammatory drugs (NSAIDs) may be of benefit. Other agents, including plicamycin, gallium nitrate, or pamidronate may be administered when the hypercalcemia is severe or refractory to first-line therapy. Please refer to previous discussion for specific details on mechanism of action and dosage.

C. **Primary hyperparathyroidism**

1. The **underlying pathogenesis** is an autoimmune-stimulated excess secretion of PTH from the parathyroid glands.

2. The **specific manifestations** include those referable to the hypercalcemia itself; in addition, hypophosphatemia, and a decreased urine calcium level.

3. The **specific evaluation and management** include the steps outlined in Box 9-3 and referral to an endocrinologist and a surgeon with expertise in parathyroid surgical procedures for parathyroidectomy. Definitively, surgical resection is the treatment of choice.

D. **Vitamin D intoxication**

1. The **underlying pathogenesis** is ingestion of inappropriately large amounts of vitamin D, which results in an increase in the absorption of calcium from the GI tract and a concurrent decrease in tubular excretion of calcium and phosphorus, resulting in an increase in serum calcium and phosphorus levels. People who take large quantities of vitamins are at greatest risk for this syndrome.

2. The **specific manifestations** include those attributable to the hypercalcemia and an antecedent history of vitamin abuse. Manifestations include hypercalcemia, hyperphosphatemia, and a decreased urine calcium level.

3. The **specific evaluation and management** include the steps outlined in Box 9-3 and discontinuing vitamin D or A from nonfood sources (recall that cod-liver-oil tablets are rich in both). If levels are severely increased, the administration of a short course of steroids (e.g., prednisone, 40–60 mg in a 1- to 2-week tapering dosage) is helpful.

E. **Sarcoidosis**
   1. The **underlying pathogenesis** is an increase in the activity of vitamin D by the macrophage-like sarcoid cell in the noncaseating granulomata, which generate the enzyme vitamin D_1-hydroxylase, therefore resulting in hypercalcemia through a vitamin D–mediated (increased calcitriol) process.
   2. The **specific manifestations** include interstitial infiltrates on chest radiographs, hilar adenopathy on chest radiographs, polyarticular arthritis, erythema nodosum, and renal dysfunction. The systemic, idiopathic disorder has hypercalcemia as one of its manifestations.
   3. The **specific evaluation and management** include the steps outlined in Box 9-3, making the clinical diagnosis of sarcoidosis, and initiating **treatment** with steroids. The steroids treat not only the hypercalcemia but also the sarcoidosis itself. The management of sarcoid is beyond the scope of this text; however, because the most devastating manifestations are pulmonary, referral to a pulmonologist is indicated.

F. **Paget's disease**
   1. The **underlying pathogenesis** is of the idiopathic increase in osteoclast activity with bone resorption and secondary blast activity with bone formation—all resulting in abnormal bone. There has been some evidence that the underlying origin is the infection of the osteoclasts with paramyxovirus. The rapid resorption, highly vascular, disorganized bone expansion, which increases the bone fragility and risk of fractures. The prevalence of the disease is 2%–3% of men and women older than 50 years and 10% in patients of Northern European heritage older than 50 years.
   2. The **specific manifestations** include bone pain at sites of involvement, a significant increase in the amount of osteoarthritis in the joints adjacent to the areas of involvement; increased warmth of the skin over the bones, and fractures of vertebral or pelvis, there is often the presence of genu varus (i.e., legs bowed), there is an increased risk in osteogenic sarcoma. In addition, there is often hypercalcemia and hypercalciuria, especially in immobilized patients.
   3. The **specific evaluation and management** include the steps outlined in Box 9-3, making the clinical diagnosis, performing radiographs of the axial skeleton, and performing a bone scan to look for increased uptake at the sites of Paget's disease. Laboratory studies include increased alkaline phosphatase, increased bone alkaline phosphatase, and increased urine hydroxyproline levels. Bone biopsy of the ilium (tetracycline-labeled transiliac) will reveal the mixture of bony resorption

and abnormal disordered and disorganized bone being laid down. The specific **treatment** of Paget's disease includes:

  a. Calcitonin: This agent acts by decreasing the resorption of bone, as measured by markers for bone resorption (i.e., a decrease in alkaline phosphatase, a decrease in urinary dihydroxyproline, and a decrease in N-telopeptide of type I collagen). The dose of calcitonin is 100 IU s.c. for salmon calcitonin or 0.5 mg s.c. for human calcitonin thrice weekly. The limits of this relatively well tolerated agent include:

  i. Only a modest decrease in disease progression
  ii. Patient with tachyphylaxis
  iii. Exacerbation on withdrawal.

  b. Etidronate: This is a bisphosphonate (i.e., an analog of pyrophosphate). It inhibits remineralization of bone and therefore decreases the abnormal formation of bone. The dose of etidronate is 5 mg/kg (400 mg/day) taken on an empty stomach. The limits and side effects include hypophosphatemia and an accelerated osteoporosis.

  c. Pamidronate (Alendronate): This is a very potent bisphosphonate that inhibits osteoclastic activity at a low dose, a dose too low to inhibit remineralization, and thereby no increase in osteoporosis. There is improvement in all manifestations except the pain. Dose: 15–90 mg in 1000 mg NS infused over 4–24hr.

  d. NSAIDs: Administered concurrent with one of these **modalities,** especially the pamidronate, to afford effective analgesia. See Table 7-8 (page 393).

  4. Referral: Endocrinology.

III. Consultation

Problem	*Service*	*Time*
Primary hyperparathyroidism	Endocrine/Surgery	Required
Malignancy	Hematology/Oncology	Urgent
Sarcoidosis	Pulmonary	Required

IV. Indications for admission: Decreased levels of consciousness, evidence of intravascular volume depletion, or any concurrent electrolyte disturbances.

Hyperkalemia (Boxes 9-4 and 9-5)

The normal range for serum potassium in the extracellular fluids is 3.5–5.0 mEq/dL.

The physiologic mechanisms that maintain potassium homeostasis and prevent hyperkalemia are several.

B O X 9-4

Overall Evaluation and Management of Hyperkalemia

Evaluation

1. Screen patients at risk for development of hyperkalemia (i.e., check potassium 5–7 days after starting an ACE inhibitor, especially in a diabetic patient or a patient with renal failure.
2. If hyperkalemia is present (i.e., K^+ >5.1 mEq/dL), determine the following laboratory values:
   a. Repeat K determination within hours.
   b. Electrolytes, BUN, creatinine, and glucose, for baseline purposes and to look for concurrent problems (e.g., renal failure).
   c. Urinalysis to look for evidence of renal dysfunction (e.g., casts, hematuria).
   d. Medication profile to look for medications that could result in hyperkalemia.
   e. Volume status of the patient. Assess if the patient is hypovolemic, euvolemic, or hypervolemic.
   f. 12-lead ECG to look for any of the described changes.
   g. Discontinue, at least temporarily, any exogenous source of potassium or any exacerbating medications (ACE inhibitors, NSAIDs, KCl supplements, and sodium-free salt, which contains KCl).
   h. Assess for and treat any evidence of adrenal insufficiency (see page 495).
3. If the potassium level is >6.0 mEq/dL with or without ECG changes, or if there is any degree of hyperkalemia with ECG changes:
   a. Admit to or transfer to a telemetry bed and perform all of the tests described previously.
   b. Acute intervention is mandatory and is described in Box 9-5.

Aldosterone (i.e., mineralocorticoids)

When the serum potassium increases, the cells of the zona glomerulosa increase production of the mineralocorticoid aldosterone, which acts on the renal tubules to increase the urinary loss of potassium. This is a coarse adjustment: There may be an actual decrease in the total body stores of potassium. Thus aldosterone production is central to the body's prevention of hyperkalemia.

B O X 9-5

Acute Management of Hyperkalemia

1. Calcium gluconate
   Dose: 1–3 g i.v.
   Onset: 3–5 min
   Duration: 1–2 hr
   Mechanism of action: Membrane stabilization
2. Sodium bicarbonate ($NaCO_3$)
   Dose: 1–2 ampules i.v.
   Onset: 10–15 min
   Duration: 4–6 hr
   Mechanism of action: Extracellular to intracellular shift
   Caveat: Most effective if the patient has a concurrent metabolic acidosis
3. Glucose or glucose and insulin
   Dose: $D_{10}W$ at 100 mL/hr; add regular insulin to the infusion as needed to keep patient's serum glucose 150–200 mg/dL;
   or
   1 ampule of $D_{50}W$ as an i.v. bolus and administer regular insulin s.c. to keep the serum glucose 150–200 mg/dL
   Onset: 15 min
   Duration: 12 hr
   Mechanism of action: Extracellular to intracellular shift
4. Loop diuretic
   Dose: Furosemide, 20 mg i.v.
   Onset: 2–4 hr
   Duration: 4–6 hr
   Mechanism of action: Loss of potassium in the urine
   Caveat: Most effective if patient has concurrent volume overload
5. Kayexalate
   Dose: Oral: 15–30 g p.o. q.A.M.
   Rectal: 50 g as a retention enema; must be kept in rectum/colon for >15 min
   Mechanism of action: Cation exchange of Na^+/K^+ at the colonic mucosal surface.
6. If adrenal insufficiency is suspected, administer 4 mg dexamethasone i.v., and then, after completion of the cosyntropin (Cortrosyn) stimulation test (page 496), administer hydrocortisone, 100 mg i.v., q.6hr or methylprednisolone (Solu-Medrol), 80 mg i.v., q.8hr.
7. Dialysis, either hemodialysis or peritoneal dialysis

Renal Tubules

The kidneys have a central role in regulating the level of potassium and adjust loss in the urine to prevent hyperkalemia. This is mainly through mineralocorticoid effects. This is a coarse adjustment measure in which there can be an actual decrease in the total body stores of potassium.

Catecholamines

Epinephrine and norepinephrine both drive potassium into the cells from the extracellular fluids. This is one reason that patients after "code 4" can be hypokalemic. This is a fine adjustment. The total body potassium is unchanged; it is only moved from the extracellular to the intracellular compartment.

Insulin

Insulin, by driving glucose into the cell, also drives potassium into the cell. This is a fine adjustment. The total body potassium is unchanged; it is only moved between the extracellular and the intracellular compartments.

Acid–Base Status

An alkaline pH (>7) in the extracellular fluids will drive potassium intracellularly, whereas an acid pH (<7) will drive potassium from intracellular to extracellular spaces. This is a fine adjustment. The total body potassium is unchanged; it is only moved between the extracellular and the intracellular compartments.

I. **Underlying causes**
   Underlying causes of hyperkalemia include anything that disturbs one of the physiologic mechanisms that maintain potassium homeostasis or anything that markedly increases the release of potassium into the extracellular fluids.
   A. **Disturbances of physiologic mechanisms**
      1. Primary adrenal insufficiency [i.e., destruction or dysfunction of either or both glands (Addison's disease) or of the zona glomerulosa, the area of the adrenal gland that produces mineralocorticoids].
      2. Acute or chronic renal failure may contribute to or result in the development of hyperkalemia.
      3. The administration of medications (e.g., β-blockers, NSAIDs, ACE inhibitors, and/or K-sparing diuretics) will, in certain patients, cause hyperkalemia. A patient at highest risk for the development of hyperkalemia from an ACE inhibitor or K-sparing diuretic is one with type IV renal tubular acidosis (RTA). Type IV RTA is a form of tubular acidosis in which there is a non–anion gap metabolic acidosis and hyperkalemia (i.e., a syndrome quite similar to a hypoaldosterone state). This disease, which in the past was referred to as hyporeninemic hypoaldosteronism, is probably not rare, but

only a rarely recognized manifestation of dysfunction associated with diabetes mellitus. The patient is often asymptomatic until an exacerbating factor is added, usually a medication such as an ACE inhibitor, at which time the potassium level significantly increases.

B. States that increase the **release of potassium from the cells into the extravascular fluids**

Hemolysis, tumor lysis syndrome, and rhabdomyolysis cause cellular disruption and release of intracellular contents, rich in potassium, into the extracellular fluids. Hemolysis can occur in the process of drawing blood and therefore is a potential source of a falsely increased potassium level. Tumor lysis syndrome is a potentially catastrophic process in which a patient with a rapidly growing, usually lymphoproliferative disorder (e.g., lymphoma) receives chemotherapy. The chemotherapy destroys a significant number of tumor cells, which release large quantities of potassium, phosphorus, and purines (uric acid), resulting in severe hyperkalemia and renal failure.

II. Overall manifestations

A patient with hyperkalemia is often free of symptoms and signs until markedly increased potassium levels are present. The first signs of severe hyperkalemia may be ECG changes, which proceed to significant dysrhythmias and even ventricular tachycardia with sudden death. The ECG changes include but are not limited to:

- Diffuse flattening of the P waves
- Diffuse peaking of the T waves
- Diffuse widening of the QRS complexes
- Severe, hemodynamically compromising brady/tachydysrhythmias

The threshold for ECG changes due to hyperkalemia is different for different patients: one patient may tolerate a potassium of 6.0 mEq/dL, whereas another will have florid ECG changes at 5.5.

Once ECG changes due to hyperkalemia are present, the next rhythm potentially is asystole or ventricular tachycardia; therefore, any ECG changes are emergency findings.

III. Adrenal insufficiency

A. The **underlying pathogenesis** is one of the destruction of atrophy of the adrenal cortices, including the zona glomerulosa (mineralocorticoids), the zona fasciculata (glucocorticoids), and the zona reticularis (ketosteroids). The underlying causes of primary adrenal insufficiency include the following:

1. Autoimmune: 60%–70% of cases today; there is a slow destruction of the glands by cytotoxic lymphocytes; small glands.

2. Infections including mycobacterial disease, histoplasmosis, paracoccidioidomycosis, in which the glands are enlarged and calcified, and finally HIV infection of the glands.

3. Hemorrhage: Including meningococcemia.
4. Drugs including ketoconazole.
5. Infiltrative processes, including metastatic carcinoma, hemochromatosis, and sarcoidosis.
6. Adrenoleukodystrophy: X-linked recessive disorder; spastic paralysis, adrenal insufficiency; dysfunction of long-chain fatty acids.
7. PGA II (i.e., Schmidt's syndrome—Addison's disease and Hashimoto's disease).

   The **underlying etiologies** of secondary adrenal insufficiency include panhypopituitarism and chronic excessive steroids, with resultant decrease in adrenocorticotropic hormone (ACTH) and therefore, cortisol.

B. The **specific manifestations** include hypotension, hyperkalemia, increased BUN and creatinine, a normal anion-gap metabolic acidosis, eosinophilia, and hypoglycemia. There is also an increase in skin pigment, fevers, hyponatremia, and intravascular volume depletion. The underlying origin will also have **specific manifestations** in addition to the adrenal insufficiency manifestations.

C. The **overall evaluation and management** includes that described in Boxes 9-4 and 9-5 and performing a *cosyntropin-stimulation test*.

   1. **Cosyntropin-stimulation test**
      a. The steps in this examination include:
         i. Time = 0: Draw serum aldosterone and cortisol
         ii. Time = 0: Administer 0.25 mg (250 μg) ACTH i.v.
         iii. Time = 60 minutes: Draw serum aldosterone and cortisol
      b. **Results**

         Cortisol of >20 μg/dL rules out primary adrenal insufficiency

         Aldosterone of >5 ng/dL rules out primary adrenal insufficiency

         If a blunted increase to ACTH, consistent with adrenal insufficiency

   2. Other tests in evaluation include:
      a. Antibodies to adrenal cortex: Sensitivity, 70%; specificity, >90%
      b. Antibodies to 21-hydroxylase: Higher sensitivity and specificity
      c. **Metyrapone challenge:** Best test to differentiate primary from secondary adrenal insufficiency. Metyrapone blocks the last step in cortisol (11 β-hydroxylase). The steps include:
         • 2300 hours: 3 g metyrapone p.o.
         • 0700 hours: Measure serum 11-deoxycortisol
         • If the 11-deoxycortisol is <7.5 μg/dL, secondary/tertiary adrenal insufficiency

- If the deoxycortisol is >7.5 μg/dL, primary adrenal insufficiency

D. The **specific treatment** includes making the clinical diagnosis and starting an infusion of D5.9 N saline to replete fluids, correct any hypoglycemia, and administer dexamethasone, 4 mg i.v. Perform the cosyntropin (Cortrosyn)-stimulation test and then administer hydrocortisone, 60–100 mg i.v. q.6–8hr. The maintenance doses are
  1. Dexamethasone, 0.5 mg p.o. q.HS
     -or-
     Prednisone, 5 mg p.o. q.HS
     -and-
     Fludrocortisone, 0.1 mg p.o., q.d.
     Adjust to keep the morning ACTH level 4–18 pmol/L
  2. Hydrocortisone, 20 mg p.o. q.A.M. and 10 mg p.o. q.P.M.
     Cortisol acetate, 25 mg p.o., q.A.M., and 12.5 mg p.o., q.P.M.
  3. The patient must always receive stress (increased) doses during times of stress (e.g., infections, surgery).

IV. **Long-term management**
    Long-term management of hyperkalemia includes defining and treating the underlying cause. The clinician must be appropriately cautious in initiating any agent that may precipitate or exacerbate hyperkalemia. If such an agent is initiated, the clinician must monitor, especially early on, the potassium level quite closely. If the patient has chronic renal failure, refer to a dietitian to educate the patient on a low-potassium diet; administer $NaHCO_3$ by mouth to keep the serum HCO_3 at >15 mEq/dL; if nonacidotic or refractory to the first two interventions, administer sodium polystyrene sulfonate (Kayexalate) 15–30 mg p.o., q.A.M.; and, when necessary, initiate chronic dialysis (see section on Renal Dysfunction in Chapter 3 for details of management).

V. **Consultation**

Problem	*Service*	*Time*
Acute renal failure	Renal	Urgent/emergent
Addison's disease	Endocrinology	Emergent

VI. **Indications for admission:** Any ECG changes, a potassium level >6.0 mEq/dL, any evidence of acute renal failure, or Addison's disease.

Thyroid Dysfunctional States

The normal thyroid gland is located in the anterior neck and is ~15–20 g in total mass. The gland is soft, symmetric, bilobed, and nontender. It produces two specific hormones, calcitonin and thyroxine.

Calcitonin is produced in the parafollicular or C-cells and is involved in calcium homeostasis. An increase in plasma calcium levels will result in an increase in the production of calcitonin to decrease the calcium level back to normal. The hormone is, at most, a minor player in overall calcium homeostasis.

Thyroxine is the major endocrine product of the thyroid gland. This hormone, which requires the anion iodide for its synthesis within the thyroid gland, controls and regulates the overall baseline catabolic rate of the entire body. It is required for the sustenance of life. The hormone is produced in the tetraiodinated state (T_4; i.e., levothyroxine) in the gland. In the peripheral tissues, it is deiodinated to the most active form, triiodothyronine (T_3). The thyroid gland of the average person produces ~125 μg of thyroxine per day. As a result of its central and integral role to the biochemical machinery of the cells, an overall increase or decrease in the amount of this hormone produced will cause significant pathology. In this section, the overall approach to thyroid dysfunction, whether or not a goiter is present, the **specific manifestations,** evaluation, management, and sequelae of hypothyroidism, hyperthyroidism, and thyroid nodules are discussed (Box 9-6).

I. **Thyroid excess states (i.e., hyperthyroidism)** (Box 9-7, page 504)
   A. The **specific manifestations** of an excess of thyroid hormone, a hormone that intimately regulates the overall catabolism of the cells within the body, include heat intolerance, diaphoresis, unintentional weight loss, fine hair, lid lag (Darymple's sign), tachycardia, atrial fibrillation, and symmetric muscle weakness, greater proximally than distally. Extreme hyperthyroidism (i.e., thyroid storm) can result in death. Manifestations that may be harbingers of such a catastrophic event include hyperpyrexia, temperatures >105°F, and marked tachycardias. Of interest is that

(text continues on page 502)

B O X   9-6

Overall Evaluation and Management of Suspected Thyroid Diseases

Evaluation

1. Take a history and perform a physical examination.
   a. Tachycardia, atrial fibrillation, diaphoresis, weight loss, fine tremor, diarrhea, thin body habitus, proximal muscle weakness, and bilateral lid lag all are indicative of hyperthyroidism.

(continued)

B O X 9-6 *(continued)*

  b. Normocardia or bradycardia, dry skin, weight gain, constipation, obese body habitus, proximal muscle weakness, and coarse thick hair with loss of lateral eyebrow hair bilaterally (Queen Anne's sign) all are indicative of hypothyroidism.
  c. Further suggestive features on the history and physical examination include:
    i. A history of antecedent radiation to the neck, even in the distant past, which is associated with an increased risk of hypothyroidism and thyroid malignancy.
    ii. Scars about the neck. Query the patient regarding specific thyroid surgeries.
    iii. Assess and document features of the thyroid gland itself, including the size of the gland, the consistency of the gland, whether the gland is tender or nontender, whether any nodules are present, and, if nodules are present, their size and location within the gland.
2. Based on the clinical data gleaned from the history and physical examination, classify the patient as being clinically hyperthyroid, hypothyroid, or euthyroid.
3. History of medications and supplements is important as hyperthyroidism may be exacerbated or caused by long-term iodide ingestion (Jod Basedow) or amiodarone; hypothyroidism may result from long-term ingestion/use of lithium.
4. Determine serum electrolyte, BUN, creatinine, and glucose levels for baseline purposes and to look for any concurrent electrolyte disturbances.
5. Determine a complete blood cell count with differential for baseline purposes.
6. Perform urinalysis and, if the patient is female, a urine pregnancy test.
7. Perform thyroid-function tests (i.e., free T_4, TSH, and free T_3 assays) (see Table 9-2 for specifics on normal values and interpretation of any abnormal values).

Management

1. **Specific management** is discussed in the text. If the patient is hyperthyroid, see page 498; if hypothyroid, see page 507; if thyroid nodules are present, see page 511; if goiter is present, see Tables 9-3 and 9-4.
2. Refer to an endocrinologist.

TABLE 9-2
Thyroid Function Tests

Test	Normal Ranges	Interpretation

Free T_4	5–12 μg/dL	Increased:
		  Hyperthyroid
		Normal:
		  Normal, *or* T_3 hyperthyroid
		Decreased:
		  Hypothyroid

TSH	Highly sensitive; uses immunospecific mono-clonal antibodies
	0.5–6.0 μU/mL
		If low:[a]
		  a) Primary hyperthyroidism
		  b) Secondary hypothyroidism
		  c) Tertiary hypothyroidism
		If high:
		  a) Primary hypothyroidism
		  b) Secondary hyperthyroidism
		NOTE: If low and the free T_4 is low to normal, check the free T_3 to rule out T_3 thyrotoxicosis.

Free T$_3$	Direct measurement of the biological active hormone, via radioimmunoassay Test is rarely needed[b] in the workup of thyroid disease Normal: 80–200 ng/dL	If increased: T$_3$ hyperthyroid not necessary in all thyroid evaluations, specifically indicated in patients with a low TSH but normal free T$_4$ in order to evaluate for T$_3$ thyrotoxicosis.
Radioactive iodine uptake	Measures activity of thyroid tissue by measuring uptake of radioactive ^{131}I by thyroid tissue ^{131}I is given p.o. Images of uptake obtained at 6 and 24 hr Not to be confused with the clinically useless thyroid ^{99m}Tc or ^{131}I "scan" Normal: 30%–40% uptake at 24 hr	High uptake (>60%): a) Graves' disease b) Early Hashimoto's disease c) Endemic goiter d) Early postpartum Low uptake (<10%): a) Late Hashimoto's disease b) Jod Basedow/factitious hyperthyroidism c) de Quervain's disease d) After removal or ablation of thyroid tissue

T A B L E 9-3
Causes of Goiter

Endemic: Results from a lack of iodide salts in the diet. Endemic to the Great Lakes region of North America, the Balkan peninsula of Eastern Europe, the Andes region of South America, and east-central Asia
Thyroiditis: Diffuse, symmetric goiter; see Table 9-4 for specifics
Graves' disease: Diffuse, symmetric goiter; see text for specifics
Plummer's disease: Multinodular, symmetric to asymmetric goiter; see text for specifics
Solitary nodules: See Thyroid nodules (page 511)
Multinodular goiter: See Thyroid nodules (page 511)

(text continued from page 498)
younger patients will have many more of the classic manifestations than will older individuals.
  B. **Causes of hyperthyroidism**
    1. **Graves' disease.** This is an autoimmune disease with the constellation of hyperthyroidism with diffuse goiter; dermopathy; peau d'orange skin changes, especially on the pretibial areas; and ophthalmopathy, unilateral or bilateral with proptosis. The exophthalmus (i.e., proptosis) is specific to Graves' disease and not a part of the overall hyperthyroidism.
      a. The **specific evaluation** of Graves' disease involves making the clinical diagnosis by using the tests described in Boxes 9-6 and 9-7. The TSH will be 0.0 μU/mL, and the free T_4 and free T_3 levels will be increased. A radioactive iodide-uptake scan will show a diffuse and marked increase in the uptake of iodide, >70% at 24 hours.
      b. **Specific management** includes administering β-blockers, unless contraindicated. Further management includes the initiation and administration of antithyroid agents or radioactive iodine.
        i. Antithyroid medications decrease thyroid hormone synthesis and therefore, over time, decrease the levels of thyroid hormone present. They should be used for 6–12 months or until the patient is euthyroid.
          (a) **Propylthiouracil (PTU)** inhibits the organification of the iodide anions, thus inhibiting T_4 synthesis. Furthermore, it blocks the peripheral conversion of the relatively inactive T_4 to T_3. Side effects are hepatitis and, rarely, agranulocytosis. The starting dose is 300 mg/24 hr p.o., in a b.i.d. dosing schedule.

T A B L E 9-4
Thyroiditis

Disease	Presentation	Histopathology	Laboratory Findings	Radioactive Iodide Scan at 6 and 24 hr (Normal at 24 hr: 10%–40% uptake)	Natural History	Treatment
Hashimoto's disease	Nontender Diffuse goiter Hyper- or hypothyroid at presentation	Lymphocytic	Early: Increased, T_4 Normal TSH Positive antimicrosomal antibodies Late: Decreased, T_4 Increased TSH	Early: Increased uptake Late: Decreased uptake	Indolent, can have goiter long term; initially hyperthyroid, then hypothyroid	Early: β-blockers if symptomatic Late: Need levothyroxine replacement
de Quervain's disease	Acute onset Exquisitely tender Diffuse goiter Upper respiratory infection antedates it by 5–7 days	Granulomatous	Acutely, can be clinically and biochemically hyperthyroid; negative antimicrosomal and antithyroglobulin antibodies	No uptake diffusely	Acutely, patient is hyperthyroid, then can have 2–4-month period of hypothyroidism; long term, euthyroid	Salicylates or an NSAID If severe, can use a short course of steroids (prednisone, 60 mg p.o. q.d. in rapid taper)
Lymphocytic	Nontender Diffuse goiter during 2nd and 3rd trimester of pregnancy	Lymphocytic	Early: Increased T_4 Normal TSH Late: Normal	Contraindicated if patient is pregnant	Acutely hyperthyroid, followed by transient postpartum hypothyroidism; long term, euthyroid	Observation, symptomatic

B O X   9-7

Evaluation and Management of Hyperthyroidism

1. Perform the evaluations listed in Box 9-6.
2. Perform a urine pregnancy test.
3. Determine the underlying cause from the history and physical examination and a radioiodide uptake scan (see Table 9-4 for information on the radioiodide uptake scan).
4. Administer β-blockers, specifically propranolol, 10–40 mg p.o., q.i.d., or atenolol, 50–100 mg p.o., q.d., unless there is a contraindication, to blunt the tachycardia and other manifestations of the hypercatabolic state.
5. If the patient is in thyroid storm (i.e., here is evidence of acute severe excess of thyroid hormone with life-threatening hemodynamic instability), the clinician should:
   a. Administer a β-blocker, either in doses listed or, acutely, as an i.v. injection of 1 mg propranolol, may repeat q.1hr times 3, or metoprolol, 25 mg i.v., may repeat times 1, then oral β-blocker
   -and-
   b. Administer potassium iodide (KI) 1–2 g intravenously over 24 hours. This agent is highly effective in inhibiting release of T_4 and in inhibiting all steps in the synthesis of T_4 and the conversion of T_4 to T_3 peripherally.
   ***This regimen, β-blockers and KI, is effective also as a preoperative **modality** for patients with untreated hyperthyroidism who require a nonthyroid surgical procedure.
6. Consult an endocrinologist for assistance.

-or-

  (b) **Methimazole (Tapazole)** inhibits the organification of the iodide anions, thus inhibiting T_4 synthesis. Side effects are hepatitis and, rarely, agranulocytosis. The starting dose is 30 mg/24 hr p.o., in a once daily dosage.

  ii. Radioactive iodide 131 is the **treatment** of choice in virtually all patients with Graves' disease. The only contraindication is concurrent pregnancy. The dose of this agent is 5–15 mCi (the equivalent of 4,000–20,000 rad) to the thyroid gland itself). Graham et al. reported in a long-term,

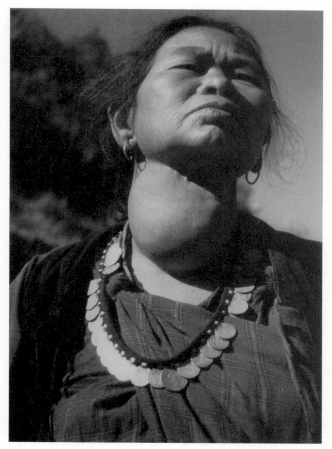

FIGURE 9-1
Endemic goiter; large symmetric goiter from iodide deficiency.

longitudinal study that there is no increased risk of secondary malignancies in patients treated with the radioactive isotope [131]I. Some reports showed an association between the administration of ^{131}I for Graves' and the future development of ophthalmopathy, so some endocrinologists recommended that if ophthalmopathy is present from the outset, non-[131]I **modalities** should be used. Overall, however, this **treatment** is clearly the most efficient and effective treatment for hyperthyroidism as the result of Graves' disease.

c. The clinician must observe the patient for the development of a **dermopathy.** The dermopathy is best treated with a topical glucocorticoid cream (e.g., triamcinolone, 1% cream, b.i.d.).

d. The clinician must observe the patient for the development of **ophthalmopathy.** The manifestations of the ophthalmopathy, like those of the dermopathy (specifically, unilateral or bilateral exophthalmos) can occur even after the hyperthyroidism has been successfully treated. The **specific evaluation and management** include performing a computed tomography (CT) scan of the orbits to document thickening of the musculature and to rule out any other space-occupying lesions. **Treatment** includes administration of lubricating eyedrops (e.g., methylcellulose 1% (Isopto Alkaline) drops o.u. t.i.d.–q.i.d.) and, if early in course, the administration of systemic steroids for 3–6 months and referral to ophthalmology for specific intervention. If the process is severe or refractory to steroids, local irradiation may be indicated and is usually quite effective. In all cases, any resultant hypothyroidism must be aggressively managed as hypothyroidism will exacerbate the ophthalmopathy.

e. Follow up thyroid-function tests as, after ^{131}I therapy, hypothyroidism will invariably occur. Replacement with levothyroxine is indicated.

f. In patients who are pregnant, the administration of PTU in doses mentioned is indicated to decrease the free T_4 levels to those appropriate for that portion of pregnancy (i.e., usually 50% above normal). **Treatment** of hyperthyroidism will decrease the risk of hyperemesis gravidarum later in pregnancy.

2. Plummer's disease. This is the development of a hyperthyroid state from a toxic multinodular goiter.

a. The **specific manifestations** include the **overall manifestations** of hyperthyroidism and an enlarged goiter with multiple discrete nodules. The goiter and the nodules are nontender. There is no associated ophthalmopathy or dermopathy.

b. The **specific evaluation** includes the overall evaluation (see Boxes 9-6 and 9-7), TSH level of 0.0, increased free T_4 level, and a radioactive thyroid uptake scan demonstrating several nodules with increased uptake. The **specific management** is similar to that of Graves' disease [i.e., a β-blocker and

T A B L E 9-5
Causes of Jod Basedow

Oral ingestion of kelp
Oral ingestion of iodide tablets
Ingestion of meats with iodide or thyroid gland present, e.g.,
  ground beef with strap muscle used in processing
Factitious use of thyroid hormone, either as a stimulant or as
  a weight reduction agent
Recurrent, long-term use of topical iodide-containing anti-
  septics

either an antithyroid agent (methimazole or PTU)
or radioactive ^{131}I].
3. **Factitious hyperthyroidism,** including Jod Basedow
   syndrome. This is the surreptitious use of thyroid hormone or iodide with a resultant hyperthyroidism. See
   Table 9-5 for potential sources of Jod Basedow.
   a. The **specific manifestations** include those of hyper-
      thyroidism, but there is invariably no goiter, oph-
      thalmopathy, or dermopathy.
   b. The **specific evaluation** includes that described in
      Boxes 9-6 and 9-7 and the presence of a TSH level
      of 0.0 and an increased T_4 level. The most specific
      component is a diffusely decreased uptake in the
      gland on radioactive iodide-uptake scan.
   c. The **specific management** includes discovering the
      source of the iodide or levothyroxine, even if it re-
      quires confronting the patient with such data. β-
      Blockers can be administered for symptomatic relief
      of the hyperthyroidism; however, antithyroid agents
      or ^{131}I ablation are contraindicated as therapeutic
      modalities.
C. **Consultation**

Service	Time
Endocrinology	Urgent

D. **Indications for admission:** Atrial fibrillation with a rapid
   ventricular response, or any evidence of imminent thyroid
   storm. The vast majority of patients with hyperthyroidism
   will be managed as outpatients.
II. **Thyroid-deficiency states (i.e., hypothyroidism;** Box 9-8)
   A. The **specific manifestations** of a deficiency in thyroid hor-
      mone, a hormone that intimately regulates the overall ca-
      tabolism of the cells within the body, include cold intoler-
      ance, dry skin, unintentional weight gain, coarse hair,
      bradycardia, symmetric muscle weakness, greater proxi-
      mally than distally, decreased reflexes, and a delayed re-
      (text continues on page 510)

B O X   9-8

***Evaluation and Management of Suspected
Hypothyroidism***

Evaluation

1. Take a thorough history and perform a physical examination, with emphasis on the previously mentioned features/manifestations.
2. Determine serum electrolyte, BUN, creatinine, and
   glucose levels for baseline purposes.
3. Determine the complete blood cell count with differential analysis, looking for any concurrent anemia,
   usually macrocytic, if present.
4. Determine serum calcium, PO_4, and albumin levels,
   looking for any concurrent hypercalcemia or hypocalcemia.
5. Perform a urine pregnancy test at baseline.
6. Perform urinalysis, looking for concurrent proteinuria.
7. Determine creatine phosphokinase level, as it often
   will be increased in patients with proximal muscle
   weakness (i.e., hypothyroid-related myopathy).
8. Obtain a 12-lead ECG if there is any evidence of
   bradycardia.
9. Determine free T_4 and TSH levels (see Table 9-2,
   page 500).

Management

1. If consciousness is significantly depressed, suggest-
   ing impending myxedema coma, perform the following evaluations:
   a. Check ABCs as appropriate according to the ACLS
      protocol.
   b. Make finger-stick glucose determinations to rule
      out hypoglycemia.
   c. Determine arterial blood gases at baseline to rule
      out hypoxemia and hypercapnia.
   d. Replete fluids i.v., usually with $D_{5.45}$ NS, as appro-
      priate.
   e. Make arrangements for admission to an ICU.
   f. If hypoglycemic, administer one to two ampules
      of $D_{50}W$ i.v.
   g. Obtain basic core of data in Boxes 9-6 and 9-8.
   h. Do not warm the patient.

(continued)

B O X 9-8 (continued)

    i. Administer vasopressor agents (e.g., dopamine)
       to maintain adequate perfusion.
    j. Administer thyroxine, 300–500 μg by i.v. push
       over a 15-minute period.
        i. Sodium levothyroxine, 500 μg/10 mg mannitol.
       ii. Mix with 5 mL of normal saline.
      iii. Administer by slow i.v. push (10–15 minutes).
       iv. Once mixed, it is quite unstable and must be
           used immediately.
    k. Hydrocortisone, 80 mg i.v., now and q.8hr until
       stable, as the patient can often be concurrently ad-
       renal insufficient.
    l. Endocrinology consultation mandated on an emer-
       gent basis.
 2. If clinically hypothyroid but not acutely ill, or after
    stabilization of a myxedematous patient:
    a. Basic core of data, Boxes 9-6 and 9-8.
    b. Initiate levothyroxine (Synthroid; i.e., T_4). The
       usual repletion dose is 75–150 μg p.o., q.d. If the
       patient is otherwise healthy, start with a dose of
       75–100 μg/day. If the patient has a significant his-
       tory of angina or ASHD, start with a very low
       dose, 12.5–25 μg p.o., q.d., and increase the dose
       slowly (25 μg q.6–8 weeks) subsequently. The
       half-life of T_4, levothyroxine, is ~7 days; therefore,
       it takes ~4 weeks to reach a steady state with any
       dose initiation or change. The dose should be ti-
       trated to a clinically euthyroid state or TSH nor-
       malization. The TSH should be checked ~4–6
       weeks after any change in levothyroxine dosage.
    c. Check for any concurrent or concomitant autoim-
       mune disease on a longitudinal basis.
    d. Screen for lipid abnormalities as there is a high in-
       cidence of hyperlipidemia in patients with hypo-
       thyroidism.
    e. Endocrinology consultation is recommended but
       not mandatory.
    f. If there is an endemic goiter, replace the iodine
       with iodinized table salt; iodine replacement is as
       effective as levothyroxine in this specific case sce-
       nario.
    g. If the patient is unable to take anything enterally
       for >10 days, administer the thyroid replacement

(continued)

B O X 9-8 *(continued)*

parenterally. The dose is 70% of the daily oral dose administered by i.v. route q.d.

h. Overreplacement with thyroxine results in the risk of accelerating atherosclerotic disease and/or osteoporosis.

3. **Subclinical hypothyroidism:** In patients who are asymptomatic and have a TSH which is >15 mIU/L, replacement with thyroxine may be of benefit. The two specific indications are such patients who have hyperlipidemia and/or a goiter. The replacement dose is 50% of the standard dose of thyroxine (50–75 μg p.o., q.d.), and recheck the TSH in 2–3 months. Adjust the replacement dose based on the TSH and clinical assessment of thyroid status.

4. **Hypothyroidism in pregnancy:** Hypothyroidism will directly affect the developing fetus and may result in low-birth-weight neonates, cretinism, and stillbirth. In addition, there is an increased risk of preeclampsia in hypothyroid pregnant women. Adequate replacement prevents these. In hypothyroid pregnant women, the clinician must check TSH and free T_4 at end of first trimester in hypothyroid patients. If TSH is normal, no change in replacement is necessary; if TSH is increased, a mild (25%) increase in thyroxine replacement dose is indicated. Recheck the TSH 6 weeks after the dose modification.

(text continued from page 507)

laxation phase of the deep tendon reflexes (DTRs). Extreme hypothyroidism (i.e., myxedema) can result in death. Manifestations that may be harbingers of such a catastrophic event include hypothermia, bradycardias, lethargy, and coma.

B. The **underlying causes** of hypothyroidism include thyroiditides (e.g., Hashimoto's, lymphocytic, or de Quervain's; see Table 9-4), iatrogenic (e.g., antecedent radiation therapy for Graves' disease, a head and neck carcinoma, or Hodgkin's disease), or surgical removal of the gland, any of which will result in hypothyroidism. Finally, endemic goiter needs to be considered. This is hypothyroidism with a diffuse goiter as the result of deficiency of iodide in the diet. It was endemic to the Great Lakes basin of North America and still is endemic to the Struma River valley of Eastern Europe, east-central Asia including Nepal, and the Andes region of South America. Certain medications may cause or exacerbate hypothyroidism. These include $FeSO_4$, which decreases the absorption of levothyroxine by the gastrointestinal tract, and lithium which directly acts on the gland to result in hypothyroidism.

C. The **specific evaluation and management** of these entities are given in Boxes 9-6 and 9-8 and Table 9-4.

D. Consultation

Problem	Service	Time
Myxedema	Endocrine	Emergent
Hypothyroidism	Endocrine	Elective

E. **Indications for admission:** Impending or present myxedema.

III. **Thyroid nodules** (Box 9-9)

Thyroid nodules are usually found in an asymptomatic patient during a routine physical examination. The vast majority of nodules are benign; however, malignant thyroid nodules occur in a small yet significant minority.

B O X 9-9

Evaluation and Management of Thyroid Nodules

Evaluation

1. Perform an overall evaluation as described in Box 9-6.
2. Assess the clinical thyroid state of the patient: hyperthyroid, euthyroid, or hypothyroid.
3. Perform ultrasonography of the thyroid. This imaging study is not mandatory, as it does not differentiate benign from malignant lesions. However, it is helpful as an adjunct to physical examination in that it helps the clinician, particularly a nonendocrinologist, to define the number and size of the nodules. Furthermore, it will define whether the nodule is cystic or solid.
4. Thyroid scans using ^{99m}Tc or ^{131}I are useless in the evaluation of thyroid nodules.
5. Assess and stratify the risk that the nodule is malignant by using the basic core of data and clinical judgment.
   a. High risk. A patient with several of the previously mentioned **risk factors** (e.g., a young male with a solitary nodule) must be referred to an endocrinologist/thyroidologist and undergo excisional bi-

(continued)

B O X 9-9 *(continued)*

opsy of the lesion by an experienced endocrine
surgeon. The patient should be staged for distant
metastases by ^{131}I body scan.
   b. Low risk. A patient with multiple **low-risk factors**
(e.g., an elderly woman with multiple nodules)
should be monitored clinically with TSH and thyroid examinations.
   c. Intermediate risk. Usually a solitary nodule without any other **high-risk factors**. Further evaluation
and management of these patients include referral to endocrinologist/thyroidologist. One of three
approaches can be used:
      i. Excisional biopsy,
         -or-
      ii. Fine-needle aspiration of the nodule and send
for cytology. If cytology is positive for malignant neoplastic cells, refer to a surgeon and
stage with ^{131}I body scan for distant metastases. If cytology is negative for malignant neoplastic cells, one cannot rule out malignancy
and thus must use another approach listed
here (e.g., a trial of suppression).
6. Attempt suppression with exogenous thyroxine (i.e.,
50–100 μg levothyroxine, p.o., q.d., for 8–12 weeks).
May increase the dose to a maximum of 100–150 μg/
day. The goal is to decrease the TSH to 0.05–0.1
mIU/L. The theory behind suppression is that by giving the patient exogenous thyroxine, there is a negative feedback on the hypothalamus/adenohypophysis
and a decrease in TSH. Most benign nodules are
quite dependent on TSH and rapidly decrease in size
when TSH is removed, whereas most malignant neoplastic nodules are significantly more autonomous
(i.e., independent of TSH for growth). Therefore if
there is a decrease in size of the nodule, continue levothyroxine dose/suppression; follow up TFTs, TSH,
and nodule size over the long term. If there is no decrease in size of the nodule after 3–6 months of suppression, excisional biopsy should be performed.

Management

The **management** of thyroid malignant lesions is described in Table 9-6.

T A B L E 9-6
Thyroid Malignancies

Type	Risk Factors	Metastases	Treatment/Comments
Papillary	Past head or neck irradiation	Lymph nodes	Surgical excision of primary tumor Exogenous thyroxine, keeping the patient biochemically mildly hyperthyroid to suppress TSH If residual tumor is demonstrated by ^{131}I body scan, ^{131}I ablation; dose: 100–150 mC; p.o.; **endocrinology consultation is mandatory**
Follicular	Neck irradiation	Hematogenous Lung Bone	Essentially same as papillary; overall poorer prognosis; **endocrine consultation is mandatory**
Medullary carcinoma	Multiple endocrine neoplasia, type IIa (Sipple's disease) Bilateral pheochromocytomas Parathyroid hyperplasia Medullary carcinoma		Surgical resection Tumor is derived from the parafollicular C-cells and can produce calcitonin, prostaglandins, and histamine
Anaplastic	Neck irradiation	Aggressive local and systemic spread	Surgical excision and chemotherapy Requires oncology and endocrinology consultations

A. **Risk factors**

   Risk factors for the development of thyroid carcinoma, and therefore factors that should increase the suspicion for malignant nodules, include:

   1. Previous irradiation to the neck, either iatrogenic or exposure to nuclear fallout (e.g., living in southern Utah in the 1950s).
   2. Solitary nodule.
   3. Young age.
   4. Male sex.
   5. Firm and fixed mass.
   6. Concurrent palpable cervical nodes.

B. **Differential diagnosis**

   The **differential diagnosis** of thyroid nodules includes multinodular goiter (i.e., an enlarged thyroid gland with multiple nodules, euthyroid clinically); Plummer's disease (i.e., multinodular goiter with hyperthyroidism); benign adenoma, euthyroid or hyperthyroid; and a malignant neoplastic lesion (see Table 9-6). Other extrathyroid causes of anterior neck masses, including branchial cleft cysts and extrathyroidal lymphadenopathy, must be included in the differential diagnosis but invariably may be excluded on physical examination.

C. **Consultation**

Problem	Service	Time
Solitary nodule	Endocrinology	Urgent
Multiple nodules	Endocrinology	Elective

D. **Indications for admission:** If and when surgical intervention is required.

Bibliography

Diabetes Mellitus

Brown MJ, Asbury AK: Diabetic neuropathy. Ann Neurol 1984;15:2.

Gerich JE: Insulin-dependent diabetes mellitus: pathophysiology. Mayo Clin Proc 1986;61:787–791.

Gerich JE: Sulfonylureas in the treatment of diabetes mellitus—1985. Mayo Clin Proc 1985;60:439.

Harati Y: Diabetic peripheral neuropathies. Ann Intern Med 1987;107:546–559.

Hodges D, et al: Management of the diabetic foot. Ann Fam Pract 1986;33:189–195.

Klein R, et al: Microalbuminuria in a population based study of diabetes. Arch Intern Med 1992;152:153–158.

KROC Collaborative Study Group: Diabetic retinopathy after two years of intensified insulin treatment. JAMA 1988;260:37–41.

Moller DE, Flier JS: Insulin resistance: mechanisms, syndromes, and implications. N Engl J Med 1991;325:938–948.

Nathan DM, et al: Non-insulin dependent diabetes in older patients. Am J Med 1986;81:837–842.

National Diabetes Data Group: Classification and diagnosis of diabetes mellitus and other categories of glucose intolerance. Diabetes 1979;28:1039.

Nelson RL: Oral glucose tolerance test: indications and limitations. Mayo Clin Proc 1988;63:263–269.

Reddi AS, Camerini-Davalos RA: Diabetic nephropathy. Arch Intern Med 1990;150:31–42.

Sherwin RS, Taborlane WV: Metabolic control and diabetic complications. In: Olesky JM, Sherwin RS, eds. Diabetes mellitus: management and complications. New York: Churchill Livingstone, 1985:108–182.

Singer DE, et al: Screening for diabetes mellitus. Ann Intern Med 1988;109:639–649.

Singer DE, et al: Tests of glycemia in diabetes mellitus. Ann Intern Med 1989;110:125–137.

Hypercalcemia

Boonstra CE, Jackson CE: Hyperparathyroidism detected by routine serum calcium analysis: prevalence in a clinic population. Ann Intern Med 1965;63:468.

Levine MM, Kleeman CR: Hypercalcemia: pathophysiology and treatment. Hosp Pract 1987;July:73–90.

Lufkin EG, et al: Parathyroid hormone radioimmunoassays in the differential diagnosis of hypercalcemia due to primary hyperparathyroidism or malignancy. Ann Intern Med 1987;106:559.

Singer FR, Fernandez M: Therapy of hypercalcemia of malignancy. Am J Med 1987;82(S2A):34–40.

Hyperkalemia

DeFronzo RA: Hyperkalemia and hyporeninemic hypoaldosteronism. Kidney Int 1980;17:118–134.

Ponce SP, et al: Drug-induced hyperkalemia. Medicine 1985;64:357–370.

Williams ME, et al: Hyperkalemia. Adv Intern Med 1986;32:265.

Thyroid Dysfunctional States

Allen ME, Braverman LE: Management of thyrotoxicosis. Compr Ther 1987;13:20–30.

Cooper DS: Antithyroid drugs. N Engl J Med 1984;311:1353–1362.

Hamberger JI: The various presentations of thyroiditis. Ann Intern Med 1986;104:219–224.

Helfand M, Crapo LM: Monitoring therapy in patients taking levothyroxine. Ann Intern Med 1990;113:450–454.

Helfand M, Crapo LM: Screening for thyroid disease. Ann Intern Med 1990;112:840–849.

Levine SN: Current concepts of thyroiditis. Arch Intern Med 1983;143:1952–1956.

Nordyke RA, et al: Graves' disease. Arch Intern Med 1988;148:626–631.

Robbins J, et al: Thyroid cancer: a lethal endocrine neoplasm. Ann Intern Med 1991;115:133–147.

Sakiyama R: Common thyroid disorders. Am Fam Pract 1988;38:227–238.

Salman K, et al: Selection of thyroid preparations. Am Fam Pract 1989;40:215–219.

de los Santos ET, Mazzaferri EL: Thyroid function tests. Postgrad Med 1989;85:333–351.

Wartofsky L: Guidelines for the treatment of hyperthyroidism. Am Fam Pract 1984;30:199–210.

—D.D.B.

Chapter 10

Male Genitourinary Tract

Prostate Dysfunction

The prostate gland is located at the inferior aspect of and immediately adjacent to the urinary bladder in males. It is an organ through which the urethra passes as it enters into the proximal penis. In the pelvis, the prostate gland is immediately anterior to the midrectum. The vas deferens from each testis also passes through this structure as it enters the urethra. In the normal state, the prostate gland produces secretions that are components of seminal fluid.

The **overall manifestations** of prostate dysfunction include the complaints of hesitancy (i.e., inability promptly to initiate a forceful urinary stream); dribbling (i.e., leakage of urine after urination); urinary tenesmus (the sensation of inadequate evacuation of the urinary bladder); hematuria; pyuria; nocturia (i.e., frequent urination at night); increased frequency of urination; and even dysuria (i.e., a burning sensation during urination). On rectal examination, the prostate gland may be enlarged and tender; on scrotal examination, the epididymides may be tender or enlarged; and in severe cases, the urinary bladder may be distended with urine, as detected by percussion of the lower abdomen (Box 10-1).

I. **Pathologic conditions affecting the prostate**

   Three discrete but overlapping and quite common pathologic conditions are discussed here: prostatitis, benign prostatic hypertrophy, and prostatic nodules.

   A. **Prostatitis:** Refer to Pyuria section, Chapter 3 (page 171).

   B. **Benign prostatic hypertrophy**

      Benign prostatic hypertrophy (BPH) is a common entity that affects all males to various degrees during their lifetimes. It is quite prevalent in the elderly.

      1. The **specific manifestations** include those attributable to the obstruction (i.e., hesitancy and frequency). These

manifestations are insidious and progressive. The symptoms can worsen precipitately when a urinary tract infection occurs. On rectal examination, the prostate gland is diffusely enlarged, nontender, about the consistency of the biceps muscle in contraction, and without nodules. The bladder may be distended. The **natural history** of this entity entails progression to the point of complications. Complications may include recurrent urinary tract infections and the development of obstructive nephropathy.

2. The **specific evaluation and management** include the steps outlined in Box 10-1, treating any concurrent UTI, and referral to a urologist. The α_1-selective agents (prazosin or terazosin) have been of some efficacy in decreasing symptoms and objective signs of obstruction and as such should be used as first-line agents. When such agents are begun, they should be administered on a q.HS regimen at the lowest dose possible to avert the untoward side effects of hypotension, particularly hypotension on arising. If the patient does not tolerate these first-line agents or if the symptoms are refractory to first-line therapy, referral to a urologist is indicated. The intervention entailing transurethral resection of the prostate (TURP) remains the surgical treatment of choice.

C. **Prostatic nodules**

Prostatic nodules are also quite prevalent, especially with increasing age. These nodules may be asymptomatic until discovered.

B O X   10-1

Overall Evaluation and Management of Suspected Prostate Dysfunction

Evaluation

1. Take a thorough history, looking for any history of hesitancy, dysuria, pyuria, hematuria, increasing nocturia, or hesitancy. See page 516 for details.
2. Perform a thorough physical examination with emphasis on the rectal and scrotal examinations:
   a. Evaluate the prostate size, consistency, and the presence or absence of tenderness. The normal gland should be smooth, without nodules, nontender, and nonboggy. A marker for firmness

(continued)

B O X 10-1 *(continued)*

is that the normal gland should be about the consistency of the contracted belly of the biceps muscle.
  b. Examination should also include palpation of the epididymides and testes for tenderness and masses. If the gland is enlarged, check for any urinary bladder distention by percussing out the superior border of the bladder above the pelvis. On percussion, the urinary bladder should not be superior to the pubis.
3. Perform a urinalysis, looking for any pyuria or hematuria (see Chapter 3, page 171 and page 136, for specifics on the evaluation and management of pyuria and hematuria, respectively).
4. Determine the urinary postvoid residual volume if there is any evidence of obstruction. In this technique, the patient voids, attempting to evacuate the urinary bladder completely. A sterile catheter is then inserted into the urinary bladder to obtain the residual urine. The normal residual volume is <50 mL. A residual volume >100 mL is distinctly abnormal and consistent with urinary-outlet obstruction.
5. Obtain a urine specimen for culture and sensitivity testing if pyuria or hematuria is present.
6. Determine serum creatinine, blood urea nitrogen (BUN), glucose, and electrolyte levels for baseline purposes.
7. Obtain a prostate-specific antigen level.

Management

1. If benign prostatic hypertrophy is diagnosed, consider the initiation of prazosin, 2 mg p.o., q.HS, or terazosin, 5 mg p.o., q.HS, and/or refer the patient to a urologist. Prazosin has been demonstrated to provide a significant amount of symptomatic relief.
2. If prostatitis is diagnosed, initiate antibiotics for a 3-week course. Empiric regimens include:
  a. Ciprofloxacin, 500 mg p.o., b.i.d., or
  b. Trimethoprim–sulfamethoxazole (Bactrim), one tablet p.o., b.i.d., or
  c. Doxycycline, 100 mg p.o., b.i.d.
3. If nodules are present (i.e., indurated palpable lesions in the gland itself), the suspicion for prostate carcinoma should be high. Refer the patient to a urologist for transrectal prostate biopsy of the nodule.

1. On **examination** these lesions are nontender, indurated (similar in consistency to the tragus of the ear), and may be single or multiple. There usually are no associated scrotal or urinary manifestations. The minimal detectable size of these lesions (i.e., the sensitivity of digital examination for nodule detection) is 1 cm.
2. The **specific evaluation and management** of prostatic nodules include the steps outlined in Box 10-1 and are based on the fact that an indurated nodule is potentially a focus of prostate adenocarcinoma. Therefore, referral to a urologist for transrectal biopsy of the lesion is indicated. A prostate-specific antigen (PSA) assay during the annual digital examination is of utility in screening (see prevention chapter 16, page 710) because an increased PSA titer increases the likelihood that the nodule is prostatic adenocarcinoma and reinforces the need for urgent invasive evaluation.

II. **Consultation**

Problem	Service	Time
Prostatic nodules	Genitourinary	Required
Benign prostatic hypertrophy	Genitourinary	Required
Chronic prostatitis	Genitourinary	Elective
Acute obstructive renal failure	Renal	Urgent
Purulent urethritis	Public Health Service	Required

III. **Indications for admission:** Renal failure, a systemic infection from urinary obstruction, or surgery. Some surgical procedures can be performed in an ambulatory surgical center, obviating an overnight in-hospital admission.

Scrotal Masses

The scrotum is a structure that keeps the sexual reproductive organs of the male in an extraabdominal space. Spermatogenesis is optimal at temperatures slightly <98.6°F; therefore, it has been postulated that the scrotum evolved to keep the testes cooler by keeping them outside the abdomen and pelvis. The contents of the scrotum include the two testes and the ducts that drain the testes into the penile urethra. The testes in the normal state are smooth, oval, nontender structures ~4 cm in longitudinal dimension and 25 mL in volume. The ducts include the epididymides, which are coiled, nontender structures applied to the posterior aspect of each testis, and the vas deferens, a tubular structure extending from the tail of the epididymis to the prostatic urethra. The vas deferens, with the spermatic vein and spermatic artery, forms the spermatic cord. The floor of the scrotum is made of the abdominal wall and is a site in which congenital and acquired hernias form. It is not uncommon for a male to develop a scrotal mass during the course of his lifetime (Box 10-2).

I. **Differential diagnosis**

The differential diagnosis of scrotal masses includes the following entities:

A. **Hydrocele**

1. The **underlying pathogenesis** of this mass is that it comprises the fluid-filled congenital remnants of the processus tunica vaginalis. The **specific manifestations** include a chronic, nontender, and transilluminable lesion. The mass may wax and wane in size; an indirect hernia may be concurrently present.

2. The **specific evaluation and management** include making the clinical diagnosis by performing the steps described in Box 10-2 and referring the patient to a general surgeon for elective repair, as clinically indicated.

B. **Inguinal hernia**

See section on Hernias in Chapter 2 (Table 2-15, page 126).

C. **Testicular carcinoma**

1. The **underlying pathogenesis** of this entity is the malignant neoplastic growth of germ cells in one of the testes. A specific risk factor for development is cryptorchidism, or the abnormal congenital retention of one or both testes within the abdomen. Cryptorchidism not only decreases spermatogenesis (warmer ambient temperature) but also, through unclear means, increases the risk of development of a germ cell malignant neoplasm. The histopathologic types of tumors are described in Table 10-1.

2. The **specific manifestations** include the development of a scrotal mass that is relatively acute, nontransillu-

T A B L E   10-1
Histopathologic Types of Testicular Carcinoma

Type	Frequency	Tumor Markers	
		AFP	β-HCG
Seminoma	40%	Negative	Negative
Embryonal cell carcinoma	25%	Positive	Positive
Teratoma	5%	Negative	Negative
Immature teratoma	25%	Positive	Negative
Choriocarcinoma	2%	Negative	Positive

B O X 10-2

Overall Approach to a Patient with a Scrotal Mass

Evaluation

1. Take the history, with an emphasis on the following features:
   a. The duration of time that the lesion has been present. Acute lesions are present for <1 week and chronic lesions are present for >1 week.
   b. Determine the presence or absence of pain.
   c. Investigate the history for trauma and sexually transmitted diseases.
2. Perform a physical examination, with emphasis on the following features:
   a. The mass is tender or nontender.
   b. The mass is transilluminable or not. Transillumination is checked by shining a light source such as a penlight into the mass. A mass that transilluminates is fluid filled.
   c. The mass is reducible or nonreducible. If the lesion is reducible (i.e., it resolves or reenters the abdominal cavity from the scrotum with application of mild force), it is consistent with an inguinal hernia.
3. Determining these three variables—acuity, tenderness, and transilluminability—in the assessment of scrotal masses is pivotal in making the diagnosis.
4. Perform urinalysis with microscopic analysis.

Management

1. If the mass is acute, tender, unilateral, and nontransilluminable, ultrasonography of the testes and referral to a urologist emergently are mandatory to rule out testicular torsion.
2. If there is any evidence of concurrent purulent urethritis, manage as for a sexually transmitted disease (see Chapter 6, page 344).

minable, usually quite small, and usually nontender. However, if the tumor is rapidly growing, it can become ischemic and, therefore, tender. Often the lesion is firm and contiguous to the testis. Very often the mass is small, nontender, and detected only on routine physical examination or monthly patient testicular self-examination. When the lesion is advanced, the patient may have weight loss.

3. The **specific evaluation and management** include the steps outlined in Box 10-2 and referral to a urologist for further evaluation and management. If there is a suspicion for one of these neoplasms, one should obtain serum tumor markers. These markers include α-fetoprotein (AFP) and β-human chorionic gonadotropin (β-HCG). Table 10-1 summarizes the utility of these markers for different histopathologic types of testicular carcinoma.

D. **Testicular torsion**

1. The **underlying pathogenesis** is a testis abnormally twisted on its spermatic cord, thus embarrassing the venous drainage and the arterial supply to the testis, resulting in swelling, pain, and ischemia of the testis.

2. The **specific manifestations** include an acute, painful, tender, and nontransilluminable lesion. The condition is most common in young males, but it can occur in any age group.

3. The **specific evaluation and management** include the steps outlined in Box 10-2 and developing the clinical suspicion that torsion is the underlying lesion. Ultrasonography with Doppler-flow studies should be performed to demonstrate a decreased flow of blood in the affected spermatic cord and testis. Emergent referral to a urologist for surgical intervention is indicated.

E. **Orchitis/epididymitis**

1. The **underlying pathogenesis** is a bacterial infection. The bacteria are either from a urinary tract source (e.g., gram-negative bacilli) or, more commonly, are sexually transmitted (i.e., *Chlamydia* spp.).

2. The **specific manifestations** include a mass that is acute in onset, tender, and nontransilluminable. The patient can have findings of systemic infection, such as fevers and tachycardia, and often reports a history of sexually transmitted diseases.

3. The **specific evaluation and management** include the steps listed in Box 10-2 and performing ultrasonography of the mass to look for an abscess cavity. If abscess is present, referral to a urologist for surgical drainage and the initiation of parenteral antibiotics is indicated. Antibiotic regimens can include ciprofloxacin 500 mg p.o. b.i.d. × 14 days or doxycycline 100 mg p.o. b.i.d. for 14 days; if severe, initiate regimen with ciprofloxacin 400 i.v. b.i.d.

F. **Varicocele**
   1. The **underlying pathogenesis** is the formation of a venous varicosity in the spermatic vein. Because the spermatic vein on the left does not drain directly into the inferior vena cava, but on the right, the spermatic vein does, there is an increased incidence of varicosities on the left side.
   2. The **specific manifestations** include a chronic, non-tender, nontransilluminable mass, usually on the left side. The lesion often has the consistency of "a bag of worms" and decreases in size with elevation of the scrotum.
   3. The **specific evaluation and management** of this lesion entail making the clinical diagnosis by performing the steps described in Box 10-2. Usually no intervention is necessary; however, if the lesion is new and on the right, a thorough examination of the pelvis should be performed to rule out any new cause for obstruction to spermatic vein blood flow.

II. **Consultation**

Problem	Service	Time
Hydrocele	General surgery	Elective
Inguinal hernia	General surgery	
Strangulated		Emergent
Incarcerated		Urgent
Reducible		Elective
Testicular carcinoma	Urology	Urgent
Testicular torsion	Urology	Emergent
Testicular abscess	Urology	Emergent
Epididymitis	Urology	Elective

III. **Indications for admission:** Strangulated or incarcerated hernia, testicular torsion or abscess, or for any elective surgical procedure.

Bibliography

Prostate Dysfunction

Catalona WJ, Scott WWW: Carcinoma of the prostate: a review. J Urol 1978;119:1.

Hill SJ, et al: New use for alpha blockers: benign prostatic hypertrophy. Am Fam Physician 1994;49:1885–1888.

Lepor H: Nonoperative management of benign prostatic hypertrophy. J Urol 1989;141:1283.

Lepor H: The emerging role of alpha-agonists in the therapy of benign prostatic hyperplasia. J Androl 1991;12:389.

O'Brien WM: Benign prostatic hypertrophy. Am Fam Pract 1991;44: 162–171.

Schwager EJ: Treatment of bacterial prostatitis. Am Fam Pract 1991;44: 2137–2141.

Scrotal Masses

O'Brien WM, Lynch JH: The acute scrotum. Am Fam Pract 1988;37:239–247.

Prater JM, Overdorf BS: Testicular torsion: a surgical emergency. Am Fam Pract 1991;44:834–840.

—D.D.B

Chapter 11

Gynecology/Breast

Breast Masses and Lumps

The physiology of the breasts is such that they are under significant control of several hormones. These hormones include:

1. **Estrogens.** These hormones stimulate the proliferation of the epithelial cells in the ducts and increase the vascularity of the breast tissue itself. The two physiologic times of estrogen excess are the follicular (proliferative) phase of the menstrual cycle and pregnancy.
2. **Progesterones.** These hormones stimulate the proliferation of acini. The states in which there is an overall increase in progesterones include the luteal (secretory) phase of the menstrual cycle and pregnancy.
3. Many other hormones, including oxytocin and prolactin, are involved in the production and release of milk from the breast in the postpartum state.

   I. **Differential diagnosis** (Box 11-1)
   A. **Fibroadenoma**
      1. The **pathophysiology** of this lesion is that it is quite probably a specific form of fibrocystic change. There is an increase in the fibrous and ductal epithelial tissue in the lesion itself. It is often associated with estrogen excess, the estrogens stimulating the ductal and vascular structures of the breast.
      2. The **specific manifestations** of this entity include the presence of a discrete solitary lesion, which quite often becomes mildly painful and tender, but will not change in size, in the follicular (i.e., high estrogen) phase of the menstrual cycle. These are invariably in a premenopausal woman, as without estrogens they will not occur.
      3. The **specific evaluation and management** include making the clinical diagnosis by performing the examina-

B O X 11-1

Overall Evaluation and Management of Breast Masses

Evaluation

1. Implement effective screening programs to detect masses and lumps within the breast tissue itself so that any lesion that is malignant (neoplastic) will be detected early in its clinical course. These screening programs include:
   a. Breast self-examination (BSE). This method should be taught to all women at the time of menarche. It should be performed by the woman on a monthly basis. A premenopausal woman should examine her breasts at approximately day 4–5 of the cycle, as this is the time frame in which the breast tissue is under the least hormonal stimulation. A postmenopausal woman should examine her breasts on the first day of each month.
   b. Annual breast examination by physician. Useful in detecting any palpable lesions. Features positively correlated with (i.e., are attributes of) breast carcinoma include:
      i. Solitary mass.
      ii. Mass induration.
      iii. A lack of tenderness.
      iv. Concurrent axillary lymph node enlargement.
   c. Bilateral mammograms. Should be performed at age 40 years for baseline, and then every other year for 10 years, and then annually after age 50 years. The mammograms complement the annual physical examination and the monthly BSE. Findings positively correlated with (i.e., are attributes of) a breast carcinoma include:
      i. Mass with irregular borders.
      ii. Clustered microcalcifications.
      iii. Overlying skin changes.
   Once a mass is discovered:
2. History is integral, including any history of hormone-related carcinoma, endometrial and/or breast; any family history of breast carcinoma.
3. Examine the patient for any concurrent findings (i.e., any nipple discharge). If nipple discharge is present, send for cytologic examination. Furthermore, examine for any concurrent axillary or supraclavicular lymph node enlargement.

(continued)

B O X 11-1 *(continued)*

4. Any suggestive lesion must have a biopsy performed
   for histopathologic diagnosis. One of two biopsy
   methods can be used:
   a. Perform a needle aspiration of the mass. If fluid
      or cells are obtained, send the specimen for cyto-
      logic examination. If malignant neoplastic, refer to
      a surgeon for definitive therapy.
      -or-
   b. Refer directly to a surgeon for excisional biopsy
      (i.e., complete resection of entire mass). A frozen
      section of the biopsy can easily and rapidly be
      performed for diagnosis of the mass. In this sce-
      nario, the patient, the primary care physician, and
      the surgeon should discuss the options for **treat-
      ment,** if indeed the lesion is malignant neoplastic,
      before the biopsy is performed. The surgical op-
      tions include:
      i. Modified radical mastectomy, which includes
         the removal of the axillary lymph nodes.
         -or-
      ii. Lumpectomy with concurrent axillary node dis-
          section—mandatory for staging purposes.

tions described in Box 11-1. The mammogram will reveal a discrete solitary mass, usually with a large clump
of calcium. Once the histopathologic diagnosis is secured, no further intervention is required.
  B. **Intraductal papilloma**
     1. The **pathophysiology** of this lesion is that it is quite
        probably a specific form of fibrocystic change, involving
        the duct only.
     2. The **specific manifestations** of this entity include the
        onset of serous or even bloody nipple discharge from
        one specific duct at the nipple. In most cases, the papil-
        loma is subareolar but nonpalpable and nontender.
     3. The **specific evaluation and management** include mak-
        ing the clinical diagnosis by performing the examina-
        tions described in Box 11-1. The mammogram may re-
        veal a solitary lesion in the subareolar area with no
        calcifications present. Once the histologic diagnosis by
        excisional biopsy is secured, no further intervention
        is required.
  C. **Fibrocystic changes (FCCs)**
     1. The **pathophysiology** has not been completely eluci-
        dated. Clearly there is a component of hormone media-

tion. Estrogen-excess states, especially those associated with luteal-phase defects and dysfunctional uterine bleeding, are highly associated with fibrocystic breast changes. The estrogens result in the exuberant growth of the ductal and vascular structures, with resultant cystic and proliferative changes within the breast. The change is quite prevalent; in fact, 90% of women will have this disorder at some time during their lifetimes.

2. The **specific manifestations** of this entity include the presence of multiple, bilateral lumps within the breasts. The lumps are quite diverse in size and can have marked variation in terms of tenderness and size during various times of the menstrual cycle. Again this process is specific to the premenopausal time frame.

3. The **specific evaluation** includes making the clinical diagnosis by performing the examinations described in Box 11-1. The mammogram will reveal multiple lesions within both breasts; usually no calcifications are present. The sensitivity and specificity of mammography and of the physical examination in the detection of malignant lesions are decreased with FCCs. One caveat is that if one lesion becomes dominant or is atypical, it should be regarded as suggestive and aggressively evaluated with aspiration. Aspiration, by using a 20-gauge needle and syringe, is an effective diagnostic tool in an atypical lesion. The lesion should be completely drained of fluid; the fluid and any tissue obtained should be sent for cytologic examination. Indications for immediate referral to a surgeon for excisional biopsy include:
   a. Recurrence after lesion drainage.
   b. Any atypical cells on the cytologic examination.
   c. Any clusters of microcalcifications on mammography.
   d. Complex cyst on mammogram.

4. The **specific management** of FCC includes instructing the patient to perform BSE on a monthly basis. Further modalities for therapy include the following:
   a. Oral contraceptives. This is particularly useful in patients with concurrent dysfunctional uterine bleeding.
   b. Danazol. In recurrent severe FCC. This synthetic androgen can be administered in a dose of 100–400 mg p.o., q.d. (in b.i.d. dosing), and is effective in significantly decreasing the manifestations in >90% of cases. The agent is contraindicated in any woman who is pregnant or any woman who desires to become pregnant in the near future. Side effects include, but are not limited to, hirsutism, secondary amenorrhea, and hepatic dysfunction.

D. Breast carcinoma

1. The **pathophysiology** is not completely known; however, several discrete **risk factors** for the development of the most common histopathologic type of breast carcinoma, infiltrating ductile adenocarcinoma, are known. These include long-term use of unopposed estrogens, early menarche, and late menopause. Additional **risk factors** include a personal history of breast carcinoma in the contralateral breast, and a family history of breast carcinoma in a first-degree female relative (mother, sister, or daughter). Finally, recent studies have uncovered a gene (BRCA1), which is also highly correlated with the development of breast carcinoma.

2. The **specific manifestations** include the presence of a unilateral, solitary, nontender, indurated lesion in the breast. It can be mobile, or if more advanced, fixed to the overlying and/or deep structures. If fixed to the overlying skin, there can be a peau d'orange appearance to the skin and/or nipple retractions, whereas if fixed to the deep fascia, it is immobile. There may be concurrent axillary and/or supraclavicular lymph node enlargement, these nodes being nontender and firm.

3. The **specific evaluation and management** include making the clinical diagnosis by performing the examinations described in Box 11-1. The mammogram will reveal a solitary lesion with irregular borders, clusters of microcalcifications, and overlying skin thickening. Clearly, referral to a surgeon for definitive therapy is indicated in an expedient manner. Staging and postsurgical therapy are discussed in the section on Breast Malignancy in Chapter 5, page 276.

II. Consultation

Problem	Service	Time
Any lesion suggestive of carcinoma	Surgeon	Urgent
Severe fibrocystic changes	Gynecology	Elective

III. Indications for admission: Specific only to therapeutic surgical interventions. Most excisional biopsies can be performed in ambulatory surgical suites, obviating admission to an inpatient service.

Contraceptive Modalities

Effective and safe modalities to prevent conception are known. The primary care physician is in a position to educate patients about these modalities. Furthermore, the primary care physician is in a position to educate patients about the specific modalities effective in the prevention of sexually transmitted diseases (STDs).

B O X   11-2

Overall Evaluation and Management of Contraception

1. Educate the patient in the various modalities.
2. Encourage the patient's sexual partner to become involved in the educational process and to instruct him
   or her as to modalities which he or she can use that
   are safe and effective.
3. Obtain a history including:
   a. Last menstrual period.
   b. Previous pregnancies and results.
   c. History of STDs and of number of partners.
   d. History of hormonally stimulated malignant neo-
      plastic lesions (e.g., endometrial carcinoma,
      breast adenocarcinoma, or ovarian carcinoma).
   e. History of deep venous thrombosis (DVT) and/or
      arterial thrombosis.
   f. Previous modalities of contraception.
   g. Current knowledge base of contraceptive and mo-
      dalities of "safer sex."
4. Pelvic examination, for baseline.
5. Urine pregnancy test, before initiating any oral contraceptive pill regimen.

Although many of the modalities for contraception are designed
for women, the responsibility for contraception, prevention of
STD, and of any failure of prevention rests equally with **both** sexual
partners (Box 11-2).

I. **Contraceptive methods**
   A. **Abstinence**
      1. The mechanism of action of this specific **modality** is
         quite straightforward: reproduction is not possible
         without heterosexual activity. This is the complete
         avoidance of contact between male genitals and female
         genitals. The efficacy of this modality is 100%. A sig-
         nificant benefit of this modality is the 100% efficacy in
         the prevention of STDs.

         Although, in its pure sense, abstinence is straightfor-
         ward (i.e., the complete inhibition of all sexual contact),
         this is relatively unrealistic. There are several variants,
         each with varying contraceptive efficacy. The vari-
         ants include:
         a. Sexual activity without male to female genital con-
            tact. Couples can have sexual activities that do not

require direct contact of the female to male genitalia. The efficacy of this **modality** is 100% for contraceptive purposes, whereas in the prevention of STDs, it is of lesser efficacy.

b. Sexual activity that involves contact of the female and male genital areas but minimizes the risk of exposure of the ovum to sperm. One example is the **rhythm method.** In the rhythm method, the couple abstains from direct female-to-male sexual contact during ovulation. This requires that the couple know the duration of the female's cycles, that the female has regular cycles, and that the couple is able to abstain from unprotected intercourse during the period 10–16 days before the onset of menstrual flow (i.e., at the time of ovulation). Because there are normal variations in the duration of cycles, there is a significant risk of conception by using this method. The effectiveness of this method is improved by increasing the ability of the individual to predict time of ovulation. This may be accomplished based on the physiologic fact that the female's temperature will increase by 1.0–1.5°F at the time of ovulation. Therefore, if the female takes her oral temperature each morning and records it, she can attempt to predict when ovulation will occur. The couple then must abstain from unprotected intercourse during the days immediately preceding the temperature increase and during it. The overall efficacy of the rhythm method, even with fastidious recording of cycles and temperatures, is only 40%–60%. Furthermore, in a nonmonogamous relationship, there is a risk of transmission of STDs.

c. Another "method" is that of **withdrawal.** Because there is direct female-to-male contact and invariably an admixture of female and male secretions, there is **no efficacy** in contraception. Furthermore, in a nonmonogamous relationship, there is a high risk of transmission of STDs. The primary care physician must educate patients and the public to the risks inherent to this commonly used method.

B. Condoms

1. The mechanism of action of this **modality** is straightforward. It is the application of a latex sheath over the external aspect of the penis, affording a barrier between direct contact of female and male genital secretions. The psychomotor skills requisite for this modality are quite simple, but should be taught to the male at the outset. The condom must be placed on an erect penis and rolled up to its base. These are available over the counter without prescription. A caveat to the use of condoms is that if lubricants are used, they should be water soluble.

2. The efficacy of this **modality** is, when used properly, 90%–95%. There are virtually no adverse side effects except for latex allergy. Finally, because there is a barrier to direct contact of genital secretions, the efficacy in prevention of transmission of disease is very high.

C. **Diaphragm**
1. The mechanism of action of this **modality** is not dissimilar from that of the cervical cap. It is the application of a latex sheath over the external aspect of the cervix, affording a barrier between male genital secretions and the cervix. The difference between this and the barrier method of condoms is that condoms afford a complete barrier to contact between male/female sexual secretions, whereas a diaphragm does not. The device is a latex rubber structure with a fixed rim, which is placed in the superior vagina. The patient is fitted for the device and is instructed in the psychomotor skills requisite to the use of this modality. The device should snugly yet comfortably cover the entire cervix from the symphysis pubis to the posterior fornix. It is placed before intercourse with spermicidal jelly and kept in place for 6–12 hours. It must remain in place for 6 hours after the last episode of sexual intercourse. A caveat to use is that, other than the spermicidal jelly, no concurrent lubricant should be used. A prescription is required for use.
2. The efficacy of this **modality** is, when used properly, 95%. Adverse side effects include an increased risk of urinary tract infections and the development of a mild vaginal odor that develops if it is in place for >12–18 hours. The patient should have a pelvic and Pap smear performed on a yearly basis, as well as refitting the diaphragm. The diaphragm should be refitted on a yearly basis, and after labor and delivery, and/or marked weight change. Finally, because there is direct contact of genital secretions, the efficacy of this modality in preventing the transmission of STDs is, in nonmonogamous relationships, low.

D. **Oral contraceptives**
1. The mechanism of action of this **modality** is hormone based. Ovulation in the physiologic setting requires the secretion of follicle-stimulating hormone (FSH) and luteinizing hormone (LH) from the adenohypophysis in general, and a midcycle surge in LH secretion in specific. The combination oral contraceptive pill (i.e., one that has both an estrogen and a progestin component) inhibits the FSH and LH secretion and the LH surge.

Although there are many different names and types of combination oral contraceptives, the dosing regimens are quite similar. The clinician should become comfortable with three or four different combination pills. There are several guidelines that one can use in dosing these agents.

a. Ascertain any contraindications to oral contraceptive use. Absolute contraindications to initiation and indications for discontinuance include:

    i. Deep venous thromboembolism.

    ii. Thrombotic cerebrovascular accident.

    iii. Myocardial infarction.

    iv. Monocular blindness, retinal arterial occlusion.

    v. Pregnancy

    vi. Hormone-mediated malignancy (e.g., breast, ovarian, or endometrial carcinoma).

b. Instruct patient to discontinue smoking, as this is an independent risk factor for the development of the adverse thrombotic effects of the oral contraceptive pill.

c. Instruct the patient that this will not protect her from STDs, and therefore, the principles of "safer sex" must be described and practiced.

d. Two first-line agents are Ortho-Novum 1/35: 1 mg of norethindrone and 35 μg of ethinyl estradiol; one tablet p.o., q.d., for 21 days, then 7 days without for withdrawal bleeding; or Ortho-Novum 7/7/7, a triphasic agent: 7 days of ethinyl estradiol, 35 μg, and norethindrone, 0.5 mg, followed by 7 days of ethinyl estradiol, 35 μg, and norethindrone, 0.75 mg, followed by 7 days of ethinyl estradiol, 35 μg, and norethindrone, 1.0 mg, and then 7 days off for withdrawal bleeding.

e. If the patient has a history of mild hypertension or significant premenstrual water retention, change to an agent with lower progesterone activity (e.g., Desogen 35 or the triphasic agent, Ortho-Novum 7/7/7).

f. If the patient develops hirsutism or acne vulgaris related to androgens, change to a progesterone agent with less androgenic activity (e.g., Demulen or Desogen).

g. If the patient misses a pill, she should take it immediately. If she forgets two to three pills on consecutive days, she should take two each morning until back on schedule and use another concurrent form of contraception for the remainder of the cycle. If she misses more than three pills, she should stop completely, have withdrawal bleeding, and restart 7 days after the first pill was missed. In the latter case, other modalities for contraception should be considered and even recommended.

2. **Efficacy**

The efficacy of this **modality** is 97%–98% when used appropriately.

3. Potential negative side effects

   a. Increased risk of DVT.

   b. Increased risk of cholelithiasis.

   c. Increased risk of the development of hypertension.

4. Potential positive side effects

   a. A decrease in risk of ovarian carcinoma.

   b. A decreased risk of endometrial carcinoma.

   c. A decrease in the symptoms of dysfunctional uterine bleeding and/or fibrocystic changes of the breast.

   d. The overall effects of combination oral contraceptives on lipids include:

      i. Estrogens. Decrease low-density lipoprotein (LDL), increase high-density lipoprotein (HDL), and increase triglycerides.

      ii. Progestins. Increase LDL, decrease total cholesterol, decrease HDL, and decrease triglycerides.

E. **Morning-after pill**

1. The mechanism of action is not completely clear. It probably accelerates the transport of the blastula to the endometrium before development of the endometrial lining, so it is unable to implant. The dose is Ovral (ethinyl estradiol, 0.05 mg, and norgestrel, 0.5 mg), two tablets p.o., q.12hr times two within 48 hours of intercourse.

2. The efficacy of this **modality** is, when used properly, 90% if administered to the patient within 48 hours of intercourse. Adverse side effects are quite minimal except for a significant amount of nausea and perhaps some vomiting after administration. There is obviously no efficacy in preventing STDs.

F. **Depo-Provera**

1. The **mechanism of action** is that it inhibits ovulation and impairs implantation. It is a long-acting progesterone agent. The dose is 150 mg i.m. q.3 months.

2. The **efficacy** of this modality is 97%–99%. Adverse side effects include weight gain and irregular menstrual bleeding.

G. **Surgical sterilization**

1. **Vasectomy**

This is the surgical ligation of both of the vasa deferens, the tubes that carry sperm from the testes into the penis. This procedure requires local anesthesia via two small incisions in the posterior scrotum and has few to no adverse effects. It takes ~2 months for the sperm already present to be absorbed; therefore, a concurrent **modality** of contraception must be used during the first 2 months after the procedure.

2. **Tubal ligation**

   This is the ligation of both of the fallopian tubes, thus preventing the sperm from reaching the proximal tube, in effect forming a permanent barrier to sperm–ovum interaction. This procedure can be easily performed via laparoscopy and entails tying off and then cutting a portion of the tubes.

II. **Consultation**

Problem	Service	Time
Any patient	Planned Parenthood	Elective
Vasectomy	Urologist	Elective
Tubal ligation	Gynecologist	Elective

III. **Indications for admission:** None. Even surgical sterilization can be performed on an outpatient basis.

Menopause

I. **Definition**

Menopause is the loss of reproductive functioning and capacity in a previously fertile woman. It is the transition between the fertile phase of a woman's life and the nonfertile phase. Although many specific manifestations occur during and after this profound transition, the most reproducible manifestation is the acquired absence, either through natural or iatrogenic means, of menstruation for a period of >1 year in a previously menstruating, currently nonpregnant woman. The average age at onset of natural menopause is 50–51 years. Iatrogenic menopause usually occurs as a result of bilateral oophorectomy with or without concurrent hysterectomy. Hysterectomy itself will result in amenorrhea but, if the ovaries are functional, not true menopause (Box 11-3).

A. **Natural menopause**

This is the primary failure and atrophy of the ovaries as a result of the loss of oocytes produced by follicles. Although there are hundreds of thousands of oocytes in the ovaries, they rapidly decay after age 35 years, resulting in a loss of all functional oocytes and their adjacent supportive structures (i.e., follicles) by age 50–55 years. The ovaries without any oocytes result in infertility, whereas the lack of follicles results in inability to produce the hormones estrogen and progesterone.

B. **Iatrogenic menopause**

This will result in a syndrome of menopause, depending on the procedure performed. If the procedure performed

B O X   11-3

Overall Evaluation and Management of Menopause

Evaluation

1. Overall history and physical must include:
   a. Date of the last menstrual period.
   b. The features of the antecedent menstrual periods (e.g., duration, regularity).
   c. The presence of any other concurrent vaginal discharge.
   d. The history of hysterectomy and/or oophorectomy.
   e. Age of the patient.
   f. The presence of hot flashes (e.g., acute manifestation of estrogen withdrawal).
   g. The presence of dyspareunia (i.e., painful intercourse) and atrophy of the vulvar/vaginal mucosa as a result of atrophic vaginitis.
   h. Pelvic examination, mandatory as a baseline examination.
2. Urine pregnancy test. This is of extreme importance, as one must rule out pregnancy as a cause of secondary amenorrhea.
3. If hysterectomy was performed but the ovaries are intact, the initial manifestations of true menopause (i.e., ovarian failure) will be hot flashes and atrophic vaginitis.
4. Plasma FSH and LH levels should be obtained. These will be increased in primary ovarian failure (i.e., true menopause).

Management

1. Assess the risk for development of osteoporosis. Specific intervention in evaluation and prevention of osteoporosis includes:
   a. Walking 1–2 miles every or every other day.
   b. Prescribing a multivitamin on an every-day basis. This will supply adequate amounts of vitamin D to prevent concurrent vitamin D deficiency.
   c. Prescribing 1.0–1.5 g of calcium carbonate per day. The patient should be instructed to take the calcium with meals, as the absorption of calcium is greatest in a relatively high-pH (alkaline) environment.

(continued)

B O X 11-3 *(continued)*

  d. Systemic estrogens. If there is no contraindication, estrogen prophylaxis regimens are based on the presence or absence of a uterus in the patient.
     i. **If patient does not have a uterus,** the regimen: conjugated estrogens, 0.625 mg p.o., q.d. for an indefinite period.
     ii. **If the patient has a uterus**, the regimen:
         Days 1–14: Conjugated estrogens (Premarin), 0.625 mg p.o., q.d.
         Days 15–24: Conjugated estrogens, 0.625 mg p.o., q.d., and medroxyprogesterone, 2.5–10.0 mg p.o., q.d.
         Days 25–28: No hormones.
         All cycled for indefinite period.
2. If hot flashes are present and severe, initiate systemic conjugated estrogen therapy unless there is a contraindication. See the preceding and text for regimens.
3. If atrophic vaginitis is present, the application of topical water-soluble lubricant (e.g., KY jelly or topical estrogens) is quite effective. The topical agent is conjugated estrogens (Premarin) to the vulvar epithelium on a q.d. or b.i.d. basis.
4. In all cases in which estrogens are used in patients who have a uterus, pelvic examinations are required on a regular basis (i.e., q.6 months). Any atypical vaginal discharge and/or bleeding must be aggressively evaluated by a gynecologic consultant with endometrial biopsy and/or curettage of the uterine endometrium.
5. In all cases in which estrogens are to be used, a baseline breast examination and mammograms are required and then repeated on a routine screening basis.

is bilateral oophorectomy, irrespective of concurrent hysterectomy, there is the sudden loss of oocytes and follicular cells; therefore it is not dissimilar from natural menopause.

In both, the hormones estrogen and progesterone are no longer produced from the ovaries, resulting in an atrophy of the uterus in general and of the uterine endometrium in specific. Therefore, there is a loss of menstruation (i.e., the development of secondary amenorrhea). Furthermore, the deficiency of estrogen and progesterone results in a marked decrease in the feedback on the adenohypophyseal hormones, i.e., an increase in LH and FSH.

II. Manifestations

The **specific manifestations** of ovarian failure include an acceleration of osteoporosis, hot flashes, and atrophic vaginitis.

A. Osteoporosis

This is the loss of bone, a process of very high prevalence in the aging population. Loss of bone markedly increases the risk of fractures of the vertebral spine and the hips and results in significant morbidity.

1. The **pathophysiology** of this process is not completely understood. Although the mechanism of disease development is unclear, several descriptive features are well known.

   a. It is a process of bone loss, both of bony matrix (i.e., the collagen and protein substrate) and of the mineral component of bone (i.e., calcium phosphate). It affects the trabecular bone (i.e., the laminar, reticulated areas within the bone) to a greater extent than the cortical bone (i.e., the compact, dense areas of ossification at the periphery of the bony structures).

   b. There are certain, quite specific **risk factors** for the development of osteoporosis. These include:

      i. **Ovarian failure** (i.e., menopause). The withdrawal of long-term estrogens from the physiologic milieu increases the rate of osteoporosis.

      ii. **Significant long-term inactivity.** There is an inverse correlation between the level of physical activity and the rate of osteoporosis development (i.e., exercise decreases the rate of osteoporosis development).

      iii. **Poor nutrition,** specifically a deficiency in vitamin D and/or calcium, will increase the risk of osteoporosis.

      iv. **Genetics.** A family history of osteoporosis is strongly correlated with accelerated osteoporosis.

      v. **Ethanol.** Excessive ingestion of ethanol is directly correlated with accelerated osteoporosis.

      vi. **Tobacco smoking.**

   c. Once present, osteoporosis is effectively irreversible, but it is a disease process that is eminently preventable.

2. The **specific manifestations** of osteoporosis include the fact that the patient is invariably asymptomatic until a fracture occurs. The most common sites include compression fractures of the thoracic spine or a hip fracture. A **compression fracture** of the thoracic vertebra can

manifest with a relatively diverse range, from the painless development of dowager's hump (i.e., the marked increase in kyphosis) to the development of severe pain starting at the specific vertebral body and radiating anteriorly (see Table 7-5, page 376). The **specific manifestations** of a **hip fracture** (Table 7-4, page 374) include the sudden onset of pain, decreased range of motion in the affected hip, and superior displacement and external rotation of the affected lower extremity at the hip itself, all precipitated by a fall, usually with only a modest amount of force.

3. The **specific evaluation and management** include that described in Box 11-3. The overall objective is to discover patients who are at high risk for the development of accelerated osteoporosis and to intervene before the process reaches the clinical level of fractures. The **specific management** includes that described in Box 11-3. Unless there is a contraindication, all women who have ovarian failure, either physiologic or iatrogenic, should receive estrogen-replacement therapy. The replacement with systemic estrogens has been demonstrated not only to slow the rate of bone matrix and mineral loss in postmenopausal osteoporosis, but also to prevent the development of atherosclerotic disease and may even retard the development of dementia. Estrogens are fraught with several potentially quite significant side effects and therefore cannot be used in all cases. These side effects include but are not limited to:

   a. An increased risk of carcinoma of the uterine endometrium. The long-term use of unopposed estrogens will result in proliferation of the endometrial tissue of the uterus. Several studies suggested a strong correlation between the long-term use of estrogens and the development of the premalignant neoplastic lesion, cystic hyperplasia, and the malignant neoplastic lesion, uterine adenocarcinoma of the endometrium. This is a moot problem in a patient without a uterus but is a concern in all other patients receiving estrogens. A major method to decrease the risk of this side effect is to cycle the estrogens, by using the physiologic model. This cycling of the hormones ensures a monthly withdrawal of the estrogens with resultant sloughing of the endometrial tissue (i.e., menstrual flow).

   b. A questionable increase in the risk of breast adenocarcinoma. There may be a slight increase in the risk of breast carcinoma; however, the epidemiologic evidence is far from complete. Any patient with an antecedent history of breast adenocarcinoma, a strong family history of breast adenocarcinoma, or a history of dysplastic breast disease should not be prescribed estrogens.

c. A slight increase in the risk of development of thromboembolic disease in premenopausal but not in postmenopausal women. However, anyone with a history of DVT/pulmonary thromboembolism (PTE) and/or a concurrent risk of hypercoagulability should not be prescribed estrogens.

4. Follow-up should be a regular pelvic examination. If there is any abnormal vaginal discharge or bleeding, immediately refer the patient to gynecology for endometrial examination. The patient must continue with regular breast examinations and mammograms.

B. Hot flashes

These are very common acute manifestations of ovarian failure. They can be markers for the onset of true menopause (i.e., ovarian failure) in a patient who has had a previous hysterectomy without oophorectomy.

1. The **physiology** of this specific process is postulated to be as the result of the sudden and precipitate decline in estrogens from the physiologic milieu. This withdrawal will lead to paroxysms of facial and/or body vasodilation.

2. The **specific manifestations** include the subjective feeling of flushing in the face and/or body, which can be quite frequent, quite severe, and extremely distracting to the patient.

3. The **specific evaluation and management** include the overall, as described in Box 11-3, and the initiation of a program of conjugated estrogens in the dosing regimens described in Box 11-3.

C. Atrophic vaginitis

1. The **physiology** of this very common sequel of menopause is the loss of estrogens, which results in a decrease in the elasticity, vascularity, and thickness of the vaginal mucosa.

2. The **specific manifestations** include dyspareunia (i.e., pain upon intercourse), a marked decrease in vaginal secretions, and atrophy/kraurosis (i.e., shrinkage of the mucosa of the vulva and vagina). The epithelium is easily traumatized, and postcoital erythema and even bleeding may occur.

3. The **specific evaluation and management** include making the clinical diagnosis, the overall evaluation and management, as described in Box 11-3, and the use of a water-soluble jelly (KY jelly) before intercourse, and/or the application of topical estrogen cream. If the patient is receiving estrogens for prophylaxis of osteoporosis, this will supplant the need for topical therapy.

III. Consultation

Problem	*Service*	*Time*
Any evidence of concurrent metabolic bone disease	Endocrine	Required
Any hip fracture	Orthopedics	Urgent
Any compression vertebral fracture	Orthopedics	Elective

IV. Indications for admission: Acute hip fractures; otherwise, management is outpatient.

Pelvic Masses

I. **Differential diagnosis of pelvic masses** (Box 11-4)
   A. **Endometrial carcinoma** (see section on Vaginal Discharge, page 553).
   B. **Leiomyomas, fibroids** (see section on Vaginal Discharge, page 551).
   C. **Pelvic inflammatory disease** (See section on Sexually Transmitted Disease, Chapter 6, page 344).
      1. The **pathophysiology** of this entity includes the development of inflammation in the fallopian tube as the result of a bacterial infection. The infection invariably begins as cervicitis and propagates proximally to involve the endometrium of the uterus and the fallopian tubes. The underlying pathogens are usually multiple and include *Neisseria gonorrhoeae, Chlamydia* spp., and anaerobic bacteria, including peptostreptococci. **Risk factors** include unsafe sex practices, multiple sexual partners, and the use of intrauterine devices (IUDs).
      2. The **specific manifestations** of this entity include unilateral pain in the right or left lower abdominal quadrant, often with associated nausea, vomiting, fevers, chills, and vaginal discharge. Examination discloses purulent cervical discharge, cervical motion tenderness, and a tender unilateral adnexal mass.
      3. The **specific evaluation and management** include making the clinical diagnosis by using the examinations described in Box 11-4. Further evaluation and management are based on the results. An ultrasound examination of the pelvis in addition to a VDRL and human immunodeficiency virus (HIV) assay is indicated. The partner must be evaluated and treated concurrent with the patient.
         a. **Antibiotic regimens include:**
            i. Ceftriaxone, 2 g i.v., q.24hr, and doxycycline, 100 mg i.v., q.12hr, for 7 days or for 48 hours after the last fever spike, whichever comes first. Then, doxycycline, 100 mg p.o., b.i.d., for the

B O X 11-4

Overall Evaluation and Management of Pelvic Masses

Evaluation

1. Query the patient regarding the time of her last menstrual period. This is important in determining whether the patient is premenopausal or postmenopausal. Furthermore, if the patient is premenopausal and there is an acquired absence of periods for more than one cycle (i.e., secondary amenorrhea), the suspicion for pregnancy should markedly increase.
2. Urine pregnancy test.
3. Query the patient regarding concurrent vaginal bleeding and/or other vaginal discharge. This is a very important aspect of the overall evaluation. If bleeding is present, it must be evaluated as described in section on Vaginal Discharge, page 547.
4. Pelvic examination in all cases.
   a. Differentiate whether the mass is primarily adnexal or uterine. Adnexal masses are more commonly the result of ovarian and/or fallopian tube processes, whereas uterine masses are more commonly either fibroids or a gravid uterus.
   b. If there is any thick and/or purulent discharge, obtain a Gram stain, culture on Thayer–Martin medium (for *Neisseria gonorrhoeae*), and a *Chlamydia trachomatis* culture.
5. Ultrasound of the pelvis.
   a. This is **emergent** in the following scenarios:
      i. Tender, adnexal mass with purulent cervical discharge.
      ii. A positive pregnancy test with any adnexal mass.
      iii. Any uterine and/or adnexal mass with associated vaginal bleeding.
   b. This is **urgent** in the following scenario:
      i. A nontender uterine mass without bleeding.

Management

1. If there is any concurrent hirsutism, refer to Table 11-1.
2. Referral to Ob/Gyn colleagues.
3. Educate the patient in safer sex methods.

TABLE 11-1
Hirsutism

Disease	Mechanism	Laboratory Findings	Treatment
Adrenal tumors (non–cortisol secreting)	Androgen dependent	Increased serum DHEAS Increased urinary 17-ketosteroids	Endocrine consultation Endocrinology consultation
Ovarian tumors and cysts (including PCO)	Androgen dependent	Increased serum free testosterone In PCO: serum LH/FSH > 3	Endocrinology consultation Gynecology consultation Consider oral contraceptive (combination-type pill)
Obesity	Androgen dependent; peripheral conversion of androstenedione to testosterone	No specific laboratory abnormalities Concurrent insulin resistance	Weight reduction
Hypercortisolism	Androgen dependent	Abnormal lack of cortisol suppression with dexamethasone (see Secondary hypertension, Box 3-3, page 147)	Endocrine consultation

                remainder of time, so that **treatment** is at least
                a total of 14 days; or

      ii. For early PID, Ceftriaxone, 250 mg i.m., and dox-
           ycycline, 100 mg p.o., b.i.d., for 10 days; or

      iii. If the patient is β-lactam allergic, one can admin-
           ister clindamycin, 600–900 mg i.v., q.8hr, and
           a concurrent aminoglycoside, either gentamicin
           or tobramycin i.v., for a total of 7–10 days.

  b. One must watch for and aggressively treat any com-
     plications of this infectious process. These include:

      i. Fitz-Hugh–Curtis syndrome. This is the devel-
          opment of perihepatitis. **Specific evaluation and
          management** include obtaining blood cultures,
          an ultrasound examination of the liver, looking
          for abscesses, and a longer duration of antibi-
          otics.

      ii. Tuboovarian abscess. This is the development
          of an actual abscess cavity in or adjacent to the
          infected fallopian tube. This will usually be
          quite easily demonstrable on pelvic ultrasound
          examination. It requires gynecologic consulta-
          tion, a longer duration of parenteral antibiotics,
          and, if severe or refractory to **treatment**, surgi-
          cal intervention.

D. Ovarian neoplasia—epithelial

  1. The **pathogenesis** of this is not completely understood.
     Several factors have been correlated with the develop-
     ment of ovarian carcinoma. The factors that increase
     the risk of ovarian epithelial neoplasia development
     include being nulliparous, having a family history (re-
     cent evidence that BRCA1 is associated with its devel-
     opment), and a history of antecedent breast carcinoma.
     Factors that decrease the risk of development of epithe-
     lial ovarian carcinoma include a history of multiparity
     and the use of oral contraceptive agents.

    a. The **histopathology** of this group of epithelial neo-
       plastic lesions is relatively diverse; however, the
       most common epithelial type is adenocarcinoma.

    b. The **natural history** of ovarian epithelial neoplastic
       lesions in general is that they originate in one ovary,
       locally enlarge, and spread contiguously to the peri-
       toneum, with peritoneal studding and the develop-
       ment of malignant neoplastic ascites. This peritoneal
       disease can become quite massive. When the lesion
       extends out of the ovary, the prognosis, even with
       aggressive therapy, is very poor; therefore early de-
       tection is of extreme importance in effective therapy.

  2. The **specific manifestations** include the fact that it is
     quite asymptomatic until late in its course. Often the

patient will be seen for a routine examination and have an adnexal mass and/or abdominal mass(es) discovered. There can be a history of slow enlargement of the abdomen, thought to be adipose by the patient. The disease can occur in premenopausal or postmenopausal women. On examination, hirsutism can be present, as well as ascites and, on pelvic examination, nontender fixed masses in the adnexa and superior aspects of the uterus.

3. The **specific evaluation and management** include developing an appropriate clinical suspicion for the lesion based on the data gathered in the overall section; please refer to Box 11-4. Several screening tests have been attempted but have been woefully inadequate. One of these is the tumor marker, CA-125. This marker is measured by a monoclonal antibody to the CA-125 antigen, an antigen present in many ovarian carcinomas. It is a marker for the detection of ovarian epithelial neoplasia, which does not have adequate sensitivity to be a screening tool. It can be, if increased, at the outset, a marker to be used for follow-up of the disease.

   a. Once a mass is discovered and is suggestive of this neoplastic lesion, **computed tomography (CT)** of the pelvis is indicated further to define the size and extent of the lesion. Invasive evaluation is based on the clinical suspicion that the lesion is a malignant neoplastic process. A **low likelihood of malignancy** includes lesions that are in the ovary and <2 cm in size and without any septa or solid components. A **high likelihood of malignancy** includes lesions >2 cm in size, with any component of septation or solid areas, or that have spread to structures extrinsic to the ovary.

   b. **Modalities for invasive evaluation** and **management** include:

      i. **Laparoscopy.** This procedure is performed by a gynecologist and involves the insertion of a tube with a fiberoptic imager into the peritoneum for direct visualization of the adnexae. Biopsy and therefore definitive histopathologic diagnosis by using this device is possible.

      ii. **Laparotomy.** Direct surgical intervention. This is the next step if the biopsy is positive for adenocarcinoma or if laparoscopic assessment is unavailable. The surgical intervention of choice includes:

         (a) Postmenopausal. Total abdominal hysterectomy and bilateral oophorectomy and biopsy of adjacent lymph nodes and adjacent peritoneal structures for staging purposes. Debulking of any and all gross tumor is also required.

    (b) Premenopausal. Cystectomy (i.e., removal of the entire lesion) and send the entire lesion for frozen-section analysis. If the lesion is benign, the procedure is complete; if the lesion is histopathologically diagnosed as malignant, total abdominal hysterectomy and bilateral oophorectomy and biopsy of adjacent lymph nodes and adjacent peritoneal structures for staging purposes are necessary. Debulking of any and all gross tumor is also required.

   c. Chemotherapeutic intervention, including therapeutic and adjuvant regimens, as indicated for metastatic or presumed metastatic disease. A discussion of these modalities is beyond the scope of this text.

E. Polycystic ovaries (PCO)

   1. The **pathophysiology** is based on a perturbation of the physiologic hormonal milieu of the premenopausal female.

     a. There is an abnormal increase in the production of 17-ketosteroid hormones, which have significant androgen activity from the ovaries, and/or adrenal glands (zona reticularis). These 17-ketosteroids may be catabolized into the even more androgenic agent estrone, by adipocytes.

     b. These ketosteroids and their catabolites (estrone) result in a negative feedback on the adenohypophysis to secrete FSH, but minimal effect on the secretion of LH. This results in overall abnormal levels of FSH and LH (i.e., an abnormal decrease in overall FSH and a concurrent, relative if not absolute increase in LH).

     c. The overall increase in LH results in an increase in the thecal cells, a further increase in progesterone and progesterone-like hormones, and an absence of ovulation. This will result in the development of one or more ovarian cysts (i.e., polycystic ovary disease). Furthermore, this anovulation may lead to not only secondary amenorrhea and infertility but also dysfunctional uterine bleeding (see section on Vaginal Discharge, page 554).

   2. The **specific evaluation** of this entity is to make the clinical diagnosis based on the data obtained in Box 11-4 and effectively to rule out any other origin of secondary amenorrhea. These include a primary ovarian tumor–producing androgen, Cushing's syndrome, hypothyroidism, or secondary hypogonadism, usually as a result of panhypopituitarism. Therefore, in addition to the specific laboratory examinations described in Box 11-4:

   a. If Cushing's syndrome is suspected, see secondary hypertension, Chapter 3, page 147.
   b. If hypothyroidism is suspected, obtain a thyroid-stimulating hormone (TSH) level. See Thyroid Dysfunctional States in Chapter 9, page 497.
   c. If secondary hypogonadism is suspected, look for manifestations of panhypopituitarism or a prolactinoma (e.g., galactorrhea, hypothyroidism, and bitemporal hemianopsia).
   3. The **specific management** includes making the clinical diagnosis and prescribing a weight-loss program. An effective weight-reduction program is central to management. Referral to endocrine and gynecology is indicated.

II. Consultation

Problem	Service	Time
Adnexal mass in pregnant woman	Ob/Gyn	Urgent/emergent
Adnexal mass, febrile	Ob/Gyn	Urgent/emergent
Adnexal mass, cystic and <2 cm	Ob/Gyn	Elective
Adnexal mass, noncystic, and/or >2 cm in size	Ob/Gyn	Required, semi-urgent
Polycystic ovary	Gyn	Elective

III. Indications for admission: Any adnexal mass in a pregnant patient, severe pelvic inflammatory disease, evidence of hemodynamic instability, and/or concurrent purulent or bloody vaginal discharge.

Vaginal Discharge

Every woman will have vaginal discharge at various times during her life. The normal vaginal discharge is scant and physiologic in the vast majority of cases (Box 11-5). There is a relation between such normal vaginal discharge and time of menstruation. Menstruation requires the normal functioning of four specific organs, the hypothalamus, the adenohypophysis, the ovaries, and the uterus. The cycle described subsequently occurs hundreds of times over the fertile life span of a woman.

1. At the beginning of each cycle, the hypothalamus produces the releasing factor for luteinizing hormone (i.e., LHRH), which results in the release of LH and FSH from the adenohypophysis.
2. The FSH and LH stimulate the ovarian follicles to develop and mature and to produce the hormone estrogen. During this phase (i.e., the follicular phase), the oocyte develops and, under the

B O X   11-5

Overall Evaluation and Management of Vaginal Discharge Suspected To Be Abnormal

Evaluation

1. History
   a. Menstrual history
      i. Last menstrual period (LMP).
      ii. Features of the menstrual cycles and of the menstruation itself.
         (a) Polymenorrhea—multiple short episodes of menstrual bleeding, each self-limited but abnormal in frequency.
         (b) Metromenorrhagia—excessive or prolonged menstrual bleeding occurring at irregular intervals.
         (c) Menorrhagia—excessive or prolonged menstrual bleeding at the normal time.
      iii. Para and gravida (i.e., the total number of antecedent deliveries and conceptions).
      iv. If postmenopausal, when menopause occurred, and if it was natural or iatrogenic. If iatrogenic, if the surgical procedure was a hysterectomy (i.e., not true menopause) or bilateral oophorectomy with or without hysterectomy.
   b. Current medications including systemic anticoagulants, oral contraceptives, and aspirin.
   c. History of systemic manifestations of bleeding (e.g., epistaxis, hematuria, hematemesis, easy bruising).
   d. Current method of contraception, if any.
2. Physical examination, looking for evidence of a systemic coagulopathy (e.g., petechiae, purpura, ecchymosis) and examination of the neck for goiter. The pelvic examination is central to all cases of vaginal discharge, bloody or nonbloody. Specific examinations include looking at the discharge itself and where it originates.
   a. Gram stain and culture of any purulent discharge either from the Bartholin's gland or from the cervix.
   b. A wet mount of any nonpurulent vaginal discharge, in which a freshly swabbed sample of the discharge is admixed in a test tube with 1–2 mL of normal saline, placed on a slide with a cover-

(continued)

B O X 11-5 (continued)

      slip, and microscopically imaged. One can visualize *Trichomonas* organisms or the clue cells of bacterial vaginosis (Fig. 11-1) by using this method.

  c. A KOH preparation of the nonpurulent vaginal discharge. By using the wet-mount specimen on the slide, place 2–4 drops of 10% KOH and warm the slide by using a match or Bunsen burner. One can visualize any *Candida* organisms.

  d. Papanicolaou smear of the cervix, looking for dysplastic cervical cells. One should use both the spatula, to obtain ectocervical cells, and the Cytobrush, to obtain endocervical cells (Table 11-2).

  e. Describe any lesion on the cervix.

  f. Palpate and describe any uterine, adnexal, cervical, or vulvar masses.

3. β-HCG in the urine to rule out pregnancy. This is requisite in all premenopausal women who have a uterus and ovaries.

4. If any bleeding, intravascular volume depletion, pregnancy test positive, or fevers, obtain a complete blood count.

5. If any evidence of a coagulopathy, obtain a prothrombin time (PT), activated partial thromboplastin time (aPTT), and platelet count.

6. If any suspicion for hypothyroidism, obtain TSH, refer to Chapter 9, page 497.

7. Urinalysis, to look for a concurrent pyuria or hematuria (i.e., another site of bleeding).

8. Obtain an ultrasound of the pelvis. This is especially important in patients with any abnormal bleeding, any evidence of a pelvic mass on examination, or a positive β-hCG.

direct influence of estrogens, results in proliferation of the endometrial tissue. Therefore, this phase is also known as the proliferative phase.

3. At the midpoint of the cycle (i.e., on approximately day 14), the estrogen level peaks, which results in a surge of LH from the adenohypophysis and precipitates the forceful extrusion of the oocyte from the ovary into the abdominal cavity (i.e., ovulation).

4. At the time of ovulation and LH increase, the follicular cells remaining in the ovary evolve, under the direction of LH, into a corpus luteum. This is called the luteal phase. The corpus

T A B L E   11-2
Cervical Pap Smear Results, Bethesda Classification

Findings	Recommended Next Step
Within normal limits	Routine periodic screening

Benign epithelial changes
  a. Infection, GC cervicitis
  b. Reactive
	Repeat cervical smear after treating the infection if present

Atypical glandular of unknown significance	Colposcopy

Atypical squamous cells of unknown significance (ASCUS)
  a. Reactive process
  b. Inflammatory changes
  c. Premalignant changes
	If thought to be associated with an underlying infection (e.g., *Chlamydia* or *N. gonorrhoeae*, treat the infection and repeat the smear in 2 mo
	If no underlying infection, repeat the smear q.4–6 months for 2 years or until the smear is normal for 3 consecutive times
	If two ASCUS readings, refer to colposcopy

Low-grade squamous intraepithelial lesion (LSIL)
Old nomenclature:
  CIN I
  Mild dysplasia
	Repeat the smear q.4–6 mo for 2 years or until the smear is normal for 3 consecutive times
	If two LSIL readings, refer to colposcopy

High-grade squamous intraepithelial lesion (HGIL)
Old nomenclature:
  CIN II, III
  Moderate dysplasia
  Severe dysplasia
	Colposcopy

Invasive carcinoma	Colposcopy

luteum produces progesterone, a hormone that stimulates the already proliferated endometrium to evolve further and begin a secretory function, all for the goal of supporting the implantation of a fertilized oocyte. Thus this phase is also referred to as the secretory phase.

5. If fertilization and implantation do not occur, the LH/FSH and estrogen and progesterone will, at the end of the cycle (i.e., approximately day 27) precipitately decline. The sudden loss of hormonal support for the endometrium will result in sloughing of endometrial tissue (i.e., menstrual flow).

Any change in the quantity or quality of the vaginal discharge, the concurrent presence of vaginal or pelvic manifestations, or any changes in menstruation should be used as markers that the discharge may well be abnormal. Although there is significant overlap between the two groups, there are two specific categories of abnormal vaginal discharge, bloody and nonbloody.

I. **Causes of abnormal vaginal bleeding**
   A. **Fibroids** (i.e., leiomyomas of the uterus)
      1. The **pathophysiology** of this disorder is not completely known. It has a high prevalence (i.e., 30% of women will develop these benign uterine neoplastic lesions). They are the most common neoplastic lesion involving the uterus. They are single or multiple and can occur anywhere in the uterus itself. If they occur immediately deep to the endometrium (i.e., submucosal in location), they have a high propensity of bleeding.
      2. The **specific manifestations** include the development of menorrhagia and menometrorrhagia and the presence of nontender masses within the body of the uterus. Iron-deficiency anemia is not an uncommon manifestation.
      3. The **specific evaluation and management** include making the clinical diagnosis by using the evaluative tools described in Box 11-5. Ultrasound will confirm the presence of intrauterine masses. If the patient is iron deficient, give her iron and follow up hematocrits and reticulocyte counts.
         a. Premenopausal. If the patient no longer desires to be fertile, the **treatment** of choice is total hysterectomy without oophorectomy. If the patient wants to have children, other modalities may be used. One of these procedures is myomectomy (i.e., selective and specific removal of a uterine fibroid). This procedure can effectively remove the fibroid while maintaining uterine competence. If the fibroids are asymptomatic and pregnancy is not desired, follow-up every 6 months is indicated.
         b. Postmenopausal. A total abdominal hysterectomy is the intervention of choice.
   B. **Pregnancy**
      Vaginal bleeding in a pregnant female requires immediate obstetric consultation and intervention. The three most common reasons for bleeding during pregnancy are a normal delivery (i.e., labor), a spontaneous abortion, or an ectopic pregnancy. The first cause, labor, is usually expected and quite easily diagnosed; the other two can be more vexing and fraught with potentially mortal complications.

1. The **pathophysiology** of an ectopic pregnancy and of a spontaneous abortion are quite different. A ruptured ectopic pregnancy is one in which the fertilized oocyte (i.e., the products of conception) implants in a site different from the uterine endometrium. The sites of implantation include the abdomen and the fallopian tube. The risk of this entity increases if there has been any scarring of the fallopian tubes. This scarring can be as the result of a past episode of pelvic inflammatory disease or an incomplete tubal-ligation procedure. A spontaneous abortion, commonly referred to as a miscarriage, is one in which the uterus extrudes the products of conception before they are viable for extrauterine existence. If in the first trimester, it usually is as the result of a gross genotypic abnormality of the fetus, whereas if in the second trimester, it usually is as the result of an abnormality of the uterus or cervix itself.

2. The **specific manifestations** include a history of "missing a few periods" and the onset of crampy abdominal pain and bloody vaginal discharge. In most cases, the patient knows or suspects that she is pregnant. Often there will be left or right shoulder pain. This pain is referred and usually indicates peritoneal irritation. The patient can be intravascularly volume depleted and hemodynamically unstable (i.e., hypotensive and tachycardic) at the time of presentation.

   a. If a ruptured ectopic pregnancy, the vaginal discharge is usually scant, but pain can be marked. Concurrent findings include the development of Grey Turner's sign (i.e., ecchymosis about the flank) or Cullen's sign (i.e., ecchymosis about the umbilicus). If a spontaneous abortion, there is often the passage of tissue (i.e., the products of conception) concurrent with the vaginal bleeding.

3. The **specific evaluation and management** include making the clinical diagnosis by using the data derived from Box 11-5. In both cases, the β-hCG is positive, and ultrasound will reveal no intrauterine gestational sac. In an ectopic pregnancy, there often will be an asymmetry of the fallopian tubes with a unilateral mass. In a spontaneous abortion, some tissue will pass. This tissue must be saved and sent to pathology for assessment. In both cases, immediate referral to an obstetrician is clearly indicated, as well as initiating intravenous access and performing preoperative laboratory evaluations, including typing and screening of blood. Surgical intervention on an emergency basis is indicated for a ruptured or nonruptured ectopic pregnancy, whereas observation and potential uterine dilation and curettage (D&C) are indicated for a spontaneous abortion. If the

spontaneous abortion is in the second trimester, an assessment of uterine competence is indicated.

C. **Cervical carcinoma**

As a result of effective screening programs, the mortality from this specific entity has precipitately decreased.

1. The **pathophysiology** of this type of carcinoma has been outlined to the point that there are certain specific **risk factors** in its development. These **risk factors** include infection with human papillomavirus (i.e., condylomata acuminata), infection with herpes simplex virus, a history of smoking tobacco, and multiple sexual partners. The **natural history** is one of dysplasia isolated to the cervical epithelium which slowly, usually over the course of months, invades into the deeper structures of the cervix. The dysplastic cells within the cervical epithelium actually are carcinoma in situ.

2. The **specific manifestations** of this type of vaginal bleeding include postcoital spotting and dyspareunia. The bleeding is intermittent and relatively scant and usually in the premenopausal age group. On pelvic examination, there can be and often is an indurated area, with or without ulceration, adjacent to or in the os of the cervix.

3. The **specific evaluation and management** of this entity includes making the clinical diagnosis by using the techniques described in Box 11-5. Specific evaluation includes the Pap smear, which will demonstrate atypical and/or dysplastic cells (see Box 11-2). Referral to a gynecologist for cervicography and/or colposcopy is clearly indicated. Cervicography is a microscopic photograph of the cervix looking for any abnormal areas consistent with carcinoma; colposcopy is the direct microscopic imaging of the cervix and the performance of biopsies in areas suggestive of cervical carcinoma. If any evidence of carcinoma, the procedure of choice is conization of the cervix (i.e., the removal of a cone of tissue of the cervix itself), a procedure that is curative in the vast majority of cases.

D. **Endometrial carcinoma**

1. The **pathophysiology** is primarily the result of abnormal proliferation of the endometrium itself. **Risk factors** for development include those that stimulate the growth of the endometrium, including the long-term unopposed use of oral estrogens, and states in which the patient would have relatively high levels of endogenous estrogens on a chronic but physiologic basis. These factors include but are not limited to:
   a. Early onset of menarche.
   b. Late onset of menopause.
   c. Nulliparity (i.e., never having been pregnant).

2. The **specific manifestations** include the fact that this occurs in older, usually postmenopausal women. Often the bleeding is relatively scant, but in the postmenopausal setting, very disconcerting. In all cases, any postmenopausal vaginal bleeding must be aggressively and definitively addressed and defined.

3. The **specific evaluation and management** include making the clinical diagnosis and/or having a relatively high clinical suspicion as based on the overall evaluation as described in Box 11-5. In all cases, referral to a gynecologist is indicated for endometrial biopsy and assessment. The procedure of choice is D&C of the uterine endometrium and concurrent direct imaging with a hysteroscope to look for endometrial polyps. These procedures are performed by a gynecologist.

E. **Dysfunctional uterine bleeding**

A relatively common form of abnormal vaginal bleeding.

1. The **underlying pathophysiology** is based on the fact that the patient can, for whatever reason, have one or several consecutive cycles in which ovulation does not occur. Ovulation can be stymied by many different factors, including severe stress, malnutrition, anorexia nervosa, or the perimenopause. Each cycle that occurs without an effective ovulation results in several hormonal modifications.

   a. The follicular cells remain intact and functional for a longer than normal period. This results in a longer follicular phase and overall longer duration of high levels of estrogens, causing significant proliferation of the uterine endometrium.

   b. A lack of evolution of the follicular cells into a corpus luteum, resulting in a want of progesterone production. Thus the luteal phase is markedly abbreviated, if present.

   c. The next cycle begins without a significant change in estrogen levels, and because there is little to no progesterone production, there is no marked decline and therefore no significant decline in the hormone levels; therefore, no sloughing of the endometrium (i.e., no menstrual flow), which manifests as a skipped period (i.e., secondary amenorrhea).

   d. In the next normal cycle, one in which ovulation does occur, there is the development of a normal corpus luteum and, with it, normal production of progesterones. If conception does not occur, there will be, at the end of the cycle, the normal decline in estrogens and progesterones, with a resultant sloughing of the endometrium from this cycle and the excess endometrium that had accumulated from previous anovulatory cycles. This manifests with menorrhagia (i.e., an extremely heavy menstrual flow of long duration).

2. The **specific manifestations** of this cause of bloody vaginal discharge are based on the pathophysiologic description. They include irregular periods, both in terms of duration and amount of flow, with intermittent intervals of secondary amenorrhea in which one to three cycles are missed, followed by an inordinately heavy menses. The patient is infertile even when she is aggressively attempting to conceive. Manifestations of the underlying cause are commonly present.

3. The **specific evaluation and management** of dysfunctional uterine bleeding include making the clinical diagnosis based on the tests described in Box 11-5. Once the clinical diagnosis has been made and other, more malignant causes of vaginal bleeding have been excluded, therapy can be instituted. Therapy can include:

   a. If pregnancy is not desired at present, the initiation of oral contraceptive agents. These agents will essentially take over the hormonal regulation of the menstrual cycles and iatrogenically make the menstrual cycles regular. Any oral contraceptive regimen is acceptable. One example is Ortho-Novum 7/7/7.

   b. If pregnancy is desired in the near future, an attempt to make the periods regular by controlling one cycle with exogenous hormones is indicated. The specific regimen includes ethinyl estradiol, 0.05 mg p.o., 1–3 times per day for 14 days (i.e., days 1–14), followed by medroxyprogesterone (Provera), 10 mg p.o., q.d., for 7 days (i.e., days 15–21), followed by withdrawal of hormones. The withdrawal should result in a period of menstrual flow. The next and subsequent periods can then, if the **treatment** was effective, be regular.

II. **Causes of abnormal vaginal discharge, nonbloody** (i.e., vaginitis; see also Table 11-3).

   A. *Trichomonas vaginalis*

      1. **Pathophysiology**

         This eukaryotic parasitic organism is transmitted only by sexual contact. It is specific to the male and female genitourinary tracts and results in superficial infection of the urethral and vaginal mucosa. **Risk factors** include unsafe sex with multiple sexual partners.

      2. The **specific manifestations** include the onset of dyspareunia, pruritus, and intermittent dysuria. Pelvic examination discloses copious amounts of frothy fluid with a "fishy" odor. There is concurrent evidence of cervicitis, sometimes referred to as "strawberry" cervicitis. In many patients, however, the process is relatively asymptomatic.

TABLE 11-3
Syndromes of Vaginal Inflammation

Cause	Discharge	Wet Mount	Treatment
Trichomonas	Clear Frothy Copious	Mobile trichomonads present	*Metronidazole, 2 g p.o. once; concurrently treat partner
Candida	Malodorous Whitish	Negative until KOH is added, then budding yeasts are present	Clotrimazole, 100 mg per vagina q.d. for 7 consecutive nights or Fluconazole 150 mg p.o. × 1
Vaginosis	Clear Malodorous	Clue cells—epithelial cells coated with bacteria	*Metronidazole, 500 mg p.o., b.i.d., for 7 days, or Clindamycin, 300 mg p.o., b.i.d., for 7 days
Atrophic	Scant Dyspareunia Postmenopausal	No specific findings	Premarin, 0.1% cream b.i.d.

*Metronidazole is contraindicated during pregnancy.

3. The **specific evaluation and management** include making the clinical diagnosis by using the techniques described in Box 11-5 and performing a wet-mount preparation. The wet mount will clearly demonstrate the trichomonads swimming; their activity can be increased by warming the slide. **Specific treatment** includes treatment of the patient and her sexual partner(s) with a single 2-g dose of metronidazole (Flagyl). Metronidazole is contraindicated in pregnant women. There is a >90% cure rate if the patient and partner are concurrently treated. Further treatment includes educating the patient in safe-sex techniques (i.e., the use of condoms or abstinence).

B. *Candida* species

1. **Pathophysiology**

There is an abnormal overgrowth of this fungal organism, which normally colonizes the vagina. The organisms are either *Candida albicans* or *Candida glabrata*. The organism is not transmitted sexually. It is symptomatically present only if a change occurs in the normal vaginal milieu. **Risk factors** for development include the use of oral contraceptive agents, systemic glucocorticoids, or broad-spectrum antibiotics, and diabetes mellitus. The two most common reasons for an overgrowth of *Candida* are an increase in vaginal glucose levels (e.g., as the result of diabetes and/or glucocorticoids) or a decrease in the normally present bacillary bacteria, lactobacilli.

2. The **specific manifestations** include vaginal pruritus, classically worse immediately before the onset of menstruation. There can be dyspareunia and a thick, white, almost curdled-in-appearance discharge, even with whitish, thrushlike plaques.

3. The **specific evaluation and management** include making the clinical diagnosis based on the examinations outlined in Box 11-5. The wet mount will reveal few findings; therefore, the KOH is performed, which will demonstrate yeast. Once the diagnosis is clinched, the initiation of antifungal agents should be made. The basic tenets of therapy include:

   a. Check for and reverse any and all **risk factors** for development.

   b. The initiation of clotrimazole (Mycelex, others), 100-mg vaginal suppositories in a regimen of one per vagina q.HS for 7 nights; or clotrimazole, 300-mg vaginal suppositories q.HS for 3 nights.

   c. If recurrent, one can use systemic antifungal agents, (e.g., fluconazole). The regimen for fluconazole 150 mg p.o., q.d. for one dose.

(text continues on page 561)

T A B L E 11-4
Medical Problems of Pregnancy

Disorder	Pathophysiology	Manifestations: Mother	Manifestations: Fetus	Evaluation/Management
HELLP* syndrome	Multiparous >25 years of age <36 weeks of gestation Associated with preeclampsia but may have no concurrent hypertension	Epigastric pain, nausea, and vomiting Hemolytic anemia Purpura Petechiae Ecchymosis Crackles, pulmonary edema Acute renal failure Acute liver failure	Fetal death	Smear with schistocytes Increased total bilirubin Increased LDH Evidence of a consumptive coagulopathy (DIC) Azotemia Hypoxemia *Management:* Supportive and immediate delivery
Preeclampsia/Eclampsia	Failure of trophoblastic invasion into the spiral arteries of the uterus; therefore, failure of cardiovascular adaptors to increase the plasma volume and decrease the systemic vascular resistance needed for normal pregnancy These result in: a decrease in cardiac output, a decrease in plasma volume, and an increase in SVR	Headache Visual changes Epigastric pain Hypertension, mild to moderate Edema >20 weeks of gestation *Eclampsia:* Gran mal convulsions Cerebral hemorrhage Petechiae Purpura Liver failure Death	Abruptio placenta Fetal growth retardation Fetal distress/death Oligohydramnios	*Evaluation:* Serum urate >5.5 Proteinuria DIC Increased LFTs Azotemia/uremia *Management:* If mild, monitor zealously the patient's weight, blood pressure, and urine for protein If severe, deliver fetus, treat hypertension with hydralazine and magnesium sulfate

Chronic hypertension without eclampsia	Essential hypertension antecedent to pregnancy	Asymptomatic hypertension Blood pressure >140/90 mm Hg during the first 20 weeks of gestation Risk of superimposed pre-eclampsia	Abruptio placenta Fetal growth retardation Fetal distress/death Marked increase in fetal mortality when pregnant mother has a diastolic BP >110 mm Hg during first trimester	Rest Control blood pressure with: a. Labetalol, or b. α-Methyldopa (aldomet)
Hyperemesis gravidarum	Etiology unclear Increased HCG in these patients Hypothyroidism	Severe, persistent nausea and vomiting Unable to maintain adequate nutrition or even hydration Usually in second trimester, may persist into the third trimester	Fetal growth retardation Preterm labor Low birth weight	i.v. Rehydration with D5NS Antiemetics: a. Compazine b. Metoclopramide (Reglan)
Intrahepatic cholestasis of pregnancy	Etiology unclear Family history of similar events Increased risk if cholestasis occurs with oral contraceptive pill	Pruritus on the trunk, palms, and soles Jaundice Light-colored stools Dark urine	Fetal demise Increased risk of postpartum neonatal bleeding	Cholestyramine, 10–12 g/day
Acute fatty liver of pregnancy	Marked accumulation of micro-vascular fat within the hepatocytes Much more common first pregnancy; risk decreases with subsequent pregnancies	Malaise Upper abdominal pain Nausea, vomiting Jaundice Purpura/petechiae Rarely pruritus May progress to a fulminant hepatitis with encephalopathy, hepatorenal syndrome, and even death	Fetal death Maternal death	*Evaluation:* DIC panel C/W a consumptive coagulopathy Elevated bilirubin Hypoglycemia Elevated ammonia Increased LFTs *Management:* Delivery Supportive

(continued)

559

T A B L E 11-4 (continued)

Disorder	Pathophysiology	Manifestations: Mother	Manifestations: Fetus	Evaluation/Management
Hypothyroid	Underlying/preexisting hypothyroid a. Hashimoto's b. Iatrogenic	Cold Alopecia Queen Anne's sign Delayed relaxation phase of reflexes Constipated Malaise/lethargy	Spontaneous abortion Placenta abruptio Stillbirth Preeclampsia Congenital motor and cognitive dysfunction (cretinism)	*Evaluation:* Increased TSH, usually >10 Decreased free T_4 Must measure q month in women at risk *Management:* If clinically hypothyroid, replace with levothyroxine to normalize TSH; usual dose: 100–150 μg/day If clinically euthyroid, but TSH is elevated, without a lowered T_4: a. Low-dose levothyroxine replacement (i.e., 25–50 μg/d)
Hyperthyroidism	Graves' Early Hashimoto's Iatrogenic Self-medicate	Hyperdynamic symptoms: a. Tachycardia b. Palpitations Inadequate weight gain or even weight loss Lid lag	Low birth weight Premature delivery Neonatal hyperdynamic manifestations	Treatment of choice is propylthiouracil (PTU) Radioactive iodide is contraindicated β-blockers will result in intrauterine growth retardation
Asthma	Most common pulmonary disorder of pregnancy	Muscle weakness, proximal Increased maternal mortality if poorly controlled	Low birth weight Perinatal mortality increased if poorly controlled asthma Chronic use of steroids increases the risk of premature delivery and low birth weight	Inhaled β_2 agonist Inhaled corticosteroid Low-dose systemic steroids, <2 weeks' duration if possible
Deep venous thrombosis	See page 39			

(text continued from page 557)

    d. If pruritus is severe, a low-dose glucocorticoid cream (e.g., hydrocortisone 1% cream t.i.d.) can be administered to the vulva for the first 2–3 days.

C. Vaginosis (i.e., nonspecific vaginitis)

    1. The **pathophysiology** is an abnormal overgrowth of anaerobic bacterial organisms and the nonspecific organism, *Gardnerella vaginalis,* concurrent with an overall decrease in the presence of lactobacilli—the anaerobic, gram-positive bacillary bacteria normally present in the vagina. The overgrowth results in a very superficial inflammatory response. The process is not transmitted sexually. It is symptomatically present only if there is a change in the normal vaginal milieu.

    2. The **specific manifestations** include mild vaginal pruritus and a grayish to clear vaginal discharge, which has a unique, almost fishy odor. There is often the presence of diffuse, mild erythema.

    3. The **specific evaluation and management** include making the clinical diagnosis based on the examinations outlined in Box 11-5. The wet mount will demonstrate clue cells, vaginal epithelial cells with a stippled appearance on the cell surface (see Fig. 11-1). Management includes the initiation of oral antibiotics. The patient should be treated with one of the following regimens:

        a. Metronidazole, 500 mg p.o., b.i.d., for 7 days; or, if the patient is pregnant,

        b. Clindamycin, 300 mg p.o., b.i.d., for 7 days.

D. Atrophic vaginitis (see section on Menopause, page 535).

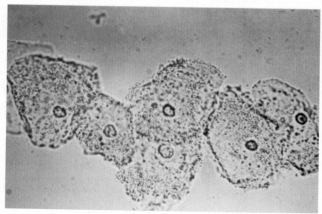

F I G U R E   11-1
Clue cells in a patient with vaginosis (nonspecific vaginitis).

III. Consultation

Problem	Service	Time
Vaginal bleeding in a pregnant patient	Ob/Gyn	Emergent
Fever with purulent vaginal discharge	Ob/Gyn	Urgent

IV. Indications for admission: Any hypotension; vaginal bleeding in a pregnant female; peritoneal signs; a tender adnexal mass and discharge from the vagina, with or without concurrent fever.

Medical Problems of Pregnancy (see Table 11-4, page 558)

Bibliography

Breast Masses and Lumps

Ernster VL: The epidemiology of benign breast disease. Epidemiol Rev 1981;3:184.

Mushlin AI: Diagnostic tests in breast cancer. Ann Intern Med 1985;103:79.

Odenheimer DJ, et al: Risk factors for benign breast disease: a case control study of discordant twins. Am J Epidemiol 1984;120:565.

Wilkinson S, Forrest AP: Fibroadenoma of the breast. Br J Surg 1985;72:838.

Contraceptive Modalities

Baird DT, Glasier AF: Hormonal contraception. N Engl J Med 1993;328:1543–1548.

Centers for Disease Control Cancer and Steroid Hormone Study: Long term oral contraceptive use and the risk of breast cancer. JAMA 1983;249:1591.

Centers for Disease Control Cancer and Steroid Hormone Study: Long term oral contraceptive use and the risk of endometrial cancer. JAMA 1983;249:1600.

Centers for Disease Control Cancer and Steroid Hormone Study: Long term oral contraceptive use and the risk of ovarian cancer. JAMA 1983;249:1596.

Mishell DR: Contraception. N Engl J Med 1989;320:777.

Rietmeijer CAM, et al: Condoms as physical and chemical barriers against human immunodeficiency virus. JAMA 1988;259:1851.

Stadel BV: Oral contraceptives and cardiovascular disease. N Engl J Med 1981;305:612.

Menopause/Osteoporosis

AACE clinical practice guidelines for the prevention and treatment of postmenopausal osteoporosis. Endo Pract 1996;2(2):157–171.

Aloia JF, et al: Calcium supplementation with and without hormone replacement therapy to prevent postmenopausal bone loss. Ann Intern Med 1994;120:97–103.

American College of Physicians: Guidelines for counseling postmenopausal women about preventive hormone therapy. Ann Intern Med 1992;117:1038–1041.

Belchetz PE: Hormonal treatment of postmenopausal women. N Engl J Med 330;1994:1062–1071.

Chapuy MC, et al: Vitamin D_3 and calcium to prevent hip fractures in elderly women. N Engl J Med 1992;327(23):1637–1642.

Grady D, et al: Hormone therapy to prevent disease and prolong life in postmenopausal women. Ann Intern Med 1992;117:1016–1037.

Leiblum S, et al: Vaginal atrophy in the postmenopausal woman. JAMA 1984;252:63.

Lufkin EG, Ory SJ: Estrogen replacement therapy for the prevention of osteoporosis. Am Fam Pract 1989;40:205–212.

Naessen T, et al: Hormone replacement therapy and the risk for first hip fracture. Ann Intern Med 1990;113:95–103.

Riggs BL, Melton LJ: Involutional osteoporosis. N Engl J Med 1986;314: 1676–1686.

Riis B, et al: Does calcium supplementation prevent postmenopausal bone loss? N Engl J Med 1987;316:173–177.

Stampfer MJ, et al: Postmenopausal estrogen therapy and cardiovascular disease. N Engl J Med 1991;325:756–762.

Pelvic Masses

Barber HRK: Ovarian carcinoma. Cancer 1986;36:149.

Crum CP, et al: Human papillomavirus type 16 and early cervical neoplasia. N Engl J Med 1984;310:880.

Eschenbach DA, et al: Polymicrobial etiology of acute pelvic inflammatory disease. N Engl J Med 1975;293:166.

Franks S, et al: Polycystic ovary syndrome. N Engl J Med 1995;333:853–861.

Richardson GS, et al: Common epithelial cancer of the ovary. N Engl J Med 1985;312:415.

Rose PG: Endometrial carcinoma. N Engl J Med 1996;335:640–648.

Wasserheit JN, et al: Microbial causes of proven pelvic inflammatory disease and efficacy of clindamycin and tobramycin. Ann Intern Med 1986; 104:187.

Vaginal Discharge

Brunham RC, et al: Mucopurulent cervicitis. N Engl J Med 1984;311:1.

Cannistra SA, Niloff JM: Cancer of the uterine cervix. N Engl J Med 1996;334:1030–1038.

Friedrich EG Jr: Vulvar pruritus: a symptom, not a disease. Postgrad Med 1977;61:164.

Goldfarb JM, Little AB: Abnormal vaginal bleeding. N Engl J Med 1980; 302:666.

Pheifer TA, et al: Nonspecific vaginitis: role of haemophilus vaginalis and treatment with metronidazole. N Engl J Med 1978;298:1429.

Richard RM: The patient with an abnormal Pap smear. N Engl J Med 1980;302:729.

Reed BD, et al: Vaginal infections: diagnosis and management. 1993;47: 1805–1816.

Medical Problems with Pregnancy

Bishnol A, et al: Thyroid disease during pregnancy. Am Fam Phys 1996;53:215–220.

Carson JL, et al: Care of the pregnant patient with medical illness. J Gen Intern Med 1992;3:577–588.

Ginsberg JS, et al: Heparin therapy during pregnancy. Arch Intern Med 1989;149:2233–2236.

Knox TA, et al: Liver disease in pregnancy. N Engl J Med 1996;335:569–576.

Levin ME, et al: Pregnancy and diabetes. Arch Intern Med 1986;146: 758–767.

Lynch CM, et al: Use of antibiotics during pregnancy. Am Fam Phys 1991;43:1365–1368.

Peterson LJ, Peterson CM: Managing the pregnant diabetic woman. Endocrinologist 1991;1:301–312.

Pitkin RM, et al: Pregnancy and congenital heart disease. Ann Intern Med 1990;112:445–454.

Schrocknadel H, et al: Hemolysis in hypertensive disorders of pregnancy. Gynecol Obstet Invest 1992;34:211–216.

Scott JR: Hypertensive disorders of pregnancy, In: Scott, JR, ed. Danforth's obstetrics and gynecology, 7th ed. Philadelphia: Lippincott-Raven, 1994:351–365.

Sibai BM: Treatment of hypertension in pregnant women. N Engl J Med 1996;335:257–265.

—K.W./D.D.B.

Chapter 12

Diseases of the Ear, Nose, and Throat

Epistaxis (Box 12-1)

The nose has a rich network of arterial supply and venous drainage. It is covered with a mucosa of stratified squamous epithelium, which is easily traumatized, leading to epistaxis. Epistaxis is bleeding from the nose. Nosebleeds can occur in the anterior or posterior aspect of the nasal passages and in either or both nasal passages.

I. **Anterior epistaxis**
   A. **Description**
      Anterior epistaxis manifests with bleeding mainly from the anterior nasal passages. The bleeding may be bilateral. Anterior epistaxis is much more common than posterior epistaxis. Although the bleeding is anterior, there may be some oozing of blood posteriorly, especially when the patient is supine. The bleeding is invariably venous, usually from the rich venous plexus termed Kisselbach's plexus.
   B. **Underlying causes** of anterior epistaxis include the following:
      1. Minor trauma to the mucosa, usually associated with or resulting from nosepicking. Although denied by patients, this habit, which has negative societal connotations, is a universal habit and a risk factor for anterior epistaxis.
      2. Nasal trauma, most commonly a fracture of the nasal bone itself, with resultant soft-tissue and vascular damage.
      3. Dry nasal mucosa, especially in the winter or in dry climates. The dry mucosa is easily traumatized and may also spontaneously crack and bleed.
      4. An acquired or genetic coagulopathy. The development of significant anterior epistaxis may herald a significant bleeding disorder. These bleeding disorders include

B O X 12-1

Overall Evaluation and Management of Epistaxis

Evaluation

1. Take a thorough history and perform a physical examination, including a history of coagulopathy or recent trauma to head or face.
2. Attempt to define the site of bleeding, anterior or posterior (see Table 12-1).

Management

1. Anterior site
   a. Patient should sit upright.*
   b. The patient or caregiver should firmly pinch the nasal ala together for 10–15 minutes.*
   c. After bleeding stops, the patient should apply sterile petrolatum gel to the nares to aid in lubrication for several days and, as a long-term measure, should use a humidifier, especially during the winter or dry season.*
   d. Examine the skin for concurrent ecchymotic or petechial lesions.
   e. Directly visualize the nasal mucosa, by using a nasal speculum and appropriate lighting, to determine the specific site of bleeding. An assistant may hold the light source or the clinician may use a headset reflector.
   f. Apply two to three drops of an α-agonist [e.g., phenylephrine (Neosynephrine)] to a cotton swab and apply it to the affected nasal mucosa, followed immediately by 10–15 minutes more of nasal alar compression. This agent immediately vasoconstricts the vessels, thereby decreasing blood flow to the area and increasing the ability to form thrombus.
   g. If bleeding continues, directly cauterize the specific sites of bleeding under direct visualization. Cauterization is accomplished by applying silver nitrate sticks to the mucous membranes.

*These are commonsense measures that the patient can be instructed to perform at home, and they may be performed in urgent care/office setting.

(continued)

B O X 12-1 (continued)

h. If bleeding continues, apply a 4% cocaine solution to the nasal mucosa, and recauterize, by using either silver nitrate or a heat probe, and pack the anterior nasal cavity with petrolatum gauze for 24 hours. Cocaine is an effective α-agonist, and thus vasoconstrictor, and is also a superb local anesthetic for the nasal mucosa, thus affording the patient effective local anesthesia when placing the anterior packing, a procedure that is quite painful. The packing is cotton gauze, which is placed into the anterior nasal chamber with some force. The packing is removed in 24 hours.

i. If a coagulopathy is suspected, perform laboratory tests including a complete blood count (CBC), prothrombin time (PT), activated thromboplastin time (aPTT), and platelet count, looking for any increase in the coagulation parameters or thrombocytopenia (see section on Excessive Bleeding States in Chapter 5, page 268).

2. Posterior site
   a. Obtain radiographs of the face, head, and cervical spine to rule out concurrent fractures.
   b. Place the patient in a cervical collar until a cervical spine fracture has been ruled out radiographically.
   c. Expedient referral to an ENT consultant is clearly indicated.

thrombocytopenia, disseminated intravascular coagulation (DIC), and iatrogenic excessive therapeutic anticoagulation with heparin or warfarin. If a coagulopathy is present, the patient usually has concurrent symptoms and signs of bleeding dysfunction, including menorrhagia, easy bruising, petechiae, purpura, or gingival bleeding.

II. Posterior epistaxis

Posterior epistaxis is uncommon and significant, usually requiring emergency **evaluation and management**. It usually occurs as a result of or associated with acute trauma to the facial bones, especially trauma causing fracture. The bleeding is usually arterial and requires immediate management of the airway, ruling out concurrent cervical spine or head trauma, admission to the hospital's ENT service for surgical intervention, and/or the placement of a posterior pack.

T A B L E 12-1
Anterior versus Posterior Epistaxis

Type	Characteristics	Site	Management
Anterior	Common Mild trauma Blood from anterior nares, unilateral or bilateral	Venous Kisselbach's venous plexus	Patient should sit up and lean forward Topical α-agonists Cautery with silver nitrate Anterior nasal packing with petrolatum gauze See text
Posterior	Rare Facial trauma, usually associated with facial bone fractures	Arterial	Airway Rule out concurrent head or cervical spine trauma ENT consultation Admission

III. Consultation

Problem	Service	Time
Uncontrolled anterior epistaxis	ENT	Emergent
Posterior epistaxis	ENT	Emergent

IV. Indications for admission: Severe coagulopathy or posterior epistaxis.

Oral Diseases (Box 12-2)

The oral cavity is the anatomic space immediately anterior to the pharynx. For the most part, it is lined with stratified squamous epithelium. Several structures in the oral cavity assist in basic functions. These unique structures are the teeth and the tongue. Although many disease states can affect the mouth, the three most common ones are dental caries, gingivitis, and oral carcinoma.

I. Simple caries

A. The **manifestations** of this common entity include acute or subacute pain referrable to one area of the mouth and even to a specific tooth. Often the decayed area will be small, but it is not uncommon to see gross decay of the tooth with parts of the tooth actually broken. In children, caries most commonly occur on the crowns, whereas in adults, caries usually occur at the gum line or adjacent to restorations (i.e., fillings).

B. The **underlying pathogenesis** is bacteria (anaerobic) production of enzymes and a slightly acid milieu that result in absorption of calcium from the tooth enamel. Once the

---

B O X 12-2

Overall Evaluation and Management of Oral Diseases

Evaluation

Perform a thorough examination of the oral structures, including direct visualization of the entire surface, including the sides of the tongue, and palpation of the mucosa of the mouth.

Management

1. Referral to dentist for any carious teeth.
2. Referral to dentist for semiannual prophylactic care.
3. Referral to ENT for any indurated lesions, especially if painful.

integrity of the enamel, the hard protective covering of the tooth, is broken, a cavity forms. The **natural history** of the disease once the cavity forms is slow, irreversible progression with dentine, the softer middle layer of the tooth, being resorbed. The cavity eventually reaches the pulp cavity, the structure that contains the blood vessels and nerves that serve the tooth. When the pulp cavity is involved, pain and abscess formation develop.

C. The **specific evaluation and management** of simple caries entail referral to a dental professional for corrective therapy and underscoring to the patient the importance of regular dental visits.

II. **Periapical abscess** (i.e. complicated caries)

A. The **specific manifestations** of complicated caries include the onset of severe pain and loss of chewing function on the entire side of the mouth ipsilateral to the involved tooth. The pain is dull, throbbing, aching, quite severe, and is often referred to other ipsilateral trigeminal nerve roots. The patient often has concurrent intolerance to hot and cold. Examination may reveal palpable swelling at the base of the tooth and in the adjacent gingival area, fevers, chills, and ipsilateral swelling of the face. There is, invariably, reproducible discomfort on percussion (i.e., tapping the diseased tooth). This is a direct result of inflammation involving the periodontal ligament. There may be a sinus tract draining of foul-smelling material the sinus forms from a periapical abscess.

B. The **underlying pathogenesis** is untreated caries that extends into the pulp cavity, resulting in infection, ischemia, and necrosis of the pulp chamber with resultant abscess formation and osteolysis at the periapical area. Causative organisms include anaerobes (i.e., peptostreptococci and *Bacteroides*) and gram-positive aerobic bacteria (i.e., streptococci, including those of the viridans group).

C. The **specific evaluation** includes examination, making the clinical diagnosis, and urgent referral to a dentist or endodontist for a drainage procedure. A radiograph of that tooth for confirmation of the diagnosis is indicated. This radiograph, obtained by the dental professional, will show lysis and/or sclerosis of the apical tooth area or of the adjacent bone.

D. The **specific management** is drainage of the tooth itself, by the classic root canal (i.e., opening the roots through the crown of the tooth and debriding the tissue) or by extraction of the tooth itself.

1. All patients should receive periprocedure antibiotics for 5 days, starting 6 hours before the procedure. The antibiotic schedule is either penicillin (VK), 500 mg p.o., q.i.d., for 5 days, or erythromycin, 500 mg p.o., q.i.d.

2. If there is any evidence of cellulitis (swelling, purulent discharge, or fevers), the antibiotics should be initiated immediately and continued for several days before the procedure for a total duration of 7–10 days. Finally, as the patient will be in significant distress, analgesics, including narcotic analgesia, should be prescribed until the procedure can be performed. A nonsteroidal antiinflammatory drug (NSAID; see Table 7-8, page 393) may be effective in pain management.

III. **Gingivitis**

A. The **specific manifestations** of this common oral disorder include bleeding from the gums when the teeth are brushed. There usually is no associated pain until late into the course of the disease. The patient may be unaware even of significant disease. Examination discloses mild swelling of the gingiva adjacent to the tooth and recession of the gingiva on the teeth, thus exposing the proximal aspects of the teeth (see Fig. 12-1). There are often a large number of caries in the areas of the teeth adjacent to the receded gingiva.

B. The **underlying pathogenesis** of this inflammation of the gingiva adjacent to the teeth is plaque. Plaque is an acquired, abnormal material coating the teeth that is quite hard and consists of bacteria. These bacteria invariably are anaerobic. The presence of plaque results directly in inflammation of the gingiva. The **natural history** is one of

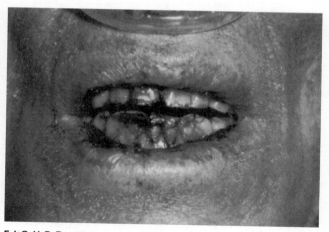

F I G U R E   12-1
Severe gingivitis. Note recession of the gingivae and purulent material on the periodontal surfaces. The gingivae bleed easily.

progressive loss of gingiva, increased risk of caries, especially adjacent to the gingiva, and tooth loss. Because this area is teeming with anaerobes, there is an increased risk of gravitational pneumonias in patients with a history of loss of gag reflex and/or decreased level of consciousness (e.g., patients with an antecedent cerebrovascular accident or ethanol abuse).

C. The **specific evaluation and management** include referral to a dental professional for therapeutic and prophylactic professional dental hygiene sessions every 4–6 months and instructing the patient to floss every day.

IV. **Squamous-cell carcinoma**

A. The **specific manifestations** of this disorder include a painless plaque, ulcer, or lump in the mucosa, mouth, tongue, or subcutaneous tissues of the neck. There is invariably a personal history of smoking tobacco (pipes, cigars, or cigarettes) or the chewing of tobacco, or ingestion of ethanol, especially in large quantities. The lesions can be asymptomatic until large. Examination includes direct visualization of the oral mucosa, palpation of the mucosal surfaces, and palpation of the cervical lymph nodes. Any lesion that is increasing in size, painless, ulcerated, indurated, or that occurs in a patient with **risk factors** for the development of carcinoma should make the clinician suspicious for a malignant neoplastic lesion.

B. The **underlying pathogenesis** is unclear. **Risk factors** that are irrefutably associated with development include smoking or chewing tobacco products and ethanol abuse.

C. The **specific evaluation and management** including having an appropriate clinical suspicion that a lesion may be malignant and, at that time, expedient referral to an ENT specialist for biopsy. The use of tobacco is proscribed.

V. **Consultations:**

Problem	Referral	Time
Caries, gingivitis, complicated caries	Dentist	Required/urgent
Oral ulcer, painless	ENT	Required/urgent

VI. **Indications for admission:** Virtually all of these conditions can be evaluated and managed on an outpatient basis.

Otalgia/Otitis

Four discrete syndromes result in ear pain and/or inflammation of the external or middle ear: otitis externa, otitis externa maligna, serous otitis media, and purulent otitis media (Box 12-3).

I. **Otitis externa**

A. The usual **manifestations** include unilateral pain in the external canal, commonly referred to as an earache. At times, the pain will extend into the ipsilateral tragus. Ex-

B O X 12-3

Overall Evaluation and Management of Otalgia/Otitis

Evaluation

1. Take a history and perform a physical examination, including palpation of the auricle and adjacent lymph nodes and visualization of the tympanic membrane looking for erythema and swelling.
2. Remove all cerumen from the canal. This is best accomplished with otologic lavage with warm normal saline or sterile water or even warm tap water. The patient is placed in an upright position and, by using a syringe with a "Christmas tree" top, the water is gently yet firmly injected into the external ear canal until cerumen is flushed out.
3. Query the patient regarding auditory and position sensation, including dizziness or vertigo, as these indicate more of an inner ear dysfunctional state.
4. Document auditory acuity, at least grossly, by using a ticking watch or rubbing fingers adjacent to the ear to ascertain any gross auditory deficit.

Management

1. If concurrent vertigo is present, see section on Vertigo in Chapter 14, page 672.
2. If an auditory deficit is present after **treatment** of common external and middle ear dysfunctional states, refer the patient to an audiologist for formal testing.

amination may reveal a significant amount of cerumen in the canal or swelling of the external canal precluding direct visualization of the tympanic membrane. Although pain and tenderness are the most common manifestations, erythema and pruritus of the affected areas are not uncommon. There may be a purulent discharge with crusting in the involved auditory canal.

A specific severe and potentially life-threatening type of otitis externa is **otitis externa maligna**. This manifests with a diffusely swollen and markedly tender auricle and can progress to a severe life-threatening infection of the face and head.

B. The **underlying pathogenesis** is a superficial infectious inflammation of the external auditory canal. Overall **risk factors** for development include ceruminous impaction, trauma due to patient attempting to clean his ears, and swimming in lake water or nonchlorinated swimming pools. This entity is most common during the summer months. Organisms that can cause otitis externa include *Staphylococcus aureus, Pseudomonas* spp., or fungi, *Candida,* or *Aspergillus.* Staphylococcal infections specifically manifest with a yellow crusty exudate; pseudomonal infections manifest with a greenish exudate.

In otitis externa maligna, **risk factors** include uncontrolled diabetes mellitus or immunosuppression with neutropenia or long-term high-dose steroids. The disease process is significantly more virulent, involves deeper structures, and the etiologic organism is invariably *Pseudomonas aeruginosa* (see Fig. 12-2).

C. The **evaluation** of otitis externa includes that listed in Box 12-3.

D. The **specific management** includes, after thoroughly cleaning and drying the external canal (see Box 12-3), the use of topical agents. The topical agent is Corticosporin (neomycin, 0.5%; hydrocortisone, 1%; and polymyxin B, 10,000 units/mL) solution or suspension in a dose of 2 drops b.i.d. to t.i.d. for 10–14 days, to the external canal. If the canal is completely obstructed, a 2- to 3-cm ribbon of cotton gauze (e.g., Nu Gauze packing strip) can be gently inserted into the canal. This forms a wick to which the

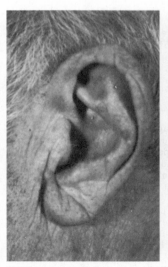
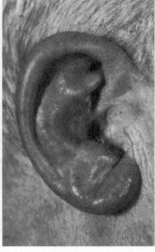

FIGURE   12-2
Left and right ears, showing otitis externa maligna in the right. Note the diffuse erythema and swelling.

topical agents are applied. If a fungal cause is suspected, clotrimazole (Lotrimin 1%) solution applied t.i.d. to the affected ear canal is indicated. Prevention by prohibiting the insertion of objects into the ear canal (e.g., Q-Tips). Furthermore, the patient should be instructed to use ear-plugs when swimming.

Otitis externa maligna mandates aggressive **evaluation and management**, for its natural history is one of rapid spread to adjacent tissues, bacteremia with resultant gram-negative rod septicemia, and mortality. These patients uniformly require admission, ENT, and infectious disease consults. The initiation of an intravenous aminoglycoside (e.g., gentamicin, 2 mg/kg i.v.), stat, and an antipseudomonal PCN or a third-generation cephalosporin is also mandatory.

II. Serous otitis media

A. The **specific manifestations** of this common entity include a mild decrease in auditory acuity bilaterally or unilaterally with an associated "popping" sensation in the affected ear(s). There may be modest pain in the affected ear(s). Often there are concurrent symptoms of nasal congestion, frontal headaches, and nonproductive cough. On examination, the tympanic membrane (TM) of the affected ear will demonstrate mild erythema and some air bubbles and fluid behind the affected TM. On direct visualization, the landmarks of the TM are not embarrassed, as one can clearly see the umbo, the pars tensa, and the pars flaccida. The reflex cone of light, however, is often decreased.

B. The **underlying pathogenesis** is nonpurulent inflammation of the middle ear as a result of (i.e., concurrent with) allergic rhinitis or a viral upper respiratory tract infection (URI). The disease is self-limited and will resolve when the underlying process, either the allergy or the viral URI, has resolved.

C. The **evaluation** is as described in Box 12-3 and making the clinical diagnosis.

D. The **specific management** is directed toward the underlying associated condition and the relief of symptoms. Acetaminophen prn and/or decongestants and/or antihistamines are clinically indicated (see Table 12-5, page 585).

Mycoplasma pneumoniae can cause a specific form of serous otitis media, bullous myringitis. Myringitis is inflammation of the TM without concurrent effusion. This form is usually associated with an atypical interstitial pneumonitis and requires, in addition to decongestants and acetaminophen, a 10-day course of erythromycin 500 mg p.o. q.i.d.

III. Purulent otitis media

A. The **specific manifestations** of this relatively common disorder include the acute onset of unilaterally decreased auditory acuity, modest to severe otalgia (i.e., pain in the affected ear) and occasionally otorrhea (i.e., the discharge of material, usually purulent, from the affected ear when the TM ruptures). Headaches and fevers may be concurrent with this process. There usually is a several-day antecedent history of rhinorrhea and scratchy sore throat. On examination often there is a bulging of the TM with loss of bony landmarks and a marked decrease in the cone of light reflex. Furthermore, the TM often is very erythematous. Finally, the patient will often have tender unilateral lymphadenopathy ipsilateral to the infected ear.

B. The **underlying pathogenesis** is a bacterial infection of the middle ear. It is not uncommon for the patient to have an antecedent serous otitis media. The pathogens that cause this disease process include *Streptococcus* spp., *Haemophilus* influenzae, and *Branhamella catarrhalis.* The most common complication is one of perforation of the TM. This perforation will acutely decrease the symptoms and will result in purulent otorrhea. This complication will, with antibiotics and conservative therapy, result in minimal sequelae. Other more malignant complications of this entity, if untreated, include the local suppurative complications of leptomeningitis, purulent labyrinthitis, brain or intracranial abscesses, and purulent mastoiditis.

C. The **evaluation** includes those items described in Box 12-3 and making the clinical diagnosis.

D. **Specific management** includes the initiation of antibiotics. Antibiotic regimens include amoxicillin, 500 mg p.o., t.i.d., for 10 days; trimethoprim–sulfamethoxazole (TMP-sulfa; Bactrim DS), 1 tablet p.o., b.i.d., for 10 days; or amoxicillin with clavulanic acid (Augmentin), 500–875 mg p.o., b.i.d., for 10 days. Any one of these regimens will effectively treat an infection due to these pathogens. Further therapy includes the prn use of decongestants and acetaminophen. It is rare that consultation with ENT is necessary unless there is evidence of recurrent disease, lack of resolution after standard first-line therapy, or perforation of the TM.

IV. **Consultation**

Problem	*Service*	*Time*
OEM	ENT	Emergent
Recurrent disease or complications of OM	ENT	Elective
Complications (except TM perforation)	Infectious diseases	Urgent

VI. **Indications for admission:** Complications of acute purulent otitis media, or any evidence of otitis externa maligna.

Pharyngitis (Box 12-4)

I. The **overall manifestations** of pharyngitis include the acute onset of sore throat, pain on swallowing (odynophagia), fevers to varying degrees, diffuse erythema of the tonsils and posterior pharynx, varying degrees of cervical lymph node enlargement, varying degrees of rhinitis and cough, and symptoms and signs specific to the underlying cause.

II. The **underlying pathogenesis** of acute pharyngitis include bacterial and viral agents. A list of these follows, along with their **specific manifestations** and **natural history**.

   A. **Streptococcus pyogenes**

   1. The **specific manifestations** of this common cause of pharyngitis include the acute onset of sore throat, present from the outset of the disease process, with concurrent fevers, chills, and intermittent night sweats. The sore throat can be of such magnitude as to cause significant odynophagia, potentially leading to mild intravascular volume depletion. Often, nausea with mild intermittent vomiting is present, but rhinorrhea, cough, and otalgia are uncommon. On examination, the tonsils and

---

B O X 12-4

Overall Evaluation and Management of Acute Pharyngitis

Evaluation

1. Take a thorough history and perform a physical examination, including direct visualization of the tonsils, posterior pharynx, and nasal mucosa and palpation of the cervical lymph nodes. A history of family members being diagnosed with specific entities in the recent past is also quite useful.
2. Formulate a ranked differential diagnosis and, based on the data gleaned from the history and physical examination, a clinical suspicion for the organism that has the greatest risk of complications, usually *Streptococcus pyogenes.*
3. Categorize the patient into one of three overall groups in regard to suspicion for *Streptococcus pyogenes*—high, low, and intermediate suspicion— before undertaking any further laboratory and therapeutic interventions. See text for specifics.

posterior pharynx are erythematous and covered with exudative material. The cervical nodes at the angle of the mandible (i.e., the jugulodigastric nodes) are invariably enlarged and tender bilaterally.

2. **Natural history**

The vast majority of cases are self-limited and resolve spontaneously within 7–10 days. There are, however, complications from this specific infectious entity. Complications occur in a small minority of patients but are potentially mortal and, with appropriate intervention, are preventable. The complications can be local or systemic.

   a. **Local** (i.e., head and neck) complications include the formation of a peritonsillar abscess (quinsy) or the formation of an abscess in, or spread of local infection to, the retropharyngeal space (Ludwig's angina).

   b. **Systemic complications** include the development of rheumatic fever (see Table 12-2 and the section on Polyarticular Arthritis in Chapter 7, page 397). A further complication is the development of immune complex–mediated glomerulonephritis.

B. **Rhinovirus and other RNA viral causes** (see also "viral rhinitis" subsequently)

1. The **specific manifestations** include a mild to moderate sore throat, usually preceded by rhinorrhea, otalgia, cough (productive or nonproductive), myalgias, and a low-grade fever. On examination, the posterior pharynx is often erythematous with minimal amounts of exudative material; furthermore, there often are some shotty, mildly tender cervical lymph nodes present.

2. The **natural history** is somewhat specific to the individual viral agent but, overall, is usually self-limited, with

T A B L E   12-2
Jones' Criteria in the Clinical Diagnosis of Rheumatic Fever

Major
    Pancarditis
    Chorea
    Polyarticular arthritis
    Subcutaneous nodules
    Erythema marginatum
Minor
    Increased ASO titer (Todd units)
    Increased Streptozyme titer (DNase-antideoxyribonuclease B)
    Increased C-reactive protein

complete resolution in 3–5 days. Specific viral agents include enteroviruses, adenoviruses, and coxsackie-viruses. Coxsackievirus A infection manifests as a distinctly painful pharyngitis with vesicles on the pharynx. This is a part of a more generalized gingivosto-matitis referred to as herpangina. Overall, there are few, if any, complications of viral pharyngitis.

C. **Infectious mononucleosis syndrome** [i.e., Epstein–Barr vi-rus (EBV)/cytomegalovirus (CMV)/acute human immuno-deficiency virus (HIV)]

1. The **specific manifestations** of this relatively common cause of pharyngitis include a prodromal phase of mal-aise and constitutional symptoms for 2–5 days, fol-lowed by the acute onset of a severe sore throat, usually with significant odynophagia. On examination, there are an exudative, approaching purulent, pharyngitis with associated petechiae on the mucous membranes of the mouth, and diffuse, tender lymphadenopathy, both cervical and generalized. Other associated findings may include a mild amount of icterus and spleno-megaly.

2. The **natural history** is dependent on the underlying cause. The three viruses that cause this syndrome are EBV, CMV, and acute infection with HIV. The natural history of EBV and CMV is that there is usually a com-plete resolution of the syndrome in 10–20 days. Com-plications can include splenic rupture, hepatitis, Coombs-positive hemolytic anemia, intravascular vol-ume depletion due to inability effectively to swallow, and thrombocytopenia as a result of sequestration asso-ciated with splenomegaly. Approximately 5% of pa-tients develop one of these acute complications of EBV infection. The natural history of HIV is as described in Chapter 6, page 320. Recall that the patient has a nega-tive HIV antibody during this syndrome but is quite viremic and therefore, highly infectious in this phase.

D. *Neisseria gonorrhoeae*

1. The **specific manifestations** of this rare form of pharyn-gitis, which can occur in patients who are at risk (i.e., those practicing fellatio or cunnilingus on an infected partner), include the acute onset of a severe sore throat. Examination reveals an exudative pharyngitis with multiple ulcer-type lesions and tender bilateral cervical lymphadenopathy. Often there is evidence of concur-rent urethritis or cervicitis.

2. The **natural history** is described in the infectious dis-ease chapter; for *Neisseria gonorrhoeae* in specific, see Chapter 6, page 340.

III. **Evaluation and management**

The **specific evaluation and management** are based on the degree of clinical suspicion that *S. pyogenes* is causing the pharyngitis.

A. **High suspicion of *S. pyogenes***

In the high-suspicion group (i.e., patients with the classic findings listed in the discussion on streptococcal pharyngitis), those with a history of rheumatic fever, or those in close contact with people with documented β-hemolytic streptococcal infections, treatment should be initiated. **Treatment** regimens include penicillin VK, 500 mg q.i.d., for 10 days; amoxicillin, 500 mg p.o. t.i.d., for 10 days; or erythromycin, 500 mg p.o., q.i.d., for 10 days. There rarely is any need for pharyngeal cultures or rapid assays in these cases. The only indication for a pharyngeal culture would be to document the disease to treat household contacts of the patient.

The **treatment** of streptococcal pharyngitis with PCN or erythromycin will decrease the development of local complications (i.e., abscesses), decrease the period of communicability, and decrease the risk of rheumatic fever. It will not decrease symptoms or the duration of the symptoms, nor will it decrease the risk of development of glomerulonephritis.

B. **Low suspicion of *S. pyogenes***

If the suspicion is low (i.e., another cause is more likely), treat supportively. There is essentially no need for pharyngeal bacterial culture. If viral or infectious mononucleosis is suspected, perform the following measures:

1. Provide analgesia and antipyretics. Acetaminophen, 500 mg p.o., q.4–6hr, as a tablet or as an elixir is best.

2. Perform a Monospot antibody test (i.e., the heterophile antibody test). The mechanism behind this test is that it measures an antibody associated with EBV infection but not the immunoglobulin M (IgM) antibody increase that occurs early in the course of EBV. The patient's serum is mixed with horse RBCs. If agglutination occurs, it is positive and caused by the presence of a heterophile antibody in the patient's serum. This test has a specificity of 99% and a sensitivity of 85% for EBV pharyngitis.

3. Provide fluids p.o. If severe odynophagia that prohibits adequate oral hydration is present, i.v. fluid replacement may be required.

4. Determine the CBC with differential. A finding of >40% atypical lymphocytes is quite specific for infectious mononucleosis in general and for EBV in specific.

5. Prescribe rest. It is very important for the patient to rest and refrain from any exercise or work-related activities.

6. If EBV is diagnosed, follow the hematocrits and perform

a baseline Coombs test to monitor for the development of a Coombs-positive hemolytic anemia.

7. If EBV is diagnosed and there is severe pain in the pharynx or inability to swallow even fluids, initiate prednisone, 40–60 mg p.o. with an initial dose of 80 mg methyl prednisolone i.v., in a rapid taper.

8. If EBV is diagnosed, closely monitor for the development of splenomegaly. The patient should be proscribed from any activity that may traumatize the abdomen during and immediately after the infection. These activities include contact sports, as the spleen can easily rupture in EBV-related splenomegaly.

9. If there is any indication of gonococcal pharyngitis, perform a pharyngeal swab with streaking of the swab on Thayer–Martin agar media. **Treatment** is discussed in the section on sexually transmitted diseases in Chapter 6, page 340.

C. **Intermediate suspicion of *S. pyogenes***

If the suspicion for streptococcal pharyngitis is intermediate, pharyngeal cultures or rapid streptococcal antigen techniques for diagnosis come into play (Table 12-3). These diagnostic techniques include the following.

1. **Pharyngeal culture.** The swab must be placed in or on the posterior pharynx and should, if possible, be plated onto medium at the time of the examination. This test has a sensitivity of 90% and a specificity of 75%–80%; however, it requires 24–48 hours to complete. Therefore, begin PCN or erythromycin if and when the cultures become positive for β-hemolytic *Streptococcus* spp.

2. **Rapid antigen detection techniques.** These are novel and effective assays for the detection of the Group A carbohydrate antigen in the streptococcal cell wall. Two of these techniques are latex agglutination and enzyme-linked immunosorbent assay (ELISA). Both are commercially available and applicable and have a sensitivity of 80%–90% and a specificity of 85%–100%. The test requires 20 minutes to complete. If positive, PCN, amoxicillin, or erythromycin in doses described above (page 580) can be initiated. If negative, treat as viral infection (see previous discussion).

IV. **Consultation**

Problem	Service	Time
Quinsy or Ludwig's angina	ENT	Emergent
Rheumatic fever	Infectious diseases	Urgent

V. **Indications for admission:** Any local complications of streptococcal infections, including quinsy and Ludwig's angina; rheumatic fever; intravascular volume depletion; and any decreased hematocrit in EBV, as a result either of hemolysis or of splenic rupture.

T A B L E 12-3
Evaluative Tests for Streptococcal Infections

Test	Sensitivity	Specificity	Time to Perform	Advantages	Disadvantages
Culture	90%	99%	24–48 hr	Easy to learn technique Minimal discomfort to patient	Time Cannot differentiate acute from chronic (i.e., infection from colonization)
Rapid screens	95%	99%	15–20 min	Time	Cost Cannot differentiate acute from chronic infection Special laboratory setup required

Rhinitis Syndromes (Box 12-5)

I. Viral rhinitis

   A. The **specific manifestations** of viral rhinitis, also known as the common cold, include the acute onset of bilateral rhinorrhea with concurrent sore throat, boggy mucous membranes, sneezing, nonproductive cough, mild watery eyes, a popping sensation in the ears, and overall malaise. It is rare to have any significant gastrointestinal manifestations, and, with the exception of viral rhinitis due to coxsackievirus A or B, these viruses rarely cause myalgias. Examination usually reveals serous otitis, a low-grade fever, usually $\leq 101.0°F$, mild erythema of the posterior pharynx, usually without exudate, and bilateral shotty, mildly tender cervical lymph node enlargement.

   B. The **underlying pathogenesis** is direct infection of the mucosal surface of the nose and the entire pharyngeal area.

B O X 12-5

Overall Evaluation and Management of Rhinitis

Evaluation

1. Take a thorough history and perform a physical examination, including querying the patient as to the onset of symptoms, any new pets, any seasonal component, and any associated lower respiratory tract manifestations.
2. Attempt to determine the underlying cause, whether viral or allergic (Table 12-4).

Management

1. Instruct the patient in basic hygiene, such as covering the nose and mouth when sneezing or coughing, washing and drying hands before touching items, and disposing of tissues with sputum or mucus on them.
2. If a new pet is in the household, perform a trial of a "pet holiday"; remove the pet from the household and observe the patient for symptomatic relief.
3. Prescribe acetaminophen and/or a decongestant prn for viral rhinitis (Table 12-5).
4. Prescribe an antihistamine and/or a decongestant prn for atopic rhinitis (Table 12-5).

T A B L E 12-4
Rhinitis Syndromes

Type	Precipitating Factors	Mechanism	Treatment
Viral	Adenoviruses Rhinoviruses Enteroviruses	Viral infection of upper respiratory tract	Decongestants Acetaminophen
Atopic	Allergens	IgE-mediated histamine release results in vasodilation and increased mucus production	Avoidance Desensitization Antihistamines Decongestants Topical steroids
Vasomotor	Odors Tear gas	Parasympathetic stimulation	Avoidance

T A B L E 12-5
Upper Respiratory Tract/Rhinitis Medications

Agent	Indications/Effects	Side Effects	Dosage
Entex LA (phenylpropanolamine and guaifenesin)	Decongestant Expectorant	Tachycardia Tremor	One tablet p.o. q.12hr prn
Drixoril (Pseudoephedrine and brompheniramine)	Decongestant Antihistamine	Dry mouth Tachycardia Urinary retention Drowsiness	One tablet p.o. q.12hr prn
Benylin DM syrup (dextromethorphan and ammonium chloride)	Antitussive Expectorant	Drowsiness (contains 5% ethanol by volume)	1–2 teaspoons p.o. q.4–6hr prn
Contac cough and sore throat liquid (acetaminophen, dextromethorphan, and guaifenesin)	Antitussive Expectorant Contains no ethanol	Tachycardia	1–3 teaspoons p.o. q.4–6hr prn
Benadryl (diphenhydramine)	Antihistamine	Drowsiness Dry mouth	25–50 mg p.o. q.6hr prn
Hisminal (astemizole)	Antihistamine	Minimal drowsiness Dry mouth	10 mg p.o. q. A.M.
Robitussin (guaifenesin)	Expectorant	Tachycardia	1–2 teaspoons p.o. q.6hr prn
Robitussin DM (guaifenesin and dextromethorphan)	Expectorant Cough suppressant	Tachycardia	1–2 teaspoons p.o. q.6hr prn
Robitussin AC (guaifenesin and codeine)	Expectorant Cough suppressant	Tachycardia	1–2 teaspoons p.o. q.6hr prn

Viral agents that cause this include enteroviruses (which include echovirus and coxsackievirus), coronaviruses, and rhinoviruses. The mucous membranes provide the source and terminus of transmission. Typical mechanisms of transmission of the virus include kissing, coughing, or sneezing, which spread the infected particles of mucus. The infected particles of mucus transmit the disease by contact with surfaces such as doorknobs or tissue paper containing the mucus. The incidence of these infections increases in the winter or spring, and epidemics often occur in families, nursing homes, schools, and dormitories. The **natural history** is one in which the classic manifestations are self-limited (i.e., last for a period of 2–5 days), followed by complete resolution.

C. The **specific evaluation** includes that described in Box 12-5.

D. The **specific management** is twofold: prevention and symptomatic relief. Prevention cannot be overemphasized. Prevention includes good hygiene (i.e., washing the hands, covering the mouth and face when coughing or sneezing, immediately disposing of tissues after use, and washing clothes and handkerchiefs in hot water). Although there is no known effective **modality** to shorten the natural course (i.e., cure the common cold), symptomatic relief can be afforded. Specific modalities include the use of decongestants, acetaminophen, and cough suppressants as necessary (see Table 12-5), the use of vitamin C in doses of ≤ 2 g/day with adequate fluids and, perhaps most effective, generous doses of Mom's chicken soup. The patient should be instructed to ingest adequate amounts of fluids and get adequate rest. The pharmacologic agents do not shorten the disease course and may have side effects. Therefore, patients should use the agents sparingly and discontinue them if any side effects occur.

II. **Atopic/allergic rhinitis**

A. The **specific manifestations** of this common disease, also known as hay fever in the autumn and rose fever in the spring, include a relatively wide variety of upper respiratory tract symptoms of varying degrees of intensity and severity. All of the symptoms and signs occur on a recurrent or even long-term basis, whenever the allergen is present. The onset of allergic-mediated rhinitis usually occurs during late childhood, adolescence, or early adulthood. Onset in neonates, toddlers, and the elderly is rare. The patient has bilateral rhinorrhea; bilateral conjunctivitis; watery, itchy, red eyes; sneezing; and nasal congestion. Rarely, if ever, are there any associated fevers, cough, myalgias, arthralgias, or gastrointestinal symptoms.

B. The **underlying pathogenesis** is a classic allergen IgE-mediated mechanism. In this mechanism, the patient is exposed to an allergen, a specific protein that causes IgE production from lymphocytes. The IgE then coats the plasma membrane of mast cells within the nasal mucous membranes. The initial exposure to the allergen will cause no mediator release and thus is asymptomatic. The next exposure, however, causes the release of IgE from lymphocytes, and the allergen cross-links with two IgE molecules on the mast cell surface to cause the mast cell to release the mediator, histamine. Histamine causes vasodilation and an increase in mucus production, the classic manifestations of allergic rhinitis.

1. The **allergens** can be any inhaled protein material but are commonly pollens, molds, dusts, hair, or danders. The specific time when the rhinitis occurs is pivotal in the diagnosis. Patients in whom disease occurs seasonally are likely to be allergic to pollens or molds. If manifestations occur in the spring or autumn, the allergen is likely to be a pollen, whereas if manifestations occur in the summer, the allergen is likely to be a mold or dust. Finally, if manifestations are mainly at a specific site (e.g., at home or after obtaining a new animal), the likely allergen is a hair type, a dander, or a form of hair spray.

2. The prevalence of this disease is between 15% and 20% of the population in the United States. The **natural history** is one of recurrence of symptoms whenever the allergen is present.

C. The **evaluation** of this disorder includes the steps outlined in Box 12-5 and making the clinical diagnosis. Further evaluation entails referral to an allergist for skin testing.

   Skin testing is not required for all patients. Specific indications for skin testing include a questionable history, young age, severe symptoms that significantly affect a patient's life, or when a specific allergen must be diagnosed and documented to optimize avoidance or attempt desensitization. The methods of skin testing are described subsequently.

1. The **scratch test** is the first one performed. Very dilute extracts of various potential allergens are placed over individual superficial scratches in the skin. A positive reaction is the development of a local wheal and flare. If positive, the patient has an IgE-mediated response to that protein. If negative or equivocal, and the clinical suspicion for that substance as an allergen to the patient is still present, an intradermal test is necessary.

2. The **intradermal test** is more sensitive than the scratch test. The specific protein extract is placed intradermally. A positive reaction is a wheal and flare.

3. These tests have a small risk of precipitating a severe allergic/anaphylactic reaction and therefore must be performed under the direction of a physician and with epinephrine readily available. Please refer to Table 4-1 (page 197) for specifics in the management of anaphylaxis.

D. The **specific management** includes the following basic principles and modalities and can be based on the clinical diagnosis. Skin-test confirmation is not necessary to initiate any of the following except desensitization.

1. **Avoidance of the allergens.** This common-sense **modality** is effective but underused by patients with allergies.

   a. Avoidance techniques for allergens that mainly occur outdoors, such as pollens and molds, include the use of central air conditioning, changing all clothes and taking a shower before retiring each night, shutting the windows in the house, and staying indoors as much as possible, especially on windy days when pollen counts are high.

   b. Avoidance techniques for allergens that mainly occur indoors, such as dust and mites, include installing a dehumidifier in the home, the installation and use of high-efficiency particle air cleaners, keeping the bed linen clean, and covering the mattress with a plastic sheet. If the allergen is due to a household pet, giving the pet away is truly effective.

2. **Prescribe antihistamines.** These agents are quite effective in the **treatment** of atopic/allergic rhinitis.

   a. The **mechanism of action** of these agents involves competition for H_1 receptors on the target cells for histamine. Thus histamine is still released from mast cells, but it is not allowed to act on its target cells in and about the upper respiratory mucosa. Therefore it is important to give the agent before histamine is released (i.e., before exposure to the allergen has occurred).

   b. Many agents are available over the counter and by prescription. Some of these agents include chlorpheniramine and diphenhydramine, both which cause sedation as a significant side effect, and astemizole, which is available only by prescription and causes less sedation. Astemizole has a potential for life-threatening ventricular tachycardia if used with erythromycin or ketoconazole. (See Table 12-5, page 585, for specifics on agents, doses, and side effects.)

3. **Prescribe decongestants.** These agents afford symptomatic relief of rhinorrhea.

a. The **mechanism of action** of these agents involves α-adrenergic receptor agonism, resulting in local vasoconstriction.

b. These agents, which are all available in over-the-counter preparations, can be applied topically as nasal sprays or taken as oral agents. Side effects include tachycardia and, especially if the spray is overused for $>3-4$ consecutive days, a paradoxic exacerbation of the rhinitis, rhinitis medicamentosa. Therefore these agents should be used for short-term **treatment** and with caution by patients with hypertension or heart disease (see Table 12-5).

4. Prescribe **intranasal steroids.** These agents have significant efficacy.

a. The **mechanism of action** of these agents involves suppression of the release of mediators and thus, on a local level, prevention of IgE- and histamine-mediated responses.

b. A commonly used agent is beclomethasone (Beconase, Vancenase) in a dose of two puffs in each nostril, b.i.d. These agents are effective when used on a long-term basis during the season when the allergen is present and are especially effective if started a week or two before the season. Side effects include mucosal atrophy and an increased risk of epistaxis.

III. **Vasomotor rhinitis**

A. The **specific manifestations** of this quite common form of rhinitis include the acute onset of unilateral or bilateral nasal edema and copious rhinorrhea that is acutely precipitated by specific odors or perfumes. Associated manifestations are the onset of watery eyes and, occasionally, a cough and scratchy throat. There virtually are never any concurrent fevers, dyspnea, or otalgia. The manifestations resolve rapidly when the inciting agent is removed from the environment.

B. The **underlying pathogenesis** is direct stimulation of the parasympathetic ganglia by the agent, which results, by a completely different mechanism from that of viral or atopic rhinitis, in local vascular dilation and rhinorrhea. The classic example is tear gas.

C. The **specific evaluation** includes making the clinical diagnosis, usually from the history alone.

D. The **specific management** is not only straightforward and easy, but it is also effective: the patient must avoid the inciting agent. No further evaluation or therapy is necessary.

IV. **Consultation**
No consultations are required.

Sinus Disease (Box 12-6)

I. The **underlying pathogenesis** of sinusitis relates to the anatomic communication of the sinuses with the ambient environment via relatively small-caliber passages in the nasopharynx. Thus any process that affects the upper respiratory system in general and the nasopharynx in specific can result in sinus dysfunction. These structures can become infected by any viral or bacterial pathogens that have infected the other portions of the upper respiratory tract. Moreover, atopic disease can directly and indirectly affect them.

   A. **Risk factors**
   Specific **risk factors** for the development of acute sinusitis include (a) a recent URI or active atopic disease, both with resultant increased formation of mucus, direct effects on the sinus respiratory mucosa, and the potential for temporary sinus obstruction; and (b) a history of trauma or the presence of a foreign body, either of which can obstruct drainage and thus increase the risk of infection.

   B. **Causative pathogens**
   The bacterial pathogens that cause acute purulent sinusitis include *Streptococcus pneumoniae, Haemophilus influenzae,* and *Branhamella catarrhalis.*

II. The **overall manifestations** of acute sinusitis include the acute onset of nasal congestion, greenish yellow/purulent nasal discharge, unilateral or bilateral facial pain that is exacerbated by leaning forward, and fever. There invariably is an antecedent

---

B O X   12-6

Overall Evaluation and Management of Acute Sinusitis

Evaluation

1. Percuss over the symptomatic sinus. If it is tender, inflammation is present.
2. Perform nasal examination with a speculum.
3. If the process is recurrent or the patient is immunocompromised, referral to ENT and/or head computed tomography (CT) are indicated.

Management

1. Initiate antibiotics, either TMP-sulfa or amoxicillin (see text).
2. Initiate a decongestant (see Table 12-5).

history of symptomatic viral or atopic rhinitis. Other manifestations are specific to the sinus involved and include the following.

A. Frontal sinusitis

Characterized by pain and tenderness to percussion over the lower forehead, unilaterally or bilaterally. There is opacification of the involved sinus on transillumination with a speculum. On nasal examination, purulent material drains from its meatus in the middle nasal turbinate.

B. Maxillary sinusitis

Characterized by pain and tenderness to percussion over the cheek bones, unilaterally or bilaterally. The pain is often referred to the ipsilateral maxillary teeth as a result of trigeminal innervation. There is opacification of the involved sinus on transillumination with a speculum. On nasal examination, purulent material drains from its meatus in the middle nasal turbinate.

C. Ethmoid sinusitis

Pain is present in the retroorbital area with associated erythema and tenderness to percussion over the upper lateral nose. Transillumination of this sinus is impossible. On nasal examination, purulent material drains from its meatus in the superior nasal turbinate.

D. Sphenoid sinusitis

This form of sinusitis is exceedingly rare unless concurrent with other sinusitides. The pain is present in the retroorbital area with associated erythema and tenderness to percussion over the upper lateral nose. On nasal examination, purulent material drains from the meatus in the superior nasal turbinate, although the superior turbinate is difficult to visualize unless a nasopharyngoscope is used.

III. Evaluation

The **specific evaluation** includes making the clinical diagnosis by using the basic techniques described in Box 12-6. Further evaluation is by CT of the sinuses and referral to ENT.

A. Radiography

Sinus radiographs are of little use in the evaluation of sinusitis; if imaging is necessary, it should be that of a CT scan of the sinuses, making plain films quite superfluous.

B. CT

CT of the sinuses is rarely required in the acute setting, but if there is any evidence of complications, or if the disease process is recurrent, or if the host is an immunocompromised host, this is the optimal imaging **modality** to visualize the sinuses for any underlying anatomic defect. Evidence of sinusitis on these radiographs includes the following findings:

1. Opacification of the involved sinus.
2. Air–fluid levels within the sinus.
3. Abnormally thick mucosa (i.e., >5 mm).

C. **Complications**

The **evaluation** and definitions of specific complications include osteomyelitis of the frontal bone, sometimes referred to as Pott's puffy tumor, in which the patient has fever, pain, swelling over the frontal bone, an increased erythrocyte sedimentation rate (ESR), and bone and gallium scans consistent with osteomyelitis (i.e., showing increased uptake). A further complication is orbital cellulitis: the patient has ptosis, eyelid edema, proptosis, conjunctivitis, and decreased range of motion of the extraocular musculature. This can rapidly progress and lead to erysipelas and death if not treated (see page 609). Finally, the most dramatic complication is cavernous sinus thrombosis, manifested by unilateral lid edema, ptosis, proptosis, and palsies of cranial nerves III, IV, and VI.

IV. **Management**

The **specific management** includes antibiotics, decongestants, antihistamines, and monitoring for the development of any complications. The antibiotics should be a 14-day course of one of the following: either amoxicillin, 500 mg p.o., t.i.d., or TMP-sulfa (Bactrim DS), one tablet p.o., b.i.d., or cefuroxime (Ceftin; a second-generation cephalosporin), 500 mg p.o., b.i.d., or ciprofloxacin, 500 mg b.i.d., or amoxicillin with clavulanic acid (Augmentin), 500–875 mg p.o., b.i.d. The use of a decongestant on a short-term basis to decrease mucus production and to decrease any swelling and obstruction about the meatus is useful. An antihistamine is of benefit if there is any evidence of allergic rhinitis (see Table 12-5). If the disease is recurrent, CT scan, a longer course of antibiotics, and referral to ENT are indicated. If there is any evidence of complications, the patient will require emergency consultation with ENT and infectious disease colleagues and admission to the hospital for parenteral antibiotics and surgical drainage of the involved sinus.

V. **Consultation**

Problem	Service	Time
Any complication	ENT	Emergent
Recurrent disease	ENT	Elective
Complication	Infectious diseases	Urgent

VI. **Indications for admission:** the development of any complication of acute sinusitis, or sinusitis occurring in an immunosuppressed host.

Bibliography

Epistaxis

Juselius H: Epistaxis: a clinical study of 1724 patients. J Laryngol Otol 1974;88:317–327.

Kirchner JA: Epistaxis. N Engl J Med 1982;307:1126.

Randal DA, Freeman SB: Management of anterior and posterior epistaxis. Am Fam Pract 1991;2007–2014.

Oral Diseases

Herr RD, et al: Serious soft tissue infections of the head and neck. Am Fam Pract 1991;44:878–888.

Hubbard TM: Periodontal disease and the family physician. Am Fam Pract 1991;44:487–491.

Johnson WT: Managing odontogenic infections. Am Fam Pract 1984;29:167–172.

Morse DR, et al: Infectious flare-ups and serious sequelae following end-odontic treatment: a prospective randomized trial on efficacy of antibiotic prophylaxis in cases of asymptomatic pulpal-periapical lesions. Oral Surg Oral Med Oral Pathol 1987;64:96–109.

Otalgia/Otitis

Bluestone CD: Otitis media in children: to treat or not to treat. N Engl J Med 1982;306:1399.

Eichenwald H: Developments in diagnosing and treating otitis media. Am Fam Pract 1985;31:155–164.

Pharyngitis

Bisno AL: Group A streptococcal infections and acute rheumatic fever. N Engl J Med 1991;325:783–793.

Brandfonbrener A, et al: Corticosteroid therapy in Epstein-Barr virus infection. Arch Intern Med 1986;146:337–339.

Centor RM, et al: Throat cultures and rapid tests for diagnosis of Group A streptococcal pharyngitis. Ann Intern Med 1986;105:892–899.

Murray BJ: Medical complications of infectious mononucleosis. Am Fam Pract 1984;30:195–199.

Raz R, Bitnun S: Dilemmas in streptococcal pharyngitis. Am Fam Pract 1987;35:187–192.

Rhinitis

Demichiei ME, Nelson L: Allergic rhinitis. Am Fam Pract 1988;37:251–263.

Druce HM, Kaliner MA: Allergic rhinitis. JAMA 1988;259:260–263.

Gwaltney JM Jr, et al: Symposium on rhinovirus pathogenesis: summary. Acta Otolaryngol 1984;413(S):43–45.

Sinus Disease

Axelson A, Brorson JE: The correlation between bacteriological findings in the nose and maxillary sinus in acute maxillary sinusitis. Laryngoscope 1973;83:2003.

Evans FW, et al: Sinusitis of the maxillary sinus antrum. N Engl J Med 1975;29:3735.

Stool SE: Diagnosis and treatment of sinusitis. Am Fam Pract 1985;32:101–107.

—D.D.B.

Chapter 13

Ophthalmology

Acute Blindness

The definitions of various types of blindness include the following. Only monocular blindness is discussed in greater detail later in this section.

Monocular denotes the complete loss of visual function of one eye, usually with dramatic results. Invariably the patient seeks immediate medical attention.

I. **Visual field deficits**
   A. **Hemianopsia** is the acute or insidious onset of blindness in one half of each visual field. There are two different types of hemianopsia.
      1. **Homonymous hemianopsia.** The blindness is in the same half of both fields, right or left. This is invariably the result of a lesion in the contralateral optic tract.
      2. **Heteronymous hemianopsia.** The blindness is in opposite halves of both fields. There are two types of heteronymous hemianopsia.
         a. **Bitemporal hemianopsia.** The outer (temporal) halves of both fields are blind. This is usually as the result of a pituitary tumor.
         b. **Binasal hemianopsia.** The inner (nasal) half or halves of one or both fields are blind. Quite rare and usually unilateral.
   B. **Quadrantic hemianopsia.** A quarter of the visual field is blind, usually the result of a lesion in the contralateral occipital or temporal cerebral cortex. Recall that the optic radiation passes through the temporal lobe en route to the occipital cortex.
II. **Monocular blindness**
    This quite dramatic loss of visual function in one eye is a medical and ophthalmologic emergency in which the patient must have aggressive and immediate **evaluation and management**. The causes of this process are quite diverse and are as follows.

A. **Retinal detachment**
1. The **specific manifestations** of this entity include an acute onset of monocular blindness. The patient reports the acute onset of blurred or blackened vision that over several hours progresses to complete or partial monocular blindness. The classic description is of a curtain being drawn over the visual field from top to bottom. The patient usually senses "floaters" and flashing lights before and at the initiation of the symptom complex. There are no concurrent pain, erythema, or conjunctival injection. Funduscopic examination reveals a gray membrane (i.e., the retina detached and flapping in the vitreous humor).
2. The **underlying pathogenesis** is a tear in the retina with the resultant production of floaters. Once a tear occurs, the vitreous crosses behind the retina with a progression of the retinal detachment. The tear usually begins at the superior temporal retinal area.

   Although it can happen spontaneously, certain **risk factors** for its development include extreme myopia as the result of an elongated eyeball length, recent trauma to the affected eye, a history of retinal detachment, lattice degeneration at periphery of retina (8% of people have this network at the ora serrata). Finally, a detachment may occur as result of vitreous bleed secondary to severe diabetic retinopathy.
3. The **specific evaluation** includes making the clinical diagnosis by performing the tests described in Box 13-1.
4. The **specific management** is to obtain an emergency ophthalmology consultation, preferably with an expert in **laser treatment**. The patient should remain supine with the head turned to the side ipsilateral to the retinal detachment. Emergency laser is indicated. The laser treatment is for the surgeon to place a hole in the sclera, drain the subretinal fluid, cauterize the hole with a laser, and then place a scleral buckle to keep the sclera and retina juxtaposed.

B. **Central retinal vein occlusion**
1. The **specific manifestations** of this entity include the acute onset of complete loss of vision in one eye. The loss of vision is painless. There usually are no associated prodromal symptoms. On examination, the only abnormality is a markedly edematous retina with multiple hemorrhages and dilated, tortuous veins, classically referred to as the "blood and thunder" appearance.
2. The **underlying pathogenesis** is occlusion of the central retinal vein, often as the result of long-standing uncontrolled systemic hypertension. Occlusion of the

B O X   13-1

Basic Ophthalmologic Examination

1. History, including any recent exposure to agents or recent trauma.
2. Inspection of the orbits and eyes themselves, looking for any gross abnormalities, the presence of proptosis, ptosis, conjunctival injection, chemosis and/or foreign bodies in the eyes or in the palpebral surfaces.
3. Examination of the extraocular musculature.
4. Examine and measure the size of both pupils at baseline.
5. Examination of the pupillary reflex to direct and consensual light and to accommodation.
6. Visual acuity with and without refraction by using the Snellen chart, in left eye (OS) and right eye (OD).
7. Visual field examination by confrontation.
8. Perform a slit-lamp examination of the cornea, conjunctiva, and anterior chamber structures. The slit-lamp examination is integral to all ophthalmologic examinations. Note and describe the cornea, conjunctivae, and anterior chamber structures.
9. Apply fluorescein dye to the affected red eye. The application procedure entails first applying a topical anesthetic to the eye (Table 13-1), and then applying two drops of fluorescein to the inferior palpebral conjunctiva. The patient is then instructed to close the eye for 10–15 seconds and then open it for irrigation with sterile saline solution. The eye is then examined by using a cobalt blue light. In the normal setting, no dye should be taken up by the cornea. If there is any uptake by the cornea, as manifested by a fluorescent green color, pathology either an infection, abrasion or ulceration is present.
10. Funduscopic examination. If any suspicion of acute glaucoma, should not use mydriatic agents.
11. Any suspected pathology mandates an emergent referral to an ophthalmologist.

central retinal vein markedly impedes venous drainage from the retina, thereby increasing venous pressure in the retina, the exudation of fluids from the venous system, retinal edema, and venous dilation.

(text continues on page 600)

TABLE 13-1
Ophthalmic Agents

Agent	Indications	Contraindications	Side Effects	Dosage
Timolol (Timoptic) (0.25% and 0.5% solutions)	Open angle glaucoma	Bronchospasm Left ventricular heart failure 2nd or 3rd degree AV block	Wheezing	1 drop of 0.25% solution b.i.d. OU, then increased to 1 drop of 0.5% solution b.i.d. OU, titrating to IOP.
Pilocarpine (Isotocarpine) (0.5%, 1%, 2%, 3%, 4%, and 6% solutions)	Open angle glaucoma Miotic agent	Allergy to agent	Rare	2 drops of the 1% to 4% solution in affected eye(s) b.i.d. to t.i.d., titrate the concn. of solution to the target IOP
Gentamicin (Garamycin) Ointment: 0.3% Solution: 0.3%	Dacrocystitis Hordeolum Conjunctivitis Keratitis	Allergy to agent	Rare	Ointment: apply b.i.d. to t.i.d. Solution: 1 drop q.4hr
Tobramycin (Tobrex) Solution: 0.3%	Dacrocystitis Hordeolum Conjunctivitis Keratitis	Allergy to agent	Rare	Ointment: apply b.i.d. to t.i.d. Solution: 1 drop 1.4hr

(continued)

T A B L E 13-1 *(continued)*

Agent	Indications	Contraindications	Side Effects	Dosage
Sulfacetamide (Sulamyd) Ointment: 10% Solution: 10%, 30%	Hordeolum Conjunctivitis Keratitis Trachoma*	Allergy to agent	Rare	Ointment: apply 1–2 cm ribbon q.i.d. and q.н.s. Solution: 2 drops of the 10%–30% solution into the lower conjunctival sac q.2–3hr. and q.н.s. for 5 days
Erythromycin (Ilocytin) 0.5% ointment	Conjunctivitis Trachoma*	Allergy	Rare	0.5–1.0 cm ribbon of ointment into the conjunctival sacs of the affected eye(s) q.d. or b.i.d. for 5 days
Dexamethasone (0.1% solution)	Steroid-responsive keratitis, uveitus, conjunctivitis	HSV infections Fungal infections Viral infections Allergy to agent Soft contact lenses	Posterior subcapsular cataracts Rupture of the globe	Should be used under direct interaction with ophthalmology
Cromolyn sodium (Opticrom 4% solution)	Atopic conjunctivitis		Rare	1–2 drops 4–6 times per day, OU

Agent	Indication	Contraindication	Side Effects	Dosage
Naphcon-A (naphazoline and pheniramine) solution	Atopic conjunctivitis	Allergy to agent	Rare	1–2 drops q.4–6hr OU
Isoptotears (methylcellulose) Solution: 0.5% and 1.0%	Dry eyes	Allergy to agent	Rare	2 drops q.4–6hr prn
Tropicamide (Mydriacyl) Solution: 1%	Mydriatic, for examination	Allergy to agent; Acute (closed) angle glaucoma	Photophobia and blurred vision, acutely	1–2 drops in eye to be examined
Cyclopentolate (cyclogyl) Solution: 0.5% and 1%	Actinic keratitis	Allergy; Acute (closed) angle glaucoma	Rare	2 drops OU q.6hr
Proparacaine (0.5% solution)	Topical anesthetic; lasts 15 minutes	Allergy to agent	Rare	2 drops in eye to be examined 1 min before exam
Idoxuridine (0.1% solution)	Antiviral	Allergy to agent	Rare	1 drop in affected eye q. 1–2 hr. for 5–7 days. Use only under direction of an ophthalmologist

*If trachoma is suspected, the treatment includes antibiotic eyedrops, systemic antibiotics, referral to an ophthalmologist, and reporting of the case to Public Health (see page 675).

(text continued from page 596)

The pressure can be increased to such a level as to cause arterial retinal hypoperfusion and ischemia.

3. The **specific evaluation** includes making the clinical diagnosis by performing the tests described in Box 13-1. The **specific management** is to obtain an emergency ophthalmology consultation.

C. **Central retinal artery occlusion**

1. The **specific manifestations** of this entity include the acute onset of monocular painless blindness. The patient usually has other sequelae of arterial thromboembolic disease in the past including cerebrovascular accidents (CVAs) and/or a history of atrial fibrillation and/or left ventricular failure. The funduscopic examination reveals the presence of a cherry-red spot in the macula, an optic disc that is pale relative to surrounding retinal tissue, and, when compared with the contralateral eye, the presence of retinal arteries that are significantly decreased in size. Furthermore, there may be cholesterol emboli (Hollenhorst plaques) in the arteries.

2. The **underlying pathogenesis** is one of occlusion of the central retinal artery with resultant ischemia and infarction of the retina. This usually is as the result of an arterial thromboembolic event. The **risk factors** for the development of this entity include anything associated with thrombus formation in the left heart (e.g., atrial fibrillation, left-sided endocarditis, atrial enlargement, and/or plaques in the carotid artery). Of note is the fact that these are the same **risk factors** for ischemic embolic cerebrovascular accidents.

3. The **specific evaluation** includes making the clinical diagnosis by performing the tests described in Box 13-1. The **specific management** is to obtain an emergency ophthalmology consultation. Clearly anticoagulation with heparin must be strongly considered. The dosage, goals, and management are quite similar to those for an ischemic embolic CVA (see section on Cerebrovascular Accidents, Chapter 14, page 625, for further discussion).

D. **Acute (narrow-angle) glaucoma**

See section on Red, Inflamed Eye, page 609.

E. **Temporal arteritis**

1. The **specific manifestations** of this entity include an acute onset of painless, monocular blindness. The blindness is quite often associated with a concurrent or antecedent history of generalized, predominantly proximal muscle weakness, unilateral or bilateral jaw claudication on mastication (chewing), and a recurrent unilateral throbbing headache ipsilateral to the

affected eye. On examination, the eye, including the fundus, is usually quite remarkable. There usually is tenderness to palpation over the ipsilateral temporal artery and objective moderate muscle weakness, greater proximally than distally.

2. The **underlying pathogenesis** is one of a systemic granulomatous vasculitis of the middle-sized arteries, especially branches of the external carotid artery.

3. The **specific evaluation** includes making the clinical diagnosis by performing the tests described in Box 13-1. Furthermore, an erythrocyte sedimentation rate (ESR) and biopsy of the temporal artery are indicated. The ESR will be markedly increased, at times >100 minutes, and the biopsy will show the arterial vasculitis. Because the results of these tests/procedures will take at least several hours to return, if this entity is clinically suspected, emergency empiric therapy with steroids is clearly indicated.

4. The **treatment** regimen consists of prednisone, 60 mg p.o, stat, and then 40–60 mg p.o., q.d. The dose is slowly tapered to 10–15 mg p.o., q.d., for the next 18–24 months, at which time further tapering is attempted. Weaning from steroids is titrated to the manifestations of weakness, blindness, and the ESR. Consultations with ophthalmology, ENT for biopsy of the temporalis artery, and rheumatology at presentation are indicated.

F. Trauma

1. The **specific manifestations** of this entity include a marked decrease in vision after an episode of significant blunt and/or invasive trauma to the eye. On examination, the damage is usually quite evident and can range from a retinal detachment to enucleation, a penetrating foreign body, or a hyphema (i.e., the presence of blood in the anterior chamber).

2. The **specific evaluation and management** include making the clinical diagnosis by performing the tests described in Box 13-1. Emergency referral to ophthalmology is clearly indicated.

III. **Consultation**

Problem	Service	Time
Any monocular blindness	Ophthalmology	Emergent
Any visual field blindness	Ophthalmology	Emergent
Homonymous hemianopsia	Radiology, for head CT	Urgent
Temporal arteritis	Rheumatology/ENT	Urgent

IV. **Indications for admission:** Monocular blindness, evidence of penetrating trauma to the eye, or any new visual field cut.

Cataracts

As the human lens ages, changes over time will result in the development of opacities. These acquired lenticular opacities, which are termed cataracts, can and do progressively worsen until the patient has significant visual impairment. There are two major types of cataracts, the nuclear cataract and the cortical, including the posterior subcapsular cataract. Each of these is discussed.

I. **Types of cataracts**
   A. **Nuclear cataracts**
      1. The **specific manifestations** include the insidious onset of decreased vision. The patient often reports that the visual acuity for far vision is affected more than that for near vision. Furthermore, day vision is worse than night vision. On examination by using a slit-lamp or the 4–10× on ophthalmoscopy, there is a translucent yellow discoloration in the center or nucleus of the lens. This can actually impede the ability of the examiner to visualize the fundus. One lens may be affected more than the other. The visual acuity will be objectively decreased. Two specific, unique patterns of cataracts are "sunflower" pattern of Wilson's disease and iridescent spots of myotonic dystrophy.
      2. The **underlying pathogenesis** is one in which, with increasing age, the center of the lens changes from its transparent baseline to a translucent yellowish color. The major and irreversible risk factor for development is increasing age: virtually everyone older than 70 years has a component of a nuclear cataract. Other more preventable or reversible **risk factors** include exposure to ultraviolet light and potentially the cholesterol-lowering agent, lovastatin.
   B. **Cortical including posterior subcapsular cataracts**
      1. The **specific manifestations** include the insidious onset of decreased vision. The patient often reports that the visual acuity for near vision is affected more than that for far vision. On examination, there is a translucent yellow discoloration in the central portion of the posterior capsule of the lens (i.e., it is located in the posterocentral aspect of the lens). This can actually impede the ability of the examiner to visualize the fundus. One lens can be affected more than the other. The visual acuity will be objectively decreased. These cataracts occur in a younger population than do the nuclear cataracts.
      2. The **underlying pathogenesis** has been postulated to be as the result of chronic, abnormally increased

amounts of glucose within the lens itself. The increased amounts of glucose are catabolized by an alternate pathway, by using the enzyme aldose reductase, to the molecule sorbitol. Sorbitol is quite osmotically active and increases the water in the lens, making it less transparent. The **risk factors** for development are disease processes or states that result in hyperglycemia (i.e., diabetes mellitus, Cushing's syndrome, and the long-term use of glucocorticoids).

II. Evaluation and management

The **specific evaluation and management** of a patient with a cataract include making the diagnosis by the examination techniques described in Box 13-1. The **specific management** is referral to an ophthalmologist for surgical intervention. The surgical procedures performed are included here for the purposes of edification.

A. Surgical intervention

All surgical procedures are performed under local anesthesia and with mild sedation, and virtually all can be performed on an outpatient basis. There are two types of cataract surgery, intracapsular or extracapsular extractions of the cataract.

1. **Intracapsular extraction.** The entire lens is removed in one piece. This is a procedure for the **treatment** of posterior subcapsular cataracts.

2. **Extracapsular extraction.** The capsule is opened, the contents are removed, and the posterior capsule remains. Best procedure for nuclear cataracts.

3. **Secondary cataract:** YAG-laser **treatment** (i.e., yttrium aluminum garnet laser treatment).

    Either procedure requires 6–8 weeks of postoperative eye rehabilitation. Rehabilitation includes the use of contact lenses or the use of intraocular implants. Intraocular implants are the rehabilitation **modality** of choice and must be placed at the time of surgery.

III. Consultation

Service	Time
Ophthalmology	Required

IV. Indications for admission: None.

Open-Angle Glaucoma

This is a quite common disease process. It affects 2%–3% of the population and is asymptomatic until advanced and irreversible damage to the visual fields has already occurred. Although the disease shares the same name with acute-angle glaucoma, and both processes have an increased intraocular pressure (IOP) and, if untreated, will lead to blindness, they have very few similarities.

I. The **specific manifestations** of open-angle glaucoma are quite different from those of acute-angle glaucoma (see section on Red Inflamed Eye, page 609, for manifestations of acute-angle glaucoma). They include an insidious onset of progressively deteriorating visual acuity, which remains minimally symptomatic or even asymptomatic until late in the course of disease. There is no associated pain or redness or excessive watering of the eyes.

Early in the course of disease, there are no signs, except for the presence of a modestly increased IOP. Funduscopic and visual field examinations are quite normal.

Late in the course, the IOP remains modestly increased and, on funduscopic examination, the optic cup can abnormally enlarge and deepen. The normal cup should be <30% the size of the disc diameter. If >30%, this is abnormal and consistent with open-angle glaucoma. In addition, the vessels are more prominent on the nasal side in chronic, severe, open-angle glaucoma. Furthermore, the visual fields become constricted with loss of the temporal aspects of the visual field(s) first.

II. The **underlying pathogenesis** of the increased IOP in open-angle glaucoma is unclear. Irrespective of the mechanism, the increased IOP results in damage to the optic nerve head by pressure-induced enlargement of the optic cup. The increased pressure can also result in ischemia to the retina and optic nerve and a decrease in neuronal transport flow down the dendrites and axons that compose the optic nerve. Both of these result in the loss of axons, dendrites, and neurons in and about the optic nerve and the macula. The loss of function in the macula is temporal to nasal. Thus the increased IOP damages both the macula and the optic nerve head.

Risk factors for the development of this disease include increasing age, a family history of open-angle glaucoma, male sex, African American heritage, and a history of atherosclerotic heart disease or diabetes mellitus.

III. The **specific evaluation and management** include those described in Box 13-1 and performing effective screening.
   A. **Screening**
      This disease process begs for screening. There is a long period of subclinical disease that, if untreated, results in severe visual impairment, and there are effective and relatively simple **treatment** modalities that prevent the development of this visual sequela. The screening techniques used include applanation tonometry or air-puff tonometry, either technique usually performed by an optometrist or ophthalmologist.
      1. Screening should begin at age 40 years to obtain a baseline reading. Screening should be every 2–3 years until age 65–70 years, at which time the screening

should be continued on an annual basis. Screening can be by either technique.

2. Normal IOP has a mean value of 15 mm Hg, with a range of 10–20 mm Hg.

3. If the IOP is increased (i.e., >21 mm Hg), refer to an ophthalmologist for confirmation. Concurrently, visual-field assessment and extensive funduscopic examination are indicated.

B. **Treatment for open-angle glaucoma**

1. **Topical β-blockers.** Timolol (Timoptic) solution is, unless contraindications to its use are present, a first-line agent in the therapy of open-angle glaucoma. See Table 13-1 for specifics on the agent, its contraindications, and dosage.

2. **Acetazolamide (Diamox).** This carbonic anhydrase inhibitor is an effective agent in decreasing IOP by decreasing aqueous humor production. It is a second-line agent because it has a number of potentially significant side effects including fatigue, the development of a normal anion-gap metabolic acidosis, and the development of calcium nephrolithiasis. The dosage of acetazolamide (Diamox) is 250 mg p.o., 1–4 times per day.

3. **Surgical intervention.** Referral to ophthalmology for an elective laser trabeculoplasty/iridectomy by using an Nd:YAG laser or an argon laser. The iridectomy forms a communication between the anterior and posterior chambers and, when performed in both eyes, is curative. This is an outpatient procedure.

IV. **Consultation**

Problem	*Service*	*Time*
All cases of increased IOP	Ophthalmology	Required

V. **Indications for admission:** None.

Red Inflamed Eye, Unilateral or Bilateral

This is not only one of the most common problems people in day-to-day life develop, but it is also a common reason for patients to contact a primary care physician. The overall **evaluation** is described in Box 13-1, the overall ophthalmologic examination.

I. **Hordeolum**

A. The **specific manifestations** of this entity include the acute onset of pain and swelling in the eyelid with increased tearing and redness in the involved eye. On examination there is a palpable, indurated area in the involved eyelid, which on visual inspection has a central area of purulence with surrounding erythema. Furthermore, there invariably is erythema in the adjacent conjunctiva.

B. The **underlying pathogenesis** of this quite common problem is the acute development of a small abscess within a gland in the upper or lower eyelid of one eye.

   1. There are two basic types of hordeola, internal and external.

      a. Internal hordeola are deep from the palpebral margin and are the result of inflammation and infection of a meibomian gland, with abscess formation in that gland.

      b. External hordeola are immediately adjacent to the edge of the palpebral margin and are as the result of inflammation and infection of the glands of Moll or Zeis, with abscess formation in one of these glands. This type of hordeolum is colloquially referred to as a sty.

   2. The usual pathogen for either one of these two entities is the gram-positive coccus, *Staphylococcus aureus*.

C. The **specific evaluation** includes making the clinical diagnosis by using the information described subsequently and the examination described in Box 13-1.

D. **Management**

   1. Apply warm compresses 5 times/day to the affected eye for 48 hours.

   2. Apply topical antibiotics for 5–7 days. Any of the topical drops is effective. See Table 13-1 for specific agents and dosage.

   3. If there is any evidence of concurrent cellulitis, systemic antibiotics are indicated. Specific agents include cephalexin (Keflex), 500 mg p.o., q.i.d., for 7 days, or dicloxicillin, 500 mg p.o., q.i.d., for 7 days.

   4. If there is no improvement in 48 hours, referral to ophthalmology for I&D of the hordeolum, especially if internal, is indicated.

II. **Chalazion**

A. The **specific manifestations** of this entity include the presence of a painless, indurated lesion deep from the palpebral margin. This lesion may be present for months and be of only minimal concern to the patient. When symptoms are present, as they can be on an intermittent, recurrent basis, they include pruritus and redness of the involved eye and eyelid. The patient can usually recall having an internal hordeolum affecting the same eyelid in the past.

B. The **underlying pathogenesis** is chronic inflammation of an internal hordeolum involving the meibomian gland. The chronic inflammation often becomes microscopically granulomatous but is invariably noninfectious. An internal hordeolum often antedates the development of a chalazion.

C. The **specific evaluation** includes making the clinical diagnosis by using the information described and the examination described in Box 13-1.

D. **Management**

Referral to an ophthalmologist for elective excision of the lesion is indicated. No further acute intervention is necessary.

III. **Blepharitis**

A. The **specific manifestations** of this quite common condition include erythema and scale formation on one or both eyelids. The manifestations begin and are most evident at the margin of the eyelids, involving the skin immediately adjacent to the eyelashes. There can be some mild associated pruritus and conjunctival erythema, but virtually never any pain, edema, or fevers.

B. The **underlying pathogenesis** is an infectious or noninfectious inflammation of the palpebral edge. The inflammation is self-limited and mild. It does not progress to a serious local or systemic process.

1. The infectious **etiology** results from superficial infection with *S. aureus*. Unique manifestations of this cause include superficial ulcerations of the skin adjacent to the palpebral edge and concurrent mild to moderate conjunctivitis in the affected eye.

2. The noninfectious **etiology** results from a localized form of seborrheic dermatitis. Unique manifestations of this cause include bilateral erythema of the eyelid margins, with greasy scales present. The conjunctivitis, if present, is quite mild.

C. The **specific evaluation** includes making the clinical diagnosis by using the information and the examination in Box 13-1.

D. The **specific management** includes removal of the scales and gentle scrubbing of the eyelid margins with a moistened cotton-tipped applicator each morning, followed immediately by application of a topical antibiotic in ointment form to the eyelid margins, b.i.d., for 7 days. The solution used to moisten the cotton-tipped applicator may be tap water or baby shampoo diluted by volume 50% with tap water. See Table 13-1 for a list of the topical antibiotics available. Consultations are rarely necessary.

IV. **Acute dacrocystitis** (infection of the lacrimal gland)

A. The **specific manifestations** of this relatively infrequent disorder include an acute onset of unilateral pain in the medial canthal region of the affected eye. There invariably are tenderness and warmth in the medial canthal area and, occasionally, purulent discharge from the area about the medial canthus area. There invariably are mild to moderate conjunctivitis and a significant increase in tearing in the affected eye (epiphora). The tears from the affected eye overflow.

B. The **underlying pathogenesis** is partial or total obstruction of the nasolacrimal duct/nasolacrimal sac, which then becomes secondarily infected. The nasolacrimal duct is located in the extreme lateral aspect of the medial superficial eye structures. Its orifice is in the medial canthal area. This duct, in the normal state, drains tears from the eye into the nasal structures.

1. **Risk factors** for the development of nasolacrimal duct obstruction and therefore of dacryocystis include trauma to the area, recurrent atopic disease, and a history of infections involving the area. Although there usually is an underlying reason for nasolacrimal obstruction, in some cases, especially in young children, there is a converse pathogenesis (i.e., the infection is primary with the secondary development of nasolacrimal obstruction).

2. Causative agents include the bacteria *S. aureus, Streptococcus pneumoniae,* and the Group A streptococci.

3. **Natural history**. The process can evolve into a facial cellulitis. Furthermore, even in cases that are self-limited or effectively treated in the acute setting, there may be scarring of the nasolacrimal duct, which increases the likelihood of recurrence.

C. The **specific evaluation** includes making the clinical diagnosis by using this information and the examination described in Box 13-1. Further **specific evaluation** includes performing a Gram stain and culture on any purulent discharge obtained, and clinical examination of the entire HEENT system.

D. **Management**

1. Initiate systemic antibiotics. Specific agents can include cephalexin (Keflex), 500 mg p.o., q.i.d., for 7 days, or dicloxicillin, 500 mg p.o., q.i.d., for 7 days, or erythromycin, 500 mg p.o, q.i.d., for 7 days.

2. Topical antibiotics in the form of drops can be useful as adjuvant therapy but do not replace systemic antibiotics. See Table 13-1 for specific agents and dosing schemas.

3. Referral to an ophthalmologist on an urgent basis is indicated for I&D of any pocket of adjacent pus and to relieve the obstruction surgically.

V. **Preseptal cellulitis**

A. The **specific manifestations** include the acute or subacute onset of swelling, erythema, pain, and an increased tearing in one eye. There is usually concurrent conjunctival irritation, chemosis, and an inability to open the eye completely on the affected side. There is an antecedent dacrocystitis, chalazion, or hordeolum present in the affected aye. There is no decrease in visual acuity in the affected eye.

B. The **pathogenesis** is one of an infection in the eyelids; the infection does not extend posteriorly into the orbit, as the preseptal fascial plane and tarsal plate act as barriers to its posterior progression. The pathogens include anaerobes, *Staphylococci, Streptococci,* and occasionally, *Haemophilus influenzae* in children.

C. The **evaluation and management** of this includes making the clinical diagnosis and initiating antibiotics with amoxicillin and clavulanic acid (Augmentin, 500 mg p.o. b.i.d. for 7 days), a second-generation cephalosporin [e.g., cefuroxime (Ceftin) 500 mg p.o. q.12hr], or TMP/sulfa (one tablet p.o. b.i.d. for 7 days). Referral to an ophthalmologist may be indicated.

VI. Orbital cellulitis

A. The **underlying pathogenesis** is that this is the posterior progression of the any skin/skin-structure infection past the preseptal fascia and into the orbit. There is often an antecedent preseptal cellulitis or acute hordeolum. The most common etiologic organisms include anaerobe, *Staphylococci, Streptococci,* and, in children, *Haemophilus influenzae.*

B. The **manifestations** of this entity include the presence of a red eye, proptosis of the affected eye, decreased range of motion (ROM) of the eye, and the potential for a cavernous sinus thrombosis, with acquired deficits of cranial nerves III, IV, VI, and the sensory aspects of V.

C. The overall **evaluation and management** includes the fact that this is an ophthalmologic emergency and requires a computed tomography (CT) scan of the orbit. The orbital CT will reveal ethmoid sinusitis and retrorbital edema; **treatment** includes admission to the hospital for parenteral antibiotics: cefuroxime 1.5 g i.v. q.8hr for 7 days, vancomycin, or ampicillin and sulbactum (Unasyn) 1.5 g i.v. q.6hr for 7 days. Referral to ophthalmology is indicated in all cases.

VII. Acute (Closed)-Angle Glaucoma

A. The **specific manifestations** of this relatively uncommon but dramatic cause of a red inflamed eye include the acute onset of a unilateral headache ipsilateral to the affected eye, and concurrent nausea and vomiting. The patient describes photophobia, severe pain, and significant redness in the affected eye. Furthermore, the patient will often report seeing halos. On examination, the affected eye has a moderately dilated pupil, which is minimally responsive to direct or consensual light. In addition, the clinician can shine a light source (e.g., a pocket penlight or slit lamp) at an angle into the anterior chamber from the temporal side. On the "normal" setting, no shadow will be demonstrated over the iris; in acute (closed)-angle glaucoma, a shadow is demonstrated over the nasal side of the iris. There is a markedly increased IOP when measured by Schiotz or applanation tonometry. The IOP, which normally is <15 mm Hg, is as high as 40–60 mm Hg!

B. The **underlying pathogenesis** is one of an underlying congenital defect in which there is an abnormally narrow angle in the anterior chamber. This results in a relative obstruction to flow of the aqueous humor out of the anterior chamber. The narrow chamber angle is present in <1% of the population; therefore, <1/100 of people are at risk for the development of the acute process. Mydriasis in and of itself decreases the angle, and therefore, in a patient at risk, can precipitate total obstruction to flow with the resultant marked increase in IOP. This increase in IOP will then result in decreased blood perfusion to structures, ischemia, and significant intraocular damage.

C. The **specific evaluation** includes making the clinical diagnosis by using this information and the examination described in Box 13-1.

D. **Management**
   Once the diagnosis is made or suspected, emergency therapy is indicated.
   1. Discontinue the use of any precipitating or exacerbating agent.
   2. Instill the miotic agent, pilocarpine. The dosage is one to two drops of pilocarpine, 4% solution, in the affected eye stat and repeated every 20 minutes until a surgical procedure is performed. This agent, like any miotic agent, reverses the mydriasis and decreases the degree of obstruction.
   3. Acetazolamine (Diamox), 500 mg i.v., is indicated concurrent with the other interventions. This is a weak carbonic anhydrase inhibitor, which will decrease production of aqueous humor and therefore decrease IOP.
   4. **Emergency consultation** with ophthalmology for emergency surgery is indicated. The surgical procedure of choice is laser (argon or Nd:YAG) iridectomy within hours of presentation. The contralateral eye should undergo this procedure prophylactically. The iridectomy is an acquired communication between the anterior and posterior chambers.
   5. If the surgery is delayed, mannitol, 1.5 g/kg by i.v. bolus, is indicated as a further temporizing therapeutic **modality**. This agent is osmotically active in the plasma and results in an osmotic diuresis and a decreased IOP.

VIII. Conjunctivitis

This common process affects virtually every person one or more times during his or her lifetime.

A. Viral/serous

1. The **specific manifestations** of this very common form of conjunctivitis include the acute onset of unilateral or bilateral erythema of the conjunctivae, copious watery discharge, and ipsilateral preauricular lymphadenopathy. There are usually no systemic manifestations, decreased visual acuity, or any purulence unless a bacterial superinfection occurs. On fluorescein examination there is no uptake of dye.

2. The **underlying pathogenesis** is direct infection of the conjunctivae by a virus. The most common agents are one of three different types of adenovirus, types 3, 8, or 19. The transmission is by direct contact, usually by the fingers to the contralateral eye or to other patients. It can also be transmitted in swimming pools. Adenovirus is highly contagious and can cause epidemics. It is most common in midsummer to early autumn.

3. The **specific evaluation** includes making the clinical diagnosis by using this information and the examination described in Box 13-1.

4. The **specific management** includes:
   a. Eye lavage with sterile normal saline on a twice daily basis for 7–14 days for symptomatic relief.
   b. Vasoconstrictors are of some benefit (see Table 13-1 for specific agents and dosages). Topical nonsteroidal antiinflammatory drugs (NSAIDs) may also be of benefit in addition to cool compresses.
   c. Topical antibiotics are of questionable benefit unless the discharge becomes purulent, at which time the discharge must be sent for Gram stain, culture, and sensitivity.
   d. Referral to ophthalmology should be made on an elective basis.

B. Bacterial/purulent

The discussion is limited to adult bacterial conjunctivitis. Neonatal conjunctivitis is extremely important, but one should refer to pediatric texts for **evaluation and management** of that process.

1. The **specific manifestations** of this relatively common form of conjunctivitis include an acute onset of copious, purulent discharge from both eyes. There can be some mild decrease in visual acuity and mild discomfort, but the major manifestation is marked discharge. The patient is virtually always afebrile and has few or no concurrent systemic manifestations.

2. The **underlying pathogenesis** is a bacterial infection of the conjunctiva with resultant purulence. Causative agents can be divided into two overall groups, common pathogens and rare pathogens.

   a. Common pathogens include *Streptococcus pneumoniae*, *S. aureus*, and *Haemophilus aegyptius*.

      i. The **natural history** is usually one of self-limited disease; however, in some cases, a secondary keratitis with visual impairment can occur.

      ii. The **transmission** is by direct contact of secretions and/or by autoinoculation (i.e., from one eye to the other). In these cases, fingers are the vehicles.

   b. Rare pathogens include *Chlamydia trachomatis* and *Neisseria gonorrhoeae*. Although these two agents are rare in the adult population of the United States, they deserve special mention because of the following facts:

      i. The **natural history** is one of severe conjunctivitis and keratitis with the development of permanent visual impairment.

      ii. The **transmission is** either by direct contact of eye secretions either via fingers or via contact of the eyes with water in nonchlorinated swimming pools. Furthermore, it can be spread to a neonate by vaginal delivery from an infected mother and result in neonatal bacterial conjunctivitis. In the cases of neonatal conjunctivitis, *Chlamydia* and *Neisseria gonorrhoeae* can cause the conjunctivitis. Finally, whereas chlamydial conjunctivitis is rare in the Western world, it remains endemic to the Third World.

3. The **specific evaluation** includes making the clinical diagnosis using this information and the examination described in Box 13-1.

   a. If one of the common pathogens is suspected (i.e., the vast majority of cases), a Gram stain should be performed on the discharge. The Gram stain is performed to demonstrate the presence of polymorphonuclear leukocytes (PMNs) and a predominant organism.

      Specific therapy includes the application of topical antibiotics. An especially effective topical agent is sulfacetamide, 10% solution, 2 drops OU t.i.d. for 5–7 days.

   b. If one of the rare pathogens is suspected (e.g., in a neonate or a patient in or from a Third World country, or if there is a concurrent gonococcal infection present, a Gram stain and Giemsa stain should be performed on the discharge.

    i. The Gram stain is performed to demonstrate the presence of PMNs. If chlamydial, no organisms will be demonstrated, whereas if *Neisseria gonorrhoeae,* intracellular/gram-negative diplococci will be present.

    ii. The Giemsa stain should be performed looking for PMNs and, if chlamydial (i.e., trachoma), the presence of inclusion bodies.

    iii. Specific therapy should include topical antibiotics. sulfacetamide, 10% solution, two drops OU t.i.d. for 3–5 weeks, with concurrent systemic erythromycin, 250–500 mg p.o., q.i.d., for 7 days or doxycycline 100 mg p.o., b.i.d., for 7 days. Furthermore, the case should be reported to the Centers for Disease Control, and a consultation with ophthalmology should be made.

C. Atopic/Allergic rhinitis associated

Please refer to section Rhinitis, Chapter 12, page 586.

D. Keratoconjunctivitis siccae

    1. The **specific manifestations** of this entity include a mild, recurrent, bilateral conjunctivitis. Patients often have a sensation in one or both eyes of "scratchiness" and dryness. The patient can develop recurrent corneal abrasions from incessant rubbing. In Sjögren's syndrome, the lacrimal and salivary glands are quite enlarged. Although in end stage, there are no tears present, early in the course, there may be the apparent paradox of epiphoria (i.e., the patient has dry eyes but intermittent excessive tearing) because the small glands that continuously produce oily/serous/mucus tears are damaged first, resulting in chronic dry eyes, but the lacrimal glands (i.e., those that produce copious amounts of serous tears) are relatively unaffected.

    2. The **underlying pathogenesis** is a marked decrease in the production of tears. The differential diagnosis includes Sjögren's syndrome, a syndrome of destruction of the lacrimal glands often associated with rheumatologic disorders, or as a sequela of severe superficial eye infections or burns. Radiation therapy may also result in this syndrome.

    3. The **specific evaluation** includes making the clinical diagnosis by using this information and the examination described in Box 13-1. The specifics include a thorough history for any antecedent or concurrent rheumatologic diseases, or a history of trauma, burns, or infections of the eyes.

4. **Management**

The most effective modalities in **treatment** include the use of artificial tears (see Table 13-1 for specific agents and dosages). Referral to ophthalmology is indicated if symptoms are refractory to first- and second-line therapy.

E. **Chemical burns**

1. The **specific manifestations** include an acute onset of pain, redness, burning, and tearing after exposure to or direct contact with a gas or liquid toxic to the eye. On examination, there is marked erythema of the conjunctiva with the potential for ulcer formation. Visual acuity is often decreased.

2. The **underlying pathogenesis** of the chemical-mediated damage ("burn") is damage to the eye structures and concomitant inflammation. The chemical burn has components of both keratitis and conjunctivitis and thus, if not immediately and aggressively treated, can result in permanent visual loss and dysfunction. The most common chemical burns are the result of exposure to acids and bases. Bases are more malignant than acids and can cause more sequelae; however, both must be aggressively managed.

3. The **specific evaluation and management** include a thorough history, determining the specific agent that caused the burn, and, as soon as possible, lavage of the affected eye with copious amounts of tap water or, if available, normal saline. The initial management is quite simple: lavage, lavage, and lavage! The use of anything other than water or saline is contraindicated, for if an attempt is made to neutralize the acid or base, heat is produced, with resultant thermal injury concurrent with the chemical injury.

   a. After flushing with water or saline and emergently contacting ophthalmology, the remainder of the basic evaluation as described in Box 13-1 can be completed.

   b. If the burn is significant, one can, after thorough flushing, administer mydriatic agents and initiate topical antibiotics (see Table 13-1 for specifics on agents and dosages). Application of a patch to the affected eye is indicated.

   c. Close follow-up with ophthalmology is indicated.

   d. Prevention is the key. People need to wear protective eyewear when working with chemicals or with batteries (e.g., jump-starting a car). Educate patients that if an exposure does occur, immediately begin the lavage with water!

IX. **Keratitis**

This is the nonspecific inflammation of the cornea. The normal function of the cornea is to act as a transparent window allowing light to enter the eye with high fidelity. It is, in the normal state, clear and avascular; however, with any inflammation (i.e., keratitis), opacity and ulcerations can develop in the cornea itself (See Table 13-2, page 618, for complications).

A. **Herpes simplex**

1. The **specific manifestations** of this uncommon but severe type of keratitis include the acute onset of unilateral pain, redness, and decreased visual acuity, which often is quite marked. On examination, there is an extensive dendritic pattern of gray-colored corneal ulcers. On examination with fluorescein, these ulcers stain and can be clearly demonstrated by using the cobalt blue lamp. It is not uncommon to have concurrent vesicular blepharitis, but rarely will there be any concurrent vesicular lesions in the adjacent skin.

2. The **underlying pathogenesis** is reactivation of a primary herpes simplex type I infection. The primary infection was of the oral mucosa, which then involved and remained dormant in the trigeminal ganglion. Reactivation can be precipitated by stress. Although the reactivation usually manifests as a "cold sore," a potential reactivation manifestation is of keratitis.

3. The **specific evaluation** includes making the clinical diagnosis by using this information and the examination described in Box 13-1.

4. **Management**

Once the diagnosis is made or suspected, emergency therapy is indicated.

a. An emergency consultation with ophthalmology. The care by the ophthalmologist will include gentle debridement of the ulcer. The material debrided should be sent for a Tzanck prep and viral culture.

b. The initiation of antiviral drops and antibiotic drops for 14–21 days (see Table 13-1 for specific agents and dosages).

c. Patching the affected eye.

d. A caveat is that if there is any concurrent interstitial keratitis (i.e., an immune-mediated process), the paradoxic use of topical glucocorticoids is indicated, under the direction of an ophthalmology colleague.

B. **Herpes zoster**

1. The **specific manifestations** of this relatively rare form of keratitis are classic and dramatic. They include the acute onset of a unilateral keratitis and conjunctivitis with an antecedent erythematous, painful, vesicular

rash on the ipsilateral skin in the distribution of the trigeminal nerve, specifically V1. Furthermore, there are concurrent significant ptosis and eyelid edema. If untreated, it can progress to diffuse uveitis and blindness.

2. The **underlying pathogenesis** is reactivation of the DNA-containing varicella-zoster virus. The patient has a history of primary varicella-zoster infection (chicken pox), which, after the acute infection, remained dormant in the dorsal ganglia. The recurrence is usually precipitated by a decrease in the immune system or increasing age. It occurs in any dermatome, but if in dermatome of V1, can result in herpes zoster keratitis.

3. The **specific evaluation** includes making the clinical diagnosis by using this information and the examination described in Box 13-1.

4. **Management**
   Once the diagnosis is made or suspected, emergency therapy is indicated.
   a. The immediate initiation of systemic acyclovir therapy. Systemic acyclovir will decrease the period of viral shedding and the intensity of the uveitis/keratitis when initiated early in the course of disease. The dose is 600–800 mg p.o., 5 times per day for 10 days, or, if immunosuppressed, 10 mg/kg i.v., in q.8h dosing for 7–10 days.
   b. The patient should be placed in respiratory isolation until the rash resolves, to prevent spread to people never exposed to varicella-zoster and pregnant women.

C. **Actinic**
   1. The **specific manifestations** of this not uncommon cause of keratitis include the acute onset of bilateral eye pain, photophobia, decreased visual acuity, and conjunctivitis beginning 6–12 hours after visual exposure to a source of ultraviolet light. There are usually no systemic manifestations. The slit lamp with cobalt-blue light and fluorescein will reveal punctate, superficial uptake.
   2. The **underlying pathogenesis** is a noninfectious keratitis resulting from overexposure to ultraviolet light. The patient invariably was exposed to a source of UV light without having adequate eye protection (i.e., polarizing sunglasses). The source of UV light can be a tanning salon, arc-welding flame, or sunlight. This is one of the classic problems that occurs after looking directly at the sun during a total eclipse. Recovery without sequelae occurs in 48–72 hours.
   3. The **specific evaluation** includes making the clinical

diagnosis by using this information and the examination described in Box 13-1.

4. **Management**

   Once the diagnosis is made or suspected:

   a. Initiation of cycloplegic agents [e.g., cyclopentolate (see Table 13-1 for specific agents and dosing)].

   b. Patching of the affected eye(s) for 24–36 hours.

   c. Effective prevention with polarizing sunglasses and education on how to limit exposure to UV light.

   d. If, after 24–48 hours, there is no improvement or if at presentation there are any other abnormalities, ophthalmology should be consulted.

D. **Bacterial, specifically in contact lens wearers**

   1. The **specific manifestations** of this uncommon form of keratitis include the acute onset of unilateral pain and erythema in a patient who uses contact lenses, especially the extended-wear type. On examination, there is a hazy, nontransparent cornea with a central ulcer. On fluorescein examination, any ulceration present will take up the dye. On direct and slit-lamp examination, pus can be demonstrated in the anterior chamber (i.e., a hypopyon). A hypopyon portends a poor prognosis.

   2. The **underlying pathogenesis** of bacterial keratitis in contact lens wearers is multifactorial. Factors include improper cleaning techniques, small areas of abrasion from the contact lenses, and the duration of the lens being in contact with the cornea.

      a. The incidence of bacterial keratitis in contact lens wearers is quite low. Recent studies by Poggio et al. demonstrated that the incidence per year of bacterial keratitides is 21/10,000 users of extended wear contact lenses and 4/10,000 users of soft daily contact lenses.

      b. The organisms associated with contact lens keratitis are gram-negative bacilli, including *Pseudomonas* spp., and some gram-positive organisms, especially *Streptococcus* and *Moraxella*. The protozoon *Acanthamoeba* can result in contact lens–related keratitis.

      c. The **natural history** is the development of a hypopyon, which then results in perforation of the cornea, diffuse uveitis, and blindness (Table 13-2).

   3. The **specific evaluation** includes making the clinical diagnosis by using this information and the examination described in Box 13-1.

   4. Management

      Once the diagnosis is made or suspected:

      a. Remove the contact lens.

TABLE 13-2
Complications of Keratitis/Corneal Abrasions/Ulcers

Complication	Manifestation	Management
Anterior uveitis	*Symptoms:* Pain, Photophobia, Epiphoria. *Signs:* Miosis, Perilimbic injection (circumcorneal), Cloudiness in the anterior chamber = flare	Refer to Ophthalmology. Look for underlying etiologies, which include: Rheumatoid arthritis, Ulcerative colitis/IBD-related, Trauma, Keratitis progressing into anterior chamber, Corneal ulcer
Hypopyon	Pus level within the anterior chamber. Result of severe anterior uveitis	Refer to Ophthalmology
Band keratopathy	Decrease in visual acuity in a patient. *Slit lamp:* cloudy area in the endothelium of the corneum as the result of calcium deposition	Refer to Ophthalmology. Look for underlying etiologies, which include: Sarcoidosis, Hyperparathyroidism, Hypercalcemia, Anterior uveitis

Posterior uveitis	Inflammation of the choroid and underlying retina
	Infection
	  MTB
	  Toxoplasmosis
	  Histoplasmosis
	  HSV/CMV
	Sympathetic (i.e. posttrauma/immune mediated)
		Refer to Ophthalmology

Open-angle glaucoma	Insidious loss of vision secondary to chronic increase in IOP as the result of sludging	Refer to Ophthalmology
Posterior synechiae	Adhesions between the iris and the lens capsule Thin, white bands, may distort the pupil/iris (poikiloscoria)	Refer to Ophthalmology

    b. Obtain an emergency consultation with ophthalmology. Under the direction of the ophthalmologist, the ulcer should be scraped gently and sent for Gram stain, culture, fungal culture, and *Acanthamoeba* culture.

    c. Initiate a continuous irrigation of the superficial surface of the eye, laterally to medially, with antibiotic solutions of a cephalosporin and tobramycin for 2–4 hours. This irrigation must be under the direct and intimate supervision of an ophthalmologist. This intervention is followed by administration of a topical antibiotic ointment, patching of the eye for 3–7 days, and daily follow-up with the ophthalmologist (see Table 13-1 for specific agents and dosages).

    d. The major thrust of care after immediate management is **prevention.**

        i. Underscore the need to use meticulous technique when cleaning and placing the contact lenses.

        ii. Instruct the patient to use commercially available sterile products for cleaning lenses. Tap water should never be used, as it is usually contaminated.

        iii. Remove the contact lenses at the first signs or symptoms of irritation and wear glasses for several days (i.e., a contact lens holiday).

X. Corneal abrasion/ulcer

    A. The **specific manifestations** of this relatively common problem include the acute onset of unilateral eye discomfort and erythema. The patient often will report a scratchy sensation in the affected eye. There often is a history of a foreign body on the anterior surface of the eye. Furthermore, the symptoms are exacerbated by rubbing the affected eye. On fluorescein examination, the ulcer takes on the dye. The foreign body can be virtually any small, solid substance, including a hair, a dust particle, an eyelash, or, more ominously, a piece of metal, an insect, or a wood splinter or chip.

    B. The **underlying pathogenesis** is a scratch or trauma-related erosion of the cornea. An uncomplicated abrasion resolves without sequelae in 36–72 hours.

    C. The **specific evaluation** includes making the clinical diagnosis by using this information and the examination described in Box 13-1. Further **specific evaluation** includes a thorough examination to look for any remaining foreign bodies. If there is any history that the particle was metal, one needs to obtain a radiograph of the eye, looking for an intraocular foreign body. One must examine for the development of a corneal ulcer: an ulcer is deepest and may extend to the level of the anterior chamber. If an ulcer is left untreated, corneal perforation, anterior uveitis, hypopyon, and/or blindness may result (see Table 13-2, Complications of Keratitis/Corneal Abrasions/Ulcers).

D. Management

1. The **specific management** of a simple corneal abrasion includes flushing the eye with sterile saline for 30 minutes, the administration of topical antibiotics, usually as ointment, for 5 days (see Table 13-1), and patching the eye for 24 hours.

2. Although consultation with ophthalmology is elective for an abrasion, it is required/mandatory for an ulcer or any foreign body.

XI. Consultation

Problem	Service	Time
Internal hordeolum	Ophthalmology	Required
Chalazion		Elective
Dacrocystitis		Required
Uveitis		Emergent
Acute-angle glaucoma		Emergent
Keratitis		Emergent
Corneal abrasion		Urgent
Conjunctivitis		Elective
Chemical burn		Urgent/emergent

XII. Indications for admission: Any evidence of herpes simplex or herpes zoster keratitis, a penetrating wound to the eye, acute-angle glaucoma, or any significant chemical burn. All of these admissions are to the ophthalmology service.

Bibliography

Acute Blindness

D'Amico DJ: Diseases of the retina. N Engl J Med 1994;331:95–107.
Sanders MO: Sudden visual loss. Practitioner 1977;219:43.

Cataracts

Abrahamson IA: Cataract update. Am Fam Physician 1981;24:111.

Open-Angle Glaucoma

Everitt DE, Avorn J: Systemic effects of medications used to treat glaucoma. Ann Intern Med 1990;112:120–125.
Gottlieb LK, et al: Glaucoma screening: a cost effective analysis. Surv Ophthalmol 1983;28:206.
Mosteller MW, Zimmerman TJ: The medical management of glaucoma. In: Spoor TC, ed. Modern management of ocular diseases. Thorofare, NJ: Slack, 1985:170–188.
Quigley HA: Open-angle glaucoma. N Engl J Med 1993;328:1097–1106.

Red Inflamed Eye

Baum JL: Ocular infection. N Engl J Med 1978;299:28.

Bienfang DC, et al: Ophthalmology. N Engl J Med 1990;323:956–967.

Drugs for bacterial conjunctivitis. Med Lett 1976;18:70.

Eifrig DE: A system for examining the ocular fundus. North Carolina Med J 1983;32:631–633.

Hara JH: The red eye: diagnosis and treatment. Am Fam Pract 1996;54:2423–2430.

Havener WH: Synopsis of ophthalmology, 6th ed. St. Louis: CV Mosby, 1984.

Henderly DE, et al: Changing patterns of uveitis. Am J Ophthalmol 1987;103:131.

Moutsopoulos HM, et al: Sj§gren's syndrome (sicca syndrome): current issues. Ann Intern Med 1980;92:212.

Newell SW: The management of corneal foreign bodies. Am Fam Pract 1985;31:149–156.

Shingleton BJ: Eye injuries. N Engl J Med 1991;325:408–413.

Titi MJ: A critical look at ocular allergy drugs. Am Fam Pract 1996;53:2637–2642.

Torok PG, et al: Corneal abrasions: diagnosis and management. 1996;53:2521–2529.

Victor WH: Watery eye. West J Med 1986;144:759.

White GL, et al: Contact lens care and complications. Am Fam Pract 1988;37:187–192.

—D.D.B.

Chapter 14

Neurology

Cranial Nerve VII Disorders Including "Bell's Palsy"

Cranial nerve (CN) VII is a mixed CN in that it has both motor and sensory components. The motor components include the facial musculature and thus wrinkling of the forehead, eye closing, and lip movement. It also innervates the stapedius muscle in the middle ear and controls the secretion of saliva and tears from the salivary and lacrimal glands, respectively. The sensory component is mainly of taste. The anatomy of innervation is similar to other motor nerves, central (i.e., upper motor neuron) and peripheral (i.e., lower motor neuron). A unique feature of the innervation is that the upper face and eyes receive innervation from the upper motor neuron component (central) from both sides of the brain, whereas the lower face receives innervation from the upper motor neuron component (central) from the contralateral side only. The lower motor neuron component (peripheral) innervates the entire ipsilateral side of the face. Thus the **manifestations** of CN VII palsy are variable and dependent on the location of the lesion. Therefore, given a set of findings, one can easily locate the lesion.

I. Overall manifestations and causes
   A. Central lesions
      A central (i.e., upper motor neuron) lesion will manifest with paresis (weakness) or plegia (paralysis) of the contralateral orbicularis oris muscle but not of the orbicularis oculis muscle.
      1. Overall manifestations
         The patient is able easily to close both eyes and wrinkle the forehead but is unable to smile completely. When instructed to smile, the patient is unable normally to elevate one side of the lips. This unilateral lack of a facial (nasolabial) fold on smiling is contralateral to the side of the lesion. Associated features are common (e.g., spastic hemiparesis) and are related to the underlying cause.

2. **Causes of a central CN VII palsy:**
   Causes include the intracranial processes of intracranial tumor, head trauma, or, in the vast majority of cases, a cerebrovascular accident (see section on Cerebrovascular Accidents, page 625).

B. **Peripheral lesions**
   Peripheral (lower motor neuron) CN damage results in ipsilateral paresis or plegia of all musculature of that side of the face. Thus in a peripheral CN VII palsy, the ipsilateral frontalis, orbicularis oris, and orbicularis oculis musculature are affected.

   1. **Overall manifestations** include an inability to wrinkle forehead, close eye, and smile on the side affected. Other associated features include the sensation of an acute onset of ipsilateral facial stiffness, the development of hyperacusis (i.e., increased, approaching painful, sensitivity to auditory stimuli) and, finally, dysgeusia (ie, dysfunctional taste) can and will occur. A further manifestation may be excessive tearing (epiphoria)– "crocodile tears"—during the healing phase.

   2. **Causes of a peripheral CN VII palsy:**
      a. Herpes simplex/zoster infection involving the nucleus of CN VII (Ramsay–Hunt syndrome). This is usually quite evident, given the fact that vesicles will form on the tongue and about the external ear in the disorder. It is quite rare but should be in the differential diagnosis.
      b. **Acoustic neuroma of CN VIII.** The **specific manifestations** include associated ipsilateral tinnitus and occasionally vertigo.
      c. Facial trauma can disrupt the nerve peripherally.
      d. Surgical complication, especially after a parotidectomy.
      e. **Bell's palsy.** The most common, albeit idiopathic, cause of a peripheral CN palsy, especially in young patients. Recent evidence has indicated herpes simplex virus (HSV) as the underlying cause.

II. **Evaluation and management of CN VII palsy**
    Differentiate a central from a peripheral lesion on the basis of the physical examination.
    A. If **central,** a computed tomography (CT) scan of the head is indicated, as the most likely process is a cerebrovascular accident (CVA). Neurology should be consulted. See section on Cerebrovascular Accidents, page 625, for further discussion.
    B. If **peripheral,** query patient regarding antecedent facial trauma, past facial surgeries, and carefully examine for any evidence of a herpes infection.

1. If due to trauma or iatrogenic, the patient should be instructed on how to patch the affected eye at night and should be prescribed lubricating eyedrops [methylcellulose 1% (Isopto-Alkaline drops)].

2. If herpes infection is present or suspected, initiation of acyclovir, 200 mg p.o., 5 times per day for 7–10 days, is indicated, as is referral to ophthalmology to evaluate for and aid in the prevention of herpes keratitis. See Red Inflamed Eye, chapter 13 (page 605).

3. If the diagnosis is idiopathic peripheral CN VII palsy (i.e., Bell's palsy):
   a. 60% of patients will recover complete function in the proximate future without any treatment.
   b. Patching the eye until palsy resolves is indicated to prevent trauma or severe xerosis.

III. **Consultation**

Problem	Service	Time
Herpes infection	Infectious diseases	Urgent
Herpes infection	Ophthalmology	Urgent
Central lesion	Neurology	Urgent

IV. **Indications for admission:** Cerebrovascular accident (CVA), and any patient with evidence of herpes infection with dissemination or a history of immunosuppression. Otherwise this can be evaluated and managed as an outpatient problem.

Cerebrovascular Accidents

Cerebrovascular accidents, or strokes, are a broad group of pathologic entities that are, by definition, infarction of brain tissue due to an interruption of blood flow to that area of brain. **Manifestations** can be diverse because different portions of the brain control different functions, and thus damage to a certain area will produce neurologic deficits that may be very different from the manifestations of damage/death to an area immediately adjacent. Two other reasons for differences in manifestations include the fact that there are several different mechanisms in **pathogenesis**, and that there can be some partial or even complete reversibility of the CVA manifestations.

I. The **overall manifestations** of stroke syndromes are mainly dependent on the location of the brain tissue infarction. A thorough physical examination will quite often place the lesion.

A. **Manifestations by location of brain infarction**
   1. **Occipital lobe.** This is as the visual cortex. Therefore, damage or destruction of this area will result in blindness in the contralateral visual field.
   2. **Parietal lobe.** This functions as the sensory-input area.

Therefore, damage to this area can result in decreased ability to perceive sensory data and, if on the dominant side, receptive aphasia.

3. **Frontal lobe.** This functions as the motor cortex and a site of behaviors. Therefore damage to this area, especially the posterior aspect, will result in contralateral muscle weakness.

4. **The deep white matter, internal capsule.** This is the location of axons to the spinal cord, especially from the motor cortex. Therefore damage to this area will result in contralateral muscle weakness.

II. **Categories of CVA by pathogenesis**

CVA (stroke) syndromes are best categorized by the mechanisms of **pathogenesis** as, although many of the **overall manifestations** are similar, each category has a different **pathogenesis**, some unique differentiating features, and some significant differences in **specific management.** The syndromes are categorized into three different groups: ischemic thrombotic, ischemic embolic, and hemorrhagic (Tables 14-1 and 14-2).

A. **Ischemic thrombotic CVA: 60%**

1. The **pathogenesis** of ischemic thrombotic CVAs results from atherosclerosis of the arteries leading to the brain, carotids, and/or vertebrobasilar circulation. **Risk factors** for development are the same as for other atherosclerotic disease processes: smoking, diabetes mellitus, hypertension, and hyperlipidemia (see page 1). These include the lacunar or small infarcts involving the white matter as the result of severe hypertension.

2. The **specific manifestations** of this category include an acute onset of a neurologic deficit that may resolve over the next minutes, hours, or days, to various degrees. **Transient ischemic attacks (TIAs)** are deficits that resolve within the first 24 hours; reversible ischemia **neurologic deficits (RINDs)** resolve within the first 7 days. Any defect present after 7 days is the residua of the **completed stroke.** A specific type of TIA is amaurosis fugax, in which the patient has monocular blindness that resolves in the first 6–24 hours.

   Acute reversibility is unique to this category of CVA. This feature is inductively reasonable if one recalls that this is usually a stenosis that completely occludes and then can and often does reopen. In this model, one can compare thrombotic CVAs with acute coronary syndromes. The TIA would be analogous to unstable angina, the RIND analogous to non–Q-wave infarction, and the completed CVA to a Q-wave infarct.

3. The **specific evaluation and management** of these CVAs includes the items described in Box 14-1 along with the following specifics.

(text continues on page 630)

T A B L E 14-1
Types of CVAs by Pathophysiology

Type	Risk Factors	Historical Features	TIAs
Ischemic thrombotic	Hypertension Atherosclerosis (see page 1) Vasculitis Hypotensive episodes Oral contraceptives	Sudden onset of deficit, progresses or improves over hours to days	Common
Ischemic embolic	Mechanical heart valves Mitral stenosis Atrial fibrillation Left-sided endocarditis	Sudden onset, fixed from outset	Uncommon
Hemorrhagic	Hypertension Berry aneurysms Arteriovenous malformations Thrombocytopenia Coagulopathy	Severe headache Nuchal rigidity Vomiting Steady, slow progression of deficits over 6 hours If intraparenchymal: CT positive If subarachnoid: CT negative, but blood on LP	Uncommon

TABLE 14-2
Approach to Ischemic Thrombotic TIAs, RINDs, and Complete CVAs

Type	Symptoms/Signs	Acutely	Subacutely
Vertebrobasilar	Dysarthria Dysphagia Near syncope Hemiparesis	If evolving: anticoagulate with heparin for 5–7 days If fixed or resolving: aspirin, 325 mg p.o., q.d.*	Aspirin, 325 mg p.o., q.d.* OT/PT No surgical intervention No indications for arteriography
Carotid	Contralateral hemiparesis Amaurosis fugax	If evolving: anticoagulate with heparin and continue until definitive procedure done If resolving: aspirin* If fixed: aspirin*	Carotid Dopplers Carotid arteriography or mRA CEA, if stenosis present

*If patient is allergic to aspirin, initiate the antiplatelet agent ticlopidine, 250 mg p.o., b.i.d.

B O X 14-1

Overall Evaluation and Management of Stroke Syndromes

Evaluation

1. ABCs, as outlined by basic and advanced life support, as necessary.
2. Complete blood cell (CBC) count, for baseline purposes.
3. Intravenous access for fluids, as a patient with an acute CVA syndrome should be NPO during the acute event.
4. Thorough physical examination for baseline neurologic examination, documenting any motor, sensory, or cognitive deficits.
5. Prothrombin time (PT), activated thromboplastin time (aPTT), and platelet count to determine if there is any evidence of a coagulopathy and as baseline if anticoagulation is indicated.
6. Erythrocyte sedimentation rate (ESR). If increased, can be consistent with an inflammatory process (i.e., vasculitis).
7. Pulse oximetry, for baseline purposes. Supplemental O_2 should be administered to keep O_2 sat > 92%.
8. Nothing by mouth (NPO). Very important in the acute setting, as the swallowing mechanism is often affected by a CVA.
9. Electrocardiogram (ECG), 12 lead, for baseline purposes and to look for any acute cardiac event. Furthermore, a diagnosis of the rhythm is useful, especially if the rhythm is one of atrial fibrillation, which is associated with embolic CVAs.
10. CT scan without contrast, to look for any areas of bleeding. Blood, indicative of a hemorrhagic CVA, will be demonstrable without a contrast agent. (Fresh hemorrhage is its own contrast agent.)
11. If CT of head is negative, but suspicion for subarachnoid bleed is still present, lumbar puncture is indicated. A subarachnoid bleed will often manifest with a normal head CT but a bloody cerebrospinal fluid (CSF).

(continued)

B O X   14-1 (continued)

Management

1. Maintain blood pressure in 140–160/80–90 mm Hg range.
2. Admit to monitored or intensive care unit (ICU) bed.
3. Early and aggressive physical and occupational therapy is required.
4. Prevent any gravitational pneumonia by checking the gag reflex before allowing swallowing of food/liquid; refer to swallowing specialist.
5. Enteral tube feedings to maintain nutrition may be indicated as a temporizing measure.
6. Social services and family support required for intermediate and long-term assistance.
7. Categorize CVA into **ischemic thrombotic** (page 626); **ischemic embolic** (page 631); or **hemorrhagic** (page 632). See text for specifics.

(text continued from page 626)

    a. Maintain the systolic blood pressure >120 mm Hg to keep perfusion adequate. This can be accomplished with fluids and, if indicated, pressor agents.

    b. If the CVA is evolving clinically (i.e., new deficits are developing), the patient should be, unless contraindicated, anticoagulated with heparin. The dosing is a bolus of 5,000–10,000 units i.v., followed by an 800–1,000 unit/hour drip, with a goal to keep the aPTT at 45–60 seconds.

    There is an increasing amount of evidence to support thrombolytic therapy in this set of patients. If the patient is seen within 3 hours of the onset of manifestations, **treatment** with tPA (tissue plasminogen activator) may be effective in stopping the progression or even reversing the CVA process. The dose of tPA is 0.9 mg/kg body weight; maximum dose, 90 mg; 10% of the dose is given as an i.v. bolus, and the remainder is administered i.v. over a 60-minute period.

    c. If the CVA is not evolving or is resolving, there is no indication for anticoagulation.

    d. Once the patient is stabilized, perform carotid Dopplers to image for any plaques. If any plaques are demonstrated, carotid (two-vessel) arteriography or magnetic resonance angiography (MRA) is indicated. If stenosis of >50% is present in the carotids, carotid endarterectomy is indicated (Table 14-3). If

T A B L E 14-3
Indications for Carotid Endarterectomy

1. High-grade (>50%) carotid stenosis with recent, documented TIA or RIND
2. Carotid stenosis in patients who recently required heparin anticoagulation for treatment of stroke syndrome
3. Not necessary in completed stroke if stenosis and CVA are anatomically appropriate

no plaques are demonstrated, the plaques are either intracranial or in the vertebrobasilar system, neither of which is amenable to surgery. Vertebrobasilar arteriography is not indicated for thrombotic CVAs because no intervention can be done based on that finding.

e. In all cases, unless contraindicated, aspirin, 325 mg p.o., q.d., should be started. If the patient is allergic to aspirin or if it is otherwise contraindicated, the antiplatelet agent, ticlopidine, 250 mg p.o., b.i.d., should be administered.

B. **Ischemic embolic CVA, 20%–25% of all CVAs**

1. The **pathogenesis** of ischemic embolic CVAs is thrombus (clot) forming in the left atrium, left ventricle, or on the mitral or aortic valves, or as a result of bioprosthetic valves or endocarditis, which embolize to the brain and other vital organs.

2. The **specific manifestations** with which the patient usually presents include an acute onset of a deficit that is maximal at outset but may improve slightly over time. Virtually never is any TIA or RIND associated with this mechanism.

3. The **specific management** of these CVAs includes the items described in Box 14-1, along with the following specifics.

   a. Maintain the systolic blood pressure ~120 mm Hg to keep adequate cerebral perfusion. This can be accomplished with fluids and, if indicated, pressor agents.

   b. If there are no contraindications, the patient should be anticoagulated with heparin. The dosing is a bolus of 5,000–10,000 units i.v., followed by an 800–1,000 unit/hour drip, with a goal to keep the aPTT at 45–60 seconds.

   c. A search for the source of emboli should be rapidly undertaken. This entails imaging the heart with an echocardiogram and monitoring the heart rhythm for any episodes of atrial fibrillation. If no source in the heart is found, then carotid Dopplers looking for plaques that may have associated thrombi are indicated. If the patient is febrile or at risk for endocarditis, four sets of blood cultures must be obtained, and, if clinically indicated, antibiotics of vancomycin i.v. and an aminoglycoside i.v. should be initiated.

    d. The patient may need long-term anticoagulation with warfarin after the 5–7 days of heparin. The goal is to initiate warfarin early in the heparin course and maintain an international normalized ratio (INR) in the 2.0–3.0 range. See Table 1-17 (page 46) for anticoagulation indications.

C. Hemorrhagic CVA, 15% of all CVAs

    1. The **underlying pathogenesis** of hemorrhagic CVAs is disruption or rupture of the vessels within or adjacent to the brain itself. A rupture of a vessel within the brain itself is called an **intraparenchymal bleed** and can be the result of a ruptured arteriovenous malformation (AVM) or be hypertension related. A rupture of a vessel immediately adjacent to the brain surface is a **subarachnoid bleed** and is usually the result of a ruptured berry aneurysm and/or hypertension. Intraparenchymal (Fig. 14-1) and subarachnoid bleeds are on a clinical continuum, with overlap between the two types.

    2. The **specific manifestations** include a severe headache

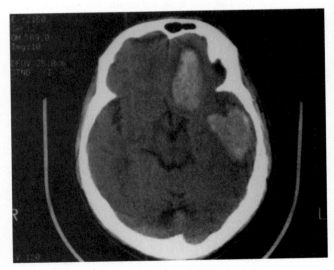

F I G U R E   14-1
CT of head without contrast agent enhancement, showing large intraparenchymal hemorrhage in the left hemisphere.

(the worst of the patient's life), nausea, vomiting, and a slow, steady progression of neurologic defects over the subsequent 2–6 hours. Virtually never is there any TIA or RIND associated with this mechanism.

3. The **specific management** of these CVAs includes the items described in Box 14-1, along with the following specifics.

 a. Any coagulopathy must be aggressively evaluated and corrected. See section on Excessive Bleeding States in Chapter 5 (page 268).

 b. If thrombocytopenic for any reason, transfuse platelets to keep >50,000/mm^3. See section on Excessive Bleeding States in Chapter 5.

 c. Calcium channel blockers, specifically nimodipine, 60 mg p.o. or n.g., q.4hr, may be of short- and long-term benefit for intracranial bleeds, especially in subarachnoid bleeds, if initiated in the first 96 hours. (The earlier, the better.)

 d. The maintenance of a stable blood pressure is of great importance (110–140/80–90 mm Hg).

 e. Further adjuvant therapy includes the initiation of stool softeners to minimize straining and the administration of acetaminophen for the relief of the headache.

 f. Once the patient is stabilized, a four-vessel arteriogram or MRA is indicated. Unlike thrombotic CVAs, it is of great importance to image the vertebrobasilar along with the standard carotid artery images to visualize the location of the ruptured aneurysm or AVM.

 g. Neurosurgical intervention for aneurysm or AVM clipping is indicated. If surgery is contraindicated for any reason, the clinician should consider referral to a radiologist or neurosurgeon for placement of an intravascular aneurysm spring device, which may be effective in preventing further bleeding.

III. **Overall prevention**

Preventive measures have dramatically decreased the overall incidence and the individual risk of cerebrovascular accidents. The impact of prevention is most clearly demonstrated in the risk factor hypertension. Unquestionably, the adequate control of hypertension has been demonstrated to decrease the risk of hemorrhagic and thrombotic CVAs. The overall prevention for all strokes includes:

1. Atherosclerotic disease risk factor modification (i.e., smoking cessation, control of hypertension, control of serum glucose in diabetes mellitus, and control of lipids in hyperlipidemias).

2. Anticoagulate patients who are at high risk for embolic CVAs. See indications listed (Table 1-17, page 46).

3. Discontinue oral contraceptives in a woman at higher risk (smokers, hypertensives, etc.).
4. Aspirin, 325 mg/day, for all patients with atherosclerotic disease. If aspirin is contraindicated, the patient should receive the antiplatelet agent ticlopidine, 250 mg p.o., b.i.d.
5. Manage asymptomatic carotid bruits. An asymptomatic carotid bruit is a prevalent finding in the older and middle-aged adult population. In all cases, unless contraindicated, aspirin, 325 mg p.o., q.d., should be administered. Carotid duplex (ultrasound and Doppler) studies should be performed. If high-grade stenosis (>50%) is found and/or if there are manifestations of TIAs in the distribution of the artery, carotid endarterectomy is indicated.

IV. **Consultation**

Problem	*Service*	*Time*
Carotid TIAs or RINDs	Vascular surgery	Urgent
Asymptomatic bruit	Vascular surgery	Elective
Any stroke	Neurology	Urgent
Any completed stroke	OT/PT	Required in most patients

V. **Indications for admission:** Any CVA. The clinician should have a low threshold for admitting directly to the ICU unless the patient is stable.

Delirium (Box 14-2)

This is an acute deterioration in mental status from a previously stable baseline. Simply put, it is an acute confusional state. Another way to state this process is the acute loss of orientation to one or more of the parameters of person (i.e., who the patient is and how she or he is related to others); place (i.e., where the patient is and its description); and time (i.e., what the date, season, and time is). This can be, but is not necessarily, associated with acute cognitive impairment, and/or a decrease in the level of consciousness (i.e., lethargy, somnolence). One cannot overstate the importance and gravity of this problem/diagnosis. It is truly a medical emergency that mandates aggressive medical evaluation and management.

I. **Overall manifestations**
This problem requires extensive history, but ironically, the patient is unable to give a good history. This is due to the very nature of delirium: the patient is a poor historian and is potentially confabulating (creating answers). Furthermore, the patient may even have concurrent aggressive, acting out type, behaviorisms. Therefore it is important to find someone, a family member or friend, who knows the patient to obtain a baseline set of parameters and to determine, if possible, when

B O X 14-2

Overall Evaluation and Management of Delirium

If it is a known diabetic patient who takes insulin, check a finger-stick glucose and administer a substance high in glucose, stat. If there is complete resolution after glucose administration and the finger-stick was low (i.e., <60 mg/dL), there is no need for further evaluation.

1. ABCs (i.e., basic and advanced life-support protocol) as necessary.
2. Establish intravenous access.
3. Administer thiamine, 100 mg i.v. or i.m., to attempt to reverse any Wernicke's disease (i.e., profound thiamine deficiency).
4. Administer one ampule of $D_{50}W$ i.v., to treat any hypoglycemia (after the thiamine is administered).
5. Administer one ampule of naloxone (Narcan) i.v., to reverse any effect of a narcotic agent.
6. Perform a finger-stick glucose.
7. Administer 0.2 mg of flumazenil i.v. to reverse any benzodiazepines ingested.
8. Laboratory examinations: serum electrolytes, blood urea nitrogen (BUN), creatinine, glucose, calcium, albumin, phosphorus, arterial blood gas, NH_4, CBC count with differential, ethanol level, urinalysis, and urine drug screen for benzodiazepines, tricyclic agents, and/or barbiturates. Abnormalities in any of these can result in delirium; therefore, they must be checked at the time of presentation.
9. Define and treat any cause discovered (see text).
10. If these **examinations and management** do not reveal the origin and/or resolve the problem, or if further investigation is clinically indicated, the following procedures should be performed:
    a. CT imaging of the head, especially in any head-trauma case or if any focal neurologic deficit is present.
    b. Lumbar puncture in every patient who has fever and delirium; this is clearly indicated.
    c. Treat the underlying cause.

the deterioration occurred. A drug- and ethanol-use history is also important, as is any medical history including diabetes mellitus, and/or recent medical history (e.g., of fevers). A history of suicide attempts or any psychiatric history is also quite helpful.

II. **Differential diagnosis**

The differential diagnosis is based on the fundamental concept that delirium is a medical problem, and therefore no psychiatric diagnoses are considered. In this problem, a psychotic reaction/psychiatric dysfunction is a diagnosis of exclusion.

A. **Medications/drugs**

Perhaps the most common cause of delirium.

1. **Ethanol.** The ingestion of excessive quantities of ethanol can cause delirium. The **specific manifestations** include the odor of ethanol on the patient's breath, decreased inhibition, cerebellar dysfunction, and a blood alcohol level usually >0.10 mg/dL. **Specific management** is to have patient discontinue the binge and to rest. Driving or operating a machine are contraindicated. The patient can usually be sent home with a family member or friend who is sober. Further details in management are outlined in the section on Substance-Abuse Syndromes in Chapter 15, Box 15-3 (page 693).

2. **Ethanol withdrawal.** Withdrawal from ethanol can result in a classic form of delirium, delirium tremens. **Specific manifestations** of delirium tremens occur after the patient abruptly discontinues ethanol ingestion after a sustained period (weeks to months) of intoxication. The patient experiences hallucinations (mainly visual) and tonic–clonic seizures during the first 48 hours, followed by delirium ~4 days after the initiation of abstinence. **Specific management** includes that in Box 14-2 and the initiation of benzodiazepines [e.g., lorazepam (Ativan), 1–2 mg p.o./i.m./i.v., q.6hr] and watching the airway. Admission to an inpatient service is required. Refer to the section on Substance-Abuse Syndromes in Chapter 15, Box 15-3 (page 693) for further details.

3. **Wernicke's syndrome.** This is the acute severe deficiency of the vitamin thiamine (B_1), most often occurring in malnourished alcoholics. The **specific manifestations** include delirium, unsteady gait, nystagmus, and reversible palsies of the extraocular musculature. This is a diagnosis/mechanism that can and will be concurrent with, but not the cause of, delirium tremens. The **specific management** is to replete thiamine, 100 mg i.m./i.v./p.o., q.d.

4. **Benzodiazepine (BZD) or narcotic withdrawal.** Analogous to withdrawal from ethanol, usually after abrupt cessation of BZD or narcotics after a long period of

significant use/abuse. **Manifestations and management** are quite similar to those of delirium tremens.

5. **BZD overdose or narcotic overdose.** An overdose of BZD or narcotic agents either accidentally or as a suicide attempt can cause delirium. The **specific manifestations** include a decreased level of consciousness and, specific to narcotics, bilateral miosis. The **specific management** includes that in Box 14-2 and supportive measures. For overdoses of BZD, the agent flumazenil, 0.2 mg, should be administered i.v. to reverse the activity of the BZD. This agent acts by competitive inhibition of the BZD receptors and can be repeated in incremental doses of 0.3 and 0.5 mg, q.3–4 minutes, to a maximum of 3.0 mg. A continuous infusion of nalaxone is sometimes required for immediate therapy. In virtually all cases, admission is indicated.

6. **PCP (angel dust).** This illicit agent is associated with a delirium with the **specific manifestations** of aggressive and acting-out behavior. The patient can harm himself and others. Management includes administration of BZDs and restraints.

7. Virtually every agent, whether medicinal or illicit, can cause delirium. This is particularly germane in the field of geriatrics. This underscores the need carefully to obtain a drug history.

B. **Electrolyte disturbances/metabolic**

Virtually every electrolyte, if abnormal to a marked degree, can cause delirium, irrespective of the underlying cause of that electrolyte imbalance. These include hypoxemia, hypercapnia, hypoglycemia, hypophosphatemia, hypocalcemia, hypercalcemia, uremia (increased BUN), azotemia (increased creatinine), and hyponatremia. The **specific management** is to normalize the electrolyte imbalance and to determine and treat the underlying cause.

C. **Acute anemia**

Delirium can result from an acute anemia, irrespective of the cause. **Specific manifestations** include intravascular volume depletion, hypotension, pale mucous membranes, and pale nail beds. Management specifics include determining the reason for the anemia, treating that cause, and, as needed, transfusion of packed red blood cells (RBCs).

D. **Hepatic encephalopathy**

This is due to an accumulation of nitrogenous catabolites that cannot be further catabolized/excreted by the liver because of hepatic failure. The **specific manifestations** include a concurrent decreased level of consciousness, asterixis, and the signs of chronic hepatic failure. Refer to the section on End-Stage Hepatic Dysfunction in Chapter 2, page 97, for further details.

E. **Fever**

Fever, especially a spiking fever, will cause delirium. The **specific management** is to determine and treat the underlying cause of the fever and to give the patient effective antipyretic agents, such as acetaminophen and/or acetylsalicylic acid.

F. **Leptomeningitis**

See section on Meningitis, page 658, for further discussion.

G. **Head trauma**

This is an overlooked cause of delirium, especially among patients with an increased risk of head trauma. This is especially true in patients who were intoxicated and then went through delirium tremens. It is not uncommon for these patients to have sustained some head trauma while intoxicated. Therefore, **specific management** in these patients is to examine for any head trauma and to obtain a CT scan of the head, without contrast, in any patient with any evidence of head trauma, any focal neurologic deficits, or an inappropriate and unexplained prolonged delirium (Fig. 14-2). The most common "silent" cause is a subdural hematoma occurring in such a scenario. If any structural defect is demonstrated on head CT, emergency consultation with neurosurgery is clearly indicated.

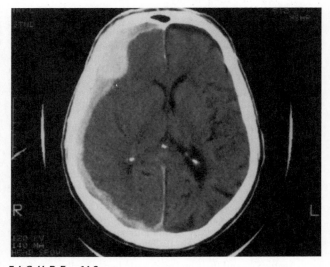

F I G U R E **14-2**
CT of the head without contrast agent enhancement, showing large subdural hematoma on the right side.

H. **Encephalitis**

This is a relatively uncommon cause of delirium, but one that should not be missed. Although there are many underlying causes, few are treatable. The most treatable causes are tertiary lues and herpes simplex. The **specific manifestations** of herpes simplex encephalitis include partial seizures, especially involving the temporal lobes, and a decreased level of consciousness. Often it occurs in young patients who are otherwise healthy. CSF protein will be markedly increased without any other abnormalities. **Specific management** includes obtaining magnetic resonance imaging (MRI), looking for temporal lobe involvement, and the empiric initiation of acyclovir, 5–10 mg/kg i.v., q.8hr for 10–14 days.

I. **Left ventricular failure**

Heart failure, especially forward failure, can manifest with delirium owing to the diffusely decreased perfusion and oxygenation of the cerebral cortex. The **specific manifestations and management** are discussed in the section on Congestive Heart Failure in Chapter 1, page 16.

J. **Hypothyroidism/hyperthyroidism**

Too much or too little thyroid hormone can result in delirium. Usually the diagnosis is clinically evident, and **specific management** is directed toward the underlying cause. For specific discussion on **manifestations and management**, see section on Thyroid Dysfunctional States, Chapter 9, page 497.

III. **Consultation**

Problem	Service	Time
Any focal deficits	Neurology	Emergent
Meningitis/encephalitis	Infectious disease	Emergent
Subdural hematoma	Neurosurgery	Emergent
Substance abuse	Addictionologist	Urgent
Suicide attempt	Psychiatry	Emergent

IV. **Indications for admission:** All cases of delirium, unless due to a rapidly reversible process (e.g., insulin-induced hypoglycemia corrected with glucose infusion).

Dementia (Box 14-3)

This is a nonspecific, insidious, progressive deterioration in intellectual and cognitive functioning. Whereas in the majority of cases, this process is irreversible, this is not necessarily always the case. The process, irrespective of the underlying cause, results in the steady loss of cortical neurons with resultant deterioration in higher brain functioning.

I. The **overall manifestations** are subtle early in the course of the disease and may not be recognized by family members or

B O X   14-3

Overall Evaluation and Management of Dementia

Evaluation

1. Thorough mental-status examination, including assessment of patient's orientation to person, place, and time.
2. Mental cognitive testing for baseline purposes.
3. Thyroid function tests, to uncover any hyperthyroidism or hypothyroidism.
4. Serum VDRL. If reactive, may be indicative of lues venereum.
5. Serum vitamin B_{12}, as a deficiency in vitamin B_{12} can result not only in megaloblastic anemia and neuropathy but also in a dementing process. If the B_{12} level is borderline, obtain a serum homocysteine level. See chapter 5, Anemia (page 253).
6. Serum electrolytes, BUN, and creatinine for baseline purposes.
7. Serum calcium, albumin, phosphorus, as hypercalcemia, hyperphosphatemia, or hypophosphatemia can manifest as or exacerbate a dementing process.
   NOTE: No other screening tests are indicated unless atypical features and/or concurrent findings are demonstrated on the history and physical examination.

Management

1. Discontinue, if possible, any medications that exacerbate dementia (e.g., the H_2 antagonist cimetidine).
2. Screen for depression by referral to a psychiatrist. Depression can often be an exacerbating factor or even the underlying mechanism for the patient's manifestations.
3. Social services consultation to outline and set in effect plans for outpatient nurse assistance and financial assistance.
4. Referral of family to support groups. Several organizations, as their primary goal, provide support to families of patients with dementing processes. The clinician must be aware of the various groups active in the community.
5. There is some evidence that cholinergic analogs (e.g., tacrine, 80 mg p.o., q.d.) may delay the manifestations of Alzheimer's disease. See text.

even by the patient. The cardinal manifestations of dementia, a deterioration in intellectual and cognitive functioning, can be demonstrated and documented by performing a thorough mental-status examination and the "mini-mental state" examination. Several other salient signs of this process can include:

A. **Frontal release signs**

These are signs of frontal lobe cortical deterioration that, when present, usually reflect moderately advanced disease. These abnormal signs include:

1. **Grasp.** Abnormal slow flexion of the patient's fingers around the examiner's fingers when examiner places fingers on patient's palm.

2. **Snout.** Abnormal puckering and protrusion of the patient's lips when the examiner rubs on the patient's lips medially to laterally.

3. **Sucking.** Abnormal sucking activity when the lips are rubbed by an examiner laterally to medially.

4. **Apraxia.** Acquired abnormal inability of the patient to perform a motor task that he knows, wants to perform, and has no specific motor or distal neurologic defect present to prevent its performance.

B. **Loss of inhibitions**

This is a very common manifestation of dementia in which the patient performs behaviorisms (e.g., inappropriate sexual contact) or says words (e.g., curses) that would be socially unacceptable and thus inhibited. The frontal lobes are the sites of learned inhibitions, and thus destruction of the frontal lobes can decrease these inhibitions.

C. **Inappropriate jocularity**

This is the significant increase in inappropriate verbal activity.

D. **Depression**

E. **Dementia,** irrespective of the underlying cause, can be exacerbated by concurrent medical and/or psychiatric problems. One of the best examples of such an exacerbating process is the common major affective disorder, depression.

II. **Management**

Long-term intervention includes support for family members and the development of schemes to manage the patient as an outpatient and, finally, when to admit the patient to a long-term care facility. In all cases, the family should be intimately involved in decision making, and a plan for future decisions must be formulated and formalized from the outset. These decisions include assignment of power of attorney for a family member, decisions on code status, and what criteria should be used for transfer to an extended-care facility. There are many support groups throughout the United States for families of patients with dementing diseases. The families should be encouraged to avail themselves of these groups.

There is some evidence that cholinergic analogs (e.g., tacrine, an agent that acts as an acetylcholinesterase inhibitor) may delay the manifestations of Alzheimer's disease. The dose is 10 mg p.o. q.i.d., maximum dose 160 mg/day; it may result in modest cholinergic side effects.

III. Consultation

Problem	Service	Time
Huntington's chorea	Genetics counselor	Elective
Subdural hematoma	Neurosurgeon	Urgent
All cases	Support groups	Elective
Extended-care facilities and plan	Geriatrician	Elective

IV. Indications for admission: Patient is unable to care for self or family members are unable to care for patient.

Gait Disturbances with Emphasis on Parkinson's Disease

Normal gait is the activity of a person as he is walking. This very complex process requires the action, interaction, and integration of many different parts of the central and peripheral nervous systems. It involves the cerebellum, the sense of vision, the senses of proprioception and touch, the basal ganglia, and the sensory and motor cortex. Because of its highly interactive and integrative mechanism, bipedal ambulation, a process that in most other animals is crude, to be streamlined and fluid, can be refined by learning new skills, and although basically the same in all normal people, has some modifications unique to each individual. An overall description of the normal gait is one foot in front of the other with the contralateral arm synchronously moving forward with each step.

I. Pathogenesis

The dark side of a process involving so many disparate sensory, motor, and integrative processes is that damage to one area can affect the whole process of normal ambulation. With increasing age, there is an increasing incidence of damage through various mechanisms to one or more of these areas. Damage to each specific area can and will result in different gait disturbances. See Table 14-4 for specific gaits, their **specific manifestations**, and therapy. One gait disturbance, that of parkinsonism, is discussed in detail.

A. Parkinson's disease and parkinsonism

This is a progressive, chronic disorder resulting from the atrophy and/or destruction of areas within the basal ganglia. It increases in incidence with age.

1. The **underlying pathogenesis** is a decrease in the neurotransmitter, dopamine, as a result of dopaminergic neu-

ronal destruction in the substantia nigra, with a resultant imbalance of acetylcholine to dopamine within the basal ganglia. The destruction of the substantia nigra, a rich site of dopaminergic neurons, can result from any of the causes listed, but irrespective of the underlying cause, the symptoms, signs, and for the most part the prognosis are the same.

2. **Causes**

   a. **Carbon monoxide poisoning.** High levels of CO can cause destruction of these cells and thus parkinsonism. Once present, the damage and manifestations are not reversible but will not progressively worsen.

   b. **Neuroleptic drugs.** These agents, which are commonly used for major psychiatric disorders, can result in acetylcholine–dopamine imbalance and parkinsonism. This is quite reversible on discontinuation of the agent.

   c. **Postencephalitis.** This postviral infection destruction of the basal ganglia was quite common after the influenza pandemic of 1918 and occasionally can be the presumptive cause today. This type, once present, is irreversible and progressively worsens.

   d. **Idiopathic.** Idiopathic destruction of the basal ganglia and substantia nigra is the cause in the vast majority of cases. This is the true Parkinson's disease, also known as "paralysis agitans."

3. The **overall manifestations** of parkinsonism in general and Parkinson's disease in specific include the following clinical features:

   a. **Gait disturbance** is the hallmark of this disorder, which is a direct manifestation of the **bradykinesis** (slowing of movement) inherent to parkinsonism. There is a significant bilateral decrease in arm swinging, the steps are bradykinetic (i.e., slow, shuffling, with a slightly flexed neck), and finally, the inability quickly to stop walking once initiated.

   b. **Tremor** is an integral component of the **manifestations**. The tremor is best demonstrated at rest and in the distal extremities and neck. It resolves with activity and is quite fine (i.e., has a frequency of four to six cycles/second). See Table 14-5 for other tremor syndromes.

   c. **Rigidity** of all musculature is often a feature. Rigidity is an abnormally increased resistance to passive movement. This results in, at baseline, a slight amount of flexion at the elbows and knees. The clinician can demonstrate this rigidity by passively moving the legs and forearms. The rigidity is often bilateral and usually has a component of "cogwheeling."

   d. **Dementia** is an integral component.

T A B L E 14-4
Gait Disturbances

Type	Manifestations	Causes	Treatment
Spastic hemi-paresis	Flexed upper extremity Arm immobile and held close to side Plantarflexed foot Circumduction of foot with foot dragging (all unilateral and contralateral to the side of the lesion)	Contralateral cerebrovascular accident (CVA) Contralateral head trauma	See CVA section (page 625) PT/OT
Parkinson's	Stooped, head-forward position Hips and knees flexed bilaterally Arms and wrists flexed bilaterally Rigid Bradykinetic Shuffling	Parkinson's disease Iatrogenic (neuroleptics) See text	See text, page 625 PT/OT
Scissors	Stiff bilaterally Thighs cross in front Short, hesitant steps bilaterally	Bilateral CVAs to the motor cortex Bilateral head trauma	See CVA section (page 625) PT/OT

Steppage	Foot drop, unilateral or bilateral Unable to dorsiflex foot, unilateral or bilateral Unable to walk on heel(s) Needs to flex knee to lift the foot	Trauma, especially to the proximal fibula, resulting in unilateral common peroneal nerve damage Charcot–Marie–Tooth syndrome: autosomal dominant, bilateral	PT/OT
Cerebellar	Wide-based, staggering gait Patient unable to stand steady when feet are together, eyes open or closed	CVA to cerebellum Acute ethanol intoxication Multiple sclerosis Vitamin B_{12} deficiency	Discontinue ethanol CT of head B_{12} levels (serum) Treat the underlying cause PT/OT
Sensory	Wide-based gait Feet in front of body center Improves when looking at the ground Sensory deficit/neuropathy in feet Charcot joints—traumatic degenerative joint disease	Diabetes mellitus Vitamin B_{12} deficiency *Lues venereum*	Control diabetes VDRL Serum B_{12} Treat the underlying cause

T A B L E 14-5
Tremor Disturbances

Type	Manifestations	Associated Features	Mechanism	Treatment
Parkinson's	Generalized, all motor areas involved At rest Frequency of 4–6 cycles/second Exacerbated by stressors	Bradykinesis Rigidity Dementia	Decrease in CNS neurotransmitter, dopamine	See text, page 647
Essential tremor	Predominantly in hands and head; lower extremities spared At rest Decreases with ethanol ingestion Onset at any age	None	Unknown May have a hereditary component	Usually nothing is needed, but if severe, treat with β-blocker (e.g., atenolol, 25–50 mg p.o., q.A.M. or primidone, 125 mg p.o., q.d.)
Cerebellar dysfunction	Distal motor areas more affected than proximal Intention tremor (i.e., occurs during voluntary motor activity)	Past pointing Decrease in fine motor skills Dysdiadochokinesis Decreased ability to perform finger-to-nose, heel-to-shin	Cerebellar CVA Multiple sclerosis Ethanol intoxication Vitamin B_{12} deficiency	Determine the cause and treat PT/OT Ethanol level as indicated
Hyperthyroid	Distal areas (hands and feet) affected more than proximal areas At rest	Weight loss Proximal weakness Goiter Eyelid lag	Increased levels of thyroid hormone	See text, page 497, chapter 9

B O X 14-4

***Overall Evaluation and Management
of Parkinson's Disease***

Evaluation

1. Thorough history and physical examination, to diagnose and document the type of gait and any of the
   concurrent manifestations described in text. Emphasis is placed on type of gait, presence of tremor, and
   presence of rigidity.
2. Examine patient for **concurrent manifestations** of autonomic dysfunction (i.e., lack of sweating, bladder
   or bowel incontinence, urine retention, orthostasis,
   or impotence).
3. Serum electrolytes, BUN, creatinine, and glucose for
   baseline purposes.
4. Serum calcium, albumin, and phosphorus. Abnormalities in calcium or phosphorus can exacerbate some
   of the features of parkinsonism.
5. If there are concurrent focal neurologic deficits, CT of
   the head is indicated to evaluate for any structural
   defects in the brain (e.g., CVA, subdural hematoma).

Management

1. Discontinue, if possible, all neuroleptic agents. Neuro-
   leptics deplete dopamine and can exacerbate the features of Parkinson's disease. In idiopathic Parkinson's disease, any neuroleptic [e.g., haloperidol
   (Haldol)] is effectively contraindicated.
2. Early consultation with OT and PT for assistance in
   management of the patient's mobility.
3. Initiate antiparkinsonian agents. The goal is to start
   only when symptomatic, as one will develop tolerance over time to the mainstay of therapy, levodopa.
   See Table 14-6 for specifics on these agents.
4. Family support. Several groups in the community
   provide support for family members of patients with
   Parkinson's disease.
5. Neurology consultation.

    e. Other features include an immobile face (mask fa-
cies), a depressed affect, and Myerson's sign [i.e.,
when the clinician taps over the bridge of the nose,
the patient continues to blink even after the fourth
tap (Box 14-4)].

T A B L E 14-6
Medications for Parkinson's Disease

Agent	Indications/Activity	Mechanism	Dosing	Side Effects
Selegeline	Early in the course of therapy Inhibits monoamine oxidase B	May decrease the generation of free radicals by reducing the oxidative metabolism of dopamine	2.5–5 mg p.o. b.i.d.	Minimal side effects
Levodopa	Initiate agent when disability is imminent Improves all manifestations	Decarboxylated to dopamine Increases dopamine To decrease side effects and increase dosage, carbidopa is added Carbidopa does not cross the blood–brain barrier and inhibits the peripheral conversion of L-dopa to dopamine by competitively inhibiting dopamine decarboxylase The carbidopa–levodopa ratio in the agent is 1:4 or 1:10, and has the trade name Sinemet (Sinemet is 25/100 or 10/100)	Start at low doses, e.g. Sinemet, 25/100 t.i.d., and slowly increase dose	Dyskinesia Hypotension Tachycardia

Drug	Indication	Mechanism	Dosage	Side effects
Amantadine	Early in course, when mild	Unknown	100 mg p.o. b.i.d.	Restlessness
Bromocriptine	Adjunctive therapy at any time	Direct stimulation of dopamine receptors	1.25 mg p.o. b.i.d., increasing the dose q. 2 wk by 2.5 mg; usual dose is 10–20 mg/day	Hypotension Tachycardia Nausea
Anticholinergic agents	Most effective in decreasing tremor Minimally effective in decreasing bradykinesis and rigidity	Unknown	Benztropine mesylate, (Cogentin) 1 mg p.o. q.d., increase slowly to 5 mg p.o. q.d. *or* Trihexyphenidyl (Artane), 2 mg p.o. t.i.d., increase slowly to 2–5 mg t.i.d.	Xerostomia Tachycardia Mydriasis Drowsiness Exacerbation of glaucoma

II. **Consultation**

Problem	Service	Time
All cases	Neurology	Required
All cases	OT/PT	Required

III. **Indications for admission:** Very few patients require admission until very late in the course of the disease.

Headaches

Virtually everyone has headaches on an intermittent basis. The vast majority of these headaches are self-limited and/or respond to relaxation, rest, and/or over-the-counter medications. Thus these headaches are, quite appropriately, not brought to the attention of the primary care physician. Several studies, however, have placed the percentage of people with recurrent, frequent headaches at 1%–3% of the population. Although the vast majority of these headaches are benign, a small number portend a malignant, even catastrophic, course.

I. **Types of headache**
  A. **Vascular headaches**
    1. **Migraines**
       This is a quite common form of recurrent headaches. It is postulated to be due to arterial vasoconstriction followed by vasodilation, with the resultant symptomatic manifestations; the underlying reason for the vasoconstriction and vasodilation is uncertain.
       a. The **specific manifestations** include a prodromal sensation or aura, followed by an intense, throbbing, usually unilateral headache that can become generalized. The headache, without **treatment**, usually lasts from 2 to 8 hours and then slowly resolves. Other **manifestations** include nausea, vomiting, photophobia, visual "stars," photopsia (i.e., the patient sensing unformed light flashes), and/or scintillating scotomas (i.e., the transient presence of visual field defects with luminous visual hallucinations). Furthermore, the patient desires to lie flat in bed in a dark room. The aura symptoms are secondary to the vasoconstriction, whereas the headache is associated with the vasodilation phase.
       b. **Family history** is specific for the fact that the first headache occurred during puberty and that one or more first-degree relatives also have similar headaches. The headaches are recurrent and can occur with a frequency of once per day to once per year. The patient may notice that specific habits or agents precipitate these headaches. These precipitating activities can include, but are not limited to, the inges-

tion of chocolate, ingestion of ethanol, a period of stress, or a menstrual cycle.

c. There are several variants of migraine headaches, each with specific unique manifestations. These variants include:

   i. **Classic migraine** has an antecedent aura.
   ii. **Common migraine** has no antecedent aura.
   iii. **Basilar artery migraine** is a special form of classic migraine, which affects the basilar artery. The patient has an aura that consists of bilateral visual field cuts, dysarthria, tinnitus, vertigo, tingling in the trigeminal nerve (V1, V2, and V3) distribution, and delirium. The headache is throbbing and located in the occipital regions bilaterally.

d. The **specific evaluation and management** include making the clinical diagnosis, acutely treating the pain, and, as clinically indicated, initiating prophylaxis. Short-term management consists of placing the patient in a dark, quiet room. See Box 14-5 for specific therapies.

   If the headache does not resolve or if any complications or new focal neurologic deficits are manifest, CT of the head must be performed to evaluate for other causes.

e. If the patient has recurrent headaches on a frequent basis, usually defined as more than four per month, prophylactic intervention should be strongly considered. Preventive measures include avoidance of precipitating factors and pharmacologic prophylactic intervention. Some agents in prophylaxis can include:

   i. **β-Blockers.** Either propranolol, 10–20 mg p.o., q.i.d., or atenolol, 25–50 mg p.o., q.A.M., can be effective in prophylaxis. One must not use if contraindicated (bronchospasm, heart failure, etc.) and furthermore, one must closely monitor blood pressure while using these agents.
   ii. **Calcium channel blockers.** Verapamil SR, 120–240 mg p.o., q.A.M., or nifedipine XL (Procardia XL), 30 mg p.o., q.d., can be effective. Monitor blood pressure closely.
   iii. Amitriptyline (Elavil), 25–50 mg p.o., q.H.S., is quite an effective prophylaxis.
   iv. An attempt should be made every 3–6 months to wean the patient from any type of prophylactic therapy.

f. Neurology consultation should be obtained for any patient with complications or when prophylaxis is necessary. Admission to the hospital is indicated if

B O X 14-5

Medications for Acute Headache
- Cafergot, the combination of ergotamine and caffeine, 1–4 tablets p.o. or p.r., at the onset of the headache;

-or-

- Fiorcet or Esgic, the combination of butalbital, caffeine, and acetaminophen, two tablets p.o. at outset and then one tablet p.o. q.6hr;

-or-

- Sumatriptan, 25 mg p.o., at outset of headache, may repeat q.1hr times 2 (24-hour maximum, 100 mg);

-or-

- Sumatriptan (Imitrex), 6 mg s.c., at outset, may repeat q.1hr times one dose (maximum dose, 12 mg/24 hr);

-or-

- Ketorolac (Toradol), 30–60 mg i.m., at outset, and then 15–30 mg i.m. q.6hr;

-or-

- Meperidine (Demerol), 50 mg i.m.

-or-

- Chlorpromazine, 25 mg i.v.; may repeat in 30 minutes with a second dose;

-or-

- Prochlorperazine, 2.5–5.0 mg i.v., times one dose

any complications occur or if pain has not resolved with aggressive outpatient management.
2. **Cluster headaches**
   These headaches are another variant of vascular headaches.
   a. The specific **manifestations** include an acute onset, throbbing, and unilateral headaches. Rarely is there an antecedent aura. These headaches often occur at night and awaken the patient from a sound sleep. These headaches last 1–6 hours, and often the patient will have several episodes in a finite period (1–2 weeks), followed by a period of no headaches (months to years), only to have another cluster of headaches occur. The patient can develop associated nasal congestion, conjunctival injection, and even a transient Horner's syndrome concurrent with the headache. In most cases, the patient will be agitated and pacing the room during the headache.
   b. The specific **management** includes the following

features. Acutely, 100% Fio$_2$ by facial mask for 15–20 minutes is very effective. Otherwise the acute intervention is quite similar to that described in migraine headaches section (Box 14-5). The long-term management is analogous to that for migraine headaches in that pharmacologic prophylactic intervention is not necessary unless the condition is quite frequent. One of several prophylactic agents can be used.

    i. β-Blocker. Same dosing as in migraine headaches (page 651).

    ii. Calcium channel blocker. Same dosing as in migraine headaches (page 651).

    iii. Lithium carbonate. Its use is indicated in severe cases that are refractory to standard therapy. In addition to closely monitoring the lithium levels, the clinician must monitor the patient for the development of any side effects of the lithium (e.g., nephrogenic diabetes insipidus).

    iv. Prednisone. In low doses (i.e., 10 mg p.o., q.d.), can be effective in prophylaxis. The disadvantage of this **modality** of prophylaxis is that it is fraught with the side effects of long-term glucocorticoid use.

    v. One must attempt to wean the patient from any prophylactic agent each 3–6 months.

  c. Neurology consultation should be obtained for any patient with complications. Admission to the hospital is indicated if complications occur or if pain is not resolved with aggressive outpatient management.

B. Tension headaches

Tension is one of the most common causes of solitary and/or recurrent headaches.

  1. The **specific manifestations** include the subacute onset of a vague, potentially intense headache. The headache is quite often bilateral. Pain usually begins in the occipital area and then becomes generalized. The headaches can recur daily. There are usually no associated features except for a decreased attention span. Usually these headaches begin or are worse in the afternoon or evening. Other than tension or stress, other factors may be involved in their pathogenesis, including a concurrent vascular component and/or an uncorrected myopia.

  2. The **specific evaluation and management** include querying the patient for any refractory visual changes and performing a visual acuity examination to diagnose such a problem. **Specific management** includes recommending the patient obtain a neck massage from spouse or significant other or take hot baths to relax any tense occipital muscles. Pharmacologic intervention can include:

a. Acetaminophen, 500–1,000 mg p.o., now and q.4–6hr for one to two doses, or

b. NSAID: ibuprofen (Motrin, Advil, Nuprin), 400–800 mg p.o., q.8hr prn.

c. If there is any suggestion of a vascular component to the headache, a trial of one of the agents listed for acute intervention in migraines is indicated (see Box 14-5). Particularly effective agents include either ketorolac (Toradol) 30–60 mg i.m. or sumatriptan 6 mg s.c. If there is any visual refractory dysfunction, referral to an ophthalmologist for corrective lenses is indicated.

d. If the headaches are recurrent, even with adequate **treatment**, or if they progressively worsen, biofeedback and evaluation with neurology are indicated.

C. **CVA/Hypertensive emergency**

The mechanism of headache development in these processes is uncertain.

1. The **specific manifestations** include the acute onset of a severe, generalized headache. The headache in a hypertensive emergency may be the chief complaint of the patient. These headaches are quite common if the hypertensive emergency is due to a pheochromocytoma. The headache of a subarachnoid hemorrhage is of acute onset, generalized, constant, and classically described as the worst of the patient's life.

2. The **evaluation and management** of this type of headache are discussed in the section on Hypertension in Chapter 3, page 142, and in the section on Cerebrovascular Accidents, page 625.

D. **Intracranial mass**

These result in headaches that are thought to be secondary to the displacement of vascular structures by the intracranial mass itself.

1. The **specific manifestations** include that quite often it is generalized, recurrent, and, with time, progresses in intensity and severity. This type of headache will often awaken the patient from a sound sleep and, unlike cluster headaches, is not associated with agitation. Because most intracranial masses occur in middle to late ages, an onset of generalized, recurrent headaches in any patient in these age groups should increase suspicion of an intracranial mass. This type of headache is classically exacerbated by a Valsalva maneuver (cough, straining with bowel movement) and eventually will manifest with concurrent focal neurologic deficits, seizures, or syncope.

2. The **differential diagnosis** of intracranial masses includes the following:

   a. **Metastatic neoplastic disease.** Usually from adenocarcinomas with primary lesions in the lungs, breast, or colon. The lesions are usually multiple, located at the border of the gray and white matter, and ~1–2 cm. There may be adjacent edema.

   b. **Primary neoplastic disease.** Lymphoproliferative or astrocytoma or glioblastoma multiforme. These lesions are usually unilateral, have irregular margins, and have adjacent edema.

   c. **Abscesses.** These can be single or multiple. They may be due to bacterial agents, usually anaerobic bacteria, or to the opportunistic protozoan organism, *Toxoplasma gondii.*

3. The **specific evaluation and management** include aggressive **evaluation and management** if an intracranial mass is suspected.

   a. CT of the head with and without contrast with imaging of the posterior fossa is clearly indicated. Indications for CT imaging include:

      i. The onset of severe, recurrent headaches in a patient older than 35 years.

      ii. Exacerbation of the headache on a Valsalva maneuver.

      iii. The presence of any neurologic defects, fevers, papilledema, or change in mental status or level of consciousness (Fig. 14-3).

      iv. Severe headaches in an immunocompromised patient.

   b. If further imaging is required, MRI has the highest sensitivity and specificity.

   c. The bottom-line need is for tissue to diagnose the lesion. The easiest way is to look for the primary neoplastic lesion and perform a biopsy of that; however, if no extracranial primary lesion is found, biopsy of the brain lesion is indicated. The biopsy should be histopathologically examined and sent for Gram stain, bacterial cultures, and AFB cultures.

   d. If there is any evidence of edema, initiation of parenteral dexamethasone is indicated (10 mg i.v., stat, and then 2–4 mg i.v. q.4hr), as is consultation with neurosurgery.

   e. In virtually all cases in which the headache is due to an intracranial mass, admission to the hospital with neurosurgical consultation is required.

   f. If tumor is present, oncology consultation is indicated, whereas if an abscess or *Toxoplasma gondii* is present, a human immunodeficiency virus (HIV)

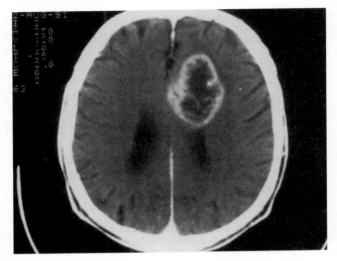

F I G U R E **14-3**
CT of the head with contrast showing a large contrast-enhancing lesion
in the left frontal/parietal areas. The differential diagnosis of contrast-
enhancing lesions includes abscesses, including those caused by
Toxoplasma gondii, lymphomas, and, as in this case, glioblastoma.

test should be performed and an infectious diseases
consultation obtained.

E. **Morning headaches**

These are headaches of uncertain **pathogenesis**, which can
be due to several discrete causes.

1. The **specific manifestations** include the fact that these
headaches are present at time of awakening and resolve
over the course of the day. Further specifics are related
to the three most common underlying causes.

   a. **Ethanol-related "hangover,"** in which the patient
   ingests ethanol the evening before and awakens with
   nausea and a generalized headache. The **specific
   management** includes instructing the patient not to
   binge drink.

   b. **Sleep apnea syndrome.** This is a syndrome in which
   the patient develops abnormally prolonged periods
   of apnea during sleep. These episodes of apnea are
   usually the result of excessive pharyngeal tissue,
   which occurs predominantly in obese patients.
   These periods of apnea lead to episodes of hypercapnia, hypoxemia, and a lack of restful sleep. The associated **manifestations** include severe snoring and

falling asleep at inappropriate times during the day. The patient can fall asleep during a routine conversation or even while driving an automobile. The **specific evaluation and management** include a formal sleep study and consultation with pulmonary medicine.

   c. **Nocturnal exposure to carbon monoxide:** older homes with older heating systems increase the risk of CO exposure.

F. **Tic douloureux** (trigeminal neuralgia)

This is the dysfunction, often idiopathic, of the peripheral component of CNV. CNV supplies sensation to the face via three branches: V1, to the forehead; V2, to the maxillary skin; and V3, to the mandibular skin.

   1. The **specific manifestations** include the acute onset of severe, lancing pain that begins at the mouth and radiates to the ipsilateral eye and ear. Virtually always unilateral, it usually involves V2 and V3 more than V1 (i.e., below the eye more than above the eye). This will spontaneously resolve only acutely to return several times in a short period. There can be and often are extended periods without symptoms. However, with increasing age, there is a decrease in the interval between episodes, and the episodes increase in intensity, duration, and frequency.

   2. The **specific evaluation and management** include making the clinical diagnosis. Further evaluation can include MRI of the posterior fossa to look for a small glioma in that area, which could be surgically resected. Refraining from agents/activities that can precipitate the symptoms (e.g., touching the overlying skin, chewing ice) is very important. Pharmacologic intervention includes initiation of carbamazepine (Tegretol) 100 mg p.o. b.i.d., on a long-term basis. If still symptomatic, ablation of the trigeminal nerve/ganglion may be indicated. Therefore, consultations with neurology and a pain-care specialist are indicated.

G. **Carious teeth, sinusitis, and leptomeningitis**

These conditions will also cause headaches. Each is discussed in separate sections pages 569, 590, and 658, respectively).

II. **Consultation**

Problem	Service	Time
Vascular headaches	Neurology	Urgent/emergent
Neurologic deficits	Neurology	Urgent/emergent
Intracranial masses	Neurosurgery	Urgent/emergent

III. **Indications for admission:** New focal deficits, CT-proven intracranial masses, or any evidence of leptomeningitis.

Meningitis

Leptomeningitis is the nonspecific inflammation of the leptomeninges themselves, including the dura mater, the arachnoid mater, and the pia mater. The dura mater is the thick, fibrous layer immediately adjacent (deep) to the bones of the skull and vertebral column. The pia mater is a thin, pliable layer of tissue intimately apposed to the spinal cord and surface of the brain. In between is the lacy and fine connective-tissue layer of the arachnoid mater. There are two spaces of anatomic importance: the subdural space, between dura mater and bone, and the subarachnoid space, between the pia mater and arachnoid mater. The subarachnoid space is filled with CSF and is the space from which CSF is obtained during a lumbar puncture (Box 14-6).

I. The **overall manifestations** at presentation include a decrease in the level of consciousness, even to the point of coma, delirium, convulsions, recurrent fevers, headaches, neck stiffness, nausea, and vomiting. Presenting signs include nuchal rigidity, Kernig's sign (abnormal involuntary flexion of the neck on passive extension of the knee when the patient is supine with the hip flexed), and/or Brudzinski's sign (abnormal flexion of the hips on passively flexing the patient's neck with the patient supine).

II. **Causes**

The causes are quite diverse and are best divided into categories of bacterial, viral, neoplastic, and mycobacterial causes.

A. **Bacterial**

Bacterial infections cause acute leptomeningitis, which if untreated, will result in the death of the patient. Each of the following organisms discussed can cause acute leptomeningitis in adults.

1. *Neisseria meningitidis.* This gram-negative coccus causes a severe meningitis and systemic illness.

a. The **specific manifestations** include the overall manifestations (see the preceding) in addition to acquired petechiae, purpura, menometrorrhagia, bleeding gingivae, and epistaxis, all as a result of an acquired consumptive coagulopathy specific to *Neisseria meningitidis*. The **natural history** of untreated disease entails sepsis and rapid death of the patient.

b. The **laboratory evaluation** (Box 14-6) includes the peripheral white blood cell (WBC) count, which usually is increased. If the WBC is inappropriately low, it can be a harbinger of impending septic shock. The CSF will have an increased protein, a decreased glucose, and an increased WBC, usually with predominance of polymorphonuclear (PMN) cells. Gram stain of the CSF shows PMN cells and gram-

B O X 14-6

*Overall Evaluation and Management
of Suspected Leptomeningitis*

Evaluation

1. ABCs (i.e., basic and advanced life support protocol), as needed.
2. Establish intravenous access in preparation for imminent administration of parenteral antibiotics.
3. Blood cultures are clearly indicated, as the pathogen can be grown from the blood in a significant minority of cases.
4. Complete blood cell count with differential for baseline purposes. In most cases of leptomeningitis, there is a significant leukocytosis and a left shift in the differential count.
5. PT, aPTT, platelets, and fibrinogen are important for baseline purposes as certain etiologies of leptomeningitis, specifically *Neisseria meningitidis,* can cause a severe consumptive coagulopathy.
6. Serum electrolytes, calcium, albumin, and PO_4 for baseline purposes.
7. Lumbar puncture—mandatory (see Table 14-7 for laboratory examinations performed on the CSF and their normal values).

Management

1. If a bacterial etiology is suspected:
   Ceftriaxone 2 g i.v.
   -or-
   Chloramphenicol 12.5 mg/kg i.v.;
   -and-
   Vancomycin 1 g i.v.
   -and-
   Dexamethasone 0.4 mg/kg i.v.
2. Admit to an inpatient service.

negative cocci. Latex agglutination of the CSF will be positive for *Neisseria meningitidis* capsular antigen. A disseminated intravascular coagulation (DIC) panel (platelets, PT, PTT, and fibrinogen) should be performed to determine whether a consumptive coagulopathy is present.

  c. **Management** includes the basics as described in Box 14-6 and aggressive, intensive, and immediate anti-

T A B L E   14-7
Cerebrospinal Fluid: Routine Tests and Normal Values

Test	Normal Value
Cell count with differential	0–5 WBCs per hpf, all mononuclear
Protein level	15–45 mg/dL
Glucose level	40–80 mg/dL (1/2 of serum glucose)
Gram stain	No cells, no organisms
AFB smear	No AFB
VDRL	Nonreactive
Latex agglutination for capsule antigens in *Streptococcus pneumoniae*, *Haemophilus influenzae*, and *Neisseria meningitidis*	None detectable
Bacterial culture	No growth
Mycobacterial culture	No growth
Cytology	No cells

biotic therapy. This is a disease process that mandates emergency antibiotics. The essential element is time. Immediate therapy is of the essence. Regimens include:

  i. Ceftriaxone 2 g i.v. q.12hr or, if the patient is penicillin allergic, chloramphenicol 12.5 mg/kg i.v., q.6hr. In addition, the patient should receive vancomycin 1 g i.v. q.12hr and dexamethasone 0.4 mg/kg i.v. q.12hr for four doses.

All regimens must be continued for 10 days or until patient is afebrile for 5 concurrent days (whichever is longer). Further principles of therapy include fluid management, **treatment** of DIC (see section on Excessive Bleeding States in Chapter 5, page 268), and placing the patient in respiratory isolation.

  d. **Prevention** is of great importance, as this disease can have morbid and even mortal outcomes, even with effective therapy early in the course. Prevention consists of placing patient in respiratory isolation, as the transmission of this pathogen is by respiratory secretions, and the prescription of rifampin, 600 mg p.o., b.i.d., for 2 days (10 mg/kg b.i.d. for 2 days in children) to any exposed contacts (e.g., members of the household, day-care members, or nursing home residents).

e. Complications of this specific form of meningeal infection include, in addition to death, the following entities: neurosensory deafness, which is usually transient; intracranial abscess formation; DIC; hydrocephalus; and/or adrenal insufficiency as a result of Waterhouse–Friderichsen syndrome.

2. *Haemophilus influenzae*
   This gram-negative coccobacillus, usually of the capsular type b, will cause a severe leptomeningitis.

   a. The **specific manifestations** include the basic symptoms and signs as described after an antecedent period of upper respiratory symptoms. This form of meningitis is much more common in young children than in adults, but still must be considered in the differential diagnosis of adult leptomeningitis.

   b. The **laboratory evaluation** (Box 14-6) includes the peripheral WBC count, which usually is increased. If the WBC is inappropriately low, it can be a harbinger of impending septic shock. The CSF will have an increased protein, a decreased glucose, and an increased WBC, usually with predominance of PMN cells. Gram stain of the CSF shows PMNs and gram-negative coccobacilli. Latex agglutination will be positive for *Haemophilus influenzae* capsular antigen.

   c. Management includes the basics as described in Box 14-5 and antibiotics. Antibiotic regimens include:
   Ceftriaxone, 2 g i.v., q.12hr; or
   Chloramphenicol, 12.5 mg/kg i.v. q.6hr and dexamethasone 0.4 mg/kg i.v. for four doses.
   Either regimen is given for 10 days.

   d. Prevention is also a major concern in this disease. Although it has fewer complications than *Neisseria meningitidis,* it can cause hydrocephalus and death. Preventive measures include:
   i. *H. influenzae* type b polysaccharide vaccine in all children aged 2–5 years (irrespective of exposure), and
   ii. Contacts should be given rifampin, 600 mg p.o. q.d for 4 consecutive days.

3. *Streptococcus pneumoniae.* This gram-positive diplococcus causes an acute meningitis.

   a. The **specific manifestations** include the **overall manifestations** as described along with, in virtually all cases, an antecedent otitis media, lobar pneumonitis, or upper respiratory tract infection. A **specific risk factor** for the development of this and other streptococcal infections is the presence of asplenia and/or hypogammaglobulinemia.

   b. The **laboratory evaluation** (Box 14-6) includes the peripheral WBC count, which usually is increased. If the WBC count is inappropriately low, it can be a harbinger of impending septic shock. The CSF will have an increased protein, a decreased glucose, and an increased WBC, usually with predominance of PMN cells. Gram stain of the CSF shows PMNs and gram-positive diplococci. Latex agglutination will be positive for *S. pneumoniae* capsular antigen.

c. Management includes the steps listed in Box 14-6 and initiation of antibiotics. Specific antibiotic regimens include:

Ceftriaxone, 2 g i.v., q.12hr and vancomycin 1 g i.v q.12hr and dexamethasone 0.4 mg/kg i.v. q.12hr for 2 days.

Either regimen is given for 10 days.

d. Prevention is important, as severe morbidity and mortality can result, even in optimally treated cases. Observation of patient contacts and early **treatment** is probably the most effective.

4. ***Listeria monocytogenes.*** This gram-positive rod can cause a leptomeningitis in adults.

a. The **specific manifestations** of this type of meningitis include fewer classic findings and thus a more subacute presentation. Many patients have mild mental status changes associated with a low-grade fever. Nuchal rigidity and the classic findings of meningeal irritation often are not present until late in the course. Groups at particularly high risk for this pathogen include alcoholics and patients receiving long-term steroid therapy.

b. The **laboratory evaluation** (Box 14-6) includes the peripheral WBC count, which usually is increased. If the WBC count is inappropriately low, it can be a harbinger of impending septic shock. The CSF will have an increased protein, a decreased glucose, and an increased WBC count, usually with predominance of PMN cells. Gram stain of the CSF shows PMNs and, rarely but diagnostically, gram-positive rods. Latex agglutination will be negative for capsular antigens. The diagnosis is presumptive until cultures return. The clinician must use care not to overlook this pathogen, as it can be confused with "diphtheroids" (i.e., contaminants). Therefore, the clinician must interpret test results in the context of the patient.

c. Management includes the steps listed in Box 14-6 and antibiotics, usually broad-spectrum antibiotics until cultures return with diagnostic confirmation. Regimens to treat *Listeria monocytogenes* include:

Ampicillin, 2 g i.v., q.4–6hr or TMP-sulfa (TMP 5 mg/kg) i.v. q.6hr.

Either regimen is given for 10–14 days.

d. Prevention is essentially having a clinical suspicion in patients with appropriate **manifestations** who are in high-risk groups and proscribing the use of unpasteurized products by patients at high risk.

B. **Viral meningitis**

Also referred to as "aseptic meningitis," this can be caused by many of the RNA viruses, including enteroviruses and picornaviruses.

1. The **specific manifestations** include an antecedent, several-day history of malaise, fever, mild neck stiffness, myalgias, and upper respiratory symptoms and signs. The neck stiffness gradually worsens and becomes associated with headache, nausea, and intermittent vomiting. This is quite seasonal, and epidemics are not uncommon in late summer and early autumn.

2. The **laboratory evaluation** includes the steps listed in Box 14-5. In the peripheral WBC count, there usually is a mild leukocytosis with lymphocyte predominance. The CSF will have a normal glucose, mildly increased protein, and a mild increase in WBCs, all of which are mononuclear. Gram stain is negative for PMNs or organisms. Latex agglutination is negative for capsular antigens.

3. Management is supportive. Antibiotics are not indicated unless suspicion of a bacterial cause is relatively high or the patient is immunosuppressed. If the patient is delirious or if HSV encephalitis is in the differential diagnoses, start acyclovir i.v. This is the only form of meningitis in which the patient can, if stable, be managed as an outpatient.

C. **Meningeal carcinomatosis**

This is a type of leptomeningitis in which the infiltrate is not as a result of infection and its resultant inflammatory response but of malignant neoplastic cells.

1. The **specific manifestations** are usually quite insidious but, once present, can consist of the classic findings of meningitis. The patient usually has acquired CN defects, especially a peripheral CN VII palsy. Many patients have a history of malignant metastatic neoplastic disease, especially adenocarcinomas of the lungs, breast, or colon, or leukemias or lymphomas.

2. The **laboratory evaluation** includes the steps listed in Box 14-5. The CSF reveals a normal glucose and a markedly increased protein. Gram stain of the CSF is negative for organisms, cell count usually with "atypical cells" present, and cytologic examination is positive for ma-

lignant cells. MRI is indicated, especially of the posterior fossa, to demonstrate the extent of leptomeningeal and adjacent structural involvement.

3. The **management** of this process is beyond the scope of this text. A consultation with oncology is indicated. Cranial irradiation or intrathecal chemotherapy (methotrexate) is indicated, under the direction of the oncologist.

D. **Mycobacterial** (See also Chapter 6, see Table 14-16, page 246, for mycobacterial treatment)

This organism can spread from lungs to extrapulmonary sites either in primary (if miliary) or reactivation mycobacterial disease.

1. The **specific manifestations** of this entity can be very insidious and consist of headache, constitutional symptoms, and moderate recurrent nausea and vomiting. Nuchal rigidity and the classic features of meningeal irritation develop only late in the course of disease. Cranial nerve deficits can also develop, especially of CNs VII and/or XII.

2. The **laboratory evaluation** includes the steps listed in Box 14-6. The CSF will have a normal glucose, a markedly increased protein that may and often does exceed 500 mg/dL, at times >2 g protein, and an increase in WBCs, the majority of which are mononuclear. Gram stain is negative for organisms but shows mononuclear cells. Latex agglutination is negative. AFB smears and cultures are positive for *Mycobacterium hominis*. Urinalysis with AFB smear/culture and chest radiography are mandatory components of the evaluation, as the primary location—pulmonary or urologic—can thus be uncovered.

3. **Management** includes placing the patient in respiratory isolation if the patient has active pulmonary disease. A course of four antimycobacterial agents is indicated:
   a. Isoniazid, 300 mg p.o., q.d.
   b. Rifampin, 600 mg p.o., q.d.
   c. Ethambutol, 15 mg/kg/day p.o.
      All three for 24 consecutive months;
      -and-
   d. Streptomycin,* 1 g i.m., q.d. for 2 weeks, and then twice per week for 10 weeks;
      -or-
   e. Pyrazinamide, 25 mg/kg/day p.o., in a q.d. dosing for 24 months.

   If CN deficits are present or developing, steroids are indicated: prednisone, 60 mg p.o., q.d. As this is a chronic disease, nutritional support must be optimized.

E. **Subarachnoid hemorrhage**
This catastrophic event can manifest with acute meningeal

manifestations. See section on Cerebrovascular Accidents, page 625, for further discussion.

III. Consultation

Problem	Service	Time
Bacterial meningitides	Infectious diseases	Urgent/emergent
Mycobacterial	Infectious diseases	Urgent
Meningeal carcinomatosis	Hematology/oncology	Urgent

IV. Indications for admission:
Bacterial meningitis, aseptic meningitis if unable to maintain volume orally, mycobacterial or neoplastic meningitis.

Seizure Disorders

A seizure is any uncontrolled abnormal activity of the brain. It can have a variety of findings ranging from a blank stare to generalized clonic activity to repetitive, automatic movements. The differential diagnosis, workup, and management are essentially the same for all seizure types, irrespective of the presenting features and manifestations (Box 14-7).

I. Overall manifestations

A. Convulsions
A convulsion is a specific form of seizure in which the **manifestations** include uncontrolled motor activity. The tonic–clonic convulsion is the classic example that is the type the general public usually thinks of when describing a seizure.

1. **Tonic.** A convulsion in which the major motor component is profound rigidity (i.e., the tone of the musculature is markedly and uncontrollably increased). This can occur alone or as a prelude to clonic activity. The classic tonic convulsion is opisthotonus, in which the patient is rigid and has a hyperextended neck. A tonic convulsive seizure is uniformly generalized.

2. **Clonic.** A convulsion in which the major motor component is rapid repetitive uncontrolled activity. This often is associated with tonic activity. A clonic convulsive seizure is uniformly generalized.

B. Epilepsy
The presence of recurrent seizures of any kind, classically idiopathic. This is a colloquial term for seizures and/or convulsions.

C. Status epilepticus
The onset of a seizure that does not spontaneously resolve, requiring emergency medical intervention. Any uncontrolled seizure, irrespective of **manifestations** or cause, must be treated aggressively as status epilepticus. The

B O X 14-7

Overall Evaluation and Management of Status Epilepticus and Seizures

Evaluation

1. ABCs (i.e., basic and advanced life support protocols), as necessary. During the seizure, maintenance of an airway is fundamental.
2. Intravenous access must be obtained for the potential administration of glucose, benzodiazepines, or antiseizure medications.
3. Basic laboratory studies, stat:
   a. Arterial blood gases.
   b. Serum calcium, albumin, magnesium, and PO_4.
   c. Serum glucose.
   d. Serum electrolytes.
   e. Antiseizure drug levels (see Table 14-9 for normal levels).
   f. Blood ethanol level.

Management

1. Thiamine, 100 mg i.v., followed by one ampule of $D_{50}W$ i.v.
2. Benzodiazepines to control the seizure immediately, either lorazepam (Ativan), 2–3 mg i.v., stat, repeated as necessary in 15–20 minutes; or diazepam (Valium), 5–10 mg i.v., stat, repeated as necessary in 15–30 minutes.
3. Initiate long-term therapy as clinically indicated with phenytoin (Dilantin), 800–1,000 mg i.v. loading dose, in one of the following protocols.
   a. 20 mg/min, usually by slow i.v. push of 8–10 100-mg prefilled syringes, each administered over 5 minutes, or
   b. 1,000 mg in 250 mL of 0.45 NS i.v. drip over 1 hour.
4. If patient is still actively seizing, add phenobarbital, 10–15 mg/kg (700–1,000 mg) by slow i.v. push at a rate of 50 mg/min.
5. CT scan of the head without contrast is especially important if there is any history of trauma or any evidence of papilledema or of new focal neurologic deficits.

(continued)

B O X 14-7 *(continued)*

6. Lumbar puncture if there is any evidence of or suspicion for leptomeningitis. See section on Meningitis, page 658.
7. Serum VDRL to evaluate for lues venereum. If reactive, should be performed on CSF.
8. EEG, to be performed under the guidance of a neurologist after admission and stabilization of patient.
9. Neurology consultation.

acute **evaluation and management** of this state are discussed subsequently.

II. **Causes**

The differential diagnosis of seizures, irrespective of **manifestations**, is essentially the same. The most likely causes for new-onset seizures are different for young adults (i.e., age 15–45 years), when compared with middle-aged and older adults (i.e., age older than 45 years). Each of the following lists is by order of frequency in each age group.

A. **Causes in younger adults**
1. **Head trauma.** Individuals in this group are usually quite active and at risk for head trauma through contact sports, motor vehicle (especially motorcycle) accidents, and ethanol-related falls.
2. **Withdrawal** from drugs, especially withdrawal from ethanol.
3. **Acute ingestion of agents,** especially tricyclic antidepressants, in a suicide attempt.
4. **Space-occupying lesions** in the cranium. These can be neoplastic (benign or malignant) or, especially in immunocompromised patients, due to infectious agents. The two most common infectious agents are anaerobic bacteria and *Toxoplasma.*
5. **Leptomeningitis.** See section on Meningitis, page 658.
6. **Idiopathic.** This is a diagnosis of exclusion; occasionally the cause of recurrent seizures (epilepsy) cannot be determined.

B. **Causes in older adults**
1. **Space-occupying lesions** in the cranium. These are usually neoplastic lesions, either malignant primary lesions (e.g., glioblastoma multiforme) or metastatic lesions. Lesions that commonly metastasize to the brain are colon, breast, and lung cancers and malignant melanomas.

2. **CVAs** may result in a seizure disorder.
3. **Metabolic or electrolyte abnormalities.** These conditions significantly increase in frequency in the elderly population as patients are given medications (e.g., insulin, diuretics) that can significantly affect electrolyte balance. At baseline, patients may be at increased risk for electrolyte or metabolic disorders that can precipitate seizures. Examples of such electrolyte or metabolic causes include:
   a. Hypokalemia.
   b. Hypocalcemia.
   c. Hypophosphatemia.
   d. Hyponatremia.
   e. Hypoxemia.
   f. Hypoglycemia.
4. **Leptomeningitis.** See section on Meningitis, page 658.
5. **Withdrawal from drugs,** especially withdrawal from ethanol.

III. **Classification of seizure disorders** (modified from the International League Against Epilepsy criteria, see Table 14-8).
   A. **Partial seizures**
      These are seizures in which only a small portion of the cerebral cortex has uncontrolled activity. The **manifestations** can be diverse and are specific to the area involved. Any partial seizure can become, either acutely or longitudinally, a generalized seizure disorder. There are two subtypes of partial seizures, simple and complex.
      1. The **specific manifestations** of simple partial seizures are distinct from those of other seizures in that the

T A B L E 14-8
Classification and General Management of Seizures

Type	Symptoms and Signs	Treatment
Partial Simple Complex	Automatisms Mania/delirium Deja vu	Carbamazepine (Tegretol)
Generalized, absence (petit mal)	Acute onset of blank stare Incontinence Decreased postural tone	Valproic acid (Depakene)
Generalized, tonic–clonic (grand mal)	Aura, followed by tonic motor activity, followed by clonic motor activity, with a period of lethargy after cessation of motor activity	Phenytoin (Dilantin)/ Phenobarbital

patient does not lose consciousness. These seizures can manifest with focal motor activity (location, motor cortex), tactile sensation/hallucination (location, sensory cortex), perception of deja vu (perception that time at present has been lived or experienced before, even on a recurrent basis; location, lower cerebral cortex), and automatic behaviorisms (e.g., snapping the fingers, mania, or delirium; location, temporal cortex).

2. The **specific manifestations** of complex partial seizures include loss of consciousness. Complex partial seizures can be associated with the **manifestations** described for simple partial seizures either before or after the event and can, like partial simple seizures, become secondarily generalizable.

3. Although the **evaluation and management** of these seizures are similar for all seizure types (see Box 14-7), several caveats are in order. The clinician must look for an intracranial structural defect if the seizure is partial. If a partial seizure is localized to the temporal region, herpes simplex encephalitis is in the differential diagnosis. **Treatment** specifics include the initiation of antibiotics for leptomeningitis, the use of acyclovir in a dose of 10 mg/kg i.v. q.8hr, for 14 days, and MRI of the temporal lobes if herpes simplex encephalitis is suspected.

B. **Generalized seizures**

These are seizures in which the entire cerebral cortex is involved. They may begin as partial seizures or may be the first indication of a seizure disorder. In all generalized seizures, there is a loss of consciousness with amnesia for the seizure itself. There are two major types of generalized seizures, absence type and tonic–clonic type.

1. The **specific manifestations of absence (petit mal)** seizures include an abrupt onset and termination, and lack of any prodromal aura or postictal lethargy. These seizures manifest with a slight decrease in postural tone, incontinence of urine or stool, a decrease in the level of consciousness, and often a "blank stare" noticeable to people interacting with the patient. These seizures may last from seconds to long periods (status epilepticus). The EEG shows bilateral, diffuse, synchronous 3-Hz spikes and domes; the pattern is pathognomonic.

2. The **specific manifestations of tonic–clonic (grand mal)** seizures include an abrupt onset and termination, and both an antecedent aura and a significant period of postictal lethargy. The classic features are an aura of

variable duration, followed by 1–2 minutes of tonic motor activity, followed by clonic activity for 2–4 minutes. The patient experiences complete loss of consciousness, incontinence of urine and stool, tongue biting, and a period of postictal lethargy. If during the postictal period there is focal weakness (paresis or plegia), the condition is described as Todd's paralysis, and the cause is a structural or anatomic lesion. Laboratory findings in the postictal phase of any tonic–clonic seizure, irrespective of cause, include an increased serum creatine phosphokinase (CPK), a high anion-gap metabolic acidosis (secondary to lactate), leukocytosis without a left shift, and an increase in serum prolactin levels.

3. The **evaluation and management** of generalized seizures include the steps listed in Box 14-7 and the following specific features. If a cause is determined from the **overall evaluation**, **treatment** is directed toward that cause. **Specifics** include antibiotics for leptomeningitis; the use of acyclovir in a dose of 10 mg/kg i.v., q.8hr for 14 days, and MRI of the temporal lobes, if herpes simplex encephalitis is suspected; the use of dexamethasone (Decadron), 4 mg i.v., q.6hr, and consultation with neurosurgery for any space-occupying lesions with adjacent edema; the correction of any electrolyte disorders; the administration of thiamine and BZD for the treatment of withdrawal seizures; and consultation with neurosurgery if head trauma or a subdural hematoma is present.

In most cases in which a specific, treatable, reversible cause is demonstrated, long-term pharmacologic therapy is not necessary.

If no **specific diagnosis** is determined, an EEG should be performed and long-term therapy continued. Further imaging techniques including MRI should be considered if the potential for a dysmyelinating disorder (multiple sclerosis), HSV encephalitis, or small structural abnormality still exists after an initially negative evaluation.

IV. **Long-term therapy**

Long-term therapy includes antiseizure medications (Table 14-9), support of the patient and patient's family emotionally, and instructing the patient in life-style modification. These modifications may include abstinence from ethanol, phenothiazines (these agents can lower the seizure threshold), and restricting driving and pilot privileges.

A. **Indications for the withdrawal** of antiseizure medications include:

1. **Ethanol-related seizures.**

TABLE 14-9
Common Antiseizure Medications: Ragimens, Indications, Levels, and Side Effects

Agent	Indications	Dose	Level	Side Effects
Phenytoin (Dilantin)	Generalized tonic-clonic	100–300 mg p.o. q.d. (usually 300) (Dose range: 5–15 mg/kg/day)	10–20 μg/mL	Cerebellar Nystagmus Ataxia Macrocytosis Positive ANA Peripheral neuropathy
Phenobarbital	Generalized tonic-clonic	100–200 mg p.o. q.d. (Dose range: 4–8 mg/kg/day)	10–40 μg/mL	Nystagmus Ataxia Hyperactivity (exacerbation of attention deficit disorder)
Carbamazepine	Partial Generalized tonic-clonic	600–1,200 mg/24 hr (300–600 mg b.i.d. to q.i.d. (Dose range: 10–25 mg/kg/day)	6–12 μg/mL	Nystagmus Hepatitis Dysarthria Leukopenia
Valproic acid	Generalized petit mal (absence) Generalized tonic-clonic	Dose range: 15–40 mg/kg/24 hr q.8hr, divided doses	50–100 μg/mL	Thrombocytopenia Tremor Alopecia
Clonazepam (Klonopin)	Generalized petit mal (absence) Myotonic epilepsy Lennox–Gaustaut syndrome	Dose range: 0.025–0.1 mg/kg/24 hr in b.i.d. to t.i.d. divided doses	20–80 ng/mL	Ataxia Exacerbation of generalized tonic–clonic seizures

2. No seizure for >2–3 years in an otherwise stable patient. This should be performed under the guidance of a consulting neurologist and consists of a slow, careful discontinuation of the antiseizure medication(s).

V. **Consultation**

Problem	Service	Time
All patients	Neurology	Urgent/emergent
Meningitis	Infectious diseases	Urgent/emergent
Subdural hematoma	Neurosurgery	Emergent

VI. **Indications for admission:** New onset or increased frequency of seizures. All patients with status epilepticus need emergency admission, usually to an ICU.

Vertigo (Box 14-8)

Vertigo is the sensation in the patient of rotatory disequilibrium. The patient senses that the body or its surrounding environment is moving in a rotatory fashion. The classic example is "bed spins" described by acutely intoxicated people who lie flat in bed.

I. **Causes**

The causes of vertigo are diverse. The discussion here is limited to the most common or treatable/reversible causes (Table 14-10).

II. **Consultation**

Problem	Service	Time
Recurrent vertigo	Neurology	Urgent
Intracranial mass	Neurosurgery	Urgent

B O X 14-8

Overall Evaluation and Management of Vertigo

Evaluation

1. Thorough history and physical examination, with particular attention placed on duration, time of onset, exacerbating features, and concurrent features (Table 14-10).
2. Perform the Dix-Hallpike–Bàràny maneuver (Table 14-11) to differentiate benign positional vertigo from other forms of vertigo.
3. Trial of specific antivertigo medications (see Table 14-12, for specific agents and their dosages).
4. CT or MRI of the posterior fossa if vertigo is recurrent or if any atypical features are present.

T A B L E   14-10
Causes of Vertigo

Etiology	Pathogenesis	Manifestations	Evaluation/Management
Benign positional vertigo	Idiopathic May be viral or postviral in origin	Acute onset on assuming a supine position Each episode is transient and self-limited Recurrent, change-in-position–related episodes Concurrent nausea, vomiting Concurrent nystagmus Never any tinnitus Never any auditory deficits	Dix–Hallpike–Bàràny test reproduces the symptoms/Tell patient to lie flat acutely and recurrently to decrease the severity of symptoms Meclizine, 12.5–25 mg p.o., t.i.d., prn is useful
Meniere's disease	An abnormal excess of endolymph in the membranous labyrinth of the vestibular and cochlear apparati of the inner ear. This results in damage to these structures	Acute onset of severe vertigo that becomes recurrent; each episode lasts several hours and has intervening periods without vertigo of various intervals Unilateral/bilateral tinnitus Uni(bi)lateral decrease in auditory acuity Horizontal nystagmus Tinnitus is antecedent to the vertigo Severe nausea and vomiting during each episode	Audiometry Low-frequency hearing loss/Low-sodium diet Thiazide diuretics, HCTZ, 25–50 mg p.o. q. day Meclizine prn ENT referral

(continued)

673

T A B L E 14-10 *(continued)*

Etiology	Pathogenesis	Manifestations	Evaluation/Management
Labyrinthitis	Actual inflammation of the vestibulocochlear apparatus; usually after a viral upper respiratory tract infection	Bilateral tinnitus Vertigo Nausea and vomiting Horizontal nystagmus Rarely any significant auditory deficit Antecedent URI All manifestations are self-limited and resolve in 1–4 days	Rest Fluids Meclizine, 12.5–25 mg p.o., t.i.d., prn

Acoustic neuroma	A neoplastic growth of Schwann cells in the cranial nerve eight (i.e., at the cerebello-pontine angle). High risk in patients with neurofibromatosis
	• *Type 1 neurofibro-matosis* Chromosome 17
	
	• *Type 2 neurofibro-matosis* Chromosome 22
		Chronic vertigo
		Cafe-au-lait spots
		Lisch nodules
		Neurofibromata
		Unilateral tinnitus
		Unilateral auditory deficit
		Bell's palsy if advanced
		• Unilateral acoustic neuroma
		  Cafe-au-lait spots
		  Neurofibromata
		  Crowes' sign
		  Lisch nodules
		• Bilateral acoustic neuroma
		  Other gliomas/schwannomas
			Audiometry: High-frequency loss/MRI/CT of posterior fossa: tumor of nerve will be demonstrable
			Referral to neurosurgery

| Brainstem CVA (Wallenberg's syndrome) | Infarction of the area of brainstem supplied by the vertebrobasilar artery
Unilateral
Damage to the lateral medulla | Acute onset of severe
Ataxia
Tinnitus
Dysarthria
Dysphagia
Diplopia
Nausea and vomiting
Ipsilateral Horner's syndrome
Ipsilateral dysdiadochokinesia
Ipsilateral loss of fine touch and proprioception
Contralateral loss of pinprick and temperature | CT/MRI of posterior fossa. See CVA, page 625 |
| Otosclerosis | Sclerosis and significant decrease in mobility of the stapes
Age of onset: 30 years | Significant decrease in conductive auditory acuity
Recurrent unilateral vertigo | Make the clinical diagnosis
Refer to ENT for further management |

T A B L E   14-11
Dix–Hallpike–Bàràny Maneuver

1. The patient is placed supine with the head in ~30° of extension and turned to the right or left, for 30–90 seconds.
2. The patient assumes a sitting position for 5 minutes.
3. Repeat the test with the patient's head turned to the contralateral side.

Interpretation: This test is positive if the patient develops vertigo and nystagmus within 30 seconds of being placed in a new position. The nystagmus, which has the rapid component to the side of the head inferiorly placed, resolves within 30 seconds. A positive test is consistent with benign positional vertigo.

T A B L E   14-12
Medications in the Symptomatic Therapy of Vertigo/Motion Sickness

Meclizine (Antivert), 12.5–25 mg p.o. t.i.d. prn
   or
Dimenhydrinate, 50 mg p.o. q.6hr, prn
   or
Scopolamine patch applied to skin q.72h.

Bibliography

Bell's Palsy

Adour KK, et al: The true nature of Bell's palsy: analysis of 1000 consecutive patients. Laryngoscope 1978;88:787–801.

Ohye RG, Altenberger EA: Bell's palsy. Am Fam Pract 1989;40:159–166.

Cerebrovascular Accidents

Brook RH, et al: Carotid endarterectomy for elderly patients: predicting complications. Ann Intern Med 1990;113:747–753.

Chambers BR, Norris JW: Outcome in patients with asymptomatic neck bruits. N Engl J Med 1986;315:860–865.

Day AL, Salcman M: Subarachnoid hemorrhage. Am Fam Pract 1989;40: 95–105.

Fields WS: Aspirin for prevention of stroke. Am J Med 1983;84:61.

Fisher CM: Clinical syndromes in cerebral thrombosis, hypertensive hemorrhage, and ruptured saccular aneurysm. Clin Neurosurg 1975;22:117–147.

Hart RG, Miller VT: Cerebral infarction in young adults: a practical approach. Stroke 1983;14:110–114.

Hobson RW, et al: Efficacy of carotid endarterectomy for asymptomatic carotid stenosis. N Engl J Med 1993;328:221–227.

Meissner I, et al: The natural history of asymptomatic carotid arterial occlusive lesions. JAMA 1987;258:2704−2707.

North American Symptomatic Carotid Endarterectomy Study in Symptomatic Patients with High-Grade Carotid Stenosis: Beneficial effect of carotid endarterectomy in symptomatic patients with high-grade carotid stenosis. N Engl J Med 1991;325:445−453.

Scherokman BJ, Hallenbeck JM: Management of acute stroke. Am Fam Pract 1985;31:190−199.

Welin L, et al: Analysis of **risk factors** for stroke in a cohort of men born in 1913. N Engl J Med 1987;317:521−526.

Delirium

Dilsaver SC: The mental status examination. Am Fam Pract 1990;41:1489−1496.

Inouye SK, et al: Clarifying confusion: the confusion assessment method. Ann Intern Med 1990;113:941−948.

Lindberg MC, Oyler RA: Wernicke's encephalopathy. Am Fam Pract 1990;41:1205−1209.

Lipowski ZJ: Delirium (acute confusional states). JAMA 1987;258:1789−1792.

Dementia

Black KS, Hughes PL: Alzheimer's disease: making the diagnosis. Am Fam Pract 1987;36:196−202.

Erkinjutti T, et al: Dementia among medical inpatients. Arch Intern Med 1986;146:1923−1926.

Katzman R: Alzheimer's disease. N Engl J Med 1986;314:964.

Van Horn G: Dementia. Am J Med 1987;83:101−110.

Gilman S: Advances in neurology. N Engl J Med 1992;326:1608−1616.

Gait Disturbances/Parkinson's Disease

Ahlskog JE, Wilkinson JM: New concepts in the treatment of Parkinson's disease. Am Fam Pract 1990;41:574−584.

Hallett M: Classification and treatment of tremor. JAMA 1991;266:1115−1117.

Hough JC, et al: Gait disturbances in the elderly. Am Fam Pract 1987;35:191−196.

Lees AJ: L-Dopa treatment and Parkinson's disease. Q J Med 1986;59:535.

Headaches

Black PM: Brain tumors. N Engl J Med 1991;324:1471−1476.

Kumar KL, Cooney TG: Vascular headache. J Gen Intern Med 1988;3:384−395.

Linet MS, Stewart WF: Migraine headache: epidemiologic perspectives. Epidemiol Rev 1984;6:107.

McKenna JP: Cluster headaches. Am Fam Pract 1988;37:173−143.

Schulman EA, et al: Symptomatic and prophylactic treatment of migraine and tension-type headache. Neurology 1992;42(suppl 2):16−21.

Walling AD: Drug prophylaxis for migraine headaches. Am Fam Pract 1990;42:425−432.

Meningitis

Gellin BG, Broome CV: Listeriosis. JAMA 1989;261:1313−1320.

Gorse GJ, et al: Bacterial meningitis in the elderly. Arch Intern Med 1984;144:1603−1607.

Lefrock JL: Drugs of choice for bacterial meningitis. Am Fam Pract 1986;33:285–291.

El-Mallakh RS: CSF evaluation in neurologic disease. Am Fam Pract 1987;35:112–118.

Quagliarello V, et al: Bacterial meningitis: **pathogenesis**, pathophysiology, and progress. N Engl J Med 1992;327:864–872.

Shapiro ED: Prophylaxis for bacterial meningitis. Med Clin North Am 1985;69:269.

Tarber MG, Sande MA: Principles in the treatment of bacterial meningitis. Am J Med 1984;76(suppl 5A):224.

Seizure Disorders

Delgado-Escueta AV, et al: The treatable epilepsies. N Engl J Med 1983;1508:1576.

Drugs for epilepsy. Med Lett 1986;28:91–94.

Hopkins A, et al: The first seizures in adult life. Lancet 1988;1:721-726.

Jubbari B: Management of epileptic seizures in adults. Am Fam Pract 1985;31:162–172.

Ojemann LM, Ojemann GA: Treatment of epilepsy. Am Fam Pract 1984;30:113–128.

Schuer ML, Pedley TA: The evaluation and treatment of seizures. N Engl J Med 1990;21:1467–1474.

Vertigo

Drachman DA, Hart CW: An approach to the dizzy patient. Neurology 1972;22:323.

Lehrer JF, et al: Identification and treatment of metabolic abnormalities in patients with vertigo. Arch Intern Med 1986;146:1497–1500.

Snow JB Jr: Positional vertigo. N Engl J Med 1984;310:1740.

—D.D.B.

Psychiatry

Mood Disorders Including Depression

Depression is a very common syndrome that can affect any individual at any time (Box 15-1). It has been estimated that up to one fourth of patients in the outpatient setting and up to one third of medical inpatients have some clinical manifestations of depression. Although quite prevalent, depression can easily be overlooked and therefore undertreated. The syndrome of depression has many different manifestations and a diverse set of causes, each origin with a different pathogenesis. Furthermore, depression of any origin exacerbates many concurrent medical problems and/or is exacerbated by concurrent medical, psychiatric, and/or substance-abuse syndromes. One can clearly see why depression can be a slippery syndrome to evaluate and manage.

I. The **overall manifestations** of depression include the presence of a depressed mood (i.e., the subjective manifestations of feeling "blue" or "down in the dumps") and a despondent affect (i.e., the objective observation that the patient looks depressed by an experienced examiner). Other overall vegetative manifestations of depression include:
   A. **Change in sleep pattern**
      This is often a symptom of depression. This change can be excessive sleeping compared with baseline or insomnia, classically early morning awakening with inability to return to sleep.
   B. **Change in appetite**
      There is usually a decrease in appetite in patients with depression, which can result in weight loss.
   C. **Anhedonia**
      A significant decrease in the desire and perceived need for pleasure is very common in patients with depression.
   D. **A feeling of hopelessness**
      The patient has no aspirations and looks forward to nothing but an unchanging, bleak, cold existence.

B O X 15-1

Overall Evaluation and Management of Depression

Evaluation

1. Obtain a history with emphasis on:
   a. The **overall manifestations** of depression.
      i. Sleep disturbances.
      ii. Somatic complaints (e.g., chest pain, abdominal pain).
      iii. Delusional thoughts.
      iv. Libido disturbances.
      v. Appetite disturbances.
      vi. Depressed mood.
   b. Any concurrent or antecedent events (e.g., bad news, divorce, loss of employment, death of spouse).
   c. A history of mania, depression, and/or substance abuse.
   d. Current use of any therapeutic agents and agents for alteration of mood.
   e. Assess the patient for suicide risk potential (see Box 15-2, page 683).
2. Perform a physical examination, looking for objective evidence of a despondent affect, manifestations of hyperthyroidism or hypothyroidism, manifestations of muscle weakness/muscle atrophy, and/or documented weight loss.
3. Obtain the following laboratory parameters:
   a. Serum electrolytes, looking for hyponatremia or hypernatremia, which can exacerbate preexisting depression or manifest as a syndrome of depression.
   b. Serum calcium, as hypercalcemia can exacerbate preexisting depression or manifest as a syndrome of depression.
   c. Serum phosphorus, as hyperphosphatemia can exacerbate preexisting depression or manifest as a syndrome of depression.
   d. Thyroid-stimulating hormone (TSH) levels, to screen for hypo-/hyperthyroidism, either of which can exacerbate preexisting depression or manifest as a syndrome of depression.
   e. ECG, 12 lead, for baseline purposes, if any antidepressant agent is considered to be initiated.

(continued)

B O X 15-1 *(continued)*

4. Categorize and define the syndrome of depression by using these data.
   a. If **major depression:** Initiate an antidepressant agent (see Tables 15-1 and 15-2) and psychotherapy.
   b. If **bipolar disorder:** Initiate lithium, an antidepressant agent (see Tables 15-1 and 15-2) and psychotherapy.
   c. **Dysthymic, cyclothymic,** and **reactive depression:** Initiate psychotherapy.
   d. If **physiologic:** Treat the underlying condition.
5. Treat any concurrent, exacerbating factors or diseases, especially any chemical abuse/dependency.
6. Admit all patients with suicidal/homicidal ideation or risk and any and all patients with active psychosis.

E. **A significant decrease in libido**
   The patient's interest in developing and evolving intimate interrelationships with fellow human beings, including sex, is markedly embarrassed.
F. **A significant decrease in interactions with fellow human beings**
   This is a corollary to the decrease in libido, in that there often is a withdrawal from others, including family members and close friends. The patient will often decrease attendance at or even completely avoid social/family gatherings. Furthermore, attendance at work and/or school can become markedly compromised.
G. **Recurrent thoughts of death, suicide, and/or homicide**
   See Box 15-2 for **specific risk factors** in suicide.
H. **A marked increase in somatic complaints**
   These complaints include but are not limited to myalgias, arthralgias, abdominal pains, and chest pains. These somatic manifestations can be severe, and often the patient will have had several unremarkable medical evaluations for these specific complaints. In patients with major depression, the somatization can be so marked as to result in delusions of decay or rot in the chest, muscles, or abdomen.
I. **A change in psychomotor activity**
   This can be either agitation (i.e., irritation, restlessness, hyperactivity) or retardation (i.e., slow motor movements, lethargy, and increased sleepiness).
J. In severe cases, there can be delusional thoughts that reach psychotic proportions.

Agent	Sedation	Anticholinergic Side Effects*	Other Side Effects	Dosage, Initial/Maximal
Amitriptyline (Elavil)	Strong	Severe	QRS and QTc prolongation Orthostatic hypotension	25 mg p.o. t.i.d./300 mg/24 hr
Nortriptyline (Pamelor)	Minimal	Mild	QRS and QTc prolongation Minimal orthostatic hypotension	25 mg p.o. q.d./150 mg/24 hr
Trazodone (Desyrel)	Strong	None	Little to no ECG or hypotensive changes Priapism	50 mg p.o. t.i.d./600 mg/24 hr
Fluoxetine† (Prozac)	Moderate	None	No ECG or hypotensive effects	20 mg p.o. q.d./80 mg/24 hr
Buspirone‡ (Buspar)	Moderate	Minimal	Minimal side effect profile	5 mg p.o. tid; maximum: 20 mg p.o. t.i.d.
Nefazodone† (Serzone)	Moderate	Minimal	Minimal	100 mg p.o. b.i.d.; maximum: 200 mg p.o. t.i.d.
Lithium	Dose dependent	None	Granulocytopenia Mild hypothyroidism Tremor Diabetes insipidus	300 mg p.o. t.i.d./Therapeutic window: 0.6–1.5 mmol/liter

* Anticholinergic side effects include tachycardia, urinary retention, xerostomia.
† Serotonin-reuptake inhibitor.
‡ Benzodiapezine.

B O X 15-2

> **Factors in the Assessment of Suicide Risk**
>
> 1. Sex of patient: Women attempt 3 times more often than men. Men are successful 3 times more often than women.
> 2. Age of patient: Highest risk in young (i.e., teenagers) and in older, age >50 years, patients.
> 3. The presence of a syndrome of depression, acute or chronic.
> 4. A history of previous suicide attempts.
> 5. A history of substance abuse/dependency in general, and ethanol in specific.
> 6. The presence of a thought process disorder (i.e., the patient is delusional).
> 7. No social support (i.e., no job, no family).
> 8. The presence of an organized plan for completing the deed.
> 9. The lack of a significant other is a very powerful marker in increasing suicide risk.
> 10. The presence of an acute or symptomatic chronic physical illness, especially if the symptom is one of pain.
>   Each factor is given 1 point.
>   Any patient with a score of >5: Admit.
>   2–5: Watch closely, as an inpatient or outpatient.
>   <2: Watch closely, outpatient.
>   (From Patterson WM, et al: Evaluation of suicidal patients: The SAD persons scale. Psychosomatics 1983;24:343–349.)

II. Causes

The causes of depression are diverse and are best stratified into three groups, *reactive* (i.e., as the result of a loss due to death or divorce), those that are *primarily physiologic*, and those that are *primarily psychiatric*. As alluded to, depression can be and often is multifactorial with more than one of the following causes contributing to or exacerbating the syndrome of depression.

A. **Reactive depression**

This is the most common type of depression among all individuals. Every person will, at various times during life, experience reactive depression.

1. The **specific manifestations** include the development of mild to severe depression after an acute stressful

T A B L E 15-2
Substances of Abuse—United States, 1998

Category	Specific Agents	Types of Dependency	Effects	Sequelae/Side Effects
Sedatives	Ethanol Benzodiazepines (BZD) Barbiturates Marijuana—The dried flowering tops of the hemp plant Hashish—Resinous extract of the hemp plant	Physiologic: marked Psychologic: marked	Decreased inhibitions Sense of well-being Mild euphoria Barbiturates/BZD: profound relaxation	Withdrawal syndrome upon abstinence; **death** Ethanol: a) Cirrhosis b) Pancreatitis c) Wernicke–Korsakoff syndrome BZD: a) Hypoventilation secondary to poor airway Cannabis (smoked) a) increased risk of bronchogenic carcinoma
Narcotics	Heroin Morphine Codeine	Physiologic: marked Psychologic: marked	Euphoria Relief of tension Analgesia	Decrease in function of all physiologic drives (appetite, libido) Withdrawal syndrome upon abstinence; **death**

Stimulants	Cocaine Crack, rock or "Roxanne"; 90% pure (Cocaine + ammonia + baking soda, baked)—this is smoked Free-base, 90% pure, extracted by using ether Amphetamines Methamphetamine, speed, crack, ice, crystal	Physiologic: minimal Psychologic: marked	Perception of increased energy Euphoria Decreased appetite Decreased need for sleep Perception of increased efficiency	Marked tolerance until doses required result in severe tachycardia and hypertension Insomnia Increased aggressive behaviorisms Sudden cardiac **death**
Hallucinogen	D-lysergic acid (LSD) Phencyclidine (PCP) Ecstasy—structure similar to LSD	Physiologic: negligible Psychologic: minimal	Vivid hallucinations, usually visual but also tactile, auditory, and olfactory are possible	"Bad trips" (i.e., nightmarish hallucinations) "Flashbacks" (i.e., a hallucination occurring years to decades after the last use of the agent) Increased aggressive/assaultive behaviorisms **Death**
Inhalants	Solvents Amyl nitrate Hydrocarbons	Physiologic: minimal Psychologic: marked	Euphoria, "head rush" Mild relaxation	Tolerance Sudden cardiac **death** Central nervous system destruction; dementia and **death**

685

event in the patient's life. This event is usually one of a loss of a person near and dear to them. This loss can be as the result of divorce, travel, or death. The reactive depression that occurs after a loss is called grief. Another common event that precipitates such depression is that of a loss of one's employment or failure to attain a level long desired. There can be significant disturbances in libido, appetite, and sleep, and the manifestations can include some delusional thinking. This can be, in severe forms, not dissimilar from major depression. The natural history is one of it being self-limited as the patient slowly, steadily works through the pain of the loss. Duration is usually <6 months; if the duration is >6 months, the diagnosis of major depression must be seriously entertained. The risk of suicide is moderate.

2. The **specific evaluation and management** include those described in Box 15-1 and effectively determining the precipitating/exacerbating factor. Clearly an assessment of risk for suicide as described in Boxes 15-1 and 15-2 must be determined. **Specific management** includes the elective referral to a psychiatrist for psychotherapy. The patient must work through the grief realistically to recover from it. Although it is relatively uncommon for antidepressant agents to be necessary for **treatment**, if used, they must be for a fixed time.

B. **Physiologic**

Occurs as the result of a medical diagnosis. Many of these etiologies can be defined and even can be reversed. The most common include:

1. **Endocrinopathies.** These include hypothyroidism, hyperthyroidism, and states of hypercortisolism, either iatrogenic or as the result of Cushing's syndrome. The **specific manifestations** of these disorders, as well as their **specific evaluation and management**, are discussed in Box 15-1 and in Chapter 9. Of note is that hyperthyroidism in the elderly can paradoxically be seen with weakness and depression (i.e., "apathetic hyperthyroidism.")

2. **Electrolyte disturbances.** These include hypercalcemia, hypophosphatemia, hyperphosphatemia, hyponatremia, or hypernatremia. The **specific manifestations** of the most common of these disorders as well as their **specific evaluation and management** are discussed in Box 15-1 and in Chapter 9.

3. **Degenerative central nervous system processes.** These include dementia, parkinsonism, tertiary lues venereum, and multiple sclerosis. The **specific manifestations** of the most common of these disorders as well as their **specific evaluation and management** are dis-

cussed in Box 15-1 and Chapter 14 (parkinsonism, dementia) or Chapter 6 (lues venereum).

4. **Intracranial events.** These include the development of space-occupying lesions (e.g., neoplasia or any CVAs). The **specific manifestations** of the most common of these disorders as well as their **specific evaluation and management** are discussed in Box 15-1 and in Chapter 14.

5. **Chemical agents, either illicit or iatrogenic.** Virtually any chemical either prescribed for therapeutic purposes or used for mood-altering purposes can result in depression. The most common of these agents include benzodiazepines, β-blockers, barbiturates, and ethanol. The **specific manifestations** of the most common of these disorders as well as their **specific evaluation and management** are discussed in Box 15-1 and in the section on Substance-Abuse Syndromes and Table 15-2 in this chapter.

C. **Psychiatric causes**

These are again quite diverse in manifestations, natural history, evaluation, and management.

1. **Major depression**

This is the quintessential origin of depression with which all other syndromes of depression are compared.

a. The **specific manifestations** include those described in the **overall manifestations** section. The patient will manifest many if not all of the **overall manifestations**. There can be and often are delusions, at times psychotic delusions, and suicidal ideation is quite common. This etiology/syndrome of depression is quite pernicious in that it has a slow, insidious onset and, once present, the natural history is one of waxing and waning, with periods of minimal manifestations and normal activity to severe manifestations and marked embarrassment of normal activities. The duration is months to years and can be lifelong.

b. The **specific evaluation and management** include those described in Box 15-1 and effectively ruling out other primary or exacerbating factors. Clearly an assessment of risk for suicide, as described in Boxes 15-1 and 15-2, must be determined. **Specific management** includes the initiation of an antidepressant medication (Table 15-1) and referral of all patients to a psychiatrist for adjunctive psychotherapy. If the patient has severe depression refractory to intensive antidepressant therapy and psychotherapy including inpatient therapy, electroconvulsive **treatment** (ECT) should be considered.

2. **Bipolar affective disorder**
   This very severe affective disorder is, when diagnosed and aggressively treated, imminently and eminently treatable.
   a. The **specific manifestations** include alternating periods of major depression with periods of severe mania. The patient will, for various periods, have major depression, which then resolves only to develop into mania. The mania manifests with an increase in activity (i.e., many activities being performed, all at a harried and frenetic pace). The efficiency in performing these activities, however, is markedly compromised. The manic patient also has a rapid, forced speech and a significantly impaired judgment, going on spending sprees and taking inappropriate risks. Furthermore, the patient with mania may develop delusions, usually of grandiose schemes or of perceived increased prowess in sexual activity or business activity. Psychotic delusions can and often do occur during the depressed and the manic phases of the disease process. The **natural history** is one of recurrent alternating episodes of depression and mania of varying duration. The duration of the syndrome is years to lifelong.
   b. The **specific evaluation and management** include those described in Box 15-1 and effectively ruling out other primary or exacerbating factors. Clearly an assessment of risk for suicide, as described in Boxes 15-1 and 15-2, must be determined. **Specific management** includes the initiation of lithium, an antidepressant medication (Table 15-1), and referral of all patients to a psychiatrist for adjunctive psychotherapy.

3. **Dysthymic disorder**
   a. The **specific manifestations** include some of those described in the **overall manifestations**, but of mild intensity. This syndrome is chronic, mild, and with minimal to negligible effect on appetite, sleep, energy level, motor activity, and functioning within society. The patient is chronically morose and can develop mild to moderate self-pity. The **natural history** is one of chronicity; the patient usually can maintain employment. The duration is usually lifelong. There is little to no increased risk of suicide, and the patient is never delusional.
   b. The **specific evaluation and management** include those described in Box 15-1 and effectively ruling out other primary or exacerbating factors. Clearly an assessment of risk for suicide, as described in Boxes 15-1 and 15-2, must be determined. **Specific management** includes the elective referral to a psychia-

trist for psychotherapy. Rarely, if ever, will antidepressant agents be necessary in therapy.

4. **Cyclothymic disorder**

   a. The **specific manifestations** are a mild version of bipolar disorder, in that there are alternating periods of mild depression and mild increased activity with periods of normalcy between. The mild depression is identical to that described in dysthymic syndrome. The increased activity is mild and without any grossly decreased judgment. The natural history is one of continuing alterations between decreased and increased mood. Duration is usually lifelong. There is little to no increased risk for suicide, and the patient is never delusional.

   b. The **specific evaluation and management** include those described in Box 15-1 and effectively ruling out other primary or exacerbating factors. Clearly an assessment of risk for suicide, as described in Boxes 15-1 and 15-2, must be determined. **Specific management** includes the elective referral to a psychiatrist for psychotherapy. Rarely, if ever, will antidepressant agents be necessary in therapy.

III. **Consultation**

Problem	*Service*	*Time*
Major depression	Psychiatry	Urgent
Bipolar disorder	Psychiatry	Urgent
Suicidal	Psychiatry	Emergent
Cyclothymic	Psychiatry	Required
Dysthymic	Psychiatry	Required
Reactive	Psychiatry	Elective

IV. **Indications for admission:** Suicidal or homicidal ideation or risk, mania, or psychotic delusions.

Substance-Abuse Syndromes

The syndrome of chemical substance abuse is epidemic in the United States. This is demonstrated not only by the prevalence of substance abuse, but also by the enormous expense of this problem in economic and, most important, human terms. The prevalence of substance abuse has been estimated to be 10%–15%. Based on this discussion, the syndrome of substance abuse is one of the gravest problems facing society in general and health care delivery, in specific, in the United States today. Several definitions cogent to any discussion of substance-abuse syndromes must be discussed herein.

Dependence is the overt physical and/or psychological, nontherapeutic need for a specific substance or activity. This is a broad definition in that human beings can develop dependence on activities or items other than chemical substances. These include compulsive gambling, eating, sexual activities and what will be discussed at length herein, chemical-substance abuse. One of the integral features of these abuse syndromes is a loss of control. In a discussion specific to chemical-substance abuse, several terms can be used to describe dependence.

Addiction (i.e., physical dependence). Actual physiologic changes occur in the body to make the patient require the substance to maintain a new homeostasis.

Withdrawal. The **manifestations** that develop on discontinuing a chemical agent to which a patient is addicted. These are pathophysiologically as the result of abstinence from the agent. The development of a withdrawal syndrome on abstinence from a specific chemical effectively defines addiction.

Habituation (i.e., psychological dependence). A compelling need, want of, lust for the specific substance to reexperience its effects. A patient can have psychologic dependence without physical dependence.

Tolerance. The need for increasing amounts of the specific chemical to derive the same effect. The amount increases until there is the development of significant and further dose-limiting side effects.

I. **Substances of abuse**

Specific substances abused today in the United States and worldwide are quite varied in chemical type, potential for physical dependence, potential for psychological dependence, and in sequelae. In all cases, however, the natural history of dependence on one or more of these agents, also referred to as mood-altering drugs, will lead to marked embarrassment in the quality of the patient's life and, in virtually all cases, markedly decrease the life span of the patient. **Specific substances** abused are described in Table 15-2. Ethanol, unquestionably the most commonly used and, unfortunately, abused chemical substance in the United States today, is described in Table 15-2 and expanded on in the discussion to follow.

II. **Ethanol abuse**

Ethanol abuse and dependency are endemic in our society. Recent estimates clearly delineate the prevalence and the human and economic burden of this dependency syndrome. These estimates include the fact that in 1985, >10 million Americans had the syndrome of ethanol dependence. Furthermore, >\$100 billion per year is lost as the result of ethanol abuse/dependency in the United States. Finally, the human cost is enormous: 30%–40% of hospital admissions have ethanol abuse either as the primary or a secondary diagnosis, 30%–50% of all suicides involve patients with ethanol abuse, 50% of all motor vehicle accidents and motor vehicle accident deaths have ethanol as a primary or contributing factor, 50% of all homicides involve ethanol as a contributing factor, and

3/1,000 live births in the United States today have fetal alcohol syndrome.

A. **Reporting**

Although the numbers are striking, this remains a syndrome that is quite underrecognized and therefore undertreated by the health care profession in general and physicians in specific. This is clearly evidenced by the fact that although 30%–40% of all admissions had ethanol as a primary or major contributing factor, only a small percentage have the diagnosis of ethanol dependence described in their medical records. The reasons for such underreporting and/or underrecognizing are not completely known, but several postulates include:

1. The social acceptability of ethanol as a drug.
2. The perceived benign nature of ethanol by society and by many health care professionals.
3. The high prevalence of ethanol abuse/dependency among health care professionals in general and physicians in specific.

   All of these reasons decrease the physician's sensitivity in describing the problem and making the diagnosis of ethanol abuse/dependency.

B. **Pathogenesis**

The **underlying pathogenesis** for the development of an ethanol abuse/dependency syndrome is not completely clear, but certain risk factors for development have been described.

1. **Genetic** (i.e., an increased propensity for ethanol abuse as the result of the patient's genetic make-up). Several studies using adopted monozygotic twins indicated that there may well be a genetic predisposition in the development of ethanol-abuse syndromes.
2. **Social environment.** Adults who grew up in broken, dysfunctional families, and/or are currently in broken, dysfunctional family relationships are at higher risk of developing a syndrome of ethanol abuse/dependency. Of clear interest is the fact that individuals with healthy family relationships have a markedly lower incidence of ethanol abuse.
3. Concurrent and/or antecedent **DSM-IV Axis I psychological dysfunctional states** (e.g., bipolar affective disorder, major depression, or schizophrenia). It has been estimated that up to one third of all patients with ethanol-abuse syndromes have such diagnoses.
4. Concurrent and/or antecedent **abuse or dependency on other chemical agents** (see Table 15-2). Clearly, dependence on one substance is a risk factor for the development of dependence on another substance. Any syndrome of addiction, whether it be to a chemical or to an activity (e.g., compulsive gambling), all of which have central to them a loss of self-control and of self-

esteem, is a risk factor in the development of concurrent dependency states.

5. Certain professions have a higher prevalence of ethanol abuse than other professions. A profession with one of the highest prevalence rates of ethanol abuse/dependency is that of physicians themselves.

C. **Evaluation** (Box 15-3)

The **overall evaluation** of an ethanol abuse/dependency syndrome is to make the diagnosis. Making the diagnosis is clearly pivotal to therapy, as the earlier the diagnosis is made, the better the chances for effective therapy and of ethanol-related sequelae prevention. The diagnosis is made best by performing a thorough history and physical examination.

1. The history must be from various sources, not only the patient himself or herself, but also collateral sources (e.g., spouse, significant other, other family members, friends and roommates). Not only can collateral sources of information provide objective data regarding the patient's substance-abuse potential, but they also can provide the clinician with insight into the patient's social milieu and to what extent the ethanol abuse/dependency is affecting that social milieu.

2. Several screening instruments have been developed to detect ethanol-abuse/dependency syndromes. Two of the best and both internally and externally valid instruments include the CAGE and MAST screening tests.

   a. **CAGE screening tool.** CAGE is a mnemonic for four specific questions, all of which should be asked of all new patients (ready to screen for an ethanol-abuse syndrome (Table 15-3). A positive response to any one of the CAGE queries correlates well with ethanol abuse. The positive predictive value for ethanol abuse/dependency of two positive responses is 82%, of three positive responses is 99%, and of four, 100%.

   b. **Michigan Alcoholism Screening Test (MAST)** uses a moderately short questionnaire to assess the patient for ethanol abuse/dependency. The questions are tailored to assess any decreased control of ethanol intake, problems with employment, and/or problems with social relationships including family and the law. The MAST has a standardized scoring system and can, with other information, be used to screen for and even to diagnose ethanol dependency and abuse syndromes.

3. **Ethanol dependence** is diagnosed from:

   a. Consumption of 0.135 ounces of pure ethanol/kg/day (i.e., ~one fifth of hard liquor for ≥30 consecutive days), and/or

(text continues on page 698)

B O X 15-3

Overall Evaluation and Management of Suspected Ethanol Abuse/Dependency

Evaluation

1. Obtain a thorough history. This must include a history from the patient and from collateral (e.g., family, friends) sources. Specific details should include:
   a. The patient's present ethanol-consumption habits, including quantity and duration.
   b. The patient's past ethanol-consumption habits.
   c. Any history of withdrawal.
   d. Any history of admission for an ethanol-related disease.
   e. Any history of blackouts (the patient cannot recall anything of a specific binge), and/or brownouts (the patient can recall events during a binge but they are fuzzy).
   f. Any history of driving under the influence of ethanol or ethanol-related motor vehicle accidents.
   g. Any history of morning tremors that resolve with ethanol use.
   h. Any history of recurrent falls and/or fractures.
   i. Any history of abusive behavior to family members and/or to others.
   j. The current relationships the patient has and how constructive (i.e., supportive) or destructive (i.e., detrimental) the relationships are.
   k. If the patient is not currently intoxicated, perform a CAGE (Table 15-3) and/or MAST evaluation.
2. Perform a thorough physical examination, with emphasis on:
   a. The presence of tremor and tachycardia at rest are indicative of impending withdrawal.
   b. Examine for palsies of extraocular muscles, ataxic gait, bilateral nystagmus, and confusion, all of which are **manifestations** of Wernicke's encephalopathy (i.e., related to acute thiamine deficiency).
   c. Examine the odor of breath, as the presence of ethanol can be easily detected by an experienced examiner.
   d. Examine patient for any signs of chronic hepatic disease/dysfunction (see section on End-Stage Liver Disease, Chapter 2, page 97).

(continued)

B O X   15-3 (continued)

3. Categorize the patient into one of three groups, one group being those patients who are acutely intoxicated or acutely abstaining from ethanol after a long binge, a second group being those who have ethanol dependence, and a third group being those patients who have ethanol abuse.
   a. **Acutely intoxicated or acute abstinence.** These patients require acute intervention. In virtually all cases, this intervention must be as an inpatient. The reason for inpatient intervention is that the risk for development of a withdrawal syndrome is quite high. The **specific manifestations** of withdrawal are diverse and can range from a mild tremor to hallucinations to generalized tonic–clonic seizure activity. Although withdrawal can occur anywhere between 36 hours and 14 days after ingestion of the last ethanol beverage, the vast majority of cases occur in the 36–72 hour range. The **specific evaluation and management** of withdrawal include:
      i. Administer thiamine (vitamin B₁), 100 mg i.m./i.v., stat to replenish thiamine stores and to treat and prevent Wernicke's encephalopathy.
      ii. Perform the following laboratory tests:
         (a) Serum glucose. Patients can be hypoglycemic after a binge as the result of a shutdown of gluconeogenesis in the liver.
         (b) Serum electrolytes, especially potassium, magnesium, and phosphorus. The patient is quite often deficient in these specific ions and will require repletion.
         (c) ECG, 12 lead, if any significant tachycardia is present.
         (d) Liver-function tests, if the patient has any evidence of hepatic dysfunction (e.g., any signs of hepatic disease or icterus), looking for gross increases of enzymes that would be consistent with acute ethanol hepatitis. (See section on Hepatitis in Chapter 2 for specifics on hepatitides.)
         (e) Urine for drug screen for other chemicals of abuse.
      iii. Initiate therapy with benzodiazepines. These agents will decrease the intensity of the excit-

(continued)

B O X 15-3 *(continued)*

atory **manifestations** including tachycardia, tremor, and anxiety. They will, furthermore, decrease the risk of withdrawal seizures. There are many different agents on the market, two of which are described in Table 15-4. The agent of choice is lorazepam (Ativan). The dosage should be scheduled and modified to keep the patient comfortable and sleepy, but without compromise of airway. The usual dosage is ~2 mg lorazepam p.o./i.m./i.v., q.4–6hr scheduled. The patient is then weaned from the lorazepam by decreasing the dose by 25% each day. Therefore, by day 5, the patient is taking lorazepam in an as-needed dosage.

iv. Adjuvant therapy including β-blockers or clonidine may have a role in some mild to moderate cases, but certainly these are not first-line agents.

v. Phenytoin is required only if the patient has another reason for seizures (i.e., phenytoin is not necessary in the **treatment** of seizures exclusively as the result of ethanol withdrawal).

vi. Nutrition should be optimized. Consultation with a dietitian may be of benefit, as well as prescription of a multivitamin, one tablet per day, and thiamine, 100 mg p.o., q.d.

vii. When sober and through withdrawal, ethanol-rehabilitation therapy can begin, best performed by referral to an addictionologist.

b. Alcohol dependent/abuser

i. Initiate inpatient or outpatient ethanol rehabilitation with the assistance of or by referral to an addictionologist.

T A B L E 15-3
CAGE Queries

C: Attempting to cut back on drinking?
A: Annoyed at criticisms regarding drinking habits?
G: Feeling guilty about drinking habits?
E: Using ethanol as a morning "eye-opener"?

(From Mayfield D, et al: The GAGE questionnaire. Am J Psychiatry 1974;131:1121.)

T A B L E 15-4
Agents Used in the Treatment of Acute Withdrawal from Ethanol

Agent	Half-life	Catabolites	Mechanism of Action	Dosage Regimen
*Lorazepam (Ativan) *Lorazepam is the agent of choice in the treatment of withdrawal syndromes.	14–16 hr	Conjugated, inactive	Binds to BZD receptors in CNS which act to release chloride anion into the neurons and inhibit activity; this is mediated by the molecule γ-aminobutyric acid (GABA) Decreases activity throughout the entire CNS, including cortical and autonomic systems Prevents seizures, decreases autonomic activity	2 mg p.o./i.m./i.v. q.4–6hr, scheduled
Chlordiazepoxide (Librium)	6–18 hr	Oxidized, active Half-life of the active catabolites is 50–100 hr	Same as lorazepam	25–100 mg p.o./i.v., q.6hr, scheduled

β-Blockers (atenolol)	6–10 hr	Not catabolized, excreted intact in urine	Competitive antagonist of β-catecholamine receptors Decreases effects of catecholamines from autonomic nervous system Decreases tremor, tachycardia Adjunctive to BZD, if no contraindication to its use: a) 2° or 3° AV nodal block b) Reversible airway disease c) Systolic heart failure	50 mg p.o., q.d., for duration of withdrawal
Clonidine (Catapres)	6–24 hr	Hepatic, inactive	A central α_2-receptor antagonist which decreases the release of norepinephrine from the autonomic nervous system Mild sedation	0.1 mg p.o., q.d. for duration of withdrawal

(text continued from page 692)

> **b.** A MAST score of ≥6, and/or
> **c.** The development of any physiologic disease as the result of ethanol and/or
> **d.** The continued use of ethanol in the face of a medical contraindication, and/or
> **e.** The development of withdrawal on abstinence from ethanol use, and/or
> **f.** The development of tolerance to ethanol, as manifested by:
> > **i.** Blood alcohol level (BAL) of >0.15 mg/dL without symptoms.
> > **ii.** BAL of >0.3 mg/dL at any time.
>
> **4.** Ethanol abuse is diagnosed from
> > **a.** A MAST score of 3–5 and consumption of >2 ounces of pure ethanol per day (i.e., ~five ethanol beverages/day), or
> > **b.** A MAST score of ≥2 and consumption of >4 ounces of pure ethanol per day (i.e., ~10 ethanol beverages/day.

D. Management

The **overall management** of a patient with an ethanol-abuse/dependency syndrome is extremely complicated, quite labor intensive, requires involvement from multiple disciplines, and is for the duration of the patient's life. The patient may relapse at any time, requiring the clinician to, in effect, start from scratch. The management schemas can best be stratified into short- and long-term phases.

1. Short-term. The patient is acutely intoxicated and/or acutely abstaining after a significant binge of ethanol. These patients are at high risk for withdrawal and require inpatient therapy. Please refer to Box 15-3 and Table 15-4 for specifics in **short-term evaluation and management**.

2. Long-term, rehabilitative. The patient is no longer intoxicated and has had resolution of any withdrawal syndrome. This is very complex, long-term, and labor intensive. Although there can be frustrations inherent to long-term therapy of such patients, the rewards of success can be marvelous to the patient, to his family, to society, and therefore are quite gratifying to the clinician. The discussion here is only a brief description of some of the basic tenets of long-term ethanol dependence rehabilitative therapy.

> **a.** Treatment is most effective in patients who are diagnosed early, who have strong family support, and who have a tangible acute loss if ethanol is restarted, or, better still, a tangible, reproducible, and positive gain if abstinence is continued. An employer who is supportive is clearly of benefit to the therapy.
>
> **b.** Successful therapy is taking each day as it comes

for the rest of the patient's life. The patient must be motivated for the rest of his (her) life to maintain successful therapy (i.e., abstinence from all chemicals). One of the best methods to reinforce this and to keep motivation optimal is to have the patient interact on a regular basis with other patients with alcohol dependency. The best example of this is Alcoholics Anonymous (AA).

c. The clinician must confront, with an empathic yet firm method, any and all defenses (e.g., denial: denying that there is a problem; and projection: blaming someone else for what the patient is doing). One method is gently but firmly to confront the patient with evidence from collateral sources regarding the ethanol habit and effects.

d. The social supportive environment in general and the patient's family in specific must be integrated into the **treatment** scheme. A social worker with experience in treating alcoholics and the families of alcoholics is extremely important in the overall therapy. Another useful support group is Alanon, a group for family members of ethanol and substance-abuse patients.

e. **Disulfiram** (Antabuse) is a **modality** that may be useful in a small, selected group of patients. This is aversion therapy in which the agent disulfiram causes severe flushing, nausea, and vomiting immediately after the ingestion of any ethanol.

   i. The **mechanism of action** of the agent is by inhibiting the enzyme, hepatic aldehyde NAD-oxidoreductase. The inhibition of this enzyme results in abnormal concentrations of the molecule acetylaldehyde in the serum whenever any ethanol is ingested. The acetylaldehyde will result in remarkable flushing, nausea, and vomiting.

   ii. This **therapy** can be attempted in only a selected group of patients who have ethanol-dependency states. These include:

      (a) Total sobriety.
      (b) Total commitment to therapy.
      (c) Intelligent patient who understands the ramifications of the therapy.
      (d) A patient without any major affective disorder, as disulfiram can exacerbate depression.

   iii. **Dose:** 250 mg p.o., q.HS.

f. Referral to and/or consultation with an addictionologist (i.e., an internist, family practice physician, or psychiatrist with postresidency training in the field of addiction/substance abuse) is indicated in virtually all cases.

T A B L E 15-5
Anxiety Disorders

Syndrome	Manifestations	Therapy
Panic disorder	Sudden, unexpected, intense attacks of apprehension or anxiety Results in physiologic manifestations (i.e., tachycardia, tremor, diaphoresis) Women > men Agoraphobia: Marked fear of being in public places (crowds, elevators) from which easy escape is difficult Men > women in agoraphobia Lesion in locus cereleus and pontine nuclei	Imipramine: Response in 8–12 weeks, see Table 15-1 -or- Alprazolam (Xanax) 1–2 mg p.o. t.i.d. (max 8 mg p.o. 24hr) -or- Fluoxetine (Prozac), see Table 15-1
Generalized anxiety disorder	Habitual worrying Motor tension, autonomic hyperactivity Apprehension Irritability, insomnia Less overwhelming but longer lasting than panic disorder	Buspirone (Buspar), see Table 15-1 -or- Tricyclic antidepressants, see Table 15-1 -or- Alprazolam (Xanax) 0.5 mg p.o. t.i.d. (max 4 mg p.o. 24hr)

Simple phobias	Persistent irrational fears
	Avoid object:
	  Date
	  Speaking
	  Social phobia
	Men > women
		β-blockers, e.g., atenolol 25 mg p.o.
		q.day

Obsessive–compulsive disorder	Recurrent intrusive and disabling thoughts (obsessions) and repetitive stereotypical behaviors (compulsions). Tourette's syndrome *Lesion:* Decrease in caudate nuclei The personality trait is less severe–perfectionism and stubborn	Fluoxetine (Prozac), 20–80 p.o. mg/day

Posttraumatic stress syndrome	Follows exposure to a traumatic stressor
	Reexperiencing the trauma
	Numbing and avoidance
	Hyperarousal
	Examples:
	  Rape
	  Warfare
	  Disaster
		Tricyclic antidepressants, see Table 15-1

III. Consultation

Problem	Service	Time
Any concurrent Axis I* diagnosis	Psychiatrist	Urgent
All cases of substance abuse	Addictionologist	Urgent

IV. **Indications for admission:** Hypotension as the result of tachy-dysrhythmias, problems with airway maintenance, acute alcohol-related hepatitis, acute ethanol-related pancreatitis, hepatic encephalopathy, cocaine-related chest pain, any BAL of >300 mg/dL, or any evidence of impending severe withdrawal. In all cases, admission should be to an inpatient internal medicine service. Indications for admission to a detoxification unit include evidence of acute intoxication (i.e., BAL 100–300 mg/dL and/or evidence of mild withdrawal).

Bibliography

Mood Disorders Including Depression

Green SA, et al: Management of acute grief. Am Fam Pract 1986;33:185.

Koenig HG: Depressive disorders in older medical inpatients. Am Fam Pract 1991;44:1243.

Michels R, et al: Progress in psychiatry. N Engl J Med 1993;329:628–638.

Patterson WM, et al: Evaluation of suicidal patients: the SAD PERSONS scale. Psychosomatics 1983;24:343–349.

The Medical Letter: Choice of an antidepressant. 1993;35:25–26.

Wise MG, et al: Anxiety and mood disorders in medically ill patients. J Clin Psychiatry 1990;51(suppl 1):27–32.

Substance-Abuse Syndromes

Jellinek E: The disease concept of alcoholism. Newark, NJ: Hillhouse Press, 1960.

Lerner WD, et al: The alcohol withdrawal syndrome. N Engl J Med 1985;313:951.

Mayfield D, et al: The CAGE questionnaire. Am J Psychiatry 1974;131:1121.

Petrakis PL, ed: Sixth Special Report to the Secretary of Health and Human Services. Rockville, MD: National Institute on Alcohol Abuse and Alcoholism, 1987.

Selzer ML: The Michigan Alcoholism Screening Test. Am J Psychiatry 1971;127:1653.

Anxiety

Brown CS, et al: A practical update on anxiety disorders and their pharmacologic treatment. Arch Intern Med 1991;151:873–884.

—D.D.B.

*Axis I diagnoses: Schizophrenia; major affective disorder, including bipolar disorder or major depression.

Prevention in Primary Care

Prevention, in the context of clinical medicine, can be conceptualized as an intervention that will prevent a morbid event from occurring in a patient's future life. These interventions are typically performed in individuals who are asymptomatic for the disorder that we are trying to prevent. Examples of preventive interventions include immunizations, screening tests, modification of and counseling in unhealthy behaviors (e.g., smoking, drinking, sedentary lifestyle). Preventive interventions can be targeted to large segments of the population (e.g., screening for phenylketonuria and hypothyroidism among all newborns, childhood vaccinations, sickle cell tests in African Americans, breast and colorectal cancer screening), as well as to special segments of the population. Examples of tests for specific populations include tests in patients at high risk for complications of an existing condition (e.g., yearly funduscopy for the early detection of retinopathy in diabetics), tests for the carrier state of a transmissible disease in people at high risk (e.g., PPD among immigrants), or tests for people in occupations that require "perfect health" (e.g., electrocardiogram and symptom-limited stress test for airplane pilots).

Depending on when the intervention happens, the target disorder might have not occurred at all (vaccination for the prevention of polio and measles, smoking cessation for the prevention of lung cancer and heart disease), in which case, the intervention is considered **primary prevention.** If the intervention uncovers a disease in its asymptomatic stage (e.g., breast and colorectal cancer screening), it is considered **secondary prevention.** Finally, if the intervention is aimed at preventing progression of a disorder that has already manifested clinically [e.g., the use of β-blockers and angiotensin-converting enzyme (ACE) inhibitors for postmyocardial infarction or aspirin for patients with symptomatic carotid artery disease], then it is considered tertiary prevention. Further specific discussion of primary, secondary, and tertiary preventive measures will follow in this chapter.

The implementation of preventive interventions is variable. Certain interventions are mandated by law; examples are the fluoridation and chlorination of water, wearing seat belts while driving, and using helmets while on a motorcycle. Other preventive interventions are done in physician offices, commonly as a consequence of recommendations by medical organizations. Examples include cervical, breast, and colorectal cancer screening recommendations promulgated by the American Cancer Society and the American College of Physicians, among other organizations. Finally, preventive interventions can occur in public spaces, such as mass screening for hypertension, hyperlipidemia, and glaucoma at shopping malls.

Practicing physicians can implement preventive interventions in a number of ways. The periodic health examination refers to a comprehensive history and physical examination accompanied in the same visit by counseling if unhealthy behaviors are detected, immunizations if required, and performance of indicated screening procedures such as a cervical Papanicolaou smear, breast examination, or flexible sigmoidoscopy. A second approach, endorsed by the Canadian Preventive Task Force, entails performing a limited number of preventive interventions at each patient visit; this strategy is known as case finding. Advocates of the latter strategy believe that a primary care physician's patient load is too high to allow the physician to perform a periodic health examination adequately in a large number of patients, and that the general population visits a physician office often enough that preventive interventions can be provided over time at several office visits.

Physicians practicing in primary care specialties (internal medicine, family medicine, ob/gyn, pediatrics) have the unique opportunity to implement a variety of primary, secondary, and tertiary preventive interventions, depending on what segment of the population they treat. This chapter reviews interventions applicable to the adult population.

Primary prevention is truly the quintessential form of disease prevention. It actually goes to the known or suspected factor in the pathogenesis of a disease and attempts to remove or modify that factor before the disease develops. Examples include immunizations to prevent infectious diseases (Table 16-1), cessation of cigarette smoking to prevent atherosclerotic disease and carcinomas (see Box 16-1), the use of safety belts in motor vehicles, and cessation of the use of chewing tobacco in the prevention of oral carcinomas. Further primary prevention recommendations are listed in Table 16-2.

Secondary preventive strategies (Table 16-3) are usually accomplished by the use of screening tests. A screening intervention is one that allows the discovery of a disorder in its asymptomatic stage. An effective screening intervention should satisfy all the

(text continues on page 709)

T A B L E 16-1
Immunizations in Adults[a]

1. Influenza vaccine: Should be offered to all individuals over age 65 and to patients at high risk for significant morbidity and mortality. The latter category includes patients with diabetes mellitus, heart disease, pulmonary disease, renal disease, and immunocompromised patients. Health care personnel should also receive this vaccine. An absolute contraindication to the vaccine is a history of allergy to egg yolk. The vaccine is usually available in the fall and should be administered on a yearly basis. Side effects of the vaccine are the same as for placebo injection. The vaccine is 65%–80% effective.

2. Pneumococcal vaccine: Similar indications as for influenza vaccine. Major differences include patients with asplenia (anatomical or functional), sickle-cell disease, Hodgkin's disease, nephrotic syndrome, or alcoholism, all of whom clearly benefit from pneumococcal vaccine. The vaccine is available year round and is given once in the lifetime of the individual. There is no contraindication to vaccination in patients who are allergic to egg yolk. The vaccine is 60%–65% effective. Recent recommentations include that a booster should be administered to:
- Asplenia
- Nephrotic syndrome
- Renal transplant
- Renal failure
- Other transplants

3. Tetanus toxoid/Diphtheria: After the primary series of 3, administer the Td booster to all adults every 10 years. If a patient with a dirty wound appears between 5–10 years after the vaccine, Td booster is indicated. In all cases there is no need if < 5 years.

4. Hepatitis B vaccine: Mandatory for individuals at high risk for exposure, including health care workers, individuals working in research laboratories, sexually active homosexual men, and intravenous drug abusers. The currently available vaccine is produced by recombinant technology. Three doses are required to achieve immunity. The duration of immunity has not been clearly defined. Recent recommendations include checking a hepatitis B antibody q 5–7 years (or if immunocompromised or on hemodialysis yearly); if the antibody titer is low, administer a hepatitis B booster. The deltoid site is the preferred site. The vaccine is effective in 85%–95% of young adults.

5. MMR (Measles, Mumps, and Rubella)
   a. Measles: Individuals born after 1956 who lack evidence of immunity. Two doses of MMR (administer the trivalent agent).

(continued)

T A B L E 16-1 (continued)

 b. **Rubella:** Women of childbearing age who lack proof
of immunity. Patient must agree not to become pregnant in
the following 3 months. Pregnancy is an absolute contraindication. The Centers for Disease Control (CDC) also recommends
vaccination of health care workers, military recruits, and college students.
 6. **Hemophilus influenza type B conjugate vaccine (Hib):**
Administer to all young children and to adults only if an increased risk of asplenia or sickle cell anemia.
 7. **Poliomyelitis:** Enhanced-potency inactivated poliovaccine
(eIPV) is the primary immunization of choice. Booster vaccine
is either the eIPV or the OPV (oral polio, live attenuated) times
one is satisfactory.
 8. **For travel outside of the United States,** one must refer
the patient to a travel health service or check with the **CDC's
Health Information for International Travel** to determine
which, if any, immunizations and agents are recommended to
effect primary prevention in those countries.

[a]Assumes that the patient received primary immunizations as
a child.

T A B L E 16-2
Primary Prevention in Adults

 1. Immunizations (see Table 16-1)
 2. Cessation of cigarette smoking (Box 16-1)
 3. Safe-sex techniques, including appropriate use of con-
    doms and abstinence/monogamy
 4. Contraception to prevent unwanted pregnancies (see
    Chapter 11)
 5. Smoke detectors in home
 6. Safety belts
 7. Cessation of chewing tobacco
 8. Store any toxic agents in a secure place in home
 9. Eliminate storage of firearms or, at minimum, store in a
    secure place
10. ASA 81 mg when older than age 35 years
11. Dietary modifications
12. Exercise thrice weekly
13. Postmenopausal (see Chapter 11)
14. Brush and floss b.i.d.
15. Twice yearly professional cleaning of teeth
16. Varicella vaccine, s.c., and repeat 4–8 weeks later. For sus-
    ceptible adolescents/adults.

B O X 16-1

Outline of Cigarette Smoking–Cessation Technique

Background

1. Cessation of cigarette smoking is essential to the primary prevention of:
   a. Atherosclerotic disease in general and coronary and cerebrovascular atherosclerotic disease in specific.
   b. Bronchogenic carcinoma.
   c. Low-birth-weight infants in pregnant mothers.
2. Cessation of cigarette smoking is essential to the primary prevention of disorders attributable to passive (i.e., second-hand) smoke:
   a. Respiratory infections in children.
   b. Bronchogenic carcinoma in family members and co-workers.

Management

1. The physician must state clearly and unequivocally to each and every patient who smokes cigarettes that the patient must stop cigarette smoking. Several tips to make this statement more effective include:
   a. State the negative outcomes that may occur if smoking cessation is not effected. These may be general items such as an increased risk of heart attack, stroke, or lung and other cancers. The clinician must attempt to make this personal and tangible to the patient (e.g., if one of the patient's parents had a heart attack at a young age, stress the fact that smoking puts the patient at an extremely high risk for a heart attack).
   b. Educate the patients about the untoward outcomes of passive smoke. They should understand that their habit is not only directly jeopardizing their own life but also negatively affecting on the health of their co-workers, roommates, and family members.
   c. State the positive outcomes of the cessation of cigarette smoking. These include the decrease in risk of heart attacks, strokes, lung and other cancers, and the prolongation of life expectancy. Again the clinician must attempt to make this personal and tangible to the patient (e.g., if the pa-

(continued)

B O X   16-1 (continued)

tient has chronic cough, the cessation of smoking
may decrease the cough; if the patient has small
children at home, cessation of smoking will decrease the risk of respiratory illness in these
children).

d. Stress the importance of this behavioral modification and emphasize that, although it will be difficult, the benefits of cessation are enormous.

e. Describe the withdrawal symptoms the patient
may feel after cessation of smoking (e.g., increased irritability, increased weight, and an intense craving for nicotine). Stress the fact that
these are transient, that they are an investment in
better health for the individual and his or her family, and that they can be minimized by exercise,
fluids, and the short-term use of a nicotine substi-
tute (i.e., the transdermal nicotine patch).

The dosage of the transdermal nicotine is:

If the patient smokes >10 cigarettes/day: Habitrol or Nicoderm, one 21-mg patch each day for
30 days, followed by one 14-mg patch each day
for 15–30 days, followed by one 7-mg patch each
day for 15–30 days; or Nicotrol, one 15-mg patch
each day for 30 days followed by one 10-mg
patch each day for 15–30 days followed by 5-mg
patch for 15–30 days.

If the patient smokes <10 cigarettes/day, the
starting dose is of the intermediate strength (i.e.,
14-mg patch). *Caveat:* Habitrol and Nicoderm
patches are applied for 24-hour periods. Nicotrol
patches are applied for 16-hour periods (i.e., applied in the morning and removed at night).

f. The patch must be used only in an intense and
committed effort of smoking cessation.

g. Instruct the patient to set a date for cessation and
to resolve to abstain from cigarette smoking from
that day hence.

h. Medications may need to be adjusted when abstinence is effected. The medications include theophylline, caffeine, and other methylxanthines. After
the effective withdrawal, the level of these often
markedly increase and thus the dose must be ad-

(continued)

B O X   16-1 (continued)

 justed downward (i.e., decrease the number of cups of coffee).
 i. FDA has ruled that this is a Category C pregnancy agent (i.e., a "risk cannot be ruled out"). It is worth the potential risks if the patient cannot abstain without pharmacologic assistance and she still smokes >10 cigarettes/day.
 j. These agents are now available over the counter.
2. Complement the discussion with written materials regarding the cessation of cigarette smoking. These can be written by the clinician himself or herself for distribution or they can be brochures that are obtained free or at a nominal fee from various health organizations. Examples of these include "Calling It Quits," by the American Heart Association, and "Smart Move," by the American Cancer Society.
3. Finally, select a nurse in the clinic to spend some time on the same day to provide reinforcement of the points made by the clinician and to make follow-up appointments and telephone calls with the sole purpose of longitudinal support for cessation of cigarette smoking.
4. One may recommend or prescribe nicotine polacrilex (Nicorette gum), 2-mg piece, q.4hr, prn, for intermittent use after the cessation of smoking has been accomplished and the transdermal nicotine has been discontinued.

(text continued from page 704)
following conditions: the targeted disorder should be relatively prevalent; the screening test must be reasonably safe, inexpensive, and acceptable by the patient; the test used for screening is capable of recognizing the vast majority of patients with the target disorder (high sensitivity) while mislabeling few patients as having the target disorder (high specificity); follow-up confirmatory tests should be safe, ideally noninvasive, and affordable; **treatment** of the target disorder in its asymptomatic stage will improve patients' prognosis compared with those patients with a similar disorder that are treated only when the disease becomes symptomatic; and the ultimate outcome of the target disorder has grave consequences for the well-being of patients, in terms of either morbidity or mortality. Of these desirable characteristics, the two most difficult to evaluate and quantify are the characteristics of the candidate screening test (sensitivity and specificity) and the efficacy of available interventions for disease diagnosed in an asymptomatic stage.

T A B L E   16-3
Recommendations for Screening Tests[a]

Breast cancer: Breast examination by a physician every 1–2 years, starting at age 40. Annual mammography starting at age 50. Stop screening by age 75. Monthly breast self-examination, to be done at midcycle, is also recommended. For women with a family history of breast cancer, yearly mammography should be started at age 35. The American College of Obstetricians and Gynecologists recommends annual or biannual mammography and annual breast examination by a physician, starting at age 40.

Colorectal cancer: Currently the U.S. Preventive Task Force recommends screening only in patients at high risk for colorectal cancer (positive family history), starting at age 50. We recommend the performance of flexible sigmoidoscopy every 3–5 years, starting at age 50. The utility of fecal occult blood testing (FOBT) is under investigation. The American Cancer Society recommends yearly FOBT, starting at age 40, and flexible sigmoidoscopy performed in two consecutive years starting at age 50 and every 3 years thereafter if the initial flexible sigmoidoscopy results are normal.

Cervical cancer: Papanicolaou smears every 1–3 years from the beginning of sexual activity. Screening can be stopped by age 65 if the smears are consistently normal. Other organizations recommend starting screening at age 18 or at the beginning of sexual life, performing Pap smears annually for 3 years, and then every 3 years if the three prior Pap smears were normal. See Chapter 11, for PAP smear evaluation.

Prostate cancer: The U.S. Preventive Task Force does not recommend either digital rectal examination, serum marker assays (PSA), or transrectal ultrasonography for asymptomatic men. The American Cancer Society recommends yearly rectal examination starting at age 40.

Skin cancer: Thorough complete skin examination recommended only for patients at high risk: family or personal history of skin cancer, precursor lesions (i.e., dysplastic nevi). The American Academy of Dermatology recommends annual complete examination for all patients as well as monthly self-examination.

Ovarian cancer: No specific recommendation other than examining carefully the uterine adnexae when performing pelvic examinations. The role of serum marker assay and (CA-125) transvaginal ultrasonography is still under investigation. Patients with a family history of ovarian cancer or breast cancer in first-degree relatives might benefit from serum marker assays and transvaginal ultrasonography done sequentially as a screening modality.

(continued)

T A B L E *16-3 (continued)*

Testicular cancer: Routine examination only for patients at high risk for testicular cancer: testicular atrophy, cryptorchidism, orchiopexy. The American Cancer Society recommends testicular examination as part of the periodic health examination and monthly self-examination in postpubertal men.

Blood pressure measurement: All panels recommend measurement at each visit and at least one every two years; all ages.

Serum cholesterol (Random): Starting at age 20 years, then every 5 years; If elevated, i.e. >200 mg/dL, perform a fasting lipid panel-total cholesterol, HDL, and triglyceride level.

---

[a]Based upon U.S. Preventive Task Force, Canadian Task Force, and American College of Physicians.

Examples of interventions that have been shown not to benefit patient outcome include the following: yearly chest radiograph for the screening of lung cancer, carcinoembryonic antigen (CEA) assay for colorectal cancer screening, a battery of blood tests in asymptomatic individuals, complete routine urinalysis in nonpregnant or nondiabetic patients, and electrocardiograms in otherwise healthy individuals. Strategies currently being investigated as potentially useful screening strategies include the prostate-specific antigen (PSA) assay alone and in combination with transrectal ultrasonography for the early diagnosis of prostatic cancer, fecal occult blood testing for colorectal cancer screening, and serum markers for ovarian cancer (CA-125), alone or in combination with transvaginal ultrasonography.

Numerous preventive interventions other than those reviewed in this chapter are suggested in the report issued in 1989 by the U.S. Preventive Task Force. The scientific merit of each of those recommendations is beyond the scope of this book but is discussed in the report.

Tertiary preventive interventions (i.e., those used to prevent further progression of disease that is already extant) include the use of aspirin in patients with atherosclerotic heart disease and cerebrovascular disease, the use of β-blockers and angiotensin-converting enzyme (ACE) inhibitors in the postmyocardial infarction period, and the cessation of smoking in a patient with chronic obstructive pulmonary disease.

In summary, primary care providers are ideally positioned to provide preventive services to large segments of the population. What preventive measures are appropriate to institute depends on the characteristics of the disease to be prevented (prevalence, morbidity, mortality), currently available technology for diagnosis and treatment, cost, and the availability of screening and confirmatory tests.

Bibliography

American College of Physicians: Guide for adult immunization, 2nd ed. Philadelphia: American College of Physicians, 1990.

Kramer SE, Graham KE: Helping your patients who smoke quit for good. Postgrad Med 1991;90:233–246.

Lawrence RS, et al: Preventive services in clinical practice: Designing the periodic health examination. JAMA 1987;257:2205–2210.

United States Preventive Services Task Force: Guide to clinical preventive services. Baltimore: Williams & Wilkins, 1989.

—D.D.B.

Subject Index

Page numbers followed by *f* indicate figures; those followed by *t* indicate tables; those followed by *b* indicate boxed material.